PATHOPHYSIOLOGY
Principles of Disease

MARTHA J. MILLER, M.A.T.

Formerly Instructor
Department of Health Careers
and Nursing
Hocking Technical College
Nelsonville, Ohio

W. B. SAUNDERS COMPANY
Philadelphia/London/Toronto/Mexico City/Rio de Janeiro/Sydney/Tokyo

W. B. Saunders Company: West Washington Square
                          Philadelphia, Pa. 19105

                          1 St. Anne's Road
                          Eastbourne, East Sussex BN21 3UN, England

                          1 Goldthorne Avenue
                          Toronto, Ontario M8Z 5T9, Canada

                          Apartado 26370 — Cedro 512
                          Mexico 4, D.F., Mexico

                          Rua Coronel Cabrita, 8
                          Sao Cristovao Caixa Postal 21176
                          Rio de Janeiro, Brazil

                          9 Waltham Street
                          Artarmon, N.S.W. 2064, Australia

                          Ichibancho, Central Bldg., 22-1 Ichibancho
                          Chiyoda-Ku, Tokyo 102, Japan

Library of Congress Cataloging in Publication Data

Miller, Martha J.

Pathophysiology: Principles of Disease

Includes index.

1. Physiology, Pathological.   I Title. [DNLM: 1. Pathology.
   QZ 4 M5492i]

RB113.M533   616.07   81–40479

ISBN 0–7216–6337–0   AACR2

Pathophysiology: Principles of Disease   ISBN 0-7216-6337-0

Last digit is the print number: 9   8   7   6   5   4   3   2

To Larry
for his encouragement and support,
Robyn and Dan
for their patience and understanding

Preface

The upgrading of demands and responsibilities in the health professions has created a need for practitioners with increasingly sophisticated preparation. *Pathophysiology: Principles of Disease* was developed to service an expressed desire on the part of students to meet this need. Their wish to really understand the underlying mechanisms of disease, the rationale for designated treatments, and the complex interrelationships between critical systems provided the impetus for this text.

To fully clarify the dynamic nature of pathology, it is necessary to delve beneath superficial signs and symptoms into the conceptual basis of disease. Since organic dysfunction can ultimately be traced to underlying cellular death or disequilibrium, the mechanisms that disrupt the optimal cellular environment must be elucidated. Pathophysiology, or the study of dynamic deviation from a baseline steady state, thus lies at a very critical point at the crossroads between basic science and clinical theory. By establishing essential linkages between clinical manifestations and causative mechanisms, it serves to enhance conceptual comprehension, encourage problem solving, and facilitate independent study.

The perceived audience for this text includes all individuals who are, or who will be, dealing clinically with the human body. Appropriate for use at the basic associate degree level, it is simultaneously comprehensive enough to service the needs of students in a four-year baccalaureate program. *Pathophysiology: Principles of Disease* could be utilized in a variety of ways:

1. as a basic text in a pathophysiology course offered to associate degree or baccalaureate students in nursing, respiratory therapy, inhalation therapy or physicians' assistants programs—to name just a few.

2. as a recommended text for students who ask for a supplementary basic reference in courses requiring a more advanced pathophysiology text.

3. as a required or recommended text to enhance underlying conceptual understanding of pathophysiology in conjunction with clinical theory or clinical assessment courses.

4. as a reference for clinical practitioners who want a concise update of principles that would enhance their understanding of the disease process.

v

Organizationally, the text is divided into four units: *Unit 1* introduces the basic conceptual framework of the text. Homeostasis and cellular needs are presented as the critical baselines from which all pathology is measured. *Unit 2* elucidates the complex and specific mechanisms designed to maintain the constancy of the cellular fluid environment. Analysis of fluid and electrolyte and acid-base imbalance is thus presented early and can serve as a point of reference in clarifying symptomatic changes evidenced during dysfunction of the critical systems. *Unit 3* deals with the evolution of disease processes in several critical systems. Comprehension of inflammation, hypersensitivity, infection, necrosis, and neoplasm is reinforced initially and then applied to specific systemic disorders. In each system, disease is related back to ultimate effects upon cellular survival needs. *Unit 4* is a culminating integrative section. Emphasis is placed upon disruption of cellular needs. It is shown how diseases of vastly different etiology and origin can all interfere with the supply of a specific cellular need—hence precipitating similar clinical symptoms.

Although the material is conceptually integrated, each unit or chapter can stand on its own, thus allowing the instructor maximal flexibility in curriculum design. Periodic short summaries of quite basic material often set the stage for more difficult concepts to follow. Throughout Unit 3, for example, an introduction to normal systemic anatomy and physiology precedes the elucidation of pathology. Emphasis, of course, is placed upon those aspects of medical physiology that will most directly enhance comprehension of disease mechanisms. Although these reviews need not necessarily be incorporated directly into course content, it has been my experience that students welcome the opportunity to read a concisely designed overview of normal structure and function before plunging into the study of systemic pathophysiology.

Since the expressed purpose of this text is to clarify and conceptualize the disease process for the *basic* health career student, in-text documentation is not utilized. While readers will be alerted to some major areas of controversy, the learner with a more advanced research orientation should be referred to the extensive reading list that is provided at the end of each chapter.

Although an effort is made to define and explain new terms as they are introduced, comprehension of the material will be considerably enhanced by a previous background in anatomy, physiology, and chemistry. Study questions at the end of each chapter are designed to maximize learning, provoke thought, and test comprehension of newly presented material.

It is hoped that the information presented in *Pathophysiology: Principles of Disease* will prove to be beneficial and supportive to the health care practitioner. Expanded comprehension should serve to enhance both skill and confidence in the clinical area. Ideally, however, the study of pathology will also engender a sense of humility and awe. It is, perhaps, ultimately through an understanding of disease that one comes to fully appreciate the delicate and intricate mechanisms responsible for the maintenance of physiological health.

Acknowledgments

The creation of this manuscript was essentially a solitary effort sustained by the encouragement and support of family, friends, colleagues, and students. My thanks to all of those whose unflagging enthusiasm helped to fuel the light at the end of the tunnel.

The publication of this manuscript, on the other hand, was most assuredly a cooperative effort utilizing the many skills and talents of an exceptionally competent staff at the W. B. Saunders Company. Many thanks go, therefore, to Katherine Pitcoff, for her initial enthusiasm when the plans for this text were first being formed; Elizabeth Cobbs, who worked with limitless patience and skill to choreograph development and design of the manuscript; Laura Tarves for her work in coordinating production; Larry Ward for his preparation of the artwork; Constance Burton for her meticulous editing; and Stephany Scott and Cathy Lindline for their assistance.

In addition, I would like to thank Kathy Rude for her creative contributions to the Teacher's Manual.

Contents

PATHOPHYSIOLOGY
Principles of Disease

Chapter 1:   Homeostasis—A Cellular View

Chapter 2:   Cellular Life Needs—A Systemic Overview

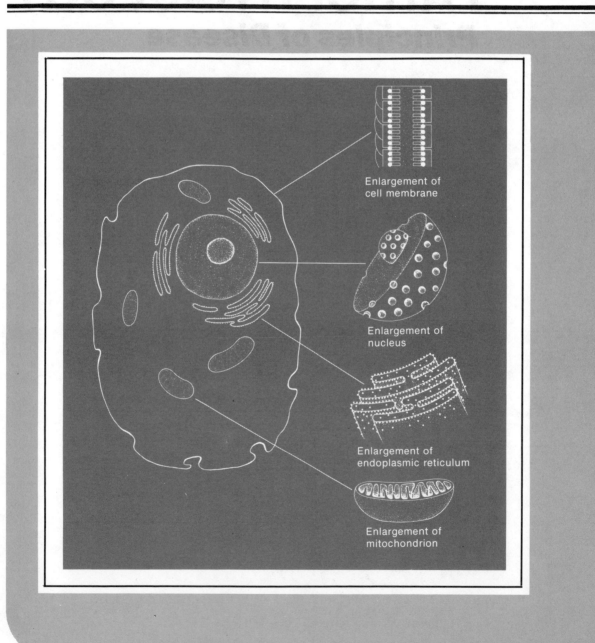

Enlargement of
cell membrane

Enlargement of
nucleus

Enlargement of
endoplasmic reticulum

Enlargement of
mitochondrion

Homeostasis

There is a tendency among health career students to view the cell as an isolated entity, unrelated to clinical concepts of health and disease in the body. As a result, the study of microscopic structures is often regarded as a necessary curricular evil. Because few students ever see the cell in proper perspective, they fail to realize that disease of the heart, lung, brain, and other structures results from death or dysfunction of the *cells* constituting these organs.

Healthy cells—healthy body is a central tenet of this text. For most students, this will be a new way of looking at pathophysiology. A conceptual approach to the underlying cellular dynamics in health and disease is emphasized. Rote learning of terminology, structural abnormalities, and clinical signs and symptoms is discouraged. As this unit unfolds, mastery of the material should help to establish a conceptual framework for developing a better understanding of pathophysiology.

Initially, the concept of homeostasis is related to the maintenance of specific cellular needs. The way in which the systems of the body work in unison to service these cellular needs is then analyzed in detail. Patience is advised in dealing with some of the preliminary material, which may seem unduly simplified. This presentation is designed to aid in the recall and review of basic information essential to the comprehension of increasingly difficult concepts.

Chapter Outline

CELLULAR ENVIRONMENT
CELLULAR SURVIVAL NEEDS
CELLULAR STRUCTURE AND FUNCTION
SERVICING CELLULAR NEEDS: A SYSTEMIC REVIEW

chapter 1

Homeostasis — A Cellular View

Chapter Objectives

At the completion of this chapter, the student will be able to:

1. Describe the structural hierarchy of the human body.
2. Describe the location of a cell with respect to interstitial fluid, capillaries, arterioles, and venules.
3. Identify and locate the three major fluid compartments of the body.
4. Differentiate between the three fluid compartments of the body with respect to function.
5. Define homeostasis.
6. Define cellular metabolism and describe its primary function.
7. Identify two wastes of cellular metabolism.
8. Identify the four basic life needs of the cell.
9. Describe the function of each primary structural component of the cell.
10. Differentiate between the four basic tissue types with respect to structure and function.
11. Differentiate between the major systems of the body with respect to basic structure and function.

CELLULAR ENVIRONMENT

There are approximately 100 trillion cells in the human body. These cells, the smallest functional units of living matter, are the building blocks of all tissues, organs, and systems. Survival of the body thus depends upon normal functioning of the cells within it. Figure 1.1 illustrates the structural hierarchy of the human body.

Under normal conditions, cells exist in a fluid environment. Blood vessels carry life-sustaining substances to the cell and remove potentially harmful waste products. In effect, the cell is an island surrounded by liquid. Substances are carried to and from this island through blood vessel pipelines. Any material traveling between cells and vessels must cross the liquid surrounding the cell. Figure 1.2 depicts the cell and the fluids critical to its survival.

Traveling through the blood vessels is *plasma*, carrying oxygen and nutrients to the cell for use in energy generation, and carrying metabolic wastes away from it. Bathing the cell is *interstitial fluid*, providing the exchange medium for substances moving between cells and capillary plasma. Within the cell membrane is *intracellular fluid*, serving as the liquid environment for chemical reactions necessary to cellular survival.

All three fluids, customarily referred to as the major *fluid compartments* of the body, are of

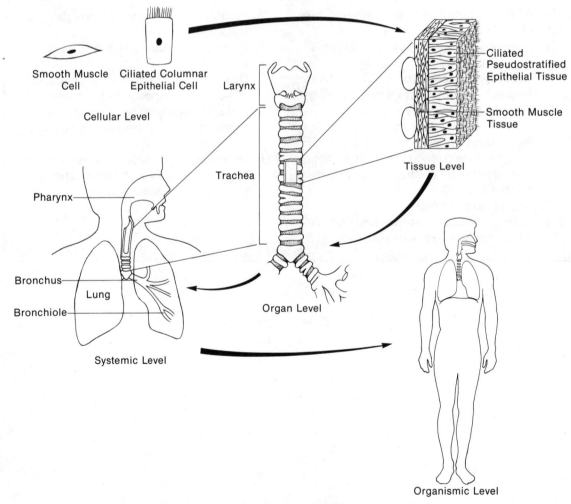

Figure 1.1 Structural hierarchy of the human body.

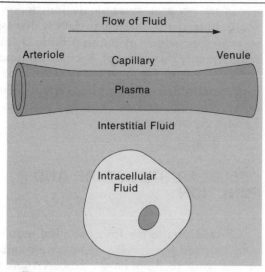

Figure 1.2 Fluid compartments of the body.

relatively constant composition. Just as human beings could not exist in the atmosphere of a foreign planet, human cells cannot survive with fluid compartments of alien composition. To insure health, body systems must function to maintain the optimal chemical composition of plasma, interstitial fluid, and intracellular fluid. Even slight deviations from normal can have serious consequences. This maintenance of fluid constancy, called *homeostasis,* is an underlying force in the function of the human body.

As indicated in this brief description of the cellular environment, ongoing dynamic exchanges are needed to support cellular health. Maintenance of homeostasis necessitates continual servicing of the interstitial fluid in several specific ways:

1. There must be a supply of the raw materials needed by cells to generate energy.

2. There must be a means of removing the wastes that are produced by cells in the process of generating energy.

3. There must be a means of maintaining the optimal cellular environment with respect to fluid volume and distribution, salt (electrolyte), and acid-base composition so as to support the energy-generating process.

It can be seen how an understanding of all aspects of homeostasis would be enhanced by a general comprehension of the energy-generating mechanism of a cell.

CELLULAR SURVIVAL NEEDS

In order for cells to grow, multiply, and perform their specific jobs in the body, they must be able to generate energy. The generation of energy enables each cell to increase in size, to repair itself, to reproduce, and to fulfill its specific function within the body. The production of this critically needed energy is achieved through intracellular chemical reactions collectively referred to as *cellular metabolism.*

A brief look at cellular metabolism reveals the basic reaction that must occur to insure cellular survival. In general, metabolism involves the chemical combination of oxygen (O_2) with certain nutrient particles to generate energy and waste products. The metabolic reactions occur inside the cell membrane, within the intracellular fluid, and are promoted by enzymes on the mitochondria. An overview of the metabolic process is provided in Figure 1.3.

Oxygen, nutrients, and intracellular enzymes are essential to cellular energy generation. Moreover, carbon dioxide (CO_2), water (H_2O), and other wastes released by the metabolic process must be eliminated if the cell is to continue to function normally. No living organism can thrive surrounded by its own excrement. The cell is no exception. Supply of the oxygen and nutrients necessary to metabolism must be coupled with removal of

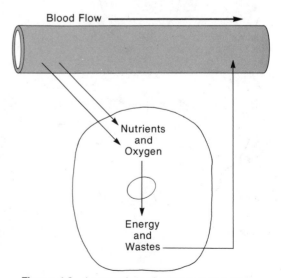

Figure 1.3 An overview of cellular metabolism.

metabolic wastes. Only in this way can health be maintained.

It must be remembered that no metabolic activity or cellular function can proceed for long without an interstitial environment of ideal composition. Hence the maintenance of fluid, electrolyte, and acid-base balance (referred to as *fluid and electrolyte balance*) is essential to cellular maintenance and survival.

As one looks at the body from this cellular view, it is possible to identify four basic *cellular survival needs,* all of which serve to maintain homeostasis. There must be a supply of (1) *oxygen* and (2) *nutrients* to feed metabolism, a means of (3) *waste elimination,* and a mechanism to maintain the (4) *fluid and electrolyte balance.* It is the function of all organs and systems in the body to service these four basic requirements of the cell. If these cellular needs are not met, systemic dysfunction will result. In fact, it is possible to classify diseases according to which of the four basic cellular requirements they disrupt. Such an approach is taken in Unit IV, in which pathologic conditions affecting (1) oxygen, (2) nutrients, (3) elimination, and (4) fluid and electrolyte balance are analyzed.

CELLULAR STRUCTURE AND FUNCTION

In addition to the four basic life requirements shared by all cells, there are a number of structural components common to most body cells. The *cell membrane* serves as an outer boundary and selectively controls the movement of substances between interstitial

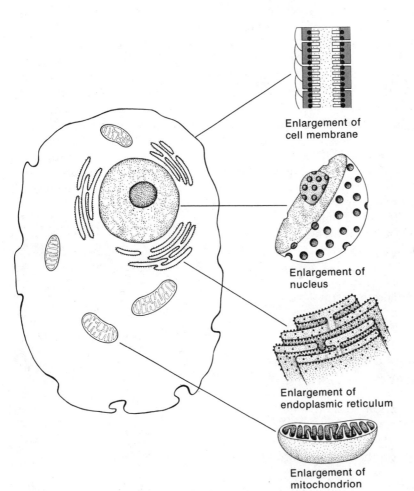

Enlargement of
cell membrane

Enlargement of
nucleus

Enlargement of
endoplasmic reticulum

Enlargement of
mitochondrion

Figure 1.4   Major structural components of the cell.

Type of Cell	Arrangement of Cells in Body	Unique Structural Adaptations	Some Select Functions
Epithelial	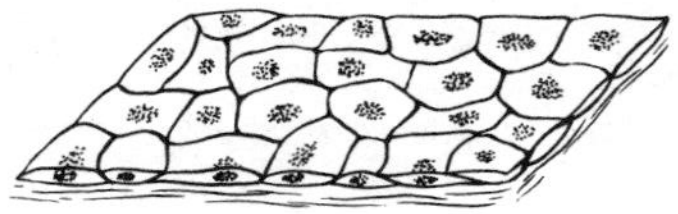 Simple squamous epithelium	Thin sheet of cells, one cell thick.	Facilitates diffusion through capillary wall and alveoli; provides smooth lining for heart and blood vessels.
	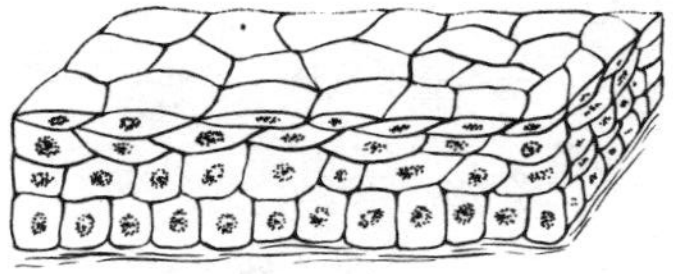 Stratified squamous epithelium	Cells arranged in several layers of thickness.	Provides protection on skin surface and in certain areas of gastrointestinal mucosa, where much abrasion occurs.
	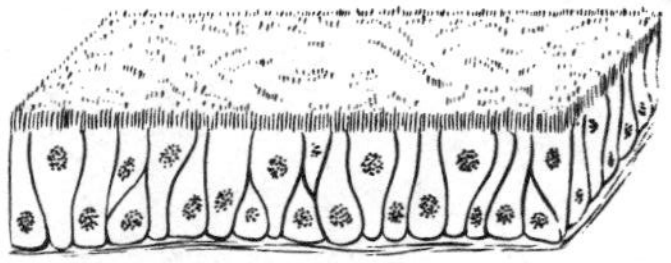 Pseudostratified ciliated epithelium	A single layer of epithelial cells resting on a basement membrane. Often interspersed with flask-shaped goblet cells and covered with tiny hairlike cilia.	Lines respiratory tract, producing mucus for lubrication and filtering inspired air.
Muscle	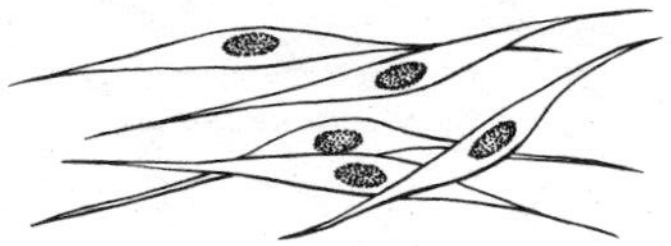 Smooth muscle	Elongated cells	Elongated shape provides potential for maximal shortening or contraction. Skeletal muscle responsible for movement of bones; smooth muscle controls contraction of internal organs.
	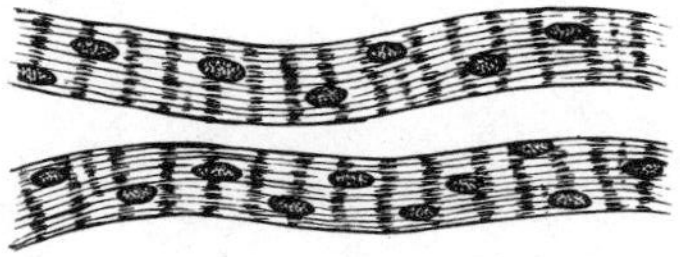 Striated muscle	Long fibrous cells	
	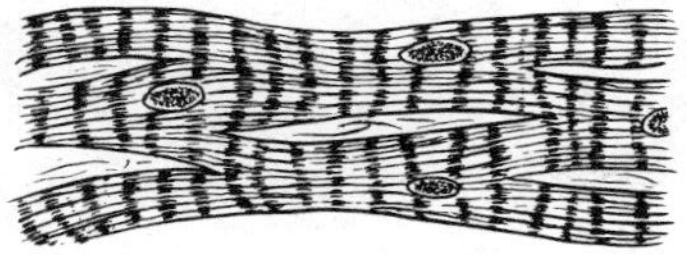 Cardiac muscle	Individual fibers interconnect to form syncytium of unified tissue.	Syncytium facilitates integrated and unified cardiac contraction.

Figure 1.5 Structural adaptation to function on the cellular level. (Bone tissue enlargement reprinted with permission from Jacob, S., Francone, C., and Lossow, W.: Structure and Function in Man, 5th ed. Philadelphia, W. B. Saunders Company, 1982.)

(Illustration continued on following page)

Type of Cell	Arrangement of Cells in Body	Unique Structural Adaptations	Some Select Functions
Nerve	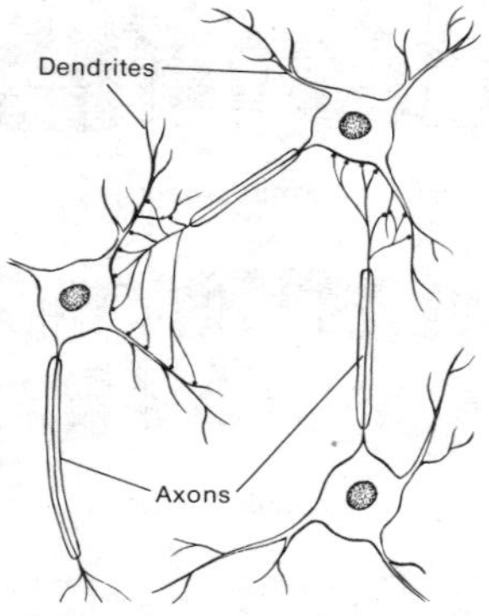 Dendrites / Axons / Three neurons synapsing	Fibrous processes extend from cell body to receive and transmit nerve impulses.	Controls integration and coordination of adaptive responses throughout the body.
Connective	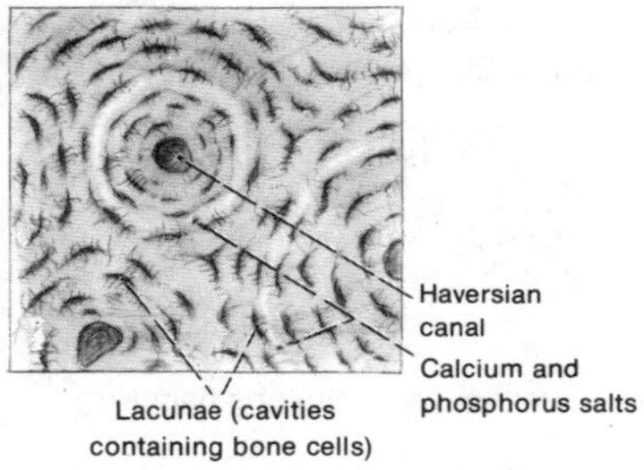 Haversian canal / Calcium and phosphorus salts / Lacunae (cavities containing bone cells) / Bone tissue enlargement	Living bone cells surrounded by nonliving calcium and phosphorus salts.	Provides firm base for the structure of the skeleton. Protects soft tissue and controls support and movement.
	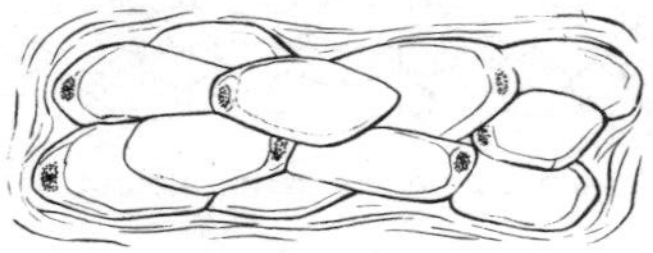 Adipose tissue	Living cells filled with yellow lipid material.	Provides layer of insulation protection and support for structures throughout the body.

Figure 1.5 *Continued.* See legend on preceding page.

and intracellular fluid. The *nucleus* helps to govern the reproductive process and insures similarity between mother and daughter cells. The *mitochondria* support enzymes essential to metabolism. The *ribosomes* are found on parallel membranes of *endoplasmic reticulum* and are the site of intracellular protein synthesis. The *intracellular fluid* provides the liquid environment necessary for chemical reactions to occur. Figure 1.4 presents some major cellular components in pictorial form.

In spite of these elements of structural similarity, cells can vary greatly in their *functions*, which include secretion, absorption, protection, contraction, and transmission. Adaptations specialize each cell for its particular role in the body. In much the same way that all people share certain essential characteristics, yet differ from one another in size, height, weight, and proportion, so do cells vary in their outward appearance. Whereas human individualities are rather haphazard and dependent upon many factors ranging from diet and exercise to personal preferences, cellular differences are designed to be adaptive in nature.

If two cells look very different from each other, one can be sure that they differ in function. If human roles were as programmed and limited as those of the cells, all chimney sweeps might be 12 feet tall with long thin arms, all auto mechanics might be born with wheels on their backs and narrow trunks, and all wood choppers might have grotesquely oversized chest and upper arm muscles. Although the human organism is not genetically designed to fit life vocations, we can cite many examples of structural adaptation to function on the cellular level. Some of these are illustrated in Figure 1.5.

SERVICING CELLULAR NEEDS: A SYSTEMIC REVIEW

The systems of the body exist to service the needs of the cells. They function together to insure that the basic cellular needs for oxygen, nutrients, elimination, and fluid and electrolyte balance are fulfilled. Before explor-

ORGANISM
(Many Systems)

SYSTEM
(Several Organs)

ORGAN
(Several Tissues)

TISSUES
(Many Similar Cells)

CELLS
(Smallest Structural Unit)

Figure 1.6 Structural hierarchy within the body.

ing the ways in which each cellular life requirement is provided for, it is necessary to review some basic functional aspects of the body systems.

Each system consists of a group of organs working together for a unified purpose. The organs are composed of several different types of tissue. Tissues, in turn, are made up of similar cells designed to perform a specific function. A pictorial review of this structural hierarchy concept can be found in Figure 1.6.

Major structures in each system work together to help maintain cellular health. No single system in the body could function alone to insure survival. Collectively, however, they succeed in providing oxygen and nutrients to the cells, eliminating metabolic wastes, and maintaining the fluid and electrolyte balance of the cellular environment. A brief introduction to each system is presented here. Elaboration with respect to structure and function will be presented in Units 3 and 4.

The *respiratory system* consists of structures designed to promote the intake of oxygen and the output of carbon dioxide. Air rich in oxygen moves from the atmosphere to many small thin-walled air sacs in the lungs through a passageway comprising the nasal cavities, pharynx, larynx (voice box), trachea (windpipe), two primary bronchi, and smaller bronchial subdivisions. Gas exchange occurs deep within the far reaches of the lungs. Here oxygen moves from air sacs (alveoli) into surrounding capillaries and is then carried by blood throughout the body to meet cellular

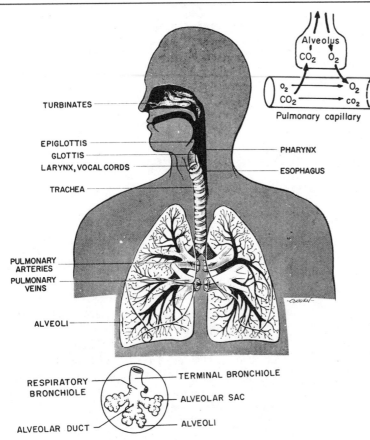

TURBINATES

EPIGLOTTIS
GLOTTIS
LARYNX, VOCAL CORDS

TRACHEA

PHARYNX

ESOPHAGUS

PULMONARY
ARTERIES
PULMONARY
VEINS

ALVEOLI

Alveolus
CO_2 O_2

Pulmonary capillary
O_2 O_2
CO_2 CO_2

RESPIRATORY
BRONCHIOLE

ALVEOLAR DUCT

TERMINAL BRONCHIOLE

ALVEOLAR SAC

ALVEOLI

Figure 1.7. The respiratory system. The diagram (upper right) shows the exchange of oxygen and carbon dioxide between the alveolus and the capillary. The inset (lower left) shows the bronchioles and alveoli. (From Guyton, A.: Physiology of the Human Body. Philadelphia, W. B. Saunders Company, 1979. Used by permission.)

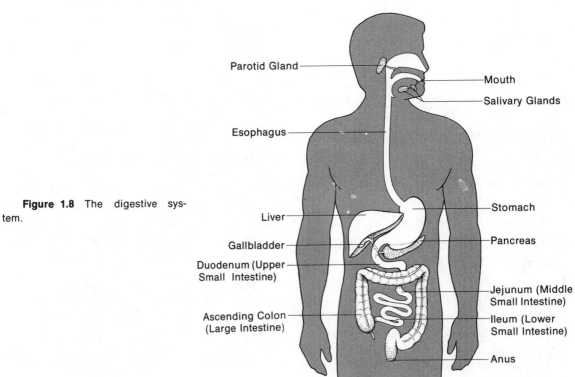

Figure 1.8 The digestive system.

Parotid Gland

Mouth

Salivary Glands

Esophagus

Liver

Gallbladder

Duodenum (Upper
Small Intestine)

Ascending Colon
(Large Intestine)

Stomach

Pancreas

Jejunum (Middle
Small Intestine)

Ileum (Lower
Small Intestine)

Anus

metabolic needs. Carbon dioxide and some water vapor are transported in the opposite direction — from capillary blood into alveoli. During expiration, these waste gases proceed back up the respiratory tree to be eliminated into the atmosphere. A pictorial summary of this system is presented in Figure 1.7.

The *digestive system* insures that ingested food is broken down into particles usable by body cells. The main digestive organs form a continuous tube through which foods pass from mouth to anus. The mouth, pharynx, esophagus, stomach, small intestine, and large intestine constitute this passageway, known as the gastrointestinal (GI) tract. Accessory organs service the system by secreting juices or enzymes that promote the breakdown of gastrointestinal contents. Included among these accessory structures are the salivary glands, liver, gallbladder, and pancreas.

The physical and chemical breakdown of food that occurs within the gastrointestinal tract is called digestion. If nutrients are digested adequately, they become small enough to be absorbed across the small intestinal wall into the bloodstream. In this way, food particles are made available to the body cells for use in metabolism. Nondigestible or undigested material is not absorbable. It continues to move through the gastrointestinal tract to

be excreted as fecal waste through the rectum. See Figure 1.8 for a summary presentation of the digestive system.

The *circulatory system* directly supports all life-sustaining processes by transporting essential materials throughout the body. This system consists of three major components: the blood, the heart, and the blood vessels. Blood, the liquid medium of transport, consists largely of a watery fluid called plasma that supports red cells, white cells, and platelets. These cellular elements of blood are responsible for transporting oxygen, fighting infection, and clotting, respectively. The plasma of whole blood carries nutrients, electrolytes, acids, bases, and other chemicals throughout the body.

Blood is pumped by the heart and travels within specially constructed vessels as it circulates to all body cells. Elastic-walled, contractile arteries carry blood rich in oxygen away from the heart. These vessels become thinner and narrower as blood approaches its cellular destination. At this point, the artery is transformed into an extremely fragile capillary with walls one cell thick. Exchange of nutrients and gases is facilitated by this structural modification. Blood leaves the site of cellular exchange depleted in oxygen and high in metabolic wastes. The vessel carrying it

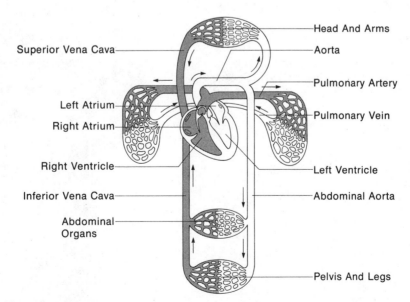

Figure 1.9 Diagram of the circulatory system. Shading indicates unoxygenated blood, and unshaded vessels carry oxygen-rich blood.

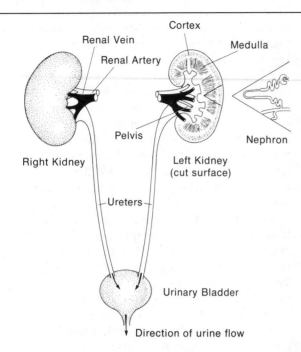

Figure 1.10 The urinary system.

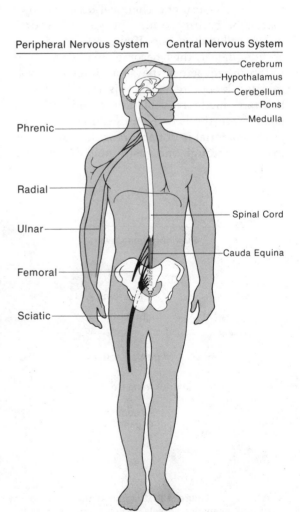

Figure 1.11 The nervous system.

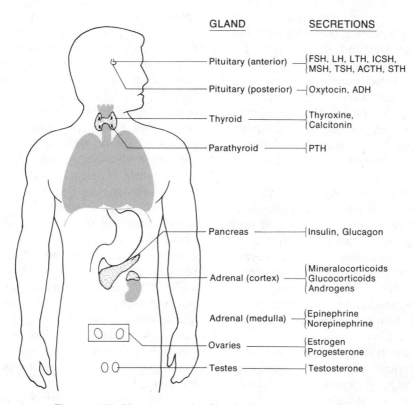

GLAND   SECRETIONS

Pituitary (anterior)   { FSH, LH, LTH, ICSH,
                          MSH, TSH, ACTH, STH

Pituitary (posterior)   —{ Oxytocin, ADH

Thyroid   { Thyroxine,
                          Calcitonin

Parathyroid   —{ PTH

Pancreas   —{ Insulin, Glucagon

Adrenal (cortex)   { Mineralocorticoids
                          Glucocorticoids
                          Androgens

Adrenal (medulla)   { Epinephrine
                          Norepinephrine

Ovaries   { Estrogen
                          Progesterone

Testes   —{ Testosterone

Figure 1.12   The major endocrine glands and their secretions.

back to the heart (the vein) is a continuation of the capillary but thicker-walled and structurally characterized by internal valves that prevent fluid backflow. It is important to remember that arteries, capillaries, and veins are continuous with each other and with the heart. The entire circulatory system forms one closed circuit, which is represented diagrammatically in Figure 1.9.

The *urinary system* functions to excrete certain metabolic wastes. The primary substances normally eliminated are water, electrolytes, and nitrogenous wastes such as urea; uric acid, and creatinine. The major components of this system are two kidneys, two ureters, the bladder, and the urethra. The kidneys manufacture urine through the activity of their functional microscopic subunits, the nephrons. The ureters transport urine from the kidneys to the bladder for storage. The urethra, in turn, carries urine from the bladder out of the body. Figure 1.10 illustrates the anatomical relationships between the component parts of the urinary system.

The *skeletal system* constitutes the hard tissue framework of the body. It is composed of 206 bones of varying size, shape, and form that support, protect, and give form to the total structure. Functionally, the red marrow contained within certain bones is an important source of blood cell production. These blood cells are needed for the transport of oxygen, the fighting of infection, and the clotting of whole blood.

The *muscular system* is composed of all skeletal (or voluntarily controlled) muscle tissue in the body. It represents a massive amount of body weight and regulates all purposeful movement. As such, skeletal muscle is involved in many activities integral to life support, such as chewing, swallowing, inspiring and expiring air, and controlling elimination of fecal and urinary wastes.

The *nervous system* can be subdivided into the central nervous system (CNS) and the peripheral nervous system (PNS). The central nervous system, consisting of the brain and spinal cord, is the master control center for many bodily functions. The cerebral cortex of the brain initiates the majority of voluntary movement and interprets most sensory infor-

mation received by the higher brain for processing. The medulla of the brain houses reflex control centers essential to the normal functioning of the cardiovascular and respiratory systems. The hypothalamus of the brain is central to many significant processes, including the maintenance of fluid and electrolyte balance.

The spinal cord extends from the base of the cranium down to the lower back, encased by bony vertebrae. It is the essential link between the brain and nerves external to the CNS, carrying information up and down the spine via well-defined tracts.

The peripheral nervous system comprises the network of nerves existing outside the CNS, carrying messages back and forth between all body structures and the CNS. Functional control over organs and skeletal muscle is maintained by the activity of these peripheral nerves. Hence they insure optimal performance of many structures essential to life support and maintenance. A diagrammatic presentation of some component parts of the nervous system can be found in Figure 1.11.

The *endocrine system* consists of many glands scattered throughout the body. These glands manufacture and release chemical secretions called hormones directly into the bloodstream. Hormones control and regulate such critical bodily functions as urinary output and composition, cellular metabolic rate, and growth and development. The maintenance of cellular survival is dependent upon the endocrine system. A brief review of some major glands and their secretions can be found in Figure 1.12.

The *reproductive system* functions to insure the continuing survival of the human race. Without the capacity to produce like offspring, any species would become extinct. Thus the reproductive organs are essential to the ongoing existence of human beings on earth. Since this system does not function in any direct way to support cellular life in the postfetal human organism, it will not be extensively discussed in this text. It must be remembered, however, that the birth of an individual with normally functioning life support systems is predicated upon the existence of normal reproductive processes.

STUDY QUESTIONS

1. What are the three major fluid compartments of the body?
2. What is the function of each of the three major fluid compartments?
3. Predict what might happen to the volume of plasma in a capillary if a blockage developed in (a) the arteriole or (b) the venule that serves that capillary.
4. A patient is suffering from chronic oxygen deficit. What might happen to his or her energy levels, and why?
5. A patient is known to have a severely elevated metabolic rate. How might this affect his or her plasma CO_2 levels, and why?
6. Which structural component of the cell is most directly involved with metabolism?
7. Which structural component of the cell is most directly involved with the manufacture of protein?
8. Explain why the following tissues are ideally adapted to their function: (a) epithelium, (b) bone, (c) blood, (d) nerve, (e) muscle.
9. Identify two or three ways in which each major system functions to service the basic cellular life needs.

Suggested Readings

Brooks, S. M., and Paynton-Brooks, N.: The Human Body, 2nd ed. St. Louis, The C. V. Mosby Company, 1980, pp. 1–9; 35–50.

Burke, S. R.: Human Anatomy and Physiology for the Health Sciences. New York, John Wiley & Sons, 1980, pp. 24–37.

Guyton, A. C.: Physiology of the Human Body, 5th ed. Philadelphia: W. B. Saunders Company, 1979, pp. 3–12.

Hole, J. W.: Human Anatomy and Physiology. Dubuque, Wm. C. Brown Company, 1978, pp. 6–11; 38–46; 88–98.

Memmler, R. L., and Wood, D. L.: The Human Body in Health and Disease, 4th ed. Philadelphia, J. B. Lippincott Company, 1977, pp. 1–9; 35–50.

Silverstein, A.: Human Anatomy and Physiology. New York, John Wiley & Sons, 1980, pp. 5–18; 39–50; 679–689.

Chapter Outline

chapter 2

Cellular Life Needs — A Systemic Overview

Chapter Objectives

At the completion of this chapter, the student will be able to :

1. Describe the significance of inspiration, diffusion, erythrocytes, and the cardiovascular system in servicing the cellular need for oxygen.
2. Identify the way in which vitamin B_{12}, folic acid, erythropoietin, and iron function to facilitate erythrocyte maturation.
3. Differentiate between cellular nutrient supply and cellular nutrient utilization.
4. Describe the significance of ingestion, digestion, absorption, and transport in servicing the cellular need for nutrients.
5. Describe the function of the liver in processing absorbed nutrients.
6. Define cellular metabolism.
7. Differentiate between the four primary steps of glucose catabolism.
8. Identify four major factors that may affect cellular metabolism and describe their significance.
9. Trace the catabolism of carbohydrates, proteins, and fats.
10. Differentiate between nondigestible and metabolic wastes.
11. Describe the processes of fecal formation and fecal elimination.
12. Identify the major metabolic wastes.
13. Describe the way in which the skin, lungs, and kidneys function to service the cellular need for elimination.
14. Describe the role played by erythrocytes in carbon dioxide elimination.

INTRODUCTION

If health is to be maintained, all cellular life needs must be met on a continuous basis. Provision for cellular oxygen, nutrients, elimination, and fluid and electrolyte balance is assured by active cooperation between the systems of the body. In fact, careful analysis of the life support mechanisms reveals that each need is met by many interacting systems. Following is a discussion of each cellular life requirement and a description of the complex manner in which it is served.

CELLULAR NEED FOR OXYGEN

When asked how the human body obtains oxygen, one immediately thinks of the respiratory system. Although it is true that oxygen does enter the body through respiratory structures, its arrival at the cell is dependent upon a much more complex process involving many body systems.

There are four essential prerequisites to an adequate supply of cellular oxygen: (1) There must be a functional means of *inspiration*. Inspiration is the movement of oxygen from the atmosphere into the lungs, and it involves cooperation between structures in the muscular, skeletal, and nervous systems. (2) There must be adequate *diffusion* of oxygen from the thin-walled alveoli (air sacs) deep within the lungs into surrounding pulmonary capillaries. Diffusion is the movement of a substance from an area of greater concentration (in this case the alveoli of the lungs) to an area of lesser concentration (in this case the plasma of pulmonary capillaries). Structural integrity of the pulmonary tissue itself and of the vessels serving the alveoli is a prerequisite to diffusion of oxygen into the bloodstream. (3) There must be a sufficient population of *erythrocytes* (RBC's) containing adequate amounts of hemoglobin. The hemoglobin within RBC's is an iron (heme)-protein (globin) complex that combines chemically with oxygen as it enters the blood. Components of the skeletal, digestive, and urinary systems must work jointly to provide the body with the RBC's necessary for oxygen transport. (4) There must be a *cardiovascular system* functioning to transport the oxygenated RBC's throughout the body. The central nervous system works in conjunction with the heart and blood vessels, to regulate and coordinate cardiac rate and vascular tone.

A closer look at each of these four factors supports the multisystemic view of cellular oxygen supply. As we elaborate in the following pages upon each of the four prerequisites listed, the critical role played by each system in supplying the cellular need for oxygen will become clear.

Inspiration

In order to take air into the lungs, the thoracic cavity must first increase in size. As the volume of the cavity is enlarged, the pressure is decreased below atmospheric pressure. Then, following a general law of physics, air will move from where it is under greater pressure (in the atmosphere), through the respiratory tree, to where it is under lesser pressure (in the lungs). The mechanism of inspiration is presented graphically in Figure 2.1.

Enlargement of the thoracic cavity is accomplished by contraction of two major muscles. The external intercostals pull the ribs up and out, thereby increasing the anterior-posterior dimension of the cavity. The diaphragm moves down, thus increasing the inferior-superior dimension of the cavity. Contraction of these muscles is dependent upon stimulation by peripheral nerves, which, in turn, receive direction from the central nervous system. The medulla, in fact, is central in determining rate and depth of respiration.

Since the nervous, muscular, and skeletal systems are integrally involved in the process of inspiration, it follows that cellular oxygen supply could be compromised by certain neuromuscular or skeletal disorders. Polio, a life-threatening disease until the development of an immune vaccine, produced iron lung victims by destroying the nerves that stimulated contraction of the respiratory muscles. Similarly, the much-publicized Guillain-Barré syndrome, contracted by certain individuals after inoculation with the swine flu vaccine, precipitated some cases of respiratory arrest and

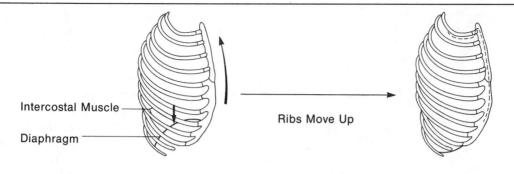

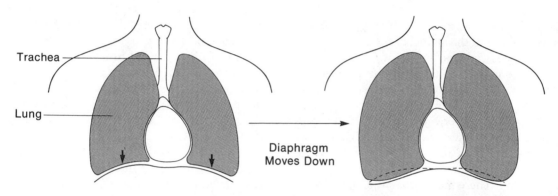

Figure 2.1 Mechanism of inspiration.

death due to paralysis of the respiratory muscles. Even a case of multiple rib fractures can interfere with inspiration by rendering thoracic enlargement painful, if not impossible.

Diffusion

Diffusion is the critical link between inspiration and oxygen transport by erythrocytes. Normally, the partial pressure of oxygen in the alveoli (pO_2) is less than that in the pulmonary capillaries. Thus, in keeping with the general laws of diffusion, oxygen molecules move from an area of higher partial pressure (in the lungs) to an area of lower partial pressure (in the plasma). This mechanism is illustrated in Figure 2.2.

If obstruction or fibrosis of pulmonary tissue should occur, as it does in emphysema or asthma, diffusion can be substantially reduced. Hence, the quantity of oxygen available to the RBC's would be decreased.

Erythrocytes

As mentioned earlier, the majority of oxygen is transported throughout the body in chemical combination with the hemoglobin

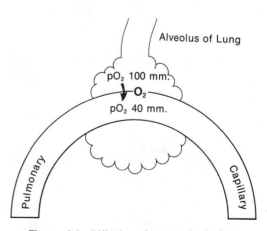

Figure 2.2 Diffusion of oxygen in the lung.

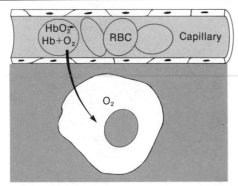

Figure 2.3 Diffusion of oxygen to metabolizing cells.

(Hb) of RBC's. Assuming adequate diffusion of oxygen out of the alveoli of the lungs (where oxygen is in high concentration), oxygen molecules then attach to the iron group of hemoglobin and are subsequently released to interstitial fluid for use by metabolizing cells (where oxygen is in low concentration). This process is presented diagrammatically in Figure 2.3.

The ability of blood to transport enough oxygen for cellular needs is dependent upon two factors. There must be a sufficient *concentration of RBC's* in plasma, and each RBC must contain an optimal *amount of hemoglobin*.

The manufacture of an adequate number of erythrocytes is influenced by the presence of three chemical factors: vitamin B_{12}, folic acid, and erythropoietin. All of these substances affect the complex process of RBC maturation that normally occurs in the red marrow of certain bones in the body.

The functional availability of vitamin B_{12} (otherwise known as the *extrinsic factor)* is dependent upon its absorption out of the gastrointestinal tract. Once freed from the confines of the small intestine, this vitamin can be stored in the liver and drawn upon by the bone marrow when its presence is required to promote erythrocyte maturation. Absorption of vitamin B_{12} is facilitated by the presence of an *intrinsic factor* normally released by the mucosal lining of the stomach. Lack of this intrinsic factor, for genetic or other reasons, results in a condition known as pernicious anemia, which affects RBC production and, secondarily, oxygen transport to body cells.

As is the case with vitamin B_{12}, folic acid availability is also linked to gastrointestinal intake. Functional in the formation of DNA, folic acid affects growth and maturation of the erythrocyte. Normally manufactured by bac-

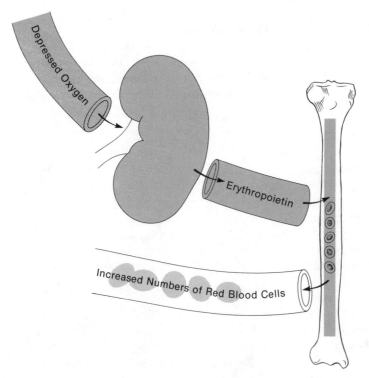

Figure 2.4 Release of erythropoietin causes an increase in production of red blood cells.

teria of the digestive tract, folic acid is also present in green leafy vegetables and liver. Along with vitamin B_{12}, folic acid promotes the development of erythrocytes in the bone marrow.

Erythropoietin is the third major factor influencing RBC maturation. Produced by the kidney and released into the bloodstream, erythropoietin is transported to the bone marrow, where it stimulates an increase in erythrocyte production. Since release of erythropoietin is triggered by depressed levels of plasma oxygen (hypoxemia), this mechanism serves as a compensatory response to decreased cellular oxygen availability. If oxygen supply should fall, the kidneys thus play a role in increasing RBC production. Hence, people living at high altitudes, where environmental oxygen levels are low, tend to show elevated erythrocyte counts. A graphic summary of the erythropoietin mechanism can be found in Figure 2.4.

Although vitamin B_{12}, folic acid, and erythropoietin promote RBC maturation and growth, they cannot insure adequate hemoglobin availability to the developing erythrocytes. As mentioned earlier, hemoglobin is fashioned from an iron and a protein group. It is the iron, or heme, portion of hemoglobin that is functional in oxygen transport. Thus, a deficit of iron (Fe) can critically diminish the supply of oxygen to body cells.

Iron for hemoglobin formation is derived primarily from two sources. It is both ingested in food and released from worn-out RBC's to be recycled into newly forming erythrocytes. Assuming normal dietary intake and absorption, it is the recycling process that becomes the largest potential stumbling block to iron availability. The mechanism of releasing iron from old RBC's is thus worth examining.

Red blood cells in the body are normally short-lived. Lacking a nucleus and the ability to reproduce, they function for about 120 days — after which time they are engulfed and destroyed by specialized *reticuloendothelial* (RE) cells found primarily in the liver, spleen, and bone marrow. With the destruction of the RBC, hemoglobin is released and split into a heme and a protein group. The heme fraction is processed by reticuloendothelial cells, and

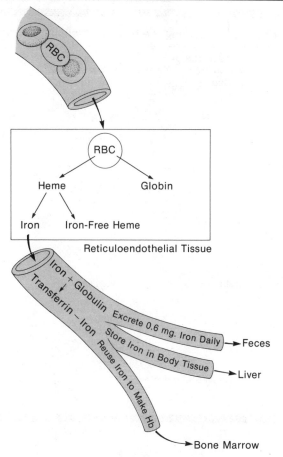

Figure 2.5 The recycling of iron in the body.

iron is liberated to be used in the manufacture of new hemoglobin. The remaining iron-free heme is converted by reticuloendothelial cells into the pigment bilirubin. Under normal conditions, bilirubin is subsequently conjugated by the liver and excreted in the form of bile. Disease of the liver, spleen, or bone marrow may, of course, disrupt this complex recycling process — as would any abnormal loss of RBC's from the body. Even excessively heavy menstrual bleeding can, over a period of time, deplete the body's pool of iron. The complicated mechanism for reusing iron is summarized diagrammatically in Figure 2.5.

Cardiovascular System

Assuming optimal concentration and composition of RBC's, it is necessary to con-

TABLE 2.1   **Meeting the Need for Cellular Oxygen**

Prerequisite to Cellular O_2 Supply	Systems Involved	Function of Systems
Inspiration	Muscular	Contraction of specific muscles causes enlargement of thoracic cavity.
	Skeletal	Ribs elevate to enlarge anterior-posterior dimension of thoracic cavity.
	Nervous	CNS controls rate and depth of respirations. PNS stimulates contraction of inspiratory muscles.
	Respiratory	Airway tubes of respiratory tract must remain open to allow for air intake.
Diffusion	Circulatory	Pulmonary capillaries receive diffusing O_2 from air sacs of lungs.
	Respiratory	Oxygen moves across walls of the air sacs into pulmonary blood.
Erythrocytes	Digestive	Involved with absorption of vitamin B_{12}, folic acid, and iron—all necessary to RBC maturation. Liver functional in recycling of iron from old RBC's.
	Urinary	Kidney functions in release of erythropoietin.
	Skeletal	Red bone marrow manufactures erythrocytes and functions in the recycling of iron.
Cardiovascular system		Heart and blood vessels pump and transport oxygenated blood.
	Nervous	CNS regulates cardiac rate and vascular tone.

sider the role of the *heart and blood vessels* in regulating the circulation of blood. Without a functional cardiovascular system, oxygenated erythrocytes will not be carried through the body. Since the nervous system controls both cardiac rate and vascular tone, it too can affect oxygen transport. Hence, cellular oxygen supply can be compromised as the result of disease of the heart, blood vessels, or nervous system. Specific disorders and their clinical manifestations are discussed in detail in Units 3 and 4.

In summary, it can be said that many different organs and systems in the body may affect the supply of oxygen to individual cells. Almost every major system plays a significant role in meeting the critical cellular need for oxygen. Conversely, then, pathological conditions of these organs and systems can result in a deficit of cellular oxygen. Certain critical diseases and their effects upon oxygen supply will be discussed in Unit 4. Table 2.1 sum-

marizes the function of each pertinent system in meeting cellular oxygen needs.

CELLULAR NEED FOR NUTRIENTS

Nutrients are needed by all cells to support metabolic reactions. The digestive system is generally thought of as central to the supply of human nourishment. The gastrointestinal tract and its accessory organs do play a significant role in meeting the cellular need for nutrients. Many other body systems, however, must also work cooperatively to insure adequate cellular nutrition.

As we analyze this cellular need for nutrients more thoroughly, it is helpful to consider two aspects of cell-nutrient interaction: (a) the *supply* of nutrients to the cell, and (b) the *utilization* of nutrients by the cell. The distinction between supply and utilization can be illustrated by a situation in which a man who has no shelter for his family is given the raw materials with which to build a house. Without the prerequisite skill and tools, however, he will make little headway in solving his problem. Success will depend upon having the necessary carpentry and masonry implements as well as the know-how to transform these basic materials into a finished product. Such is the case with the human body. Nutrients may arrive at each cell, but unless enzyme systems are available to insure adequate utilization, cellular starvation could result.

The Supply of Nutrients to the Cell

The supply of nutrients to body cells is dependent upon the interactions of four critical factors:

1. There must be a means of *ingestion*. Ingestion is the intake of food from the environment into the body. It normally involves cooperation between the skeletal (or voluntary) muscles and the nervous system as the hand and arm direct food into the mouth.

2. There must be a functional process of *digestion*. Digestion entails the physical and chemical breakdown of food within the gastrointestinal tract. It is a complex process designed to produce nutrient particles small enough to be usable by body cells. The digestive, nervous, and endocrine systems function together to insure digestion of the food we eat.

3. There must be *absorption* of digested nutrients out of the gastrointestinal tract into the blood. In this way, essential food particles are retained by the body and not lost as fecal waste.

4. There must be *transport* of absorbed nutrients by the blood, first from the gastroin-

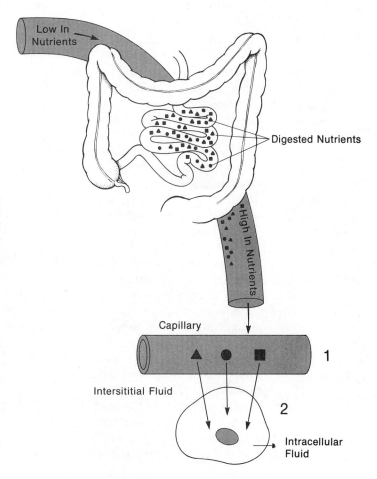

Figure 2.6 Nutrients absorbed from the digestive tract into the bloodstream initially diffuse (1) through the capillary wall into interstitial fluid and are subsequently transported (2) across the cell membrane into the intracellular compartment.

testinal tract to interstitial fluid, and second, through the cell membrane into intracellular fluid. This dual process is illustrated diagrammatically in Figure 2.6. Components of the circulatory, nervous, and endocrine systems work together to insure that food particles reach their ultimate cellular destination.

INGESTION

Ingestion of food is the essential first step in the chain of events bringing food from the environment to the cell. Functional cooperation between several key muscles in the arm and hand must be mediated by the nervous system to insure the delivery of nourishment to the mouth. Hence, certain neuromuscular disorders or alterations in state of consciousness could result in starvation unless alternate feeding mechanisms were employed. The intravenous (I.V.) introduction of nutrients into a comatose patient is an example of medically compensating for inability to ingest food naturally.

DIGESTION

The digestion of food is an essential prerequisite to its absorption. Carbohydrates (CHO), fats, and proteins, the three major nutrients, must be broken down into simple sugars, amino acids, and fatty acids and glycerol, respectively. Once reduced to smaller particles, nutrients can pass from the intestinal lumen into the bloodstream for transport throughout the body.

This reduction of nutrient molecules into more absorbable end products takes place primarily in the mouth, stomach, and small intestine. Physical breakdown involves alterations in the size and form of food particles, without any change in chemical composition. It occurs largely through muscular contractions. The coordinated activity of certain skeletal muscles responsible for grinding and chewing food in the mouth must precede swallowing. Once nutrients have passed from the oral cavity into the esophagus, contraction of smooth (involuntary) muscles in the walls of the digestive organs further facilitates breakdown. Hence the muscular system, digestive system, and nervous system (which

initiates and controls contractions) are all functional in the physical aspects of digestion.

To sufficiently reduce nutrients into absorbable form, however, *chemical* changes must accompany the physical alterations. Large-chain carbohydrates, proteins, and fats are chemically split into smaller molecular fragments in the presence of specific enzymes. The complex processes of chemical digestion are summarized in Figure 2.7.

It is important to remember that enzymatic release is partially coordinated and controlled by both endocrine and neural factors. Disorders of either of these systems could thus affect the digestive process. It is well known, for example, that certain fibers of the vagus nerve stimulate release of highly acidic digestive juices from the gastric glands lining the stomach. In certain individuals, elevated gastric acid secretions can result in erosion of the lining of the stomach or duodenum (peptic ulcer). When ulcers are intractable, or unresponsive to standard medical intervention, it is possible to obtain relief by a vagotomy. This is a surgical procedure in which those fibers of the vagus nerve that promote release of acidic gastric juice are severed. In this way, alleviation of a gastrointestinal disturbance is obtained by altering a component of the nervous system.

In summary, then, digestion involves both the physical and the chemical breakdown of ingested nutrients. The gastrointestinal tract alone cannot implement digestion. For the total process to proceed normally, cooperation between the digestive, muscular, nervous, and endocrine systems is necessary.

ABSORPTION

In order for digested nutrients to reach the cells of the body, they must first leave the confines of the gastrointestinal tract. This passage of nutrient particles from the lumen of the digestive tract into capillaries or lymph vessels is called absorption.

Although a few substances (such as alcohol and aspirin) can move readily through the stomach wall into the blood, the majority of nutrient absorption occurs in the small intestine. The small intestine is specifically

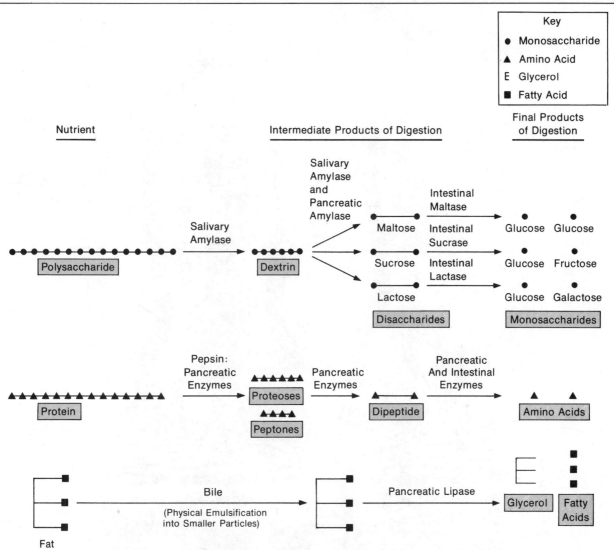

Figure 2.7 Chemical digestion of major nutrients into absorbable end products.

designed to optimize the absorptive process. Microscopic examination of the small intestinal lining reveals the presence of myriad fingerlike extensions *(villi)* projecting into the lumen of the gut. Each villus is composed of epithelial cells, which, in turn, have microvilli (brushlike borders) interfacing with intestinal contents. The surface area available for absorption is increased many times by these numerous macro- and micro-projections. The structure of the villus is presented in Figure 2.8.

To further facilitate absorption, each villus is served by both blood and lymph vessels (lacteals). Fats and fat-soluble substances are picked up by the lymph system, eventually entering the bloodstream at the junction of the left subclavian and left internal jugular veins. Most other nutrients are water-soluble and are absorbed directly into the blood. The end products of carbohydrate digestion (simple sugars) and protein digestion (amino acids), water, and most electrolytes (salts) pass through epithelial cells of the villi into the plasma of blood capillaries.

The absorptive process is summarized diagrammatically in Figure 2.9. It is dependent upon the integrity of the small intestinal

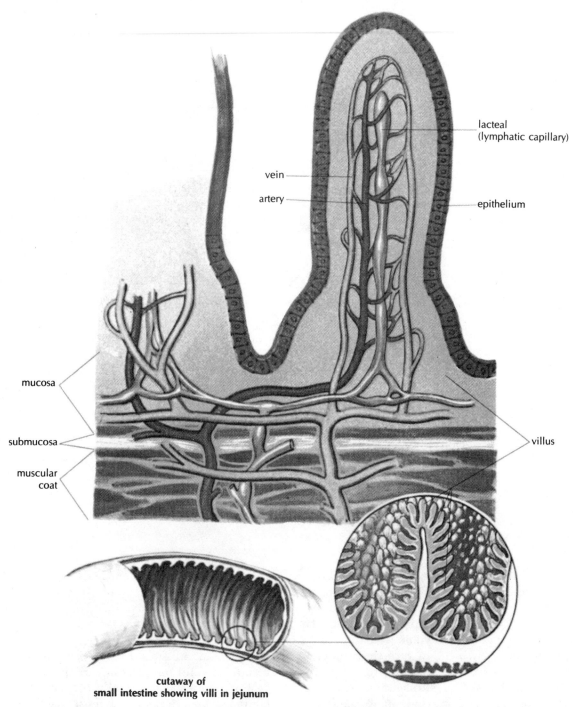

lacteal
(lymphatic capillary)

vein

artery

epithelium

mucosa

submucosa

muscular
coat

villus

**cutaway of
small intestine showing villi in jejunum**

Figure 2.8   The small intestinal villus. (From Memmler, R., and Wood, D.: The Human Body
in Health and Disease, 4th ed. Philadelphia: J. B. Lippincott Company, 1977. Used by permission.)

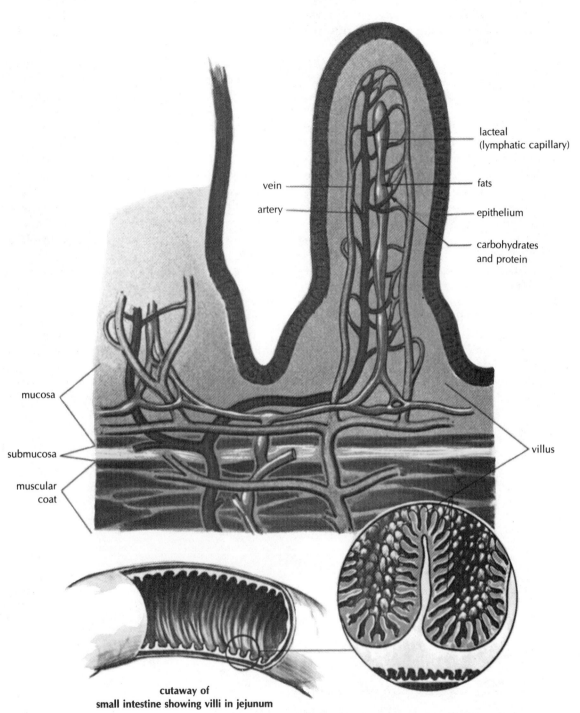

lacteal
(lymphatic capillary)

vein

artery

fats

epithelium

carbohydrates
and protein

mucosa

submucosa

villus

muscular
coat

cutaway of
small intestine showing villi in jejunum

Figure 2.9 Small intestinal absorption. (From Memmler, R., and Wood, D.: The Human Body in Health and Disease, 4th ed. Philadelphia, J. B. Lippincott Company, 1977. Used by permission.)

lining and adequate blood-lymph circulation through the villi. Hence, components of both the digestive system and the circulatory system are needed to insure adequate absorption.

TRANSPORT

Once digested particles have entered the circulatory system, they are ready for transport throughout the body. As mentioned earlier, the nutrients must first move across the capillary wall to the interstitial fluid bathing the cells and then through the cell membrane into the intracellular fluid.

Not all nutrients travel the same path from the gastrointestinal tract to the cells. Water-soluble substances (such as amino acids, simple sugars, and electrolytes) are carried by blood vessels to the portal vein and into the liver. The hepatic (liver) cells are responsible for much of the chemical processing of food. The mechanisms and significance of liver function are discussed in more detail under *The Utilization of Nutrients by the Cell.*

Fats and fat-soluble substances (such as vitamins A, D, E, and K), on the other hand, are transported from small lymphatic capillaries into progressively larger lymph vessels before finally arriving at the thoracic duct. The thoracic duct, in turn, empties lymph into venous blood. For fatty nutrients to arrive at the liver for processing, they must first pass through the heart and then be pumped to hepatic cells through arterial vessels. These nutrient transport pathways are shown in diagrammatic form in Figure 2.10.

Most food particles are thus acted on by the liver before being carried by plasma to their cellular destination. Having arrived at interstitial fluid, however, nutrients must then cross the cell membrane barrier. This is a complex selective process influenced to a large extent by the presence of certain hormones. *Insulin,* for example, is known to promote the transport of glucose and protein across the membranes of many body cells. *Growth hormone* (GH), released by the anterior pituitary gland, facilitates the movement of amino acids into intracellular fluid. An endocrine imbalance can therefore affect intracellular nutrient supplies. Diabetes mellitus, a disorder characterized by insufficient insulin output, will

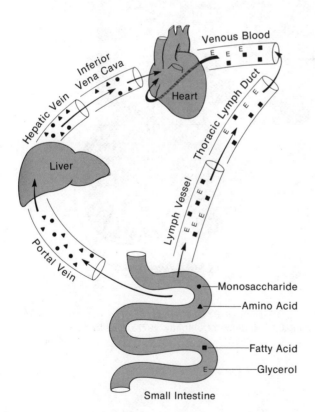

Figure 2.10 Nutrients are transported via different pathways. Water-soluble substances are carried by the blood vessels through the liver and into the hepatic vein; fats and fat-soluble substances travel via the lymphatic system into venous blood.

result in elevated blood sugar levels (hyperglycemia) as glucose unable to enter the cell accumulates in plasma. The untreated diabetic, in spite of adequate ingestion, digestion, and absorption, manifests clinical symptoms of starvation. Although food has entered the mouth, essential nutrients are not being supplied to the cell.

In summary, the nutrient transport mechanism is dependent upon interaction between components of the circulatory and endocrine systems. Failure of the heart, blood vessels, or certain glands could therefore result in cellular malnutrition.

The Utilization of Nutrients by the Cell

For the body to function normally, each cell must be able to use its supply of intracellular nutrients to generate energy for growth, repair, and functional activities. The process whereby food particles are burned in the presence of oxygen to yield energy and waste products is a two-step process:

1. For maximal efficiency, most nutrients should be processed by the liver before arriving at their cellular destination. The chemical changes caused by hepatic cells insure control over the type and amount of nutrients being carried to service cellular needs.

2. Once nutrients are inside the cell, enzyme systems must be present to support all phases of metabolism. *Enzymes* are proteins that promote the chemical reactions of metabolism without changing chemically themselves. Occasionally a nonprotein factor called a *coenzyme* is attached loosely to the enzyme to help activate it. In the body certain vitamins and minerals serve as coenzymes and are thus critical to the metabolic process. Metabolism is generally defined as the sum total of all cellular chemical reactions in the body. It involves both the building of new substances (*anabolism*) and the breakdown of nutrients to yield energy (*catabolism*). Since our primary concern is with energy generation, emphasis will be placed upon the catabolic process.

PROCESSING BY THE LIVER

As digested nutrients are absorbed into the bloodstream they are not always immedi-

ately needed by body cells to generate energy. In the liver, chemical changes can occur that enable storage of food substances until they are required for catabolism.

Carbohydrates, for example, can be stored in the body as glycogen or fats. In preparation for storage, most simple sugars (the end products of carbohydrate digestion) are first converted to glucose by hepatic cells. Glucose units can then be chemically linked into a long-chain storage molecule called *glycogen*. *Glycogenesis*, the manufacture of glycogen, occurs largely in the liver and skeletal muscle tissue. Although glycogen is the preferential storage form for carbohydrates, liver cells can also convert glucose into fats by a process called *lipogenesis*. Lipids thus generated are stored in adipose tissue depots throughout the body and mobilized when needed for catabolic reactions. Carbohydrate storage is depicted diagrammatically in Figure 2.11.

The end products of fat digestion are primarily glycerol and fatty acids. During absorption, the glycerol and fatty acids recom-

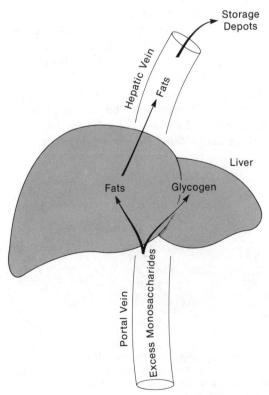

Figure 2.11 Carbohydrate storage.

bine in intestinal epithelial cells to form larger lipid molecules. When cellular metabolic needs are low, these lipids are stored in fatty tissue deposits until needed.

Amino acids, the end products of protein digestion, are used primarily for building and repairing body tissues. Thus the majority of absorbed amino acids are carried to individual cells, where they are chemically linked by intracellular ribosomes to yield essential body proteins. It is through this anabolic process that the three primary plasma proteins are manufactured by the liver. Albumin, globulin, and fibrinogen owe their existence to hepatic protein synthesis activity. They, in turn, are critical to the maintenance of fluid balance, immunity, and clotting ability, respectively. Some excess amino acids, on the other hand, can be converted in the liver to glycogen or fat. Any fat thus generated is carried to adipose tissue for storage. Glycogen remains primarily in the liver. Both glycogen and lipids wait for metabolic needs to call them into action.

It is clear that the liver plays a central role in processing, converting, and storing absorbed food particles. The functional interrelationships between the liver and the three major nutrients are shown in Figure 2.12.

The mechanisms of nutrient storage described thus far can help explain why overeating leads to obesity. Food intake in excess of the amount required for metabolic needs — whether it be of a carbohydrate, fat, or protein nature — will eventually be stored primarily in the form of lipids. The adipose tissue accepting these fats, moreover, is distributed throughout the body. About 50 per cent is found directly under the skin (subcutaneous), and the remainder is located around major organs, such as the kidney, and between muscles. If an individual maintains a reasonable level of physical activity, many of these stored lipids will be drawn upon and burned for energy. If, on the other hand, a very sedentary lifestyle is followed, the amount of adipose tissue remains stable or increases. The description of an overweight person as "fat" thus truly reflects an anatomical reality.

Not only are hepatic cells critical in regulating nutrient storage, they are also essential to *mobilizing* food for use by metabolizing body cells. Not all molecules can be used equally efficiently to feed the catabolic process. The liver serves as a factory controlling the quantity and quality of raw materials supplied to the intracellular metabolic machinery.

When energy demands increase, the body must respond by supplying more nutrients to service catabolic reactions. The ideal cellular food is glucose, with fats second best, and amino acids least desirable. In preparing these three major nutrients for cellular use, the liver again plays a central role.

To mobilize carbohydrates, glycogen is split in the liver from a long-chain molecule back into smaller glucose subunits. This process, called *glycogenolysis*, increases glucose availability to catabolizing cells and facilitates metabolic reactions.

Before fats can be used for intracellular metabolism, the larger lipid molecules must first be degraded to glycerol and fatty acids. This process, called *lipolysis*, occurs primarily in the liver. The *glycerol* released can then be directly metabolized by body cells or converted by hepatic cells into glucose by a process called *gluconeogenesis*. Fatty acids, on the other hand, are converted by the liver primarily into chemicals called *ketone bodies*. Most ketone bodies then enter plasma to be used directly in the cellular metabolic cycle. In the event that carbohydrates are limited in number or unavailable for cellular catabolism, fat mobilization increases and ketone bodies accumulate in the plasma and interstitial fluid compartments. Since ketones are slightly acidic by nature, clinical symptoms of ketosis and aci-

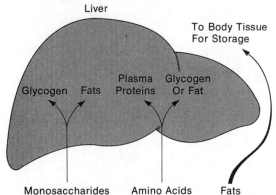

Figure 2.12 Metabolic functions of the liver: processing and storage of nutrients ingested in excess of metabolic needs.

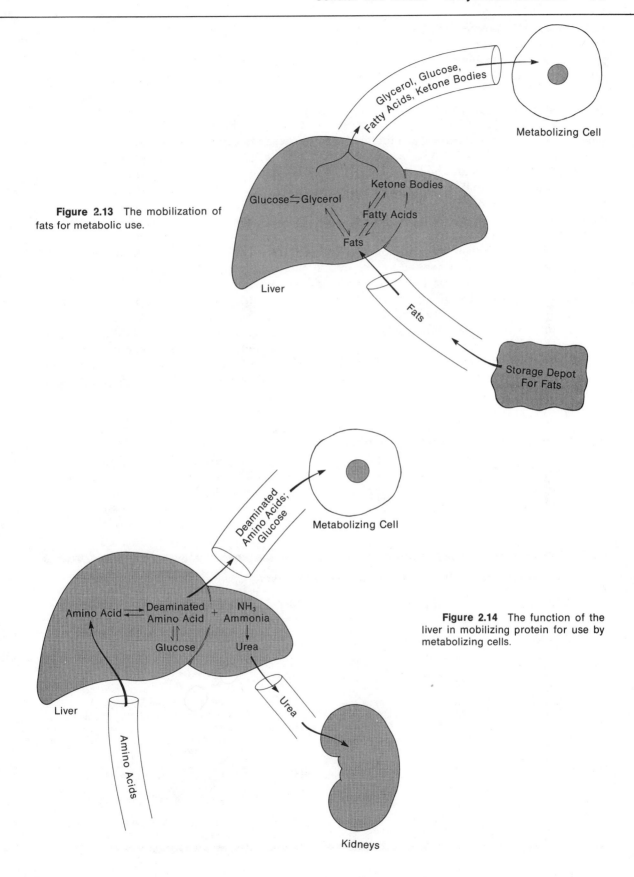

Figure 2.13 The mobilization of fats for metabolic use.

Figure 2.14 The function of the liver in mobilizing protein for use by metabolizing cells.

dosis ensue. This situation is illustrated vividly by a case of diabetes mellitus, in which glucose is not able to enter body cells owing to insufficient insulin. Lack of ability to catabolize glucose results in accelerated processing of fats for metabolism, with a concomitant rise in plasma ketone bodies. The process whereby fats are mobilized for metabolic use is shown in Figure 2.13.

Although proteins are the least preferred energy source, at times it is necessary for them to supply metabolic needs. In those cases the characteristic amino group (NH_2) must first be removed from amino acids in the liver by a process called *deamination*. The ammonia liberated by this reaction is converted to *urea* by hepatic cells and then released to the blood for excretion in the urine. The remaining deaminated protein fragment can either be liberated into plasma for use by the intracellular metabolic machinery, or be converted by the liver to glucose via *gluconeogenesis*. The function of the liver in protein catabolism is presented in Figure 2.14.

The liver is critical to the total processing of nutrients in the body. Hepatic cells stand at the crossroads of nutrient storage and utilization. They aid in the supply, conservation, and regulation of food particles. The liver's function in meeting the need for cellular nutrition is summarized in Table 2.2.

The complexities of hepatic function necessitate sensitive and well-defined controls. Hepatic metabolic activity is coordinated to a large extent by components of the endocrine and nervous systems.

Glycogenolysis, for example, is promoted by both endocrine and neural mechanisms. Glucagon, a hormone released by specialized alpha cells of the pancreas when blood sugar levels are low, stimulates the breakdown of glycogen into glucose. It is thus responsible for returning plasma glucose concentration toward normal. A similar result can be achieved by the central nervous system in response to stress or hypoglycemia. Under such conditions the *hypothalamus*, via messages carried by the peripheral nervous system, can trigger the release of *epinephrine* and *norepinephrine* from the adrenal medulla. Hence glucose is made more available at times of heightened metabolic demand. A summary of some of the major hormones influencing metabolic activity of the liver is presented in Table 2.3.

CELLULAR METABOLISM

Once hepatic processing of absorbed nutrients has occurred, most food particles are ready to be utilized by body cells. Although it is possible to use nutrients for building and

TABLE 2.2 **Storage and Mobilization of Nutrients by the Liver**

Nutrient	Storage	Mobilization
Carbohydrates	Conversion of carbohydrates into glycogen or fats. Lipids are subsequently deposited in storage depots throughout the body.	Glycogenolysis, with the release of simple sugars into the bloodstream.
Proteins	Utilization of amino acids for the manufacture of plasma proteins. Conversion of excess amino acids into glycogen or fats for storage.	Deamination of amino acids. Conversion of liberated ammonia into urea. Conversion of some deaminated amino acids into glucose.
Fats	Most excess fats are deposited in storage depots external to the liver.	Splitting of mobilized fat into fatty acids and glycerol. Conversion of some glycerol into glucose. Conversion of fatty acids into ketone bodies.

TABLE 2.3   Some Hormones Affecting Hepatic Metabolic Activity

Hormone	Site of Release	Effect on Metabolic Activity in the Liver
Glucagon	Alpha cells of pancreas	Promotes glycogenolysis and gluconeogenesis Promotes lipolysis
Insulin	Beta cells of pancreas	Stimulates glycogenesis Promotes lipogenesis
Epinephrine and norepinephrine	Adrenal medulla	Promotes glycogenolysis and gluconeogenesis Promotes lipolysis
Glucocorticoids	Adrenal cortex	Promotes lipolysis Promotes gluconeogenesis of amino acids Promotes glycogenolysis
ACTH	Anterior pituitary	Stimulates release of glucocorticoids, thereby promoting lipolysis and gluconeogenesis
Growth hormone (GH)	Anterior pituitary	Promotes mobilization of fats Promotes lipolysis
Thyroxine	Thyroid gland	Promotes gluconeogenesis of amino acids Promotes lipolysis Promotes use of protein for energy if carbohydrate or fat unavailable (liver must first deaminate the amino acids)

repairing body tissues (anabolism), the primary emphasis here is on the *catabolic aspects* of metabolism. The intracellular chemical combination of small nutrient particles with oxygen to yield energy and waste products is alternatively referred to as catabolism, cellular respiration, or cellular oxidation.

METABOLISM: A GENERAL OVERVIEW   The chemical reactions of catabolism are extremely complex and critical to cellular survival. As such, they merit further study. To demonstrate the mechanisms of intracellular oxidation, it is most helpful to trace a molecule of glucose through a cycle of cellular respiration. The catabolism of glucose, a preferred metabolic nutrient, proceeds through four primary steps: (1) glycolysis, (2) conversion to acetyl CoA, (3) Krebs cycle (citric acid cycle), and (4) storage of energy.

Glycolysis   Glycolysis is the breakdown of glucose into pyruvic acid. This chemical change can proceed in the absence of oxygen and is thus described as *anaerobic*. Glycolysis itself generates very little energy for cellular use. Breakdown must proceed to step 3 (the

Krebs cycle) in order for energy production to maximize. For pyruvic acid to eventually feed into the Krebs cycle, oxygen is necessary. In the absence of sufficient oxygen, pyruvic acid will convert to lactic acid and remain in this storage form until the oxygen deficit is corrected. With the reversal of low oxygen conditions, lactic acid will change back into pyruvic acid, thus enabling catabolism to proceed. A diagrammatic summary of glycolysis is presented in Figure 2.15.

The reversibility of the pyruvic acid-lactic acid relationship is illustrated by examination of the effect of high energy demands upon skeletal muscle cells. During periods of heavy physical exertion, catabolism to support contraction proceeds faster than oxygen can be supplied. At these times, the energy to shorten muscle fibers must be derived from glycolysis. Owing to inability to service the cells with sufficient oxygen at a rapid enough rate, lactic acid accumulates. This acid acts as an irritant, causing localized pain and soreness and a feeling of muscle fatigue. As the intensity of physical activity declines, the accumulated lactic acid can be converted back into

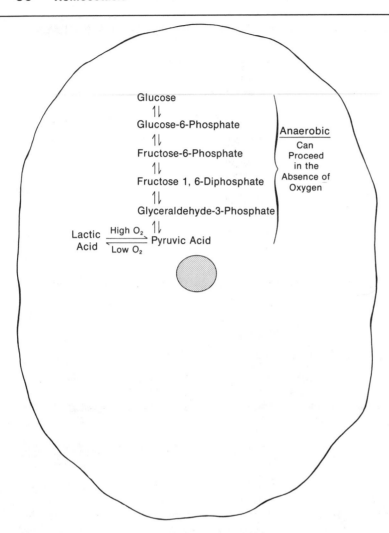

Glucose

Glucose-6-Phosphate

Fructose-6-Phosphate

Fructose 1, 6-Diphosphate

Glyceraldehyde-3-Phosphate

Lactic Acid $\xrightleftharpoons[\text{Low O}_2]{\text{High O}_2}$ Pyruvic Acid

Anaerobic
Can Proceed in the Absence of Oxygen

Figure 2.15 Glycolysis: the breakdown of glucose into pyruvic acid under anaerobic conditions.

pyruvic acid. This conversion necessitates the intake of increased levels of oxygen. Hence, increased respiratory rate usually follows heavy physical exertion and facilitates the removal of accumulated lactic acid.

Conversion to Acetyl CoA   If oxygen supply is adequate, the pyruvic acid generated by glycolysis can then be converted into a transitional substance known as acetyl CoA. Acetyl CoA, a breakdown product of pyruvic acid, is the chemical that feeds directly into the Krebs cycle.

Krebs Cycle   The Krebs cycle, or citric acid cycle, is a series of chemical reactions that completely oxidize acetyl CoA into carbon dioxide and water. The cycle is oxygen-dependent and thus described as *aerobic*. During the stepwise breakdown of acetyl CoA

into progressively smaller fragments, much energy is released. While approximately 60 per cent of the energy generated is used to maintain internal body temperature, the remaining 40 per cent is stored for use in functional work. The Krebs cycle is presented in Figure 2.16.

Storage of Energy   The generation of energy by the Krebs cycle depends largely upon the release of negatively charged particles called *electrons* from the intermediary breakdown products of the cycle. These electrons, in turn, are picked up and eventually transported to oxygen by a series of stepwise transfers in which chemicals called *cytochromes* play a major role. Cytochromes are proteins with an iron component that is specifically functional in alternately receiving and donating electrons. It is during the process of electron transfer between cytochromes that the majority of catabolic energy is released.

Some of the released energy is dissipated as body heat. The remainder can be trapped and stored in select intracellular molecules. When circumstances dictate, these storage molecules are broken down to release energy for cellular use.

One of the best storage forms for energy is the molecule ATP (adenosine triphosphate). This substance is composed of an adenosine fragment attached to three phosphate (PO_4) groups. Its structure can be represented as follows: A—P—P~P. ATP is formed from a substance called adenosine diphosphate or ADP (A—P—P) by the addition of energy and one phosphate group: A—P—P+ P+ energy → A—P—P~P. The terminal phosphate group of ATP is attached to the remainder of the mol-

ecule by a high energy bond (~). When ATP is degraded to ADP, the terminal bond is broken and stored energy is released: A—P—P~P→ A—P—P+ P+ energy.

The cellular oxidation of one molecule of glucose generates enough energy for the formation of 38 molecules of ATP. Of these 38 molecules, only two are formed during glycolysis. The remaining 36 are generated by the energy released during the Krebs cycle and subsequent electron transfers. The relationship of ATP formation to the catabolism of glucose is presented in Figure 2.17.

Factors Affecting the Metabolic Process It is clear that cellular respiration is a very complex process. The entire pathway of glucose breakdown is shown in Figure 2.18. Many factors can influence and affect the mechanisms of nutrient oxidation. Numerous vitamins and minerals, for example, are essen-

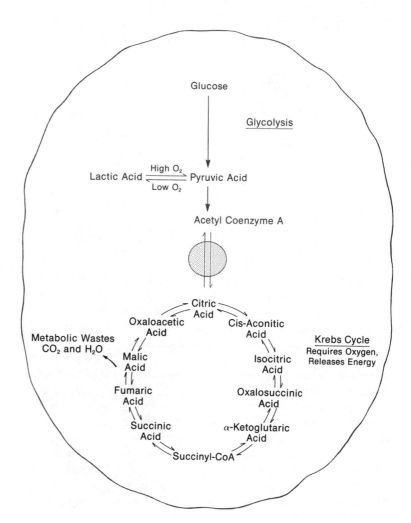

Figure 2.16 The Krebs cycle (lower half of pathway only).

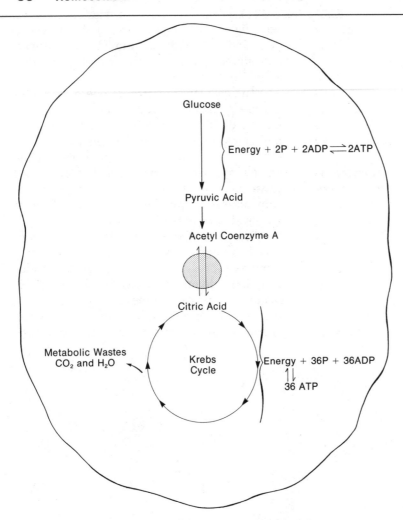

Figure 2.17 ATP formation. A total of 38 molecules of ATP are formed through cellular oxidation of one glucose molecule. Two molecules of ATP result from glycolysis, and 36 molecules are formed by the Krebs cycle.

tial to the regulation of metabolism. They serve as enzymes, coenzymes, and factors essential to the manufacture of enzymes and coenzymes in the body. The enzymes and coenzymes, in turn, are needed to facilitate the chemical reactions of catabolism. Hence, the digestive system must provide adequate intake, processing, and absorption of these nutritional components. Deficiency can result in serious metabolic derangements. Some of the vitamins and minerals essential to cellular respiration are presented in Table 2.4.

Assuming normal metabolic functioning, various factors can affect the *rate* of cellular oxidation. Among these are age, body temperature, level of physical activity, and endocrine and neural components.

It is known, for example, that newborns and young children have a much higher meta-bolic rate than do middle-aged or older individuals. This is probably due in part to the higher levels of cellular chemical activity accompanying growth and development. Fever and physical exertion also stimulate increased metabolic rate. A rise in body temperature of 10°C., for example, would increase metabolic rate by about 130%.

Several hormones are also responsible for increasing the rate of cellular catabolism. These include *thyroxin* released by the thyroid gland, *growth hormone* (GH) released by the anterior pituitary, and *epinephrine* released by the adrenal medulla. Endocrine imbalance resulting in hypersecretion of any of these substances can have serious consequences, if not checked.

Changes in metabolic rate can also be caused by the nervous system. Mobilization of

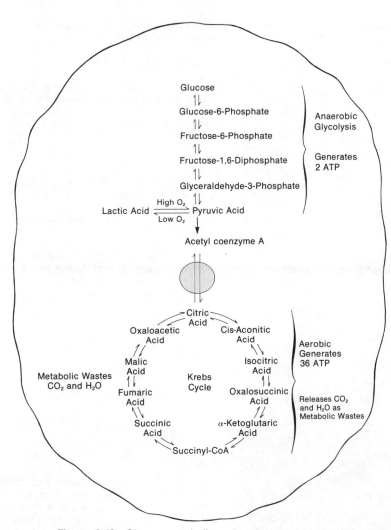

Figure 2.18 Glucose catabolism: the complete pathway.

TABLE 2.4 **Some Vitamins and Minerals Essential to Cellular Respiration**

Substance	Metabolic Significance
Vitamin B₁ (thiamine)	Serves as coenzyme for 24 different enzymes of the Krebs cycle.
Vitamin B₂ (riboflavin)	Component of certain coenzymes involved in carbohydrate and protein metabolism.
Niacin (nicotinamide)	Component of certain coenzymes involved in cellular energy generation.
Vitamin B₆ (pyridoxine)	Coenzyme in amino acid metabolism.
Panthothenic acid	Essential for conversion of pyruvic acid into acetyl COA; gluconeogenesis of amino acids and lipids.
Biotin	Serves as one coenzyme in breakdown of pyruvic acid via Krebs cycle.
Phosphorus	Component of ATP and ADP; essential to energy storage.
Iron	Component of cytochromes; involved in electron transfer and energy generation via Krebs cycle.
Iodine	Component of hormone thyroxin, which helps to regulate metabolic rate.
Magnesium	Critical constituent of some coenzymes.

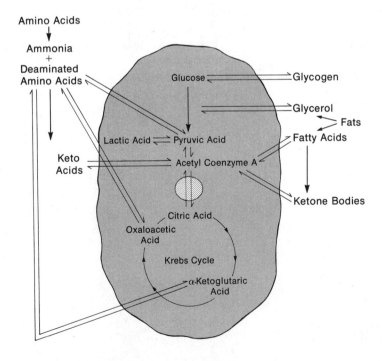

Figure 2.19 Carbohydrate, fat, and protein utilization: shared metabolic pathways. Note that products of amino acid and fat breakdown may be fed into the glucose catabolic pathways to service cellular nutrient needs.

the sympathetic nervous system, for example, is known to stimulate cellular catabolic activity. *Sympathetic nerves,* which are a specialized component of the peripheral nervous system, regulate the activity of glands and involuntary organs. They are activated primarily at times of stress or emergency to gear up the body for a "fight or flight" response. Under these circumstances, cellular energy requirements are increased. Thus the sympathetic nervous system provides a functional pathway to accommodate heightened metabolic needs.

METABOLISM: THE CATABOLISM OF SPECIFIC NUTRIENTS Having traced the metabolic fate of glucose through glycolysis and the Krebs cycle, one should now

remember that fats and amino acids can also be burned by cells to generate energy. Carbohydrates, of course, are the preferred metabolic fuel, but lipid and protein particles can also be fed into the catabolic pathway.

Carbohydrates In brief review, glucose normally proceeds through a series of intracellular chemical reactions that initially convert it, anaerobically, into pyruvic acid. In the presence of sufficient oxygen, pyruvic acid is changed to acetyl CoA and then fed into the Krebs cycle to be degraded into carbon dioxide and water. Energy generated by the oxidation of acetyl CoA in the Krebs cycle is either dissipated as heat or stored in molecules such as ATP.

Fats Before lipids can be fed into the

TABLE 2.5   **Meeting the Cellular Need for Nutrients**

Supply of Nutrients	Systems Involved	Function of Systems
Ingestion	Muscular	Contraction of voluntary muscles necessary for food intake.
Digestion	Digestive	Organs involved with mechanical and chemical breakdown of food.
	Endocrine	Regulates release of certain digestive enzymes.
	Nervous	Regulates contraction of walls of gastrointestinal tract to aid physical breakdown. Releases certain digestive juices to promote chemical breakdown.
Absorption	Digestive	Structural integrity of small intestinal wall important to absorption.
	Circulatory	Blood capillaries and lymph vessels pick up nutrients.
Transport	Circulatory	Lymph vessels and blood vessels aid in transport to body cells.
	Endocrine	Certain hormones help to regulate movement of food particles from blood into cells.

Utilization of Nutrients

Processing by the liver	Digestive	The liver must function to process nutrients for cellular use.
	Endocrine	Certain hormones regulate liver function as a nutrient processor.
	Nervous	Can help regulate liver processing function.
Metabolism	Digestive	Certain nutrients essential to metabolism as enzymes or coenzymes.
	Endocrine	Certain hormones regulate rate of metabolism.
	Nervous	Autonomic nerves modify metabolic rate.

Krebs cycle, they must first be broken down into glycerol and fatty acids. This breakdown occurs primarily in the liver. Glycerol can then be fed directly into the glycolysis pathway or be converted to glucose for metabolic use. Most fatty acids, on the other hand, are converted by the hepatic cells into ketone bodies. These ketone bodies then enter the Krebs cycle via conversion into acetyl CoA.

Proteins Although proteins are not a preferred energy source, some amino acids can enter the metabolic pathway after deamination by the liver. Alanine, for example, can be converted into pyruvic acid, while aspartic acid and glutamine feed directly into the Krebs cycle at specific points.

It is significant to note that all nutrients must in some way enter the *glucose* catabolic pathway in order to be oxidized intracellularly. Fats and amino acids do not have their own metabolic mechanisms. Rather, lipids and proteins are processed to feed into glycolysis or into the Krebs cycle. They thus share the carbohydrate pathway, at least in part. The metabolic interrelationships of the three nutrients are summarized in Figure 2.19.

The Cellular Need for Nutrients: A Systemic Overview

The preceding pages make it clear that many systems are needed to service the cellular need for nutrients. Digestive organs perform only part of the total function of providing for the cellular supply and utilization of food particles. Components of the circulatory, muscular, endocrine, and nervous systems are also significant. The roles of various systems in servicing the cellular need for nutrients are presented in Table 2.5.

CELLULAR NEED FOR ELIMINATION

In the process of producing energy for cellular use, many nonfunctional and potentially harmful waste products are generated. In order to maintain health, the body must have mechanisms for elimination of these wastes.

Wastes arise at two distinct stages of nutrient processing: (1) wastes resulting from digestion, and (2) wastes resulting from metabolism.

Nondigestible Wastes

Food ingested during any single meal is not uniformly useful. A number of substances, for example, are either undigested or nondigestible. They are not or cannot be broken down sufficiently to be absorbed and thus never contribute to intracellular oxidation. These foods simply pass through the gastrointestinal tract to be eliminated as feces.

Products high in fiber or cellulose content, such as bran, certain cereals, lettuce, and apples, serve as bulk or roughage in the digestive tract. They promote normal contractility of the colon and regularity in emptying of the bowels.

FECAL FORMATION

Feces are normally formed in the lower colon by two processes: (1) absorption of water from the gastrointestinal lumen back into the bloodstream, and (2) bacterial activity.

ABSORPTION OF WATER When food moves within the gastrointestinal tract from the small into the large intestine, it is usually in a semiliquid state called *chyme*. Once in the colon, water is absorbed from the intestinal contents back into the blood. This process helps to retain fluid that would otherwise be lost from the body and aids in the solidification of fecal material. When food remains in the large intestine for a protracted period, excessive water absorption can result in hardening of stools and constipation. If, on the other hand, food passes through the colon too quickly, fecal material remains liquefied and diarrhea results.

BACTERIAL ACTIVITY Simultaneous with absorption, bacteria that normally live in the gastrointestinal tract act upon food substances in the intestinal lumen. Bacterial activity aids in the breakdown of nonabsorbed nutrients remaining in the digestive tract.

Carbohydrates, for example, are fermented, with the release of hydrogen, carbon dioxide, and methane gases. It is these gas products that can cause bloat, discomfort, and feelings of indigestion if formed too rapidly or eliminated too slowly.

Bacteria also help to convert any remaining proteins into amino acids, indole, skatole, and hydrogen sulfide. The characteristic odor of feces is caused largely by the indole and skatole that are eliminated in fecal waste. Bacteria also act upon the bilirubin pigment of bile, converting it into material that gives feces their brown color. This explains why biliary disease, with obstruction of bile flow into the gastrointestinal tract, can result in abnormal pasty or clay-colored stool.

FECAL ELIMINATION

Assuming normal formation of feces, fecal elimination depends upon two primary factors: (1) nerve-mediated mass peristaltic waves of the colon, and (2) dilation of the internal and external sphincter muscles that guard the exit from the gastrointestinal tract.

MASS PERISTALSIS Unique to the colon is a special kind of muscular contraction known as mass peristalsis. This type of contraction functions in the bulk movement of a large amount of fecal material toward the rectum. It usually occurs only two to three times a day, and is caused primarily by a neural reflex triggered by filling of the duodenum. Thus, adequate nutrient ingestion and a functional nervous system are essential prerequisites to mass peristalsis.

SPHINCTER MUSCLES Once fecal matter has moved into the rectum and anus, circular rings of muscle known as the internal and external sphincters must open to allow defecation. Stretching and pressure normally

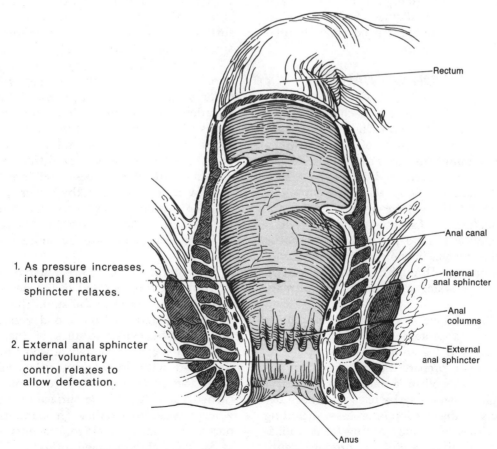

1. As pressure increases, internal anal sphincter relaxes.

2. External anal sphincter under voluntary control relaxes to allow defecation.

Rectum

Anal canal

Internal anal sphincter

Anal columns

External anal sphincter

Anus

Figure 2.20 Defecation. (From Tortora, G., and Anagnostakos, N.: Principles of Anatomy and Physiology, 2nd ed. New York, Harper & Row, 1978. Used by permission.)

initiate automatic reflex relaxation of the internal sphincter. The external sphincter, on the other hand, is under voluntary control. Nerve messages originating at the cerebrum result in relaxation of this muscle. The timing of defecation can thus be dictated by comfort and convenience. Hence, components of the muscular and nervous systems play critical roles in the control of fecal elimination. The process of defecation is elucidated diagrammatically in Figure 2.20.

Metabolic Wastes

While defecation plays an important role in the elimination of nondigestible nutrients, an alternate route must be available to rid the body of metabolic wastes. In the process of metabolizing nutrients to generate energy, several nonuseful or potentially harmful substances are produced. These nonfunctional products must be removed from the cellular environment and excreted from the body if health is to be maintained. Several systems cooperate to aid in the transport and elimination of metabolic wastes.

IDENTIFICATION OF WASTES

As we have seen, the mechanism of catabolizing nutrients intracellularly is a complex one. Small amounts of energy can be generated under anaerobic conditions via glycolysis. If low-oxygen conditions persist, substantial amounts of lactic acid can accumulate, some of which will be eliminated by the excretory organs. Essentially, however, it is the oxidation of food particles via the Krebs cycle that results in the major production of cellular energy. Through this process, carbon dioxide and water are generated as primary wastes.

Although glucose is the preferred cellular fuel, fat and protein particles can also be processed and fed into the Krebs cycle. As hepatic cells prepare noncarbohydrate nutrients for catabolism, a number of secondary metabolic wastes may be released. These by-products of the metabolic process, including *ketone bodies* (generated during fat mobilization in the liver) and *urea* (produced sub-

sequent to amino acid deamination), must be regularly eliminated if homeostasis is to be maintained.

ORGANS OF ELIMINATION

The removal of potentially harmful metabolic wastes from the body necessitates a functional circulatory system. Wastes are transported by the blood away from metabolizing cells toward appropriate excretory organs.

The primary excretory organs of the body are the skin, the lungs, and the kidneys. Because of their significance, it is worth examining briefly the regulatory mechanisms of each of these organs of elimination.

THE SKIN The skin is particularly adapted to provide for waste elimination by two independent means. Some water passes directly through epidermal cells by diffusion and is thereby excreted directly on the skin surface. Alternatively, fluid can be eliminated as perspiration by activity of the sweat glands.

Diffusion Surprisingly, more water is normally excreted by diffusion than by perspiration during any 24-hour period. Unlike perspiration, the volume of fluid eliminated by diffusion remains constant in spite of activity levels and external temperature conditions. Thus, the loss of water by diffusion is an ongoing, inflexible process that is modified only by factors affecting the integrity of the outer epidermal cells. If the external skin layer is denuded for any reason, fluid output via diffusion could increase by more than ten fold.

The Sweat Glands Sweat glands are specialized structures located in the dermis and subcutaneous layers of the skin. The content of sweat is derived from blood vessels surrounding the coiled tubules of the gland. Perspiration consists largely of water and salts combined with some urea, uric acid, and other metabolic wastes. Once formed it is carried via a duct to the surface of the skin, where it is eliminated through openings called pores. The anatomical components of the sweat gland are illustrated in Figure 2.21.

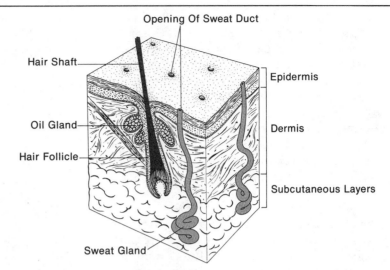

Opening Of Sweat Duct

Hair Shaft

Oil Gland

Hair Follicle

Epidermis

Dermis

Subcutaneous Layers

Sweat Gland

Figure 2.21 The sweat gland.

Although elimination of wastes is one function of the sweat glands, their most significant role is in temperature regulation. When the body is overheated, large quantities of perspiration are produced. This liquid is deposited on the skin surface and draws body heat for evaporation. Hence, the greater the output of sweat, the greater the drop in internal temperature.

The rate and quantity of sweat production are regulated largely by peripheral nerves of the autonomic nervous system carrying messages from the hypothalamus of the brain. During periods of cold weather and low activity, perspiration output is limited. With increasing exertion or elevation of environmental temperature, sweat production rises.

THE LUNGS During expiration (exhalation), the lungs normally eliminate small quantities of water vapor and the majority of waste carbon dioxide from the blood.

Water Vapor The elimination of water vapor by the lungs is largely dependent upon the exhalation of humidified air. Air taken into the respiratory tree is moistened by water derived primarily from mucus lining the nasal passages. It then travels, moisture-laden, to the air sacs of the lungs and is expelled with its water content upon expiration.

Carbon Dioxide The excretion of carbon dioxide is dependent upon four primary factors. These factors parallel those listed under Cellular Need for Oxygen as prerequisites to cellular oxygen supply, but in reverse order.

For the lungs to eliminate carbon dioxide, there must be:

1. A functional *cardiovascular system* to carry wastes from metabolizing cells to the pulmonary air sacs.

2. An adequate number of *erythrocytes* to aid in carbon dioxide transport.

3. Sufficient *diffusion* of carbon dioxide from pulmonary capillaries into the air sacs of the lungs.

4. A functional means of *expiration* to move gas from the lungs into the atmosphere.

The relationship of three of these factors to cellular oxygen supply has already been examined. Therefore, the following discussion deals primarily with the way in which the cardiovascular system, erythrocytes, diffusion, and expiration service the need for carbon dioxide elimination.

THE CARDIOVASCULAR SYSTEM: To insure removal of metabolic wastes, a functional cardiovascular system is essential. If wastes cannot be swept out of the interstitial fluid toward excretory organs, they will remain to cause pathological changes in the body.

The heart and blood vessels, however, cannot function effectively in this capacity without the aid of the nervous system. Reflex adjustments made by the medulla insure adaptive changes in cardiac rate and vascular capacity when cellular metabolic activity (and waste production) increase. Hence, the circulatory system is rendered responsive to the ongoing needs of the body.

ERYTHROCYTES: Once carbon dioxide is in the blood, it must be carried to pulmonary air sacs for elimination. Transport of carbon dioxide is a complex process that depends indirectly upon an adequate number of functional RBC's.

Carbon dioxide can be carried through the blood in several forms. A small percentage is simply dissolved in the water of plasma. Another limited amount diffuses into the erythrocyte to combine chemically with the protein portion of hemoglobin. Since oxygen normally combines with the iron (heme) group of hemoglobin, the two gases can be carried simultaneously by the hemoglobin molecule without competing for the same attachment site.

The majority of carbon dioxide moves into the RBC and is converted chemically into *bicarbonate* (HCO_3^-) as follows:

$$\underset{\substack{\text{enzyme} \\ \text{carbonic} \\ \text{anhydrase}}}{H_2O + CO_2 \; \leftrightharpoons \; H_2CO_3 \; \rightleftharpoons \; H^+ + HCO_3^-}$$

Most of the bicarbonate formed in the erythrocyte then moves out into the plasma and is carried in this form to the lungs. To maintain electrical balance, as plasma gains a negatively charged bicarbonate ion, a negatively charged chloride (Cl^-) particle diffuses from plasma *into* the RBC. This phenomenon is known as the *chloride shift*. The majority of carbon dioxide is, thus, transported in the form of bicarbonate, as illustrated in Figure 2.22.

When blood reaches the lungs, reverse chemical reactions free carbon dioxide from its bicarbonate transport form. Carbon dioxide can then diffuse from where it is in greater concentration (the pulmonary capillaries) to where it is in lesser concentration (the air sacs of the lungs), thence to be expired.

Although erythrocytes are linked to cellu-

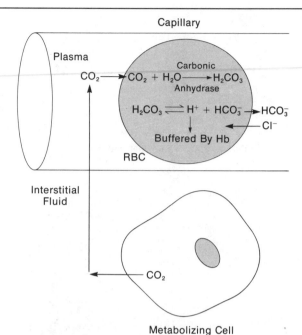

Figure 2.22 The conversion of carbon dioxide to bicarbonate within the red blood cell.

lar oxygen supply, it can be seen that they also play a role in the transport of carbon dioxide. Since the carbonic anhydrase enzyme, which indirectly facilitates bicarbonate formation, is carried within erythrocytes, these cells become potentially important in carbon dioxide elimination. Thus, all factors previously enumerated as significant to RBC production can indirectly affect carbon dioxide transport as well.

DIFFUSION: In order for carbon dioxide to be excreted by the lungs, it must first diffuse from capillaries into pulmonary air sacs. Thus, any obstruction of blood flow or tissue fibrosis will result in decreased ability to eliminate carbon dioxide from the bloodstream. Diseases such as emphysema and pneumonia may therefore cause carbon dioxide to accumulate in the plasma, resulting in a condition known as hypercapnia.

EXPIRATION: Assuming normal transport and diffusion of metabolic wastes into pulmonary air sacs, elimination ultimately depends upon *expiration* — the movement of gases from the lungs out into the atmosphere.

In order to expire air, the thoracic cavity volume must first decrease, causing pressure in the cavity to simultaneously increase. When intrapulmonic pressure becomes greater than environmental pressure, air will move from the area of greater pressure (the air sacs) to the area of lesser pressure (the atmosphere).

As with inspiration, the skeletal, muscular, and nervous systems all function to bring about essential thoracic changes. The diaphragm relaxes and moves up, thereby decreasing the superior-inferior dimensions of the cavity. The internal intercostal muscles contract, pulling the ribs down and thus decreasing the anterior-posterior dimensions of the cavity. These mechanisms of expiration are shown in Figure 2.23.

The nervous system plays an important role in coordinating respiratory muscle contractions. Neuromuscular disorders can thus interfere with carbon dioxide elimination, resulting in the development of hypercapnia.

The Kidneys The kidneys are two bean-shaped organs located just above the waist and attached to the posterior wall of the abdominal cavity. They are essential to the maintenance of homeostasis and the elimination of metabolic wastes.

The kidneys eliminate urine, which contains water and several metabolic products, including urea, uric acid, creatinine, lactic acid, and ketone bodies. Cellular health depends upon the continuous output of urinary wastes. When renal failure occurs, the accumulation of toxic wastes in the blood can result in coma and eventual death. Hence the ongoing manufacture of urine is a critical process that warrants further elucidation.

Urine is actually made and processed by functional subunits of the kidneys called *nephrons*. Each of the approximately 2 million

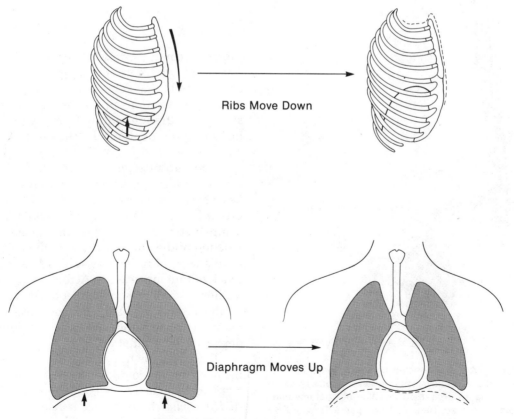

Ribs Move Down

Diaphragm Moves Up

Figure 2.23 Mechanism of expiration.

nephrons in the body receives a plasma-like filtrate from a specialized capillary network known as a *glomerulus*. The conversion of this filtrate into urine by the nephron proceeds by a series of complex steps that will be explained in Unit 2. It is important to note, however, that the entire mechanism of urine manufacture is strongly influenced by components of the circulatory, nervous, and endocrine systems.

The first step of urine formation involves filtration of material out of the blood into the nephron. Since blood pressure is a driving force for filtration, any alteration in cardiac activity, vascular tone, size of vessels feeding the nephron, or blood volume can affect urine formation. Thus, a sudden drop in blood

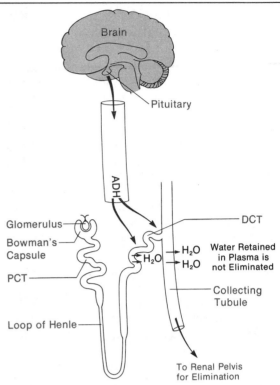

Figure 2.25   The effect of ADH upon urinary output.

pressure could seriously impede filtration. This is illustrated by the anuria (lack of urinary output) that often accompanies cardiac arrest. The relationship of the cardiovascular system to filtration of fluid from the glomerulus into the nephron is shown in Figure 2.24.

The cardiovascular system does not function in a vacuum, however. Activities of the heart and blood vessels are affected to a large extent by neural and endocrine controls. The sympathetic nervous system causes constriction of the arterioles serving the nephron. In this way, filtration pressure is reduced and renal output decreased. Acting in a similar fashion is the hormone epinephrine, released by the adrenal medulla. Epinephrine secreted naturally, or administered as a drug, can thus depress urine formation.

Once filtrate has effectively moved into the nephron, its composition and volume continue to be affected by endocrine influences. *ADH (antidiuretic hormone)* is released by the posterior pituitary gland and helps to regulate

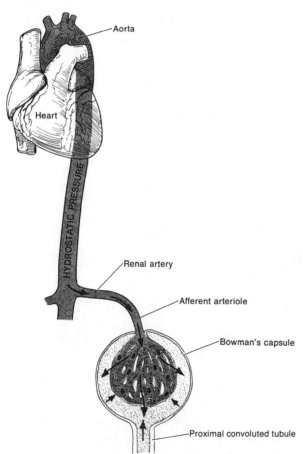

Figure 2.24   Relationship between glomerular filtration and the cardiovascular system. (From Tortora, G., and Anagnostakos, N.: Principles of Anatomy and Physiology, 2nd ed. New York, Harper & Row, 1978. Used by permission.)

the volume of urinary output. By stimulating the reabsorption of water out of the nephron back into surrounding capillaries, it helps to conserve fluid that would otherwise be excreted in urine. Hence the fate of water generated by cellular metabolism is significantly affected by ADH output. Depressed ADH secretion, as seen in diabetes insipidus, results in the loss of large amounts of body water as copious volumes of dilute urine are excreted. A simplified scheme of the effect of ADH upon urinary output is presented in Figure 2.25.

Cellular Need for Elimination: A Summary

It can be seen that many systems work in cooperation to service the cellular need for elimination. Nondigestible wastes are excreted as fecal matter by the lower gastrointestinal tract. Metabolic wastes are eliminated by the sweat glands, lungs, and kidneys. In each case, however, the primary organs of elimination depend upon interaction with other structures in the body for optimal functioning. A summary of the many systems involved in waste elimination is presented in Table 2.6.

CELLULAR NEED FOR FLUID AND ELECTROLYTE BALANCE

Each cell in the body can be likened to a tiny island floating in a sea of interstitial fluid. To insure cellular survival, the liquid bathing the cell must contain certain constituents in relatively fixed concentrations. Deviations from the optimal composition can result in cellular dysfunction or death.

TABLE 2.6   **Meeting the Cellular Need for Elimination**

Substances	Systems Involved	Function of Systems
NONDIGESTIBLE WASTES	Digestive	Formation of feces in lower gastrointestinal tract.
	Nervous	Stimulation of mass peristalsis to promote fecal elimination.
	Muscular	Voluntary control of defecation.
METABOLIC WASTES	Circulatory	Transport of wastes to organs of excretion.
	Integumentary	Elimination of water, electrolytes, and some nitrogenous wastes via diffusion and perspiration.
	Nervous	Control over sweat production, expiration, and filtration pressure in the nephron.
	Endocrine	Control over sweat production and water reabsorption in the nephron.
	Respiratory	Essential to the expiration of CO_2 and water vapor by the lungs.
	Muscular	Muscles of respiration promote expiration: sphincters maintain voluntary control over urination.
	Skeletal	Necessary for production of erythrocytes that are functional in CO_2 transport; aids in altering thoracic cavity volume to facilitate expiration.
	Renal	Kidneys manufacture and excrete urine containing water, salts, and other metabolic wastes.

It must be remembered that adequate oxygen supply, nutrient supply, and waste removal cannot in themselves insure cellular health. Like an artist who is given all necessary equipment and materials, yet is unable to "create" in an alien environment, the cell is a temperamental entity. In order for metabolic and other cellular activities to proceed normally, the optimal fluid and electrolyte balance of the extracellular environment must be closely maintained.

Fluid and electrolyte balance involves the regulation of a wide range of factors, including fluid volume, fluid distribution, electrolyte composition, and acid-base composition. Since an understanding of these difficult concepts is so important to comprehension of pathophysiology, a large portion of Unit 2 is devoted to the fluid and electrolyte regulatory mechanisms.

Suffice it to say here that many systems work jointly to insure that interstitial fluid does not deviate too far from its optimal composition. In this way, the cell is provided with a compatible environment for growth and metabolism.

STUDY QUESTIONS

1. In each of the following hypothetical cases, describe how or why disruption of homeostasis could result:
   a. Paralysis of respiratory muscles.
   b. Pulmonary disease characterized by depressed diffusion.
   c. Severe anemia.
   d. Extensive damage to the gastric lining, with decreased production of intrinsic factor.
   e. Renal failure, with decreased production of erythropoietin.

2. Why would each of the following disrupt cellular nutrient supply or utilization or both?
   a. A stroke, with extensive muscular paralysis.
   b. Gastrointestinal disease characterized by malabsorption.
   c. Obstruction of the portal vein.
   d. Extensive hepatic disease.
   e. Insufficient secretion of insulin.

3. After intake of a high-Calorie meal, excessive nutrients are most likely to be stored in which form(s)?

4. Why do ketone bodies often accumulate in plasma when fats are mobilized for utilization as cellular fuel?

5. Describe the way in which proteins are mobilized for metabolic use.

6. Why does lactic acid often accumulate in plasma when oxygen deficiency exists?

7. Briefly describe the Krebs cycle.

8. Why is oxygen deficit likely to cause feelings of weakness and tiredness?

9. What role do vitamins and minerals play in the generation of metabolic energy?

10. Why is constipation characterized by the formation of hard stools?

11. What role do lower gastrointestinal bacteria play in fecal formation?

12. Identify two or three metabolic wastes that are normally eliminated by: (a) the lungs, (b) the skin, and (c) the kidneys.

13. Describe the way in which most carbon dioxide is transported through the body.

Suggested Readings

Anthony, C. P., and Thibodeau, G. A.: Textbook of Anatomy and Physiology, 10th ed. St. Louis, The C. V. Mosby Company, 1979, pp. 471–501; 506–529.

Beck, R. R.: Hormonal regulation of intermediary metabolism. *In* Selkurt, E. E. (ed.): Basic Physiology for the Health Sciences. Boston, Little, Brown & Company, 1975, p. 317.

Cohen, A.: Handbook of Cellular Chemistry. St. Louis, The C. V. Mosby Company, 1975.

Guyton, A. C.: Physiology of the Human Body, 5th ed. Philadelphia, W. B. Saunders Company, 1979, pp. 47–52; 397–411.

Guyton, A. C.: Textbook of Medical Physiology, 5th ed. Philadelphia, W. B. Saunders Company, 1976, pp. 904–935.

Hole, J. W.: Human Anatomy and Physiology. Dubuque, Wm. C. Brown Company, 1978, pp. 496–528.

Knoebel, L. K.: Energy metabolism. *In* Selkurt, E.

E. (ed.): Basic Physiology for the Health Sciences. Boston, Little, Brown & Company, 1975, p. 265.

Landau, B. R.: Essential Human Anatomy and Physiology, 2nd ed. Glenview, Scott, Foresman and Company, 1980, pp. 385–390; 515–526; 541–563; 580–587; 589–619.

Lechtman, M. D., Roohk, B., and Egan, R. J.: The Games Cells Play. Menlo Park, The Benjamin/Cummings Publishing Company, 1979.

Martin, D. B.: Metabolism and energy mechanics. *In* Frolich, E. D. (ed.): Pathophysiology: Altered Regulatory Mechanisms in Disease. Philadelphia, J. B. Lippincott Company, 1976, p. 365.

Pflanzer, R. G.: The blood. *In* Selkurt, E. E. (ed.): Basic Physiology for the Health Sciences. Boston, Little, Brown & Company, 1975, p. 325.

Soergel, K. H., and Hofmann, A. F.: Absorption. *In* Frolich, E. D. (ed.): Pathophysiology: Altered Regulatory Mechanisms in Disease. Philadelphia, J. B. Lippincott Company, 1976, p. 499.

Tortora, G. J., and Anagnostakos, N. P.: Principles of Anatomy and Physiology, 2nd ed. New York, Harper & Row, 1979, pp. 508–531; 538–570; 578–595.

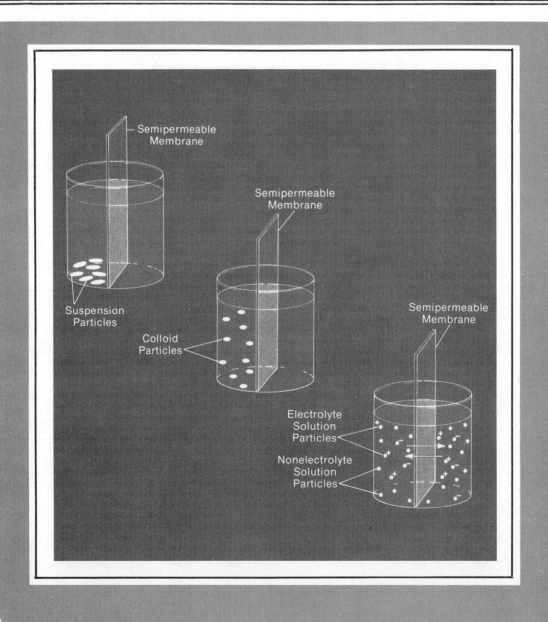

The Cellular Need for Fluid and Electrolyte Balance

The study of fluid and electrolyte balance has traditionally been considered a difficult area to master. The underlying chemical concepts, control mechanisms, and complex interrelationships are often a source of anxiety for even the most avid learners. Since an understanding of fluid and electrolyte balance is central to the comprehension of all systemic disorders, the following five chapters are devoted to this subject.

Experience has shown that learning is facilitated by first dealing with body fluids as if they were pure water, and then introducing the fluid components. Thus, fluid composition is *not* described until the principles governing fluid volume and distribution have been clarified. In this way, students can see how and when the major fluid components modify the general laws governing fluid behavior.

For the purposes of this Unit, and in keeping with tradition, the fluid components analyzed include small electrically charged particles called *electrolytes,* and chemicals classified as *acids* or *bases.* Normal function, regulation, and imbalances are discussed. Clinical examples are used with regularity to clarify and illustrate major points.

Throughout this Unit, it is important to keep in mind that the maintenance of fluid and electrolyte balance is insured by the cooperation of many systems in the body. Once again a major cellular need is met by a wide variety of organs and structures. It thus follows that disorders of diverse origin could disrupt the cellular need for fluid and electrolyte balance. The development of fluid-electrolyte and acid-base imbalances is analyzed in Chapters 6 and 7.

Chapter Outline

chapter **3**

Fluid Volumes and Distribution

Chapter Objectives

At the completion of this chapter, student will be able to:

1. Given the weight of an adult patient, calculate the fluid weight in pounds.
2. Describe the effect of age and sex upon per cent fluid weight in the body.
3. Distinguish between the obese and the normal-weight individual with respect to per cent fluid weight.
4. Differentiate between intracellular, interstitial, and plasma fluid compartments with respect to relative volume and approximate per cent of total body weight.
5. Identify the barriers that separate (a) interstitial fluid from intracellular fluid, and (b) interstitial fluid from plasma.
6. Define extracellular fluid.
7. Identify the primary sources and average daily volume of fluid intake and fluid output by the body.
8. Describe the causes and symptoms of hypervolemia and hypovolemia.

FLUID VOLUME AND DISTRIBUTION: AN OVERVIEW

A superficial look at the human body can be remarkably deceptive, suggesting that it is composed primarily of solid tissues with little liquid content. The surprising reality, however, is that the body of the average adult male contains approximately 60 per cent fluid weight. More than half of his total poundage is accounted for by liquids that are internally sealed beneath the skin. Only examination of underlying structures reveals the fluid components that are integral to our physical makeup.

Total Fluid Volume

Although the average fluid weight of an adult male is 60 per cent, it is important to realize that this figure can vary considerably as a function of factors such as age and sex.

AGE

At birth, the fluid composition of the body is as high as 80 per cent, leveling off to a norm of 60 per cent by the early teens, and decreasing to about 40 to 50 per cent in old age. These variations in fluid content can help to explain why geriatric patients are more seriously affected by the fluid losses of diarrhea and vomiting than a younger adult would be. Their relatively low fluid content renders them particularly susceptible to dehydration, even after minor episodes of water loss.

Infants also are vulnerable to disruptions in fluid balance. A characteristically high metabolic rate (with associated rapid turnover of water) renders them particularly prone to dehydration. Loss of fluid through the skin is specifically facilitated by their disproportionately elevated surface area relative to body weight. Clearly, any excessive fluid drain, as would happen during an episode of intestinal flu or as a result of food allergies, could pose a critical threat to homeostasis.

SEX

Sex as well as age can be a determining factor in fluid level differences among individuals. The mature female has relatively more adipose (fat) tissue than the average male. This is primarily due to the influence of the feminizing hormones secreted from puberty to menopause. Estrogens and progesterone promote the deposition of subcutaneous fat that softens, curves, and rounds out the female shape. Since adipose tissue is decidedly low in water content, the postadolescent female can have considerably less fluid in her body than the average male.

By the same reasoning, it follows that the obese male and female are relatively fluid-deprived. The greater the proportion of adipose tissue in their bodies, the less their per cent fluid levels. In cases of extreme obesity, it is possible for body fluid content to be reduced by as much as 50 per cent. This phenomenon renders the obese individual extremely vulnerable to dehydration. The use of diuretics (medications promoting excessive urination) in an attempt to lose weight could thus threaten fluid balance and should be carefully monitored.

Fluid Distribution

Fluid in the body is not isolated into any one vast pool. It is distributed primarily among three major areas called fluid compartments, as follows:

1. *Intracellular fluid,* consisting of all liquid within the cell membranes of the body, is the largest fluid compartment. It contains approximately 25 liters of fluid and accounts for about 40 per cent of body weight.

2. *Interstitial fluid* consists of all fluid bathing the body cells. Any material entering or leaving the intracellular compartment must cross the interstitial fluid pool, which contains a total of 12 liters by volume and accounts for approximately 15 per cent of body weight.

3. *Plasma* is the liquid component of whole blood. It is contained within the vascular system and contributes a total of 3 liters to the fluid pool, accounting for 5 per cent of body weight.

The relationship between these three compartments is depicted in Figure 3.1.

As can be seen, there is an actual physical barrier between the three fluid compartments. The *capillary wall* separates plasma from inter-

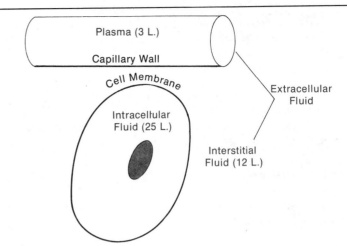

Figure 3.1 Fluid distribution in the body.

stitial fluid, while the *cell membrane* separates interstitial from intracellular fluid. Despite these barriers, fluid can flow relatively freely between the three compartments. The laws governing intercompartmental fluid flow will

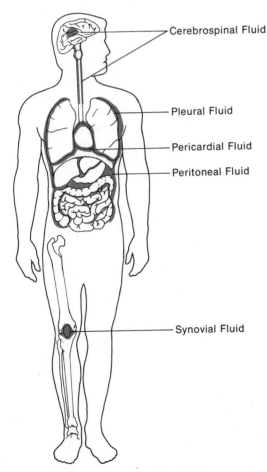

Figure 3.2 Extracellular fluid spaces.

be discussed in Chapter 4. Meanwhile, it is important to realize that the term "compartment" does not imply isolation.

Since water and most of its components can flow with particular ease between plasma and interstitial fluid, these two compartments are often referred to as the *extracellular fluid (ECF) compartment*. Extracellular fluid, in truth, consists of all body fluid external to the cell membrane. It thus technically includes a number of spaces and cavities that commonly contain fluid or could potentially fill with fluid. The pleural cavity, peritoneal cavity, pericardial cavity, joint spaces, and ventricles of the brain are typical examples. Some of these areas, and the fluid they contain, are depicted in Figure 3.2.

While the maintenance of total fluid volume is very important, the ideal distribution of fluid throughout the body must also be preserved. Any drastic change in total water content or distribution of fluid can cause severe clinical problems.

The shift of vast amounts of fluid out of the capillaries into the interstitial spaces, for example, would precipitate a severe drop in blood pressure followed by shock, unless rapidly checked. The accumulation and trapping of excessive amounts of fluid in the peritoneal cavity would have similar results. Many such problems will be analyzed in detail in this Unit. At this point, suffice it to say that optimal fluid distribution is essential to cellular health. Physiological disharmony invariably results from abnormalities in the distribution of body fluid.

MAINTENANCE OF NORMAL FLUID VOLUME

In order to insure normal fluid balance and distribution, it is important that adequate total volume be maintained. To avoid excessive gain or loss of water, daily fluid intake must approximate daily output.

Fluid Intake

Water is normally supplied to the body through two primary avenues: (1) ingestion, and (2) cellular oxidation.

INGESTION

Oral intake of water normally ranges between 1650 and 2750 ml. every 24 hours. It includes the water in liquid as well as the fluid trapped in solid food. Meats and vegetables, for example, can contain anywhere from about 60 to 95 per cent water, much of which is released during digestion and absorbed into the blood through the lining of the small intestine.

CELLULAR OXIDATION

Cellular oxidation is an additional, but less significant, source of body water. Nor-mally generated at the rate of about 250 ml. per 24 hours, it is formed as a waste product of nutrient catabolism and released into the bloodstream. Fluid volume generated via metabolism can be estimated by approximating 10 ml. of water for every 100 Calories of burned nutrients. Thus, total dietary intake will affect to some extent the oxidative water released.

SUMMARY

In brief, the total 24-hour fluid intake will approximate 1800 to 3000 ml., with variations dependent upon such factors as age, diet, size, and activity. A tabular summary of the sources of fluid intake is presented in Figure 3.3.

Fluid Output

Fluid is normally eliminated from the body by four primary pathways: insensible water loss, sweat, feces, and urine.

INSENSIBLE WATER LOSS

Insensible water loss encompasses those avenues of fluid exit we are not consciously aware of. Included in this classification are the water lost by diffusion through the skin and the water expired by the lungs.

Although most of us are aware of water lost through perspiration, few realize that we

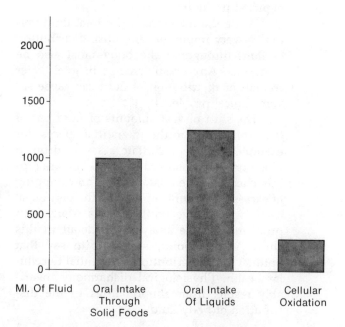

Figure 3.3 Sources of fluid intake: comparative volumes.

are constantly losing 300 to 400 ml. of fluid a day by simple diffusion through skin cells. The epidermis normally protects us from an even greater water loss through this route, but any thinning of this tissue (as occurs with aging) or loss of epidermis (as occurs with burns) can expose the system to excessive fluid depletion.

As mentioned earlier, insensible water is lost through the lungs as well as through the skin. Dry air taken into the respiratory tree is rapidly humidified by water vapor derived largely from mucus lining the nasal passages. This fluid, which moistens the air on its way into the lungs, remains in the respiratory passages to be eliminated with gases returning from the alveoli during expiration.

About 350 ml. of fluid are lost daily in this way, with considerable variation due to such factors as respiratory rate, atmospheric humidity, and body temperature. Physical exertion or increased body temperature, both of which stimulate increases in respiratory rate and depth, promote greater insensible water loss through the lungs.

SWEAT

Sweat production is another means of fluid elimination. The average loss, by perspiration, at temperatures of 68° F., is 100 ml. daily. This figure can vary considerably, of course, and is influenced by such factors as body temperature, physical exertion, and atmospheric conditions. A febrile patient, for example, with excessively high perspiration output, must be monitored carefully for possible signs of dehydration.

FECES

Although some fluid is eliminated in fecal material, the volume is usually a negligible 150 to 200 ml. daily. It is important to remember that in the process of fecal formation, most water is absorbed out of the colon back into the blood. This is a means of conserving fluid and solidifying gastrointestinal contents in preparation for elimination. If feces are not processed adequately, diarrhea can result, with loss of excessive water in the feces.

URINE

Urination is by far the most significant mechanism of fluid exit from the body. Approximately 1000 to 1500 ml. of urine are excreted daily, with variations influenced primarily by circulatory and endocrine factors. Although output can vary considerably, the cellular need for elimination will not be

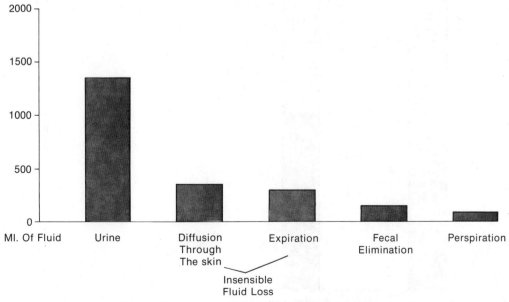

Figure 3.4 Avenues of fluid loss: comparative volumes.

met if urinary volume falls below 400 ml. in 24 hours. Depression below this level is labeled anuria and results in serious physiological imbalance. The intricacies of renal functioning will be explored more extensively in Chapter 5.

SUMMARY

As can be seen by review of the preceding pages, fluid output is regulated by several different structures. The integumentary, respiratory, digestive, and renal systems all work together to insure adequate elimination of body water. Figure 3.4 summarizes the primary avenues for fluid exit.

Fluid Intake and Output: A Summary

The maintenance of optimal fluid volume and distribution is one very important aspect of homeostasis. As long as fluid intake remains equivalent to output, the body will not experience a net gain or loss of total water content. Comparison of the normal fluid intake and output volumes reveals that the two are, in fact, equal. The total daily fluid supplied by ingestion and cellular oxidation is usually balanced by the fluid eliminated in 24 hours by the organs of excretion. A summary of normal intake and output volumes is presented in Figure 3.5.

FLUID VOLUME IMBALANCES

Any deviation from the balanced norm can, of course, affect body water content. *Hypervolemia*, or fluid excess, is seen in cases in which input is increased or output decreased or both. Conversely, *hypovolemia*, or fluid deficit, is caused by decreased intake or increased output or both. This concept is presented diagrammatically in Figure 3.6.

It is significant to note that in all cases of fluid volume imbalance, deviations from the norm affect both the plasma and the interstitial compartments. Excesses or deficits are reflected rather uniformly throughout the extracellular fluid compartment, resulting in predictable increases or decreases in plasma and interstitial fluid volumes.

The intracellular fluid compartment, on the other hand, will remain relatively unaffected unless volume changes are accompa-

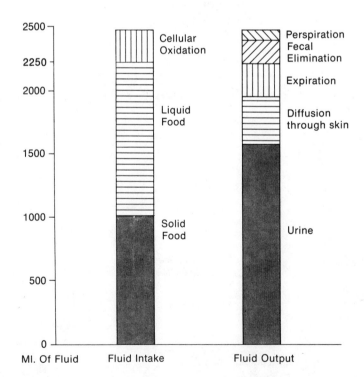

Figure 3.5 Fluid intake and output: comparative volumes.

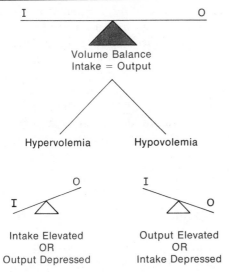

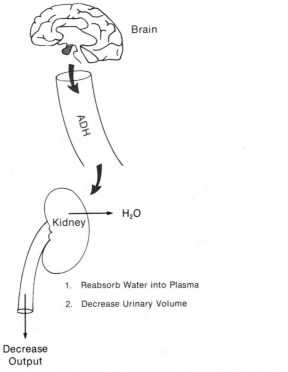

Figure 3.6 Fluid volume imbalance.

nied by alterations in electrolyte concentrations. Since electrolyte imbalance further complicates the clinical picture, at this point we will concern ourselves only with the manifestations of deviations in fluid volume. The effects of altered fluid composition are described in Chapters 5 and 6.

Hypervolemia

As mentioned earlier, cases of extracellular fluid excess can be precipitated by increased intake or decreased output of fluid or both.

INCREASED INTAKE

Examples of increased intake may be found in cases of excessive administration of intravenous (I.V.) fluids, or in instances of psychotic drinking episodes, often associated with certain types of mental illness.

DECREASED OUTPUT

Hypervolemia more commonly results from decreased output, as noted during renal failure or with specific endocrine imbalances.

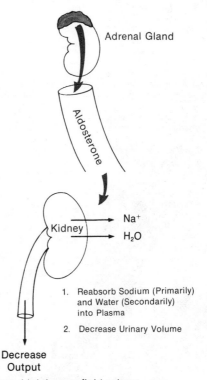

Figure 3.7 The effects of ADH (left) and aldosterone (right) upon fluid volume.

The hormones ADH (antidiuretic hormone) and aldosterone in particular affect the balance between fluid retention and urinary output. By acting directly upon the nephrons of the kidney, they promote the reabsorption of water from the nephrons back into the plasma. Their mode of action, elucidated in Chapter 5, is briefly summarized in Figure 3.7. It can be seen that both ADH and aldosterone ultimately affect fluid balance by increasing extracellular fluid volume at the expense of urinary output. Excessive secretion of either hormone will predictably induce hypervolemia.

Hypersecretion of aldosterone is typically noted in cases of adrenal cortical tumor and congestive heart failure. By stimulating the reabsorption of sodium and the secondary movement of proportional amounts of water from the nephron back into the bloodstream,

aldosterone favors fluid retention. Elevated aldosterone levels can also be seen in cases of liver disease. Since hepatic cells are primarily responsible for degrading excess aldosterone and rendering it inactive, liver disease may trigger heightened aldosterone activity as hormone levels build up in the blood.

Many steroid drugs, such as cortisone, which are often prescribed for arthritis and chronic respiratory allergies because of their anti-inflammatory activity, affect sodium and water reabsorption in a manner similar to that of aldosterone. Hence, patients on these medications should be monitored carefully for any indications of fluid excess. Hypersecretion of ADH will also characteristically result in hypervolemia. Acting directly on the nephron to facilitate water retention, ADH is often abnormally elevated in some pathological conditions, including certain malignancies and ce-

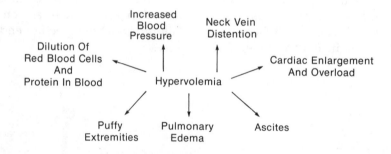

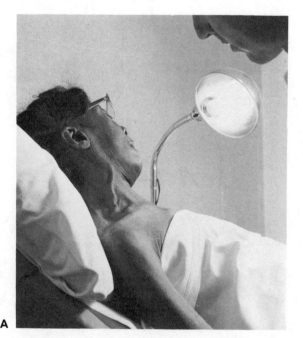

Figure 3.8 Effects of hypervolemia. *A*, Distended external jugular vein. (Reprinted with permission of the American Heart Association.) *B*, Acute pulmonary edema secondary to left ventricular failure, with moderately enlarged heart. (Reprinted with permission of Fraser, R., and Paré, J.: Diagnosis of Diseases of the Chest, 2nd ed. Philadelphia, W. B. Saunders Company, 1978.) *C*, Dependent edema of the lower legs. (Reprinted with permission of Robbins, S., and Cotran, R.: Pathologic Basis of Disease, 2nd ed. Philadelphia, W. B. Saunders Company, 1979.) *D*, Ascites with cardiac failure. (Reprinted with permission of Delp, M., and Manning, R.: Major's Physical Diagnosis, 9th ed. Philadelphia, W. B. Saunders Company, 1981.) *Illustration continued on opposite page.*

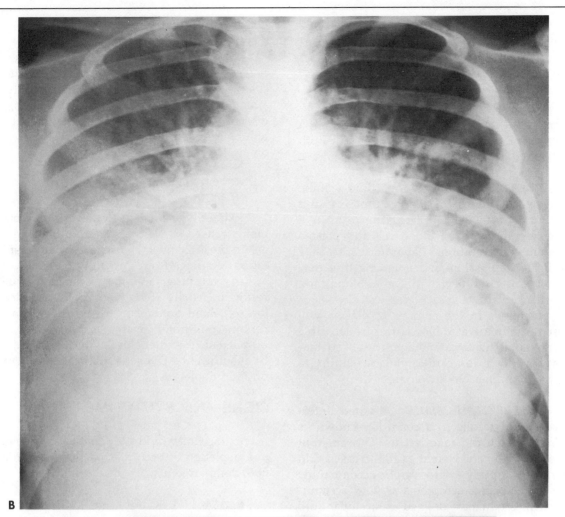

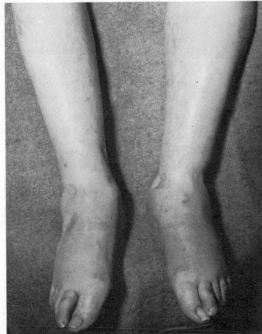

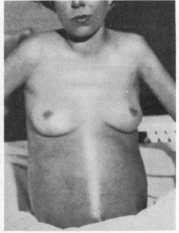

Figure 3.8 Continued. See legend on opposite page

rebral disorders, stress, surgical trauma, and pain.

SIGNS AND SYMPTOMS

Regardless of precipitating factors, patients with extracellular fluid excess present a clinical picture that reflects overload in both interstitial fluid and plasma compartments.

PLASMA Elevated plasma fluid volume effectively dilutes the large proteins and erythrocytes in whole blood. The result is a decrease in both red blood cell and plasma protein concentrations. Laboratory slips thus indicate depression in hematocrit (the percentage of erythrocytes in whole blood) and plasma protein values.

Increases in the amount of plasma will also result in elevated blood pressure, possible neck vein distention, and a potential "circulatory overload" as cardiac muscle strains to adjust to higher blood volume.

INTERSTITIAL FLUID Elevated interstitial fluid results in a condition known as *edema*, which can manifest itself throughout the body. General weight gain, increased skin turgor, and puffy eyelids can be accompanied by more specific symptoms as fluid accumulates in certain more defined extracellular fluid spaces.

Pulmonary edema, for example, can develop as fluid collects in the alveoli of the lungs, bringing symptoms of coughing, difficulty in breathing (dyspnea), and bloody sputum. *Ascites* may occur if fluid collects in the peritoneal cavity, accompanied by symptoms of abdominal pain, discomfort, and diminished inspiratory capacity.

Extracellular volume excess can be characterized by many and varied signs and symptoms, some of which are shown in Figure 3.8.

Hypovolemia

Extracellular fluid depletion can technically result from any disorder causing a decrease in fluid intake, an increase in fluid output, or both.

DECREASED INTAKE

Although decreased fluid intake will cause changes in body water content, such changes will usually be accompanied by alterations in electrolyte concentrations. Thus, a discussion of this aspect of volume depletion will be reserved for Chapter 6, which focuses on electrolyte imbalance.

INCREASED OUTPUT

Extracellular fluid depletion is most commonly caused by fluid losses from the skin or gastrointestinal tract. Hence, excessive perspiration, drainage from burns or abscesses, diarrhea, vomiting, and gastric suction could result in deficits of body fluid. In addition, loss of blood volume by hemorrhaging and certain conditions causing excessive urinary output (such as diabetes insipidus triggered by insufficient ADH secretion) can also bring on fluid depletion.

SIGNS AND SYMPTOMS

Extracellular fluid loss results, of course, in a depletion of both plasma and interstitial fluid compartments.

PLASMA Loss of plasma fluid effectively concentrates the large proteins and erythrocytes remaining in whole blood. The result is an increase in both the hematocrit and the plasma protein laboratory values except when hypovolemia is caused by hemorrhage.

In addition to the specific laboratory value changes, the depression in plasma fluid volume can cause characteristic clinical signs and symptoms. Depressed plasma volume results

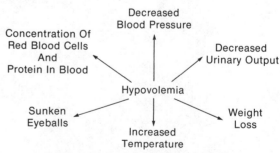

Figure 3.9 Effects of hypovolemia.

TABLE 3.1 **Fluid Volume Imbalances**

Imbalance	Causative Disorders	Clinical Manifestations
HYPERVOLEMIA	Renal failure Adrenal cortical tumor Steroid drug therapy Inappropriate ADH secretion (pain, malignancies, surgical trauma, cerebral disease)	Depressed hematocrit Decreased plasma protein concentration Elevated blood pressure Neck vein distention Circulatory overload Edema Weight gain Ascites
HYPOVOLEMIA	Excess perspiration Wound drainage Hemorrhage Diarrhea Vomiting Diabetes insipidus	Increased hematocrit* Increased plasma protein concentration* Depressed blood pressure Decreased urinary output Hypovolemic shock Decreased skin turgor Dry mucous membranes Sunken eyeballs Increased temperature Weight loss

*Except in cases of hemorrhage.

in a lowering of blood pressure. This, in turn, could decrease filtration pressure in the nephron and thus reduce urinary output. There may be indications of collapsed superficial veins, and, if blood volume falls sufficiently, hypovolemic shock could ensue.

INTERSTITIAL FLUID   The depletion of interstitial fluid is reflected by certain characteristic signs and symptoms. One could expect to see decreased skin turgor, dry mucous membranes, sunken eyeballs, and weight loss. Often, fluid loss is also accompanied by elevations in body temperature. The increase

is presumably caused, in part, by the direct effect of depressed volume upon the hypothalamic temperature regulatory center. Many of the signs and symptoms that may accompany extracellular volume depletion are presented in Figure 3.9.

Fluid Volume Imbalances: A Summary

Fluid volume imbalances are caused by a wide range of factors. Some primary disorders and clinical manifestations of fluid excess and deficit are listed in Table 3.1.

STUDY QUESTIONS

1. Mr. Jones weighs 180 lbs. Calculate:
   a. the weight of his interstitial fluid.
   b. the weight of his plasma.
   c. the weight of his intracellular fluid.
   d. his total fluid weight.
   e. what his weight would be if he *totally* dehydrated (a purely hypothetical situation).
2. Tommy Karlson, aged four months, is admitted to the hospital with intestinal flu. Why are the physicians so worried about possible dehydration?
3. Mrs. Randall is 5'3" tall, and weighs 285 lbs. She has been taking diuretics for high blood pressure. Why should she be monitored for possible dehydration?
4. Susie Powell is 5'5" tall, and weighs 120 lbs. Dan Reilly is 5'6" tall, and weighs 135 lbs. Which of the two would you expect to have the higher per cent fluid weight?
5. In each of the following situations, predict whether you would expect hypervolemia or hypovolemia to result, and why:
   a. hemorrhage
   b. adrenal cortical tumor
   c. insufficient ADH secretion (diabetes insipidus)
   d. excessive urination
   e. prolonged high fever
   f. extensive diarrhea
   g. renal failure
   h. excessive perspiration

6. Indicate whether the following are *signs* of hypovolemia or hypervolemia:
   a. elevated blood pressure
   b. high fever
   c. circulatory overload
   d. lack of skin turgor
   e. edema
   f. elevated hematocrit
   g. weight gain
   h. ascites

Suggested Readings
Books

Abbott Laboratories: Fluid and Electrolytes, Some Practical Guides to Clinical Use, 2nd ed. North Chicago, Abbott Laboratories, 1970, pp. 7–8; 48–56.

Brooks, S. M.: Basic Facts of Body Water and Ions. New York, Springer Publishing Company, 1973, pp. 1–18.

Burgess, A.: The Nurse's Guide to Fluid and Electrolyte Balance, 2nd ed. New York, McGraw-Hill Book Company, 1979, pp. 9–12; 51–55.

Burke, S. R.: The Composition and Function of Body Fluids, 2nd ed. St. Louis, The C. V. Mosby Company, 1976, pp. 1–5; 17–33.

Coleman, L.: Dehydration: When to look for it. *In:* Monitoring Fluids and Electrolytes Precisely. Nursing 79 Books. Horsham, Pa., Intermed Communications, Inc., 1978, p. 63.

Guyton, A. C.: Physiology of the Human Body, 5th ed. Philadelphia, W. B. Saunders Company, 1979, pp. 189–191; 200–203.

Hole, J. W.: Human Anatomy and Physiology.

Dubuque, Wm. C. Brown Company, 1978, pp. 680–685.

Metheny, N. M., and Snively, W. D.: Nurses' Handbook of Fluid Balance, 3rd ed. Philadelphia, J. B. Lippincott Company, 1979, pp. 1–8; 11–12; 59–63.

Stroot, V. R., Lee, C. A., and Schaper, C. A.: Fluids and Electrolytes: A Practical Approach, 2nd ed. Philadelphia, F. A. Davis Company, 1977, pp. 3–24.

Weldy, N. J.: Body Fluids and Electrolytes — A Programmed Presentation, 3rd ed. St. Louis, The C. V. Mosby Company, 1980, pp. 1–4; 69–90.

Articles

Lee, C. A., Stroot, V. R., and Schaper, C. A.: Extracellular volume imbalance. Am. J. Nurs., 75:888, 1974.

Chapter Outline

chapter 4

Intercompartmental Fluid Flow

Chapter Objectives

At the completion of this chapter, the student will be able to:

1. **List the major factors affecting fluid exchange between the plasma and interstitial compartments and describe their significance.**
2. **Identify the causes of:**
   a. Increasing capillary permeability.
   b. Decreasing capillary permeability.
   c. Increasing capillary blood pressure.
   d. Decreasing capillary blood pressure.
   e. Increasing colloid osmotic pressure.
   f. Decreasing colloid osmotic pressure.
3. **Describe the effect of the following upon fluid flow between the plasma and interstitial compartments:**
   a. Changes in capillary permeability.
   b. Changes in capillary blood pressure.
   c. Changes in colloid osmotic pressure.
4. **Identify the three primary routes whereby fluid can exit from the interstitial compartment.**
5. **List the major factors affecting fluid exchange between the interstitial and intracellular compartments and describe their significance.**
6. **Differentiate among simple diffusion, facilitated diffusion, active transport, and osmosis.**
7. **Define the terms** *isotonic, hypertonic,* **and** *hypotonic.*
8. **In each of the following cases, determine the net direction of fluid flow:**
   a. A cell surrounded by an isotonic fluid environment.
   b. A cell surrounded by a hypertonic fluid environment.
   c. A cell surrounded by a hypotonic fluid environment.

GENERAL LAWS GOVERNING FLUID FLOW

Body fluid, although distributed among specific "compartments," is not confined to a single designated area. In reality, there is constant flow and interchange between plasma, interstitial fluid, and intracellular fluid. The movement of fluid, however, is neither random nor haphazard. In general, fluid responds to a law of physics stating that substances tend to move from areas of greater concentration or pressure to areas of lesser concentration or pressure. The movement of molecules in response to these natural forces is known as *diffusion.*

We are surrounded by examples of this phenomenon. Perfume molecules sprayed in one corner of a room move to fill adjacent areas so that the odor is eventually detected several feet away. Smoke emanating from a piece of broiling meat can soon fill the kitchen. A teaspoon of sugar placed in a cup of hot coffee distributes itself uniformly through the liquid.

Body fluids behave in much the same manner. They generally flow from areas of greater concentration or pressure to areas of lesser concentration or pressure. Modifying this drive, however, is the presence of inter-compartmental barriers. The capillary wall separates plasma from interstitial fluid. The cell membrane lies between interstitial fluid and intracellular fluid. These strategically lo-

cated structures can thus impede or enhance exchange between fluid compartments.

FLUID FLOW BETWEEN PLASMA AND INTERSTITIAL COMPARTMENTS

In order to maintain cellular health, there must be a constant interchange between plasma and interstitial fluid. Blood serves as the primary transport medium for materials traveling to and from the cellular environment. Substances leaving the capillary must cross interstitial fluid before entering the cells. Conversely, material leaving the cells must move through the interstitial compartment toward plasma.

Without a mechanism to insure fluid turnover, material could stagnate in interstitial pools. Water surrounding the cells would fill with toxic wastes, and cellular death would result. To prevent this, plasma must serve as a continual source of renewal for the fluid bathing the cell.

Normal Interchange

There is an ongoing interchange between plasma and interstitial fluid. Fluid containing oxygen and nutrients normally enters the interstitial compartment at the arterial end of the capillary. Water high in metabolic wastes, on the other hand, moves into the venous end of

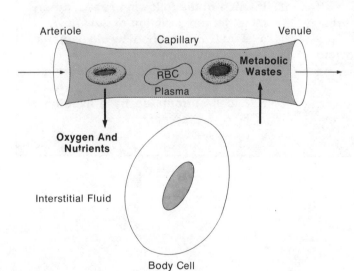

Figure 4.1 Capillary exchange.

the capillary to mix with plasma. A simplified scheme of this critical exchange is presented in Figure 4.1.

The flow of fluid between the interstitial compartment and plasma is governed by three primary factors:

1. The *permeability* of the capillary wall. Permeability, or the capacity of a structure to allow material to pass through it, is an important factor in fluid interchange. Under normal conditions the capillary is freely permeable to most physiologically significant molecules. Hence water, electrolytes, glucose, oxygen, and carbon dioxide can move readily between the interstitial and plasma compartments. Only larger molecules, such as protein, are restricted. As a result of this relatively free diffusion, most substances distribute themselves equally between interstitial fluid and plasma, driven primarily by concentration and pressure differences.

2. *Blood pressure* is the force with which blood pushes against the vascular walls. It provides the impetus for fluid to move from plasma into interstitial fluid, and it tends to push material *out* of the capillary.

3. *Colloid osmotic pressure* is the pull or draw for water exerted by protein molecules trapped within the vascular tree. It tends to attract fluid from the interstitial compartment into plasma, and thus causes material to move *into* the capillary.

Assuming integrity of the capillary wall, direction of net fluid flow between the interstitial compartment and plasma is governed

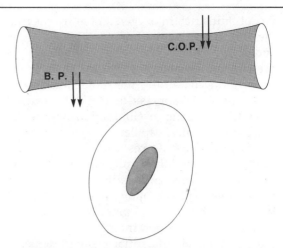

Figure 4.2 The effect of blood pressure and colloid osmotic pressure upon fluid exchange between the interstitial compartment and plasma.

primarily by the relative effects of blood pressure (B.P.) and colloid osmotic pressure (C.O.P.). If the force pushing fluid out of the capillary (blood pressure) is greater than that pulling water into the plasma (colloid osmotic pressure), net flow will be from plasma into interstitial fluid. If, on the other hand, colloid osmotic pressure is greater than blood pressure, fluid will move into the capillary from the interstitial compartment. The relative effects of blood pressure and colloid osmotic pressure upon fluid flow are summarized in Figure 4.2.

Under normal conditions, blood pressure at the arterial end of a capillary is greater than colloid osmotic pressure. This promotes the

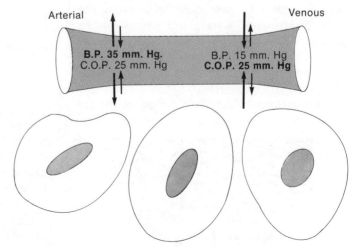

Figure 4.3 A typical capillary.

flux of fluids rich in oxygen and nutrients into the interstitial compartment. At the venous end of the capillary, however, colloid osmotic pressure exceeds blood pressure. Thus, interstitial fluid containing metabolic wastes can enter the circulatory system and be carried away for cleansing or elimination. Figure 4.3 illustrates a typical capillary.

Several other forces can also influence fluid flow across the capillary wall. For the sake of simplicity and clarity, however, emphasis will be placed upon the effects of capillary permeability, blood pressure, and colloid osmotic pressure upon interchanges between the plasma and interstitial compartments.

Capillary Permeability

To fully understand the concept of capillary permeability, it is necessary to first visualize the normal capillary structure.

Capillary walls are designed to promote interchange between plasma and interstitial fluid. This leads to optimal provision of the cellular needs for oxygen, nutrients, elimination, and fluid and electrolyte balance. Microscopic examination of the capillary wall reveals a structure only one cell thick. It is composed of many thin epithelial cells attached by a special intercellular cement. This cement is believed to contain tiny pores. Thus, passage of substances through the capillary can be effected either by movement directly through the cells or by flow through the small holes in the cement. Most physiologically significant material will take one of these two routes. Carbon dioxide and oxygen, for example, tend to pass directly through the cells. Electrolytes, water, and glucose move primarily through the pores. Protein molecules, by virtue of their large size, are denied transport. The structure of the capillary wall is illustrated in Figure 4.4.

Alterations in capillary permeability are mainly caused by factors that change the nature of the intercellular cement. By increasing the pore size, or by dissolving cement material, these factors promote the massive flux of both fluid and proteins out of plasma into the interstitial compartment.

CAUSES OF INCREASING CAPILLARY PERMEABILITY

Increases in capillary permeability are commonly caused by cellular trauma (such as burns, frostbite, and chemical irritation) and local or systemic allergic reactions.

It is postulated that both cellular trauma and allergic response promote the release of chemicals, which, in turn, produce an increase in capillary permeability. Primary among these chemicals is histamine, but other substances are also believed to contribute to increased permeability.

RESULTS OF INCREASING CAPILLARY PERMEABILITY

As capillary pores enlarge under the influence of histamine, large quantities of fluid and protein move from plasma into the interstitial compartment. The resulting increase in interstitial fluid volume is called *edema*. It is reflected clinically by enlargement and often tenderness of the affected area. Changes in capillary permeability account for much of the swelling and puffiness characteristic of burns, frostbite, and crushing injury.

It should be remembered that the interstitial fluid compartment gains fluid at the expense of plasma volume. Fluid flux out of the plasma compartment contributes to a fall in the capillary blood pressure. This decrease is aggravated by loss of plasma proteins from the vascular tree. As plasma proteins escape into the interstitial compartment, capillary colloid osmotic pressure decreases. The proteins that normally pull or draw water into the capillary proceed to attract fluid out of the tiny vessels, thus augmenting both edema and plasma loss. The effects of increasing capillary permeability are illustrated in Figure 4.5.

In summary, the two primary results of increasing capillary permeability are a loss of plasma volume and an increase in interstitial

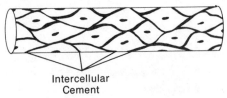

Intercellular
Cement

Figure 4.4 Capillary wall.

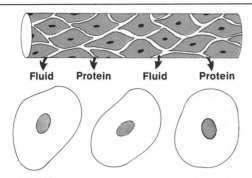

Figure 4.5 The effects of increasing capillary permeability: a conceptual diagram.

fluid. This response may be limited to a small area or may be widespread and potentially life-threatening. Its severity depends upon the degree and extent of the cellular trauma or allergic response. A mild case of poison ivy on an arm or leg, for example, will cause localized edema and discomfort but should not significantly affect systemic blood pressure. A severe systemic allergic reaction is described as *anaphylaxis*. A response of this type to penicillin, for example, precipitates massive histamine release throughout the body. Altered fluid balance and a disruption of homeostasis will result, as falling blood volume reduces the capacity of the circulatory system to supply cellular needs.

CAUSES AND RESULTS OF DECREASING CAPILLARY PERMEABILITY

In cases of severe or prolonged cellular trauma and inflammatory or allergic reactions, drugs are often administered to counteract the increases in capillary permeability. Antihistamines, steroids, and salicylates are most commonly used.

Steroids are chemicals similar in structure and function to the hormone cortisol, which is released by the adrenal cortex. Given in adequate doses, they are believed to inhibit the synthesis of histamine, thereby helping to restore capillary permeability to normal. Antihistamines are drugs that act primarily by blocking the action of histamine in the body. They are useful in counteracting certain allergic or anaphylactic responses. Salicylates, such as aspirin, are also given to combat

increased capillary permeability. Their action on histamine is similar to that of steroids, and they also counteract the pain and fever that often accompany cellular trauma.

All of these drugs help to restore capillary permeability to normal, thereby promoting the restoration of fluid balance. Thus they are examples of agents external to the body that can be used medically to help maintain homeostasis.

It should be noted that there are no instances of natural substances causing capillary permeability to decrease. Although there are clinical instances of fluid retention in the plasma compartment, they do not result from lack of capillary porosity. Rather, alterations in blood pressure and colloid osmotic pressure must be examined as possible causative factors in these cases.

Blood Pressure

Blood pressure, as defined earlier, is the force with which blood pushes out against vascular walls. It is important to remember that the blood pressure reading obtained by pumping up a cuff on the arm of a patient is a measure of pressure in the arteries. It does *not* necessarily reflect what is happening at the capillary level deep within the body. As we further analyze capillary blood pressure, it will become obvious that many factors affect the force with which blood pushes against the capillary wall.

FACTORS AFFECTING CAPILLARY BLOOD PRESSURE

Plasma volume changes will have a direct and obvious effect upon capillary blood pressure values. Excess fluid in the capillaries will create a greater outward push than will depressed fluid levels. In much the same way that a bicycle tire feels hard and firm when filled with air but soft and pliable when deflated, the outward pressure in a capillary will vary according to the amount of plasma within it.

There are several factors influencing the amount of plasma reaching the body capillaries. Obviously, extracellular fluid excesses or deficits, as discussed earlier in this Unit,

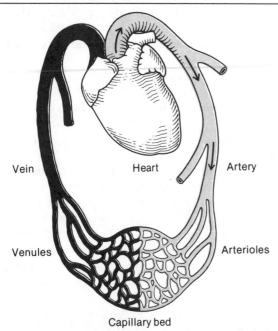

Figure 4.6 Flow of blood through the cardiovascular system. (From Hole, J. W., Jr.: Human Anatomy and Physiology. William C. Brown Company, 1978. Used by permission.)

will affect blood volume. Losses will result in depressed plasma volume and a drop in capillary blood pressure. Gains will have the opposite effect and thus contribute to a rise in capillary blood pressure.

Assuming a normal volume of blood, however, the amount of plasma contained within capillaries will be influenced by the volume of blood entering and leaving the capillary vessels at any given time. The entry and exit of capillary blood is, in turn, affected by two major factors: (1) *cardiac output,* or the volume of blood pumped by the heart per minute, and (2) the *diameter* of vessels carrying blood to and from the minute capillaries.

The significance of these factors is clarified by visualizing normal plasma transport. Blood moves in one continuous circuit from the heart into arteries, arterioles, capillaries, venules, and veins and then back to the heart. Figure 4.6 illustrates the vascular system.

CARDIAC OUTPUT With the heart serving as a pump for fluid traveling through all vessels, cardiac output can greatly influence capillary blood pressure. The complex factors affecting cardiac output warrant further

analysis and will be described in Chapter 9. At this point, suffice it to say that adult cardiac output at rest normally averages about 5 liters per minute. This figure can vary considerably, however, and mechanisms exist to adjust output so as to optimally serve cellular needs.

Physical exertion, for example, stimulates an increase in cardiac rate and strength. As a result, blood is brought more quickly to rapidly metabolizing cells. Thus, elevated quantities of oxygen and nutrients are supplied to meet energy demands, rapid waste removal is facilitated, and homeostasis is maintained.

VASCULAR DIAMETER As illustrated in Figure 4.6, blood normally moves in one continuous circuit from the heart into arteries, arterioles, capillaries, venules, and veins and then back to the heart. Once blood enters the vascular tree, its movement and distribution are largely affected by the diameter of the vessels through which it travels.

Ordinarily, blood is distributed within the circulatory system so that 5 to 10 per cent of total blood volume is found within the heart, 15 per cent in the arterial vessels, 65 to 70 per cent in the venous vessels, and only 5 to 10 per cent in the capillaries. The disproportionately large amount of blood normally encountered in the veins and venules is due primarily to the great distensibility of the venous walls. Their ability to stretch and accommodate vast quantities of fluid accounts for the rather unbalanced pattern of plasma distribution.

Deviations from the described norm result primarily from alterations in the size of the vascular lumen. Since the nervous system significantly influences the tone and status of smooth muscle within the walls of blood vessels, it can indirectly affect the volume of blood entering the capillary at any given time.

Constriction of arteries and arterioles tends to decrease blood flow into capillaries and thus to depress capillary fluid volume. Blood collects in arterial vessels, causing a rise in arterial blood pressure readings, while capillary blood pressure falls, compromising cellular needs for nutrients, oxygen, elimination, and fluid and electrolyte balance.

Venous constriction, paradoxically, can

also act to maintain low capillary blood volumes. A decrease in venous diameter is accompanied by a decrease in the normally large venous capacity for fluids. As a result, blood returns to the heart more rapidly than usual. The possibility of fluid back-up or pooling in capillary vessels is thereby reduced.

Arterial dilation, on the other hand, allows for the rapid entry of large volumes of blood into the capillary vessels. Hence with dilation of arteries or arterioles, one could expect increases in capillary fluid volumes and pressures. Simultaneous *venous dilation* could further support an elevation of capillary blood pressure. Large quantities of blood allowed to pool and remain in veins and venules would pose resistance to the exit of fluid from capillaries. Hence, plasma volume and pressure in the capillaries would predictably increase and remain elevated until venous tone returned to normal.

Capillary walls, unlike those of arteries and veins, contain no smooth muscle and thus cannot be directly affected by nerve impulses. *Precapillary sphincter* muscles (see Figure 4.7), however, which regulate the flow of blood into the capillary, may open or close in direct response to local physical and chemical influences. Low oxygen concentrations and elevated carbon dioxide levels are known to promote sphincter dilation. This mechanism facilitates the transport of greater volumes of

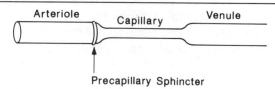

Precapillary Sphincter

Figure 4.7 The precapillary sphincter.

blood into areas where cellular needs for oxygen, nutrients, and elimination may be threatened. Release of adrenaline or exposure to cold, on the other hand, may result in sphincter constriction, with subsequent reduction in the volume of fluid entering the capillaries.

FACTORS AFFECTING CAPILLARY BLOOD PRESSURE: A SUMMARY It is important to remember that many factors influence capillary blood pressure values. The *volume of extracellular fluid, cardiac output,* and the *diameter of blood vessels* all have a major effect upon the amount of fluid reaching the capillaries. Many systems must work together to regulate capillary fluid volumes and pressures. A brief summary of some of these systems and their functions in regulating capillary blood pressure is presented in Table 4.1.

An example of the effect of many factors upon capillary blood pressure can be found by observing a person as he or she exercises.

TABLE 4.1 **The Regulation of Capillary Blood Pressure**

Regulatory Factor	Systems Involved	Functional Activity of System
Cardiac output	Endocrine and nervous	Aid in the regulation and control of cardiac rate and strength.
	Cardiovascular	Contraction of cardiac muscle serves to eject blood into the systemic arterial tree.
Extracellular fluid volume	Endocrine	ADH and aldosterone influence renal fluid reabsorption.
	Renal	The kidneys maintain an effective balance between fluid elimination and retention.
	Respiratory	Fluid is eliminated during expiration.
	Integumentary	Fluid is eliminated by diffusion and perspiration through the skin.
	Digestive	Fluid is ingested, absorbed through the gastrointestinal tract, and eliminated in feces.
Vascular diameter	Nervous and endocrine	Cause appropriate changes in vascular diameter.

Physical exertion, with the build-up of metabolic wastes in the extracellular fluid of active muscle cells, results in several adaptations. The arterioles serving the working skeletal muscle dilate. The rate and strength of cardiac contraction increase. The result is an elevation in plasma volume and blood pressure in the capillaries of skeletal muscle tissue.

At the same time that the working tissue receives an increased blood supply, nerve impulses cause the arterioles serving the skin, gastrointestinal tract, and kidneys to constrict. In this way, blood is shunted to the areas of greatest immediate need at the expense of structures that are not as metabolically stressed. It thus becomes evident that all capillaries in the body are not receiving the same amount of plasma at any given time. Very intricate mechanisms adjust blood supply so as to optimally and selectively meet cellular needs and maintain homeostasis.

CAUSES OF INCREASING CAPILLARY BLOOD PRESSURE

Capillary blood pressure will increase as a result of clinical conditions that promote (1) elevated plasma volume, (2) increased cardiac output, or (3) dilation of the vessels feeding or draining the capillaries.

ELEVATED PLASMA VOLUME A review of Chapter 3 will aid in the recall of several clinical situations that would increase plasma volume by promoting hypervolemia. Primary among these are renal failure, hypersecretion of aldosterone or ADH, liver disease, chronic use of steroid drugs, and excessive intravenous drip.

INCREASED CARDIAC OUTPUT Assuming normal plasma volume, increased cardiac output may, alternatively, cause an increase in capillary blood pressure. Higher cardiac output is most often promoted by sympathetic nervous stimulation, by the effects of the hormones epinephrine or norepinephrine, or by both.

It can thus be seen that factors promoting sympathetic nervous activity would predictably increase cardiac output. Physical exertion or emotional excitement, including fright, anger, or suspense, by triggering sympathetic

nervous stimulation can increase capillary blood pressure values.

DILATION OF BLOOD VESSELS As mentioned earlier, primary causes of increased capillary blood pressure include arterial and venous dilation. Clinically, many factors can precipitate such changes including diminished neural impulses to blood vessel walls accompanying deep anesthesia, spinal anesthesia, brain damage, strong emotional reactions, and severe pain.

Dilation of arterioles and venules is also promoted by the histamine released during allergic response to drugs, insect bites, or food. Even certain bacterial infections can indirectly cause vasodilation. Many of the harmful chemicals (toxins) released by disease-producing microorganisms are known to directly stimulate the relaxation of vascular muscles. Thus, peritonitis, gas gangrene, and certain staphylococcal and streptococcal infections can cause increases in capillary blood pressure.

FACTORS PROMOTING AN INCREASE IN CAPILLARY BLOOD PRESSURE: A SUMMARY Many factors interact to cause a rise in capillary blood pressure. A summary of

TABLE 4.2   **Causes of Increased Capillary Blood Pressure**

Causative Mechanism	Initiating Factors
Elevated plasma volume	Renal failure Hypersecretion of aldosterone Hypersecretion of ADH Liver disease Excessive intake of steroid drugs Excessive I.V. drip
Increased cardiac output	Physical exertion Emotional excitement Fright Anger
Vascular dilation	Deep anesthesia Spinal anesthesia Brain damage Severe pain Allergy-mediated release of histamine Release of certain bacterial toxins

some of the major ones is presented in Table 4.2.

It is important to remember, however, that it is the combined effect of these factors that ultimately determines capillary blood pressure values at any given time. The influence of any one determinant can always be modified by counteractive forces.

By examining the physiological effects of fright upon the circulatory system, one can derive a better understanding of this phenomenon. Fear mobilizes the sympathetic nervous system. As a result, cardiac rate and strength increase, with a subsequent rise in cardiac output. Simultaneously, however, sympathetic stimulation can cause arteriolar constriction and decrease the blood volume in many capillaries throughout the body. In these capillaries, plasma volume and blood pressure might fall, regardless of the rise in cardiac output. Hence, an accurate picture is obtained only by considering the cumulative effect of all factors influencing capillary blood pressure.

RESULTS OF INCREASES IN CAPILLARY BLOOD PRESSURE

Assuming normal capillary permeability and colloid osmotic pressure, elevated capillary blood pressure will promote a flux of fluid from the plasma into the interstitial fluid compartment.

As long as the outward push of blood pressure exceeds the inward pull of colloid osmotic pressure, there will be an accumulation of fluid in the interstitial compartment. This accumulation will be manifested by symptoms of increased skin turgor and puffiness. Simultaneously, the drain of fluid from plasma serves the purpose of bringing capillary blood pressure down toward normal. This is an example of how the laws of nature can work toward self-correction of a problem. Although this element of self-correction cannot cure the causes of elevated capillary pressure, it usually does help to modify the speed and intensity with which pathological symptoms develop.

The loss of fluid from the vascular system will continue until: (1) blood pressure falls lower than colloid osmotic pressure, or (2) fluid in the interstitial compartment builds up sufficiently to offer resistance to further out-

ward flux of fluid from the capillary. Once again, physiological forces provide a checks-and-balances mechanism, which insures that the outward flux of plasma proceeds only until capillary blood pressure values approach normal. Colloid osmotic pressure and fluid resistance forces thus guard against excessive movement of fluid out of the plasma compartment.

CAUSES OF DECREASING CAPILLARY BLOOD PRESSURE

Capillary blood pressure tends to decrease as a result of clinical conditions that promote (1) depressed plasma volume, (2) decreased cardiac output, or (3) constriction of the vessels feeding or draining the capillaries.

DEPRESSED PLASMA VOLUME A review of Chapter 3 will help to recall several clinical conditions that decrease plasma volume by promoting hypovolemia. Primary among these are excessive diuresis, diarrhea, vomiting, burns, hemorrhage, and endocrine imbalances such as diabetes insipidus.

DECREASED CARDIAC OUTPUT Many factors can affect cardiac output. We know that nervous and hormonal influences modify the rate and strength of cardiac contraction. The health and status of the heart muscle (myocardium) itself is also of primary concern in the assessment of cardiac output.

It stands to reason that a diseased heart cannot work with optimal efficiency. Hence a heart attack (myocardial infarction), congestive heart failure, valvular disorders, conduction blocks, and arrhythmias may all contribute to decreased cardiac output.

To the extent that seemingly unrelated disorders affect venous return (the volume of blood returning to the heart via the veins), they too modify cardiac output. Hence, any vascular changes that precipitate venous pooling of blood, any extracellular fluid losses, and any shift of fluid out of the plasma compartment could all technically reduce both venous return and cardiac output. We see examples of these situations in cases of extreme emotional shock, hemorrhage, and burns. A more detailed analysis of other pathological conditions affecting cardiac output is found in Chapter 9.

CONSTRICTION OF BLOOD VESSELS As described earlier, any factor causing constriction of arteries, arterioles, venules, and veins usually tends to decrease capillary blood volume and hence capillary blood pressure.

Thus, sympathetic nervous stimulation, which usually triggers vasoconstriction, can often cause decreases in capillary blood pressure. Since the sympathetic nervous system comes into play at times of physical exertion, depressed oxygen conditions, and emotional excitement, including fright, anger, and suspense, these circumstances could decrease capillary blood volume and pressure.

An example of the effects of sympathetic stimulation can often be found in the early stages of shock due to hemorrhage. The body attempts to compensate for falling blood volume by constriction of blood vessels. This serves to temporarily maintain arterial blood pressure in the absence of sufficient blood volume. Although effective in preventing a rapid drop in blood pressure, this vasoconstriction often causes cellular stress. Constriction of arterioles can deplete the volume of blood entering the capillaries and thus compromise the cellular need for oxygen, nutrients, and waste elimination. Often the precapillary sphincters respond to this stress by secondary vasodilation. Unfortunately, the resulting massive flow of blood into 60,000 miles of capillaries throughout the body produces temporary correction of cellular stress but simultaneously depressed venous return. As blood pools in the capillaries, it fails to return to the heart in sufficient quantity. It can thus be seen how the regulation of vascular changes, an intricate process, can have far-reaching physiological effects.

FACTORS PROMOTING A DECREASE IN CAPILLARY BLOOD PRESSURE: A SUMMARY Many factors can cause a fall in capillary blood pressure. A summary of some clinical situations that could predictably result in decreased capillary blood pressure is found in Table 4.3.

Again, it is necessary to remember that capillary blood pressure will ultimately be

TABLE 4.3 Causes of Decreased Capillary Blood Pressure

Causative Mechanism	Initiating Factors
Depressed plasma volume	Excessive diuresis Diarrhea Vomiting Burns Hemorrhage Diabetes insipidus

Decreased cardiac output	Cardiac disease:
	  Myocardial infarction
	  Congestive heart
	    failure
	  Valvular disorders
	  Arrhythmias
	Venous stasis

Vascular constriction	Physical exertion Emotional excitement Fright Anger

determined by many contributing factors. All of these must be taken into consideration in the assessment of capillary blood pressure status.

RESULTS OF DECREASES IN CAPILLARY BLOOD PRESSURE

Assuming a normal colloid osmotic pressure, a decrease in capillary blood pressure will cause a flux of fluid from the interstitial compartment into plasma. This fluid shift will continue until the plasma volume increases sufficiently to re-establish normal blood pressure.

As a result of fluid movement out of the interstitial space, tissue dehydration can occur, with symptoms of thirst, dry cracked lips, and dry mucous membranes.

Colloid Osmotic Pressure

Colloid osmotic pressure, as described earlier, is the pull or draw for water exerted by the large protein molecules trapped within the blood vessels. It tends to counteract the outward push of blood pressure and is the major impetus for fluid movement from the interstitial compartment into plasma. Since colloid osmotic pressure depends largely upon the presence of large protein molecules in plasma, alterations in plasma protein content can strongly influence colloid osmotic pressure values.

CAUSES OF INCREASING COLLOID OSMOTIC PRESSURE

Clinically speaking, there are few examples of elevated concentrations of plasma proteins, even with pathological conditions. Most commonly, increases in colloid osmotic pressure result from the intravenous introduction of large molecules into the plasma compartment for medical reasons. Albumin, mannitol, and dextran are examples of substances commonly used to elevate colloid osmotic pressure. Although mannitol and dextran are not protein by nature, they are sufficiently large structurally to remain within the confines of the capillary. They thus exert an attraction for water similar to that of the albumin and globulin plasma proteins.

RESULTS OF INCREASES IN COLLOID OSMOTIC PRESSURE

As a result of elevated colloid osmotic pressure, fluid will be drawn from interstitial spaces into the plasma compartment.

Administration of substances that increase colloid osmotic pressure values is therefore reserved for clinical situations characterized by the accumulation of excessive interstitial fluid or the loss of plasma volume. The resulting fluid shift decreases any existing edema while simultaneously elevating blood volume and blood pressure.

CAUSES OF DECREASING COLLOID OSMOTIC PRESSURE

As mentioned earlier, colloid osmotic pressure varies as a function of plasma protein concentrations. Thus a decrease in plasma production or a loss of plasma protein from the body will lead to a fall in colloid osmotic pressure values.

Decreased colloid osmotic pressure is frequently caused by liver disease (the liver is a primary producer of plasma proteins), severe malnutrition (inadequate protein intake), and kidney disease with albuminuria (loss of protein in the urine).

RESULTS OF DECREASES IN COLLOID OSMOTIC PRESSURE

Assuming the maintenance of a normal blood pressure, excessive fluid will remain in the interstitial compartment if colloid osmotic pressure is not sufficiently high to pull water back into the circulatory system at the venous end of the capillary.

This, in fact, does occur in cases of plasma protein deficiency or loss. Signs of edema develop as interstitial fluid accumulates. Blood volume and arterial blood pressure can fall if fluid retention in the interstitial compartment is sufficiently great.

Fluid Flow Between Plasma and Interstitial Fluid: A Summary

We have seen that the exchange of fluid between plasma and interstitial fluid is a complex process. Any clinical factors altering capillary permeability, capillary blood pressure, or colloid osmotic pressure will, in turn, affect fluid flux across the capillary wall.

In general, increased capillary permeability, elevated capillary blood pressure, and decreased colloid osmotic pressure tend to favor flux of fluid out of plasma into the interstitial fluid. Conversely, decreased capillary permeability, decreased capillary blood pressure, and increased colloid osmotic pressure promote fluid movement from the interstitial compartment into plasma. A summary of some of the primary clinical conditions affecting fluid fluxes across the capillary wall is found in Figure 4.8.

INTERSTITIAL FLUID ROUTES

We now know that fluid regularly moves from plasma into the interstitial compartments at the arterial end of the capillary. This process insures constant arrival of fresh water to bathe the cells of the body. It is obvious that fluid cannot continually accumulate in the intersti-

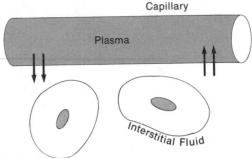

Cells Surrounded By Interstitial Fluid

Factors Promoting Shifts From Plasma to Interstitial Fluid

1. Increased capillary permeability
   burns (early stages)
   frostbite
   allergic reaction

2. Increased capillary blood pressure
   renal failure
   hypersecretion of aldosterone
   hypersecretion of ADH
   liver disease
   excessive intake of steroids
   excessive I.V. drip
   physical exertion
   emotional excitement
   anesthesia
   brain damage
   severe pain

3. Decreased colloid osmotic pressure
   liver disease
   severe malnutrition
   albuminuria

Factors Promoting Shifts From Interstitial Fluid to Plasma

1. Decreased capillary permeability (return of permeable capillary wall to normal status)
   administration of steroids
   administration of aspirin
   administration of antihistamines

2. Decreased capillary blood pressure
   excessive diuresis
   diarrhea
   vomiting
   burns (later stages)
   hemorrhage
   diabetes insipidus
   cardiac disease
   venous stasis
   fright
   anger
   physical exertion

3. Increased colloid osmotic pressure
   administration of dextran or mannitol

Figure 4.8   Factors affecting the distribution of fluid between plasma and the interstitial compartment.

tial environment without an exit route. There must be an escape valve to allow a certain volume of fluid to leave as new substances enter the interstitial compartment.

Actually, three alternative outlets are available:

1. Some fluid will *return to plasma*, drawn in at the venous end of the capillary by the pull of colloid osmotic pressure. This process was described earlier in this chapter.

2. Some fluid will enter blind-end *lymph capillaries* that are dispersed throughout the interstitial fluid compartment. These thin-walled vessels pick up extra fluid and some fluid components, returning them to blood in the area of the right and left subclavian veins. The pattern of lymph flow is presented diagrammatically in Figure 4.9.

If lymph vessels are swollen or obstructed or have been removed surgically, interstitial fluid can accumulate, with resultant swelling and reduced mobility of the affected area. This is often seen clinically when lymph nodes are swollen or blocked by spreading cancer cells or have been removed surgically to prevent further spread of a malignancy.

3. The third exit route available to interstitial fluid is movement into the intracellular compartment *across the cell membrane*. This is a complex process that merits further study. It will be analyzed in the following section.

In summary, the three alternative exit routes for fluid in the interstitial compartment provide a means of insuring balance between the three fluid compartments. These three routes are illustrated in Figure 4.10. It can be

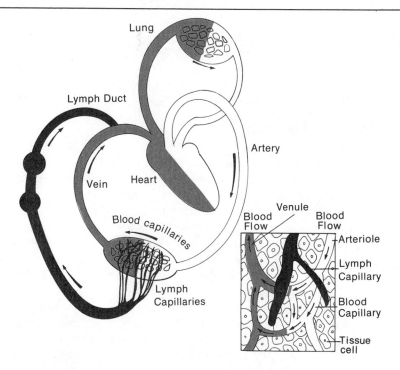

Figure 4.9 Lymphatic vessels carry fluid from interstitial spaces into the bloodstream. *Inset:* Lymphatic capillaries are very small, blind-end vessels that originate in the interstitial spaces of tissues.

seen how interstitial fluid, lying at the crossroads between capillaries and body cells, plays an important role as the middleman between the plasma and intracellular compartments.

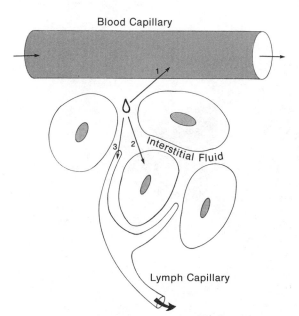

Figure 4.10 Exit of fluid from the interstitial compartment. The alternative routes available are (1) return to plasma, (2) shift into the intracellular compartment, and (3) drainage into lymph capillary.

FLUID FLOW BETWEEN INTERSTITIAL AND INTRACELLULAR COMPARTMENTS

In order to maintain homeostasis, the intracellular fluid must constantly be replenished and cleansed. Ideally, there should be ongoing interchange between intracellular and interstitial fluid to insure servicing of the cellular needs for oxygen, nutrients, and waste elimination.

Only a limited number of substances can move between the interstitial and intracellular compartments by simple diffusion. The cell membrane is structured so as to limit or modify the simple diffusion of most molecules. Hence, the majority of physiologically significant material is transported between the interstitial and intracellular compartments by a variety of specialized mechanisms. Some of these are briefly described in the following pages.

Factors Affecting Flow

To fully understand transport between interstitial and intracellular fluid, it is first necessary to visualize the major structural components of the cell membrane. The cell membrane serves as a barrier between the interstitial and the intracellular fluid compartments. It is thus in a position to modify intercompartmental flow.

CELL MEMBRANE

Structurally, the cell membrane consists of thin lipid-protein fragments lined up side by side to form an enclosure for the internal contents of the cell. These fragments are separated by small pores that carry a positive electrical charge. An illustration of this structure is provided in Figure 4.11.

Because of its structure and behavior, the cell membrane is described as being *selectively permeable*, or *semipermeable*. Unlike the capillary wall, which allows most molecules to pass through with relative ease, the cell membrane permits only a limited number of substances to diffuse freely across it. The majority of particles, therefore, must pass through the membrane driven by forces other than simple diffusion.

TRANSPORT MECHANISMS

Materials can pass in and out of the cell by a variety of mechanisms. Primary among these are: (1) simple diffusion, (2) facilitated diffusion, (3) active transport, and (4) osmosis. Transport in each of these cases accounts for the movement of specific materials between the interstitial and intracellular compartments. Each mechanism, being unique and significant, warrants further description and analysis.

SIMPLE DIFFUSION Simple diffusion is the movement of a substance from an area of greater concentration or pressure to an area of lesser concentration or pressure. In order to move freely between interstitial and intracellular compartments in response to what is called a concentration, or pressure, gradient, material must be able to pass readily through the cell membrane.

Molecules crossing the membrane barrier with relative ease must satisfy one of two prerequisites. They are either (1) *lipid-soluble* and thus able to diffuse readily through the lipid component of the membrane, or (2) *small, negatively charged* particles able to pass easily through the membrane pores.

Only a limited number of substances satisfy these criteria. Oxygen, carbon dioxide, and alcohol diffuse owing to lipid solubility; chloride and water pass through the membrane pores. The transport of water will be discussed in detail in the section dealing with osmosis.

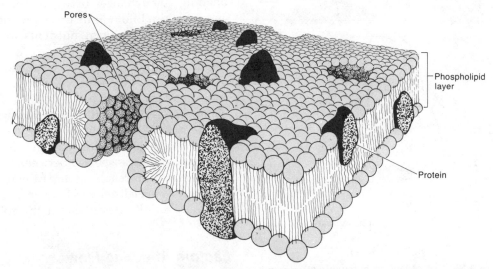

Figure 4.11 The cell membrane: a current concept of structural organization. (From Tortora, G., and Anagnostakos, N.: Principles of Anatomy and Physiology, 2nd ed. New York, Harper & Row, 1978. Used by permission.)

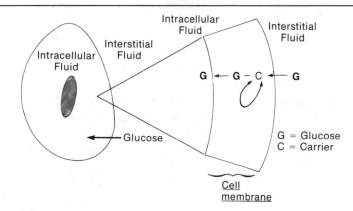

Figure 4.12 The facilitated diffusion of glucose across the cell membrane.

FACILITATED DIFFUSION Some substances cannot pass through the membrane without help. *Glucose*, for example, moves between interstitial and intracellular fluid by attaching to a phosphate carrier in the membrane, which ferries it between compartments. Once glucose is deposited at its destination, the carrier is then free to return and pick up other molecules waiting to enter. This process is illustrated in Figure 4.12.

ACTIVE TRANSPORT A number of substances can be transported against their concentration gradients (i.e., from areas of lesser to greater concentration) by an active "pump" mechanism. This pump is situated in the membrane and is driven by energy generated by cellular respiration.

Such a pump is postulated to regulate the distribution of sodium (Na^+) and potassium (K^+) within the interstitial and the intracellular fluid compartments.

Sodium is normally found primarily in the extracellular fluid, while potassium is located mainly in the intracellular compartment. If sodium attempts to leak into the cell, or potassium out, the pump drives each particle back to the compartment in which it belongs. This mechanism, which helps to insure the normal distribution of the primary fluid components, aids in the maintenance of homeostasis. The Na/K membrane pump is shown in Figure 4.13.

OSMOSIS Of all the methods by which substances can move across the cell membrane, osmosis is one of the most significant and complex. By definition, osmosis involves the transport of *water* across a semipermeable membrane from the area where water is in greater concentration to the area where it is in lesser concentration. Because this is a traditionally difficult area of study, the following section is devoted to clarifying the principles of osmosis.

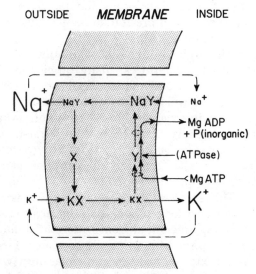

Figure 4.13 Postulated mechanism for active transport of sodium and potassium through the cell membrane, showing coupling of the two transport mechanisms and delivery of energy to the system at the inner surface of the membrane. (From Guyton, A.: Physiology of the Human Body. Philadelphia, W. B. Saunders Company, 1979. Used by permission.)

OSMOSIS: FURTHER CLARIFICATION

As mentioned earlier, substances in nature tend to move from where they are in greater concentration to where they are in lesser concentration until they are equally dispersed. Thus, sugar molecules placed into a cup of tea move within the cup in order to scatter themselves uniformly through the liquid. Ideally, when the sugar has been totally diffused, each sip of the tea should be equally sweet.

Water and other components of the body's fluid compartments are driven by the same forces of dispersal. In the body, however, barriers exist to prevent or modify simple diffusion. The cell membrane is a very selective barrier that allows few substances to pass through freely.

To facilitate a conceptual understanding of osmosis, it is helpful at this point to introduce some basic information about fluid composition. In simple terms, the interstitial fluid consists primarily of water and sodium (Na^+), whereas the major component of intracellular water is potassium (K^+). Sodium and potassium are normally present in relatively fixed concentrations within their respective compartments. Deviations too far from the normal range can precipitate cellular dysfunction or death.

Although sodium and potassium are the primary fluid particles, many other components exist in body fluids. Their source and significance will be discussed in more detail in the following chapter. It must be kept in mind that for cellular fluid balance to persist, *the total concentration of all particles in interstitial fluid must equal the total concentration of all particles in intracellular fluid.*

The reason for this becomes evident as we take a closer look at osmosis. The membrane separating interstitial from intracellular fluid is freely permeable primarily to water. Electrolytes such as sodium and potassium will not readily pass through. It has been determined that a solution of 0.9 per cent table salt (NaCl, or sodium chloride) has about the same total particle concentration as intracellular fluid. This type of solution is referred to as *isotonic.* If a solution is saltier than 0.9 per cent

NaCl, it is said to be *hypertonic;* if it is less salty, it is described as *hypotonic.* This concept of tonicity is illustrated in Figure 4.14.

ISOTONIC INTERSTITIAL FLUID   If a cell is surrounded by an isotonic solution, fluid balance is maintained. Any water molecules moving into the cell are balanced by an equal number of water molecules moving out of the cell. Thus, intravenous medication given to patients who are in a state of fluid balance must be isotonic, if they are to support homeostasis. The solution of choice may vary with the clinical situation but could include "normal saline" (0.9 per cent NaCl), "D5W" (5 per cent dextrose in water), or Ringer's solution (a combination of several particles equal in concentration to extracellular fluid).

It is important to realize that a solution isotonic to intracellular fluid does *not* have to contain the same components as intracellular fluid. It must, however, contain the same *total concentration of particles.*

If we were to determine that intracellular fluid had 100 solid particles in every 100 ml. of water, then an isotonic solution would also have to contain 100 solid particles per 100 ml. of water. However, the isotonic solution would *not* have to contain the same kind of solid particles as the intracellular fluid. Hence, normal saline and D5W are both isotonic, but one contains NaCl and water, and the other, dextrose and water. Significantly, neither solution contains the particles actually present in intracellular fluid.

HYPERTONIC INTERSTITIAL FLUID   A hypertonic solution is one that contains more solid particles per given volume of water than does intracellular fluid. Since sodium is the primary component of interstitial fluid, it is most often the particle responsible for clinical hypertonicity. As such, it will be cited in the following examples.

If a cell is put into a hypertonic environment, both water and sodium strive to cross the cell membrane in response to their respective concentration gradients. Therefore, water tends to move from the intracellular to the interstitial compartment, from where it is in greater concentration to where it is in lesser

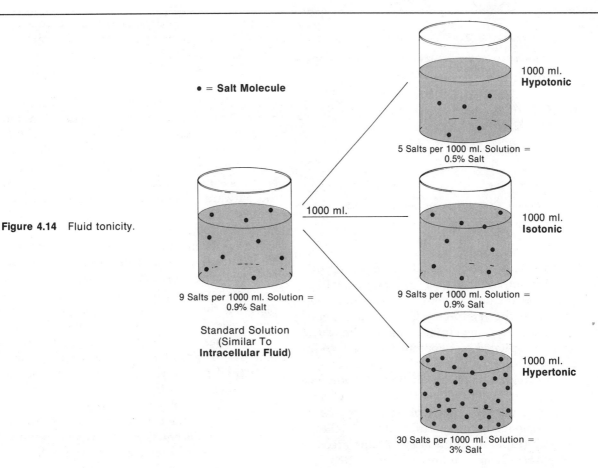

• = **Salt Molecule**

Figure 4.14 Fluid tonicity.

1000 ml.

9 Salts per 1000 ml. Solution =
0.9% Salt

Standard Solution
(Similar To
Intracellular Fluid)

1000 ml.
Hypotonic

5 Salts per 1000 ml. Solution =
0.5% Salt

1000 ml.
Isotonic

9 Salts per 1000 ml. Solution =
0.9% Salt

1000 ml.
Hypertonic

30 Salts per 1000 ml. Solution =
3% Salt

concentration. Sodium particles, on the other hand, attempt to move from interstitial to intracellular fluid to equalize their concentration. This is illustrated in Figure 4.15.

Since the cell membrane is semipermeable, it will allow only water to pass through to any measurable extent. Hence water will move from intracellular to interstitial fluid

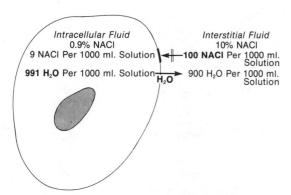

Intracellular Fluid
0.9% NACl
9 NACl Per 1000 ml. Solution
991 H₂O Per 1000 ml. Solution

Interstitial Fluid
10% NACl
100 NACl Per 1000 ml.
Solution
900 H₂O Per 1000 ml.
Solution

H₂O

Figure 4.15 Hypertonic interstitial fluid.

when the cell is surrounded by a hypertonic solution. In the process, the cellular contents will become relatively more concentrated and the fluid bathing the cell will become more dilute. Water flux thus assumes the entire burden of equalizing electrolyte concentrations.

It can be seen how a hypertonic fluid environment could damage body cells by promoting cellular water loss, or dehydration. Pathological conditions causing the development of hypertonic interstitial fluid will be discussed in Chapter 6. The clinical symptoms of these disorders are often related to problems that accompany cellular dehydration.

HYPOTONIC INTERSTITIAL FLUID A hypotonic solution is one that contains *fewer* solid particles per given volume of water than does intracellular fluid. Again, sodium will be used in the example of hypotonicity.

If a cell is put into a hypotonic environment, the drive for equalization causes water

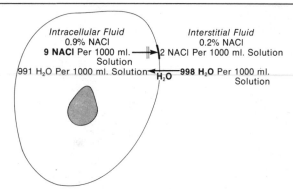

Figure 4.16 Hypotonic interstitial fluid.

to move across the cell membrane *from interstitial into intracellular fluid*. Although sodium particles attempt to move in the opposite direction, the semipermeability of the membrane prevents them from doing so. The water shift precipitated by hypotonicity is shown in Figure 4.16.

Pathological states inducing a hypotonic fluid environment will be discussed in Chapter 6. It can be seen how such disorders would cause damage by promoting cellular swelling or lysis (rupture). Clinical symptoms accompanying cellular rupture will often depend upon the cells involved. Red blood cell destruction, for example, would precipitate different problems than cerebral cellular swelling. Clinical distinctions between these different phenomena will be explored later in Unit 2.

SUMMARY

A review of Chapter 4 reveals several differences between plasma-interstitial fluid flow and interstitial-intracellular fluid flow. At

the root of these differences lies the contrast between the intercompartmental fluid barriers with respect to both structure and function.

The capillary wall, which exists as a barrier between plasma and interstitial fluid, is effectively permeable to almost all substances except large protein molecules. The retention of protein is, in turn, responsible for the maintenance of colloid osmotic pressure within the capillaries. Colloid osmotic pressure is a water-attracting force that counteracts the outward push of blood pressure. As described earlier, the direction of net fluid movement between the plasma and the interstitial compartments is determined primarily by the relative balance between blood pressure and colloid osmotic pressure.

The barrier between interstitial fluid and plasma is the cell membrane. This structure is very selectively permeable, allowing only water to pass through to any appreciable extent. The direction of water flux between the interstitial and intracellular compartments is determined primarily by the relative concentration of electrolytes on either side of the membrane. To the extent that total electrolyte concentration is equal in interstitial and intracellular fluid, neither compartment will gain or lose water. If, on the other hand, electrolyte concentrations are unequal, water will move from where it is in greater concentration to where it is in lesser concentration in an attempt to restore equilibrium.

An understanding of the nature of intercompartmental barriers is obviously important to the study of fluid flows between compartments. It is also helpful in understanding the relative distribution of fluid components within each compartment. As we proceed to Chapter 5, the information assimilated thus far should aid in clarifying the concepts related to fluid composition.

STUDY QUESTIONS

1. Trace the pathway of a hypothetical drop of fluid as it moves from the arteriole to its ultimate destination.

2. In each of the following cases, predict the net direction of fluid flow between plasma and the interstitial compartment.

a. B.P. 35 mm. Hg
   C.O.P. 25 mm. Hg

b. B.P. 20 mm. Hg
   C.O.P. 25 mm. Hg

c. B.P. 38 mm. Hg
   C.O.P. 20 mm. Hg

3. Determine what effect each of the following clinical conditions might have upon fluid flow between plasma and the interstitial compartment:
   a. severe diarrhea and vomiting
   b. adrenal cortical tumor
   c. venous dilation
   d. hemorrhage
   e. frostbite
   f. heart failure
   g. albuminuria, associated with renal disease
   h. administration of vasoconstrictor drugs
   i. bee sting
   j. severe malnutrition

4. In which of the following clinical situations could edema develop:
   a. excessive perspiration
   b. adrenal cortical tumor
   c. insufficient ADH secretion (diabetes insipidus)
   d. liver disease
   e. hemorrhage
   f. lymphatic obstruction

5. Determine which of the following would cause intracellular swelling and which would cause intracellular shrinkage, and why.
   a. administration of a hypertonic I.V. solution
   b. administration of a hypotonic I.V. solution
   c. diabetes mellitus, characterized by hyperglycemia (elevated plasma concentration of glucose)
   d. hyponatremia (depressed plasma sodium concentration)

Suggested Readings

Books

Burgess, A.: The Nurse's Guide to Fluid and Electrolyte Balance, 2nd ed. New York, McGraw-Hill Book Company, 1979, pp. 23–35.

Burke, S. R.: The Composition and Function of Body Fluids, 2nd ed. St. Louis, The C.V. Mosby Company, 1976, pp. 6–33.

Guyton, A. C.: Textbook of Medical Physiology, 5th ed. Philadelphia, W. B. Saunders Company, 1976, pp. 40–53; 386–396; 397–407.

Guyton, A. C., Taylor, A. E., and Granger, H. J.: Circulatory Physiology II. Dynamics and Control of the Body Fluids. Philadelphia, W. B. Saunders Company, 1975.

Landis, E. M., and Papenheimer, J. R.: Exchange of substances through the capillary walls. *In* Hamilton, W. F. (ed.): Handbook of Physiology. Sec. 2, Vol. 2. Baltimore, The Williams & Wilkins Company, 1963, p. 961.

Manzi, C. C.: Edema: What to do about it. *In* Hamilton, H. (ed.): Monitoring Fluids and Electrolytes Precisely. Nursing 79 Books. Horsham, Pa., Intermed Communications, Inc., 1978, p. 55.

Metheny, N. M., and Snively, W. D.: Nurses' Handbook of Fluid Balance, 3rd ed. Philadelphia, J.B. Lippincott Company, 1979, pp. 98–105.

Reed, G. M., and Sheppard, V. F.: Regulation of Fluid and Electrolyte Balance: A Programmed Instruction in Clinical Physiology, 2nd ed. Philadelphia, W. B. Saunders Company, 1977, pp. 23–39; 91–101.

Strand, F. L.: Physiology, A Regulatory Systems Approach. New York, Macmillan Publishing Company, 1978, pp. 46–60.

Twombly, M.: Shift to third space: When to expect it. *In* Hamilton, H. (ed.): Monitoring Fluids and Electrolytes Precisely. Nursing 79 Books. Horsham, Pa., Intermed Communications, Inc., 1978. p. 49.

Weldy, N. J.: Body Fluids and Electrolytes — A Programmed Presentation, 3rd ed. St. Louis, The C.V. Mosby Company, 1980. pp. 11–24.

Articles

Capaldi, R. A.: A dynamic model of cell membranes. Sci. Am., *230*:26, 1974.

Gill, J. R.: Edema. Ann. Rev. Med., *21*:273, 1970.

Guyton, A. C., Taylor, A. E., Granger, H. J., and Coleman, T. G.: Interstitial fluid pressure. Physiol. Rev., *51*:527, 1971.

Chapter Outline

chapter 5

Fluid Components

Chapter Objectives

At the completion of this chapter, the student will be able to:
1. Define the term *mixture*.
2. Differentiate between a suspension, a solution, and a colloid and give examples of each.
3. Define the term *electrolyte* and differentiate between an anion and a cation.
4. Describe the significance of the term *milliequivalent*.
5. Identify the major components in each of the three fluid compartments.
6. Explain the function of intercompartmental barriers in determining the relative distribution of fluid components.
7. Differentiate between ADH and aldosterone with respect to:
   a. Site of formation and release.
   b. Regulation of secretion.
   c. Function.
8. Describe the normal distribution, regulation, and physiological significance of:
   a. Water
   b. Sodium
   c. Potassium
   d. Chloride
   e. Calcium
   f. Phosphorus

INTRODUCTION

In order to maintain homeostasis, the composition of extracellular fluid must remain relatively constant. All substances dissolved or suspended in body water are, of course, subject to fluctuations. If cellular health is to be maintained, however, the alterations and variations must be kept to a minimum. Many systems and mechanisms work jointly to insure normal fluid composition. It is the purpose of this chapter to elucidate some of the primary fluid components, their distribution, regulation, and function.

Mixtures

To understand fluid composition, it is necessary to know something of the nature of mixtures in general.

By definition, mixtures are a combination of two or more substances that are not chemically combined. A "simple mixture" consists of two components. The substance present in greater amount is called the "dispersing phase"; the substance present in lesser amount, the "dispersed phase." Mixtures are often classified according to the size of the "dispersed phase" particles within them.

If the dispersed phase particles are large enough to settle as a result of gravity and will not pass through filter paper, the resulting mixture is called a *suspension*. Examples include calamine lotion, milk of magnesia, a combination of water and sand, or water and iron filings.

If the dispersed phase particles are very small (of molecular or atomic size), pass through filter paper, and mix uniformly with the dispersing phase, the mixture is called a *solution*. In a solution, the dispersed phase is alternatively referred to as the *solute* and the dispersing phase as the *solvent*.

Solute particles dispersed in water fall into one of two categories. Some solute particles carry a positive or negative electrical charge when dissolved in water. They are called *electrolytes* and include sodium, potassium, chloride, calcium, and magnesium. These charged particles are alternatively referred to as *ions*. They are called *cations* if

positively charged and *anions* if negatively charged.

Small solute particles that do not carry an electrical charge when dissolved in water are referred to as *nonelectrolytes*. Examples of non-electrolytes are the simple sugars glucose, fructose, and galactose.

The third type of mixture is called a *colloid*. A colloid is a mixture in which the dispersed particles are smaller than those of a suspension but larger than those of a solution. The particles do not settle with gravity but are too large to pass through a semipermeable membrane. Oil globules or protein molecules mixed with water are examples of colloidal mixtures.

As we study body fluids and their components, it is helpful to keep in mind the differences between these three types of mixtures. Figure 5.1 presents a comparison of solutions, suspensions, and colloids.

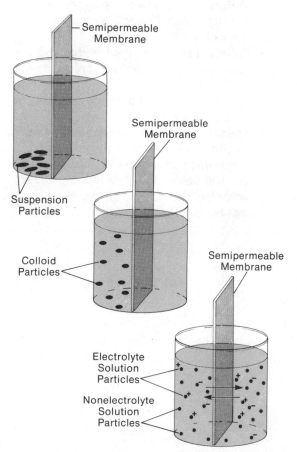

Figure 5.1 Mixtures: a comparative summary. Note that only solution-size particles can pass through the semipermeable membrane.

Relative Composition of Fluid Compartments

The three major fluid compartments of the body differ not only in volume but also in composition. Several of the differences reflect the nature of the intercompartmental barriers, as discussed in Chapter 4.

PLASMA AND INTERSTITIAL FLUID

Plasma contains both colloidal and solution-sized particles. The primary colloids are the plasma proteins albumin, globulins, and fibrinogen, which are produced by the liver. Unable to pass freely through the capillary wall, they remain primarily in the plasma at a concentration of approximately 6 gm. per 100 ml. of fluid.

Solution-sized particles, on the other hand, include the nonelectrolyte simple sugars and the electrolytes sodium (Na^+), chloride (Cl^-), and bicarbonate (HCO_3^-). Ions present in relatively low concentration in plasma include potassium (K^+), calcium (Ca^{++}), magnesium (Mg^{++}), and monohydrogen phosphate ($HPO_4^=$).

Since the capillary wall is permeable to electrolytes, these substances can diffuse freely between plasma and interstitial fluid. Hence, the ionic composition of plasma and interstitial fluid is normally identical.

The preferred way of expressing electrolyte concentrations in fluid compartments is in terms of milliequivalents per liter (mEq./L.). A milliequivalent is a measure reflecting the *chemical reactivity* of an ion. Hence 1 mEq. of sodium is the amount of sodium that will react exactly with 1 mEq. of chloride. To insure the maintenance of electrical neutrality, the total milliequivalents of cations in any solution will equal the total milliequivalents of anions. This equality is displayed in Figure 5.2, which shows the concentrations of the major cations and anions in extracellular fluid.

In summary, it is important to remember that plasma and interstitial fluid contain equivalent concentrations of electrolytes. Since larger colloid-sized particles will not pass freely through the capillary wall, the two fluid compartments differ in composition, pri-

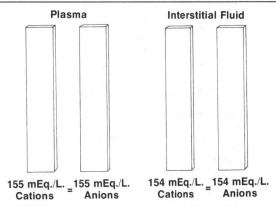

Plasma   Interstitial Fluid

155 mEq./L. _ 155 mEq./L.   154 mEq./L. _ 154 mEq./L.
Cations = Anions   Cations = Anions

Figure 5.2 The concentration of electrolytes in extracellular fluids, in milliequivalents per liter.

marily with respect to protein concentration. This difference is presented in Figure 5.3.

INTERSTITIAL AND INTRACELLULAR FLUID

The difference between the composition of interstitial and intracellular fluid is governed largely by the structure and function of the cell membrane separating them. The nature of this cell membrane barrier has been described in Chapter 4.

Largely because of selective permeability and active transport, extracellular fluid differs considerably in composition from intracellular fluid. The primary cation of intracellular fluid is potassium, normally present very sparingly in interstitial fluid. The primary anions in intracellular fluid are $HPO_4^=$ and small nega-

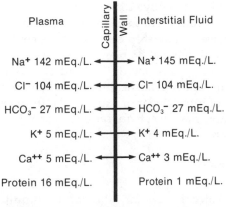

Plasma	Capillary Wall	Interstitial Fluid
Na^+ 142 mEq./L.	⟷	Na^+ 145 mEq./L.
Cl^- 104 mEq./L.	⟷	Cl^- 104 mEq./L.
HCO_3^- 27 mEq./L.	⟷	HCO_3^- 27 mEq./L.
K^+ 5 mEq./L.	⟷	K^+ 4 mEq./L.
Ca^{++} 5 mEq./L.	⟷	Ca^{++} 3 mEq./L.
Protein 16 mEq./L.		Protein 1 mEq./L.

Figure 5.3 The concentration of primary components in plasma and interstitial fluid. Note that small electrolytes are equally distributed between the two compartments. Larger protein particles, on the other hand, are selectively retained within the blood vessels.

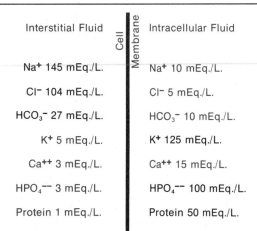

Interstitial Fluid	Cell Membrane	Intracellular Fluid
Na+ 145 mEq./L.		Na+ 10 mEq./L.
Cl- 104 mEq./L.		Cl- 5 mEq./L.
HCO₃- 27 mEq./L.		HCO₃- 10 mEq./L.
K+ 5 mEq./L.		K+ 125 mEq./L.
Ca++ 3 mEq./L.		Ca++ 15 mEq./L.
HPO₄-- 3 mEq./L.		HPO₄-- 100 mEq./L.
Protein 1 mEq./L.		Protein 50 mEq./L.

Figure 5.4 The concentration of primary components in interstitial and intracellular fluids. Because of the selective nature of the cell membrane, even small solute particles are not equally distributed between the two compartments.

tively charged protein particles referred to as proteinate. A summary of the major constituents of intracellular fluids and how they compare with the components of extracellular fluids is found in Figure 5.4.

SOME PRIMARY COMPONENTS OF FLUID COMPARTMENTS

The many constituents of fluid compartments vary with regard to distribution, function, and regulatory mechanisms governing their concentration. The following pages deal with some of the primary fluid components and their respective differences.

It is important to keep in mind that there is a close relationship between these constituents and cellular homeostasis. A significant alteration in any one of the fluid components can disrupt cellular health. Ultimately, variations of intracellular or extracellular fluid composition may result in serious systemic disorders.

Water

Water is, by far, the most ubiquitous constituent of all fluid compartments. It acts as the dispersing phase, or solvent, in plasma, interstitial fluid, and intracellular fluid. Since most physiologically significant chemical reactions proceed only in the presence of water, this substance is critical to cellular functioning. Without water, both anabolism and catabolism would cease, and cells would be unable to grow, to repair, or to generate energy.

Total water volume in the body is regulated primarily by the hormones ADH and aldosterone. ADH (antidiuretic hormone) and aldosterone act specifically upon the nephrons of the kidney to modify and control body water content.

ANTIDIURETIC HORMONE

ADH is manufactured in the hypothalamus of the brain and released by the posterior pituitary gland. It acts primarily upon the distal convoluted tubules and collecting ducts of the nephrons to stimulate the reabsorption of water. It thereby promotes a simultaneous increase in extracellular fluid volume and decrease in urinary output.

Under normal conditions, ADH output varies with the solute concentration or volume of extracellular fluid or both. Feedback mechanisms insure that ADH output increases when the concentration of plasma solutes rises (as in cases of elevated plasma sodium or plasma glucose) or when extracellular fluid volume falls. Conversely, depression of plasma solute concentrations or elevation of extracellular fluid volume will trigger a decrease in ADH release.

The responsiveness of the ADH release mechanism to changing cellular needs is, of course, critical to the maintenance of homeostasis. When plasma solute concentration is elevated, extracellular fluid becomes hypertonic to intracellular fluid. As a result, there is a flux of water out of body cells. When specialized osmoreceptor cells in the hypothalamus shrink owing to this water loss, they cause an increased output of ADH from the posterior pituitary gland. Under conditions of depressed solute concentrations, the situation is reversed. Extracellular fluid is then hypotonic to intracellular fluid, and there is flux of water into body cells. Swelling of the hypothalamic osmoreceptor cells results in decreased stimulation of the posterior pituitary with sub-

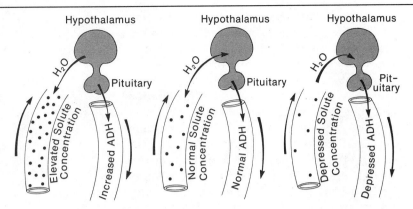

Figure 5.5 Effect of plasma solute concentration upon the secretion of ADH.

sequent decrease in ADH release. This mechanism is depicted in Figure 5.5.

Working in conjunction with the osmoreceptors of the hypothalamus are stretch and pressure receptors located in the blood vessels. When these specialized nerve endings detect falling blood volume or pressure, they send neural messages to the hypothalamus, causing increased release of ADH. The effect of greater ADH output is an increased retention of water, which, in turn, causes a rise in blood volume and pressure. Conversely, as blood volume or pressure increases, the hypothalamus releases less ADH. This, of course, favors higher urinary volume with less fluid retention. The feedback effect of blood volume and pressure upon ADH output is illustrated in Figure 5.6.

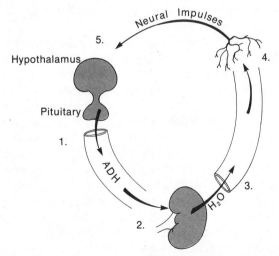

Figure 5.6 Feedback regulation of ADH secretion: 1. ADH secretion. 2 Renal reabsorption of water. 3. Increase blood volume and blood pressure. 4. Stimulate stretch and pressure receptors. 5. Depress ADH secretion.

In conditions of health, ADH release is keyed to cellular needs and directed toward the maintenance of homeostasis. Under certain circumstances, however, ADH can be released abnormally or inappropriately, with resulting pathological symptoms. These cases will be discussed in Chapter 6 as examples of fluid and electrolyte imbalance.

ALDOSTERONE

Working with ADH to affect water level in the body is the hormone aldosterone. Aldosterone, secreted by the cortex of the adrenal gland, acts directly on the tubules of the nephron to promote primary reabsorption of sodium. It affects body water only secondarily.

The mechanisms regulating aldosterone release are discussed in the following section, which deals with sodium and potassium in the body. The elevation in plasma sodium caused by aldosterone secretion creates an osmotic pull, causing water to move secondarily from the nephron into the plasma fluid. With high sodium concentrations stimulating thirst and causing increased fluid intake, it is easy to see why aldosterone promotes increases in extracellular fluid volume.

Sodium and Potassium

Sodium, the primary cation in extracellular fluid, is present in a concentration of 136 to 145 mEq./L. The maintenance of a normal concentration and distribution of sodium ions is, in fact, essential in insuring the isotonicity of extracellular fluid. The presence of sodium is also necessary to provide the electrochemical environment necessary to support muscular contractions and neural transmission. Since the tubule cells of the nephron exchange hydrogen for sodium during urine formation, renal reabsorption or secretion of sodium can indirectly affect hydrogen ion concentration and acid-base balance in the body.

Potassium ions, unlike sodium, are found mainly in the intracellular fluid, where they contribute to normal cellular functioning. Although present in limited concentrations of 3.5 to 5.6 mEq./L. in extracellular fluid, they are nevertheless critical to the maintenance of normal muscular contractility and neural transmission. In fact, one of the most devastating effects of potassium imbalance is the severe cardiac arrhythmias that can result from altered cardiac muscle activity.

The primary regulator of both sodium and potassium levels in the extracellular fluid is the hormone *aldosterone*. Aldosterone acts directly upon the renal tubule cells to promote sodium reabsorption in exchange for potassium or hydrogen secretion. This exchange of positively charged ions in the nephron helps to maintain electrical neutrality in the plasma. As a positively charged sodium ion is pulled into plasma, a positively charged potassium or hydrogen ion is simultaneously moved out of plasma to be excreted in the urine. This exchange mechanism is illustrated in Figure 5.7.

The ongoing release of aldosterone is helpful in regulating sodium, potassium, and water levels in the body. As plasma Na^+ concentration falls, or plasma K^+ concentration rises, aldosterone output is directly stim-

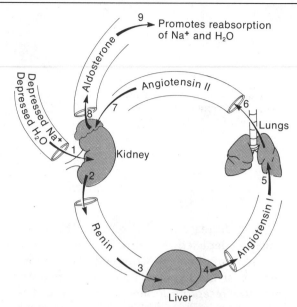

Figure 5.8 The renin-angiotensin mechanism. 1, Depressed Na^+ concentration and/or fluid depletion trigger the release of renin from the kidneys. 2. Renin is transported through the bloodstream to the liver. 3. Renin acts upon a plasma protein in the liver to cause the formation of angiotensin I. 4. Angiotensin I is released into the bloodstream. 5. Angiotensin I is converted into angiotensin II in the lungs. 6 and 7. Angiotensin II is transported to the adrenal glands through the bloodstream. 8. Angiotensin II triggers the release of aldosterone by the adrenal glands. 9. Aldosterone ultimately acts upon the kidneys to promote the reabsorption of Na^+ and H_2O.

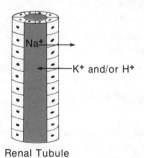

Figure 5.7 The exchange between sodium and potassium/hydrogen in the nephron. To maintain electrical neutrality, a positively charged potassium or hydrogen ion is secreted for every sodium ion that is reabsorbed.

ulated. This, of course, helps to bring the electrolyte levels back toward normal and promotes homeostasis.

Aldosterone output is also modified by a specialized renin-angiotensin mechanism that is specifically sensitive to alterations in extracellular fluid volume and plasma sodium levels. As extracellular fluid volume or plasma Na^+ concentration decreases, specialized cells in the kidneys are stimulated to release the enzyme renin into the blood. Renin, in turn, acts upon a plasma protein in the liver to produce a substance called angiotensin I. Angiotensin I is subsequently transported to the lungs, where it is converted to angiotensin II. Angiotensin II simultaneously serves two purposes: (1) It acts as a vasoconstrictor, thereby promoting the elevation of arterial blood pressure. (2) It acts as a stimulant to the release of aldosterone. Hence, the wheel comes full circle as newly released aldosterone helps to bring both fluid volume and sodium levels back toward normal. This complex mechanism is illustrated in Figure 5.8.

Chloride

Chloride, the primary anion in extracellular fluid (96 to 106 mEq./L.) functions to maintain electrical neutrality in plasma and interstitial fluid. Passively attracted to positively charged cations, chloride ions balance the positively charged electrolytes in extracellular fluids.

Since chloride ions are highly concentrated in both gastric secretions (as a component of hydrochloric acid) and perspiration, it is important to monitor upper gastrointestinal losses and diaphoresis (sweating) as potential routes of excessive chloride loss.

Of even greater clinical significance, however, is the role chlorides play in the maintenance of acid-base balance. In the establishment of electrical neutrality, chloride competes with bicarbonate (HCO_3^-) for affiliation with the cations in extracellular fluid. Thus, any decrease in chloride must be accompanied by an increase in bicarbonate, if electrical neutrality is to be maintained. Conversely, an increase in chloride should be balanced by a reduction in bicarbonate levels.

Since bicarbonate is an alkaline, or basic, electrolyte, it can be seen how increases in extracellular fluid concentration would cause alkalosis (an excess of plasma alkalinity) to develop. Conversely, depressions in bicarbonate concentrations will precipitate acidosis (a deficit of plasma alkalinity). Chloride levels are thus integrally involved with acid-base balance in the body.

Extracellular fluid chloride levels are regulated primarily by factors influencing plasma sodium concentration. In the process of maintaining electrical neutrality, chloride anions tend to passively follow sodium cations. Thus, increases in sodium levels are usually accompanied by elevated chloride concentrations, and vice versa. Hence, aldosterone, which directly stimulates the reabsorption of sodium ions out of the renal tubules into plasma, simultaneously elevates chloride concentration. Conversely, depressed aldosterone out-

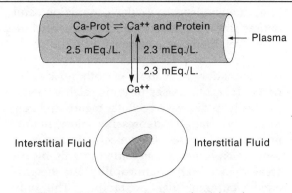

Figure 5.9 The distribution of calcium in extracellular fluid. Note that calcium can exist in the protein-bound (Ca-Prot) and the ionized form (Ca^{++}). Only ionized calcium may cross the capillary wall to distribute equally between plasma and interstitial fluid.

put tends to reduce both sodium and chloride plasma levels.

Calcium and Phosphorus

Calcium, although present in relatively small amounts (4.5 to 5.5 mEq./L.) in extracellular fluid, plays a major role in several physiologically critical processes.

To fully understand the function of calcium in the body, it is important to realize that approximately 99 per cent of this mineral is trapped in the hard crystal salts of bone. Only 1 per cent of total body calcium is distributed in the extracellular fluid. It is this 1 per cent that is measured or evaluated during standard laboratory testing.

Of this 1 per cent, moreover, close to half is bound to plasma protein (2.5 mEq./L.), and the remainder (2.3 mEq./L.) exists in a freely ionized form. It is only the freely ionized form of calcium that is able to pass through the capillary wall and play a physiologically active role in cellular processes. The protein-bound component remains primarily in plasma, unable to move into the interstitial or intracellular fluid compartments. The relative distribution of calcium in the extracellular fluid is illustrated in Figure 5.9.

FUNCTION OF CALCIUM AND PHOSPHORUS

In spite of its relatively low serum concentration, calcium is essential to blood clotting, bone metabolism, muscular contraction, and neural impulse transmission. Since calcium affects cell membrane permeability, it directly influences the ionic fluxes necessary to the depolarization (activation) of both muscle and nerve fibers. Increases in ionic calcium result primarily in decreased cellular membrane permeability, thereby depressing most neuromuscular responses. Conversely, decreases in ionic calcium are accompanied mainly by increased membrane permeability and heightened neuromuscular excitability. The only major exception to this rule is cardiac muscle tissue, in which calcium seems to promote contractility.

Alterations in plasma calcium levels can have far-reaching systemic effects. Calcium fluctuations can precipitate dysfunction in many diverse structures, including cardiac muscle, smooth muscle of the gastrointestinal tract, and neural tissue of the central nervous system. These effects and their clinical manifestations will be discussed in Chapter 6.

Phosphorus, although working with calcium to promote bone formation, is primarily found in the form of phosphate as an intracellular fluid electrolyte. Within cells, it works as a buffer to help maintain acid-base balance in the body. It is also a component of adenosine triphosphate (ATP) and creatinine phosphate, two molecules that serve as energy storage forms within body cells.

REGULATION OF CALCIUM AND PHOSPHORUS

Both calcium and phosphorus levels in the extracellular fluid are regulated primarily by parathormone, which is secreted by the parathyroid endocrine glands. This hormone, released in response to depressed plasma calcium, acts on bone tissue, the nephrons, and the gastrointestinal tract to modify plasma levels of calcium and phosphorus. Its overall effect is to increase the concentration of calcium and decrease the concentration of phosphorus in the extracellular fluid.

To fully understand the effect of parathormone upon calcium and phosphorus levels, it is necessary to briefly review some central aspects of bone metabolism. To build new bone tissue, bone cells called *osteoblasts* must

produce a ground substance into which calcium and phosphorus can subsequently be deposited. It is the addition of calcium and phosphorus, in the form of an inactive mineral salt, that is responsible for the hardening of bone. Conversely, to remodel or restructure bone, bone cells called *osteoclasts* promote absorption of bone tissue with release of calcium and phosphorus into circulating blood. Since parathormone stimulates osteoclastic activity, it promotes initial elevations in both serum calcium and phosphorus levels. This effect is heightened by a simultaneous increase in calcium and phosphorus absorption out of the small intestine into the blood, stimulated by parathormone.

Paradoxically, however, the action of parathormone upon the nephron enhances the calcium increase but cancels the phosphorus elevations caused by osteoclastic activity and gastrointestinal absorption. Parathormone acts upon the renal tubules by stimulating calcium reabsorption and phosphorus excre-

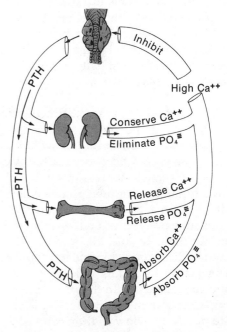

Figure 5.10 The effects of parathormone (PTH) upon the concentration of Ca^{++} and $PO_4^{\equiv}$ in extracellular fluid. Note that PTH stimulates the release of both Ca^{++} and $PO_4^{\equiv}$ from the bone and gut into the bloodstream. In the kidneys, however, PTH promotes Ca^{++} retention and $PO_4^{\equiv}$ elimination. Ultimately, PTH causes Ca^{++} blood levels to increase and $PO_4^{\equiv}$ concentration to decrease in the extracellular fluid.

TABLE 5.1 **The Maintenance of Fluid and Electrolyte Balance**

Extracellular Fluid Component	Factors Influencing Concentration of Fluid Components	Functional Systems	Activity of System
Water	ADH	Nervous	Hypothalamus produces ADH.
		Endocrine	Posterior pituitary releases ADH.
		Renal	ADH triggers the reabsorption of H_2O from the nephron.
	Aldosterone	Renal	Kidneys release renin, which helps to regulate aldosterone secretion.
		Endocrine	Adrenal glands produce and release aldosterone.
		Renal	Aldosterone triggers the primary reabsorption of sodium and secondary reabsorption of water in the kidneys.
Sodium, potassium, and chloride	Aldosterone	Renal	Kidneys release renin, which helps to regulate aldosterone secretion.
		Endocrine	Adrenal glands produce and release aldosterone.
		Renal	Aldosterone promotes the reabsorption of sodium and chloride and the secretion of potassium in the kidneys.
Calcium and phosphate	PTH	Endocrine	Parathyroid glands produce and release PTH.
		Skeletal	PTH promotes the absorption of bone and release of Ca^{++} and $PO_4^{=}$ into plasma.
		Digestive	PTH promotes the absorption of Ca^{++} and $PO_4^{=}$ from the gastrointestinal tract.
		Renal	PTH promotes the reabsorption of Ca^{++} and secretion of phosphate by the nephron.
	Vitamin D	Digestive	Vitamin D is ingested and absorbed through the gastrointestinal tract.
		Integumentary	Vitamin D is manufactured by skin, in the presence of sunlight.

tion. As a result, the cumulative effect of parathormone secretion is to *increase* the concentration of calcium and *decrease* the concentration of phosphorus in the extracellular fluid. A summary of the activity of parathormone is presented in Figure 5.10.

In conjunction with parathormone, both calcitonin (a hormone released by specialized cells in the thyroid gland) and vitamin D help to regulate blood calcium levels.

Calcitonin, released in response to elevated blood calcium levels, inhibits osteoclastic activity in the bone and thus partially antagonizes parathormone activity. Its exact mode of action is unknown, but it does help maintain normal calcium concentration through a direct feedback mechanism.

Vitamin D, on the other hand, promotes parathormone activity by facilitating both gas-

trointestinal absorption of calcium and osteoclastic breakdown of bone. It is normally either ingested or synthesized in the skin under the influence of the ultraviolet rays of the sun. Once activated by certain chemical reactions in the liver, it then supports parathormone activity in the body. In the absence of vitamin D, parathormone cannot function normally and calcium imbalances can result.

SUMMARY

A review of Chapter 5 reveals the complexity of body fluid composition. Each of the major electrolyte components is regulated by intricate mechanisms designed to insure the maintenance of optimal concentration and distribution. In Table 5.1 you will find a summary of the organs and systems functional in maintaining fluid and electrolyte balance.

It can be seen that many disparate structures work together to service the cellular need for fluid and electrolyte balance. Conversely, a disorder of any one of these structures can precipitate electrolyte disturbances. These major deviations from homeostasis are the focus of the following chapter.

STUDY QUESTIONS

1. Identify each of the following mixtures as a suspension, solution, or colloid:
   a. sugar water (glucose in water)
   b. erythrocytes in water
   c. salt water (Na^+ and Cl^- in water)
   d. albumin in water
   e. milk of magnesia

2. Label the following particles as anions or cations:
   a. Na^+
   b. Cl^-
   c. PO_4^{-3}
   d. K^+

3. If you knew that a given mixture contained 230 mEq. of cations, could you estimate how many mEq. of anions would be needed to maintain electrical neutrality?

4. Arrange the following electrolytes as they would normally exist in extracellular fluid, from highest to lowest concentration: Cl^-, K^+, Na^+, Ca^{++}.

5. From what you know about aldosterone, predict the effect of hypersecretion upon:
   a. plasma potassium levels
   b. total fluid volume in the body
   c. plasma chloride levels
   d. blood pressure

6. From what you know about the function of ADH, predict the effect of hyposecretion upon:
   a. total fluid volume in the body
   b. urinary volume

7. Determine the effect of each of the following upon the concentration of free calcium (Ca^{++}) in extracellular fluid:
   a. hypersecretion of PTH (parathyroid hormone)
   b. vitamin D deficiency

Suggested Readings

Books

Beck, R. R.: Hormonal control of water and electrolytes. *In* Selkurt, E. E. (ed.): Basic Physiology for the Health Sciences. Boston, Little, Brown & Company, 1975, p. 503.

Beck, R. R.: Hormonal regulation of calcium metabolism. *In* Selkurt, E. E. (ed.): Basic Physiology for the Health Sciences. Boston, Little, Brown & Company, 1975, p. 317.

Brooks, S. M.: Basic Facts of Body Water and Ions, 3rd ed. New York, Springer Publishing Company, 1973, pp. 19–25; 26–32.

Burgess, A.: The Nurse's Guide to Fluid and Electrolyte Balance, 2nd ed. New York, McGraw-Hill Book Company, 1979, pp. 65–76.

Burke, S. R.: The Composition and Function of Body Fluids, 2nd ed. St. Louis, The C. V. Mosby Company, 1976, pp. 34–53.

Grissinger, S.: Chloride: Clue to acidity. *In* Hamilton, H. (ed.): Monitoring Fluids and Electrolytes Precisely. Nursing 79 Books. Horsham, Pa., Intermed Communications, Inc., 1978, p. 109.

Guyton, A. C.: Textbook of Medical Physiology, 5th ed. Philadelphia, W. B. Saunders Company, 1976, pp. 1000–1002; 1019–1024; 1052–1065.

Lancour, J.: Two hormones, regulators of fluid balance. *In* Hamilton, H. (ed.): Monitoring Fluids and Electrolytes Precisely. Nursing 79 Books. Horsham, Pa., Intermed Communications, Inc., 1978, p. 29.

Luckmann, J., and Sorensen, K. C.: Medical-Surgical Nursing, A Psychophysiologic Approach, 2nd ed. Philadelphia, W. B. Saunders Company, 1980, pp. 171–227.

Reed, G.: Potassium: The chief electrolyte. *In* Hamilton, H. (ed.): Monitoring Fluids and Electrolytes Precisely. Nursing 79 Books. Horsham, Pa., Intermed Communications, Inc., 1978, p. 79.

Selkurt, E. E.: Body water and electrolyte composition and their regulation. *In* Selkurt, E. E. (ed.): Basic Physiology for the Health Sciences. Boston, Little, Brown & Company, 1975, p. 487.

Stroot, V. R., Lee, C. A., and Schaper, C. A.: Fluids and Electrolytes: A Practical Approach, 2nd ed. Philadelphia, F. A. Davis Company, 1977, pp. 49–51; 63–66; 71–73; 75–77.

Thomas, R.: Calcium: The durable electrolyte. *In* Hamilton, H. (ed.): Monitoring Fluids and Electrolytes Precisely. Nursing 79 Books. Horsham, Pa., Intermed Communications, Inc., 1978, p. 97.

Weldy, N. J.: Body Fluids and Electrolytes — A

Programmed Presentation, 3rd ed. St.Louis, The C. V. Mosby Company, 1980, pp. 5–11; 31–35.

Wolfe, L.: Sodium: Controller of fluid volume. *In* Hamilton, H. (ed.): Monitoring Fluids and Electrolytes Precisely. Nursing 79 Books. Horsham, Pa., Intermed Communications, Inc., 1978, p. 89.

Articles

Lancour, J.: ADH and aldosterone: How to recognise their effects. Nursing 78, *8*:36, 1978.

Origin and action of aldosterone. Hosp. Med., *12*:6, 1976.

Chapter Outline

chapter 6

Fluid and Electrolyte Imbalances

Chapter Objectives

At the completion of this chapter, the student will be able to:

1. Define the term *isotonic imbalance* and identify some causative conditions and resulting physiological disruptions.
2. Differentiate between hypo- and hypernatremia with respect to causes and clinical manifestations.
3. Differentiate between hypo- and hyperkalemia with respect to causes and clinical manifestations.
4. Differentiate between hypo- and hypercalcemia with respect to causes and clinical manifestations.

INTRODUCTION

In spite of the many mechanisms designed to regulate fluid and electrolyte balance in the body, deviations from the norm do occur. It is the purpose of this chapter to examine fluid and electrolyte disturbances with respect to causes and results. Since it is impossible to describe every electrolyte abnormality, some of the major ones are presented, with emphasis upon clinical relevance.

ISOTONIC IMBALANCES

The term "isotonic imbalance" is used in this text to refer to alterations in extracellular fluid volume that are accompanied by a proportional gain or loss of electrolytes. If fluids are lost, electrolytes are lost proportionately; conversely, if fluids are gained, electrolytes are retained proportionately. The fluid remaining in the body in these cases is therefore *isotonic* to intracellular fluid. In keeping with

the principles of osmosis, imbalances of this type will *not* induce cellular swelling or shrinkage. Only if total particle concentration in the interstitial fluid is altered will the intracellular fluid compartment be affected. This concept is illustrated in Figure 6.1.

Although it may be difficult to find clinical examples of a pure isotonic imbalance, this type of deviation can be noted in select cases in which sodium, the primary ion in extracellular fluid, is eliminated or retained proportionately with body water. Some major examples of this phenomenon include: (1) excessive administration of a normal saline (0.9 per cent sodium chloride) I.V. solution; (2) hypersecretion of aldosterone, with resulting proportional retention of both sodium and water; and (3) loss of body fluid containing sodium and water in isotonic proportion. Examples include hemorrhage, excessive perspiration, or wound drainage.

It is important to realize that although *total* particle concentration does not change significantly during isotonic imbalances, se-

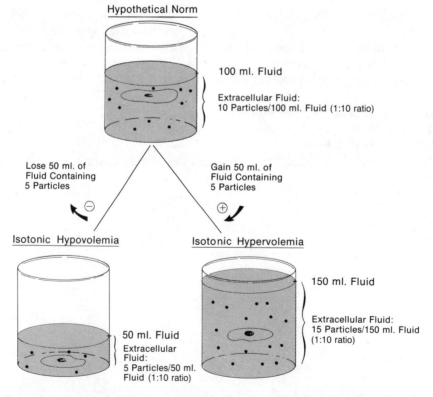

Figure 6.1 Isotonic imbalances: a conceptual presentation. Note that the gain or loss of fluid with the same particle concentration as the hypothetical norm results in the generation of isotonic hypo- or hypervolemia.

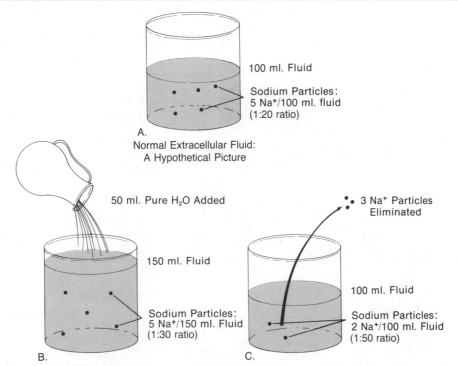

Figure 6.2 The generation of hyponatremia. Note that hyponatremia can be generated by either adding pure water (*B*) to or selectively removing Na⁺ particles (*C*) from normal extracellular fluid (*A*).

vere electrolyte deviations may nevertheless occur. In cases of extensive diarrhea, for example, it is possible to lose large quantities of potassium from the lower gastrointestinal tract. Since potassium is normally present in very small amounts in the extracellular fluid, its loss will not result in significant osmotic changes. Potassium deficit, however, can induce serious systemic disorders because of its effect upon the contractility of cardiac muscle.

Isotonic imbalances will additionally cause physiological disruption to the extent that they are associated with hyper- or hypovolemia. In these cases, characteristic symptoms of volume excess or volume deficit will be noted, as explained in Chapter 3.

SODIUM IMBALANCES

Changes in the concentration of sodium in the extracellular fluid can be effected in two primary ways: (1) by altering the amount of sodium in the fluid while keeping water levels

constant, or (2) by altering the volume of water in the body while keeping sodium levels constant.

The sketches in Figure 6.2 further elucidate this concept. Beakers A, B, and C illustrate some factors in the generation of *hyponatremia* (depressed concentration of sodium in extracellular fluid). If we assume that beaker A contains extracellular fluid of normal volume and sodium concentration, then B and C reflect two separate ways of inducing hyponatremia. In beaker B, hyponatremia is created by the addition of pure water or hypotonic sodium solution to a mixture that was originally identical to A in volume and composition. In the same way that a glass of salt water would taste less salty after the addition of plain tap water, so the fluid in beaker B would reflect depression of sodium concentration as water diluted the existing sodium ions. It is easy to see why a patient experiencing hyponatremia of this kind would present signs of both sodium depletion and fluid excess.

An alternative means of generating hyponatremia is illustrated by beaker C. In this

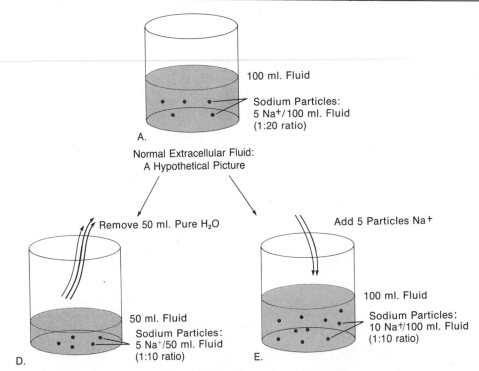

Figure 6.3 The generation of hypernatremia. Note that hypernatremia can be generated by either removing pure water (*D*) from or adding Na+ particles (*E*) to normal extracellular fluid (*A*).

case, hyponatremia is produced by selectively removing sodium from a solution that was originally identical to beaker A in volume and composition. In this instance, general fluid level remains unchanged while sodium ions are depleted. This might be difficult to envision as a laboratory exercise, but it can be seen clinically in patients with certain dietary, renal, or endocrine imbalances. Specific examples of clinical causes and symptoms of hyponatremia will be given later in this chapter.

The development of *hypernatremia* (the increase of sodium concentration in extracellular fluid) is illustrated in Figure 6.3. Again, beaker A is used as a hypothetical norm for fluid volume and sodium concentration. In this case, beakers D and E are used to illustrate two common ways of inducing hypernatremia.

In beaker E, hypernatremia is generated by the selective removal of pure water from a solution that was originally identical to A in volume and composition. This could be achieved in a laboratory by boiling the con-

tents of the beaker to evaporate water. Since sodium ions cannot evaporate, the cooled beaker would have a lower fluid volume and a higher sodium concentration. Hypernatremia clinically induced in this manner would, of course, be accompanied by symptoms of fluid deficit.

Alternatively, it is possible to induce hypernatremia by adding pure sodium, or a hypertonic sodium solution, to fluid of normal volume and composition. This is illustrated in Figure 6.3 by beaker E. Hypernatremia induced clinically in this manner would eventually be accompanied by symptoms of hypervolemia. In these cases the elevation of sodium concentration triggers a compensatory increase in ADH secretion, resulting in the retention of water by the kidneys to balance elevated sodium concentrations.

As we further explore the phenomenon of hypernatremia, it is important to keep in mind that clinical symptoms may vary considerably. An understanding of causative factors and general history will thus strongly enhance diagnostic skills.

Hyponatremia

As explained in the introductory paragraphs, hyponatremia can be caused by depression of sodium or elevation of water in the body.

CLINICAL CAUSES

Depressed sodium levels are induced by depressed sodium intake or increased sodium output. Severe nutritional deficiency could technically cause hyponatremia as could excessive renal loss due to insufficient aldosterone production. More commonly, however, clinical instances of hyponatremia are precipitated by increases in body water. These cases of increased water are, in turn, due to either decreased water output or increased water intake.

Increased water intake occurs somewhat rarely. Specific clinical instances include excessive hypotonic intravenous or tap water enema administration, excessive water consumption such as is exhibited by some schizophrenics, and abnormal fluid intake by alcoholics.

Decreased water output is more common. Excessive ADH secretion, for example, results in reabsorption of increased amounts of water from the renal tubules. This retained fluid simultaneously increases extracellular fluid volume and lowers sodium concentration in interstitial fluid and plasma. For unknown reasons, a number of disorders or conditions in the body seem to promote increased ADH output. This phenomenon, referred to as *SIADH* (syndrome of inappropriate ADH secretion), is triggered by a variety of circumstances, including certain malignant tumors, cerebral disorders, pain, surgical trauma, stress, and administration of morphine and some anesthetics.

Often, hyponatremia is precipitated clinically by simultaneously decreasing sodium and increasing water. Replacement of a water and sodium loss with pure water can occur with relative frequency. This is seen in cases in which heavily perspiring individuals, who are losing fluid with considerable sodium content, replace this fluid by drinking copious amounts of pure water. Similarly, replacing fluid lost by vomiting with pure water will dilute extracellular sodium, as will the irrigation of nasogastric tubes with pure water.

SIGNS AND SYMPTOMS

The signs and symptoms accompanying hyponatremia can vary with the causative factors. Regardless of the reasons for hyponatremia, however, depressed concentration of extracellular fluid sodium will almost always precipitate compartmental fluid shift. Water will move from interstitial to intracellular fluid in keeping with the principles of osmosis. As a result, one would expect general cellular swelling. The swelling of cerebral cells, in particular, is manifested by neural symptoms including twitching, hyperirritability, disorientation, convulsions, and coma. Swelling in other body cells will cause disruptions manifested by symptoms ranging from general weakness and muscle twitches to anorexia, nausea, vomiting, abdominal cramps, and diarrhea.

The only major exception to this general pattern of fluid shift is seen in cases in which depression in sodium concentration is due to elevated concentration of particles such as proteins, glucose, or lipids in the extracellular fluid. In these instances, the abnormally high protein, glucose, or lipid concentration in extracellular fluid serves to pull water from the intracellular into the interstitial compartment. As water flows into the interstitial fluid, it will dilute the existing sodium concentration. Referred to as cases of *hypertonic hyponatremia,* these specific disorders represent exception conditions. Hyponatremia induced in this manner is not accompanied by cellular swelling or by the characteristic neural symptoms listed previously. A presentation of hypertonic hyponatremia can be found in Figure 6.4.

When hyponatremia is specifically caused by increases in body water, the characteristic clinical picture includes symptoms of hypervolemia. In these instances, one can expect to see elevated blood pressure, weight gain, and edema.

HYPONATREMIA: A SUMMARY

It is possible to see how patients with hyponatremia can present a variety of clinical

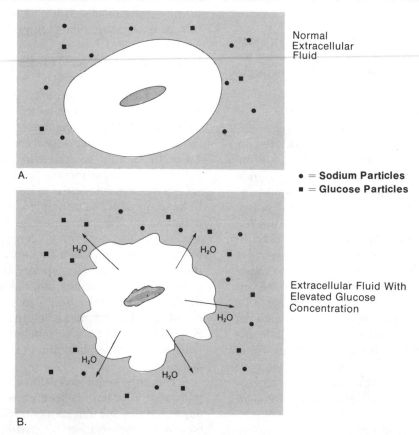

A.

● = **Sodium Particles**
■ = **Glucose Particles**

Extracellular Fluid With
Elevated Glucose
Concentration

B.

Figure 6.4   Hypertonic hyponatremia. Elevated glucose concentration draws water out of the cell, thereby diluting sodium particles in the extracellular fluid.

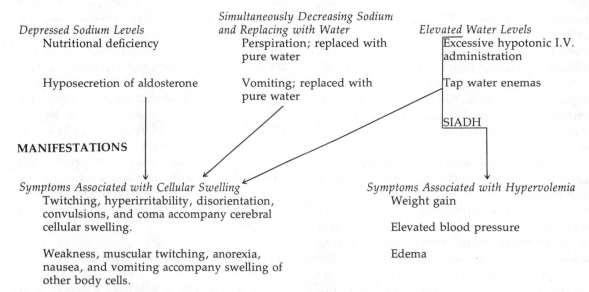

CAUSES

Depressed Sodium Levels
Nutritional deficiency

Hyposecretion of aldosterone

Simultaneously Decreasing Sodium and Replacing with Water
Perspiration; replaced with pure water

Vomiting; replaced with pure water

Elevated Water Levels
Excessive hypotonic I.V. administration

Tap water enemas

SIADH

MANIFESTATIONS

Symptoms Associated with Cellular Swelling
Twitching, hyperirritability, disorientation, convulsions, and coma accompany cerebral cellular swelling.

Weakness, muscular twitching, anorexia, nausea, and vomiting accompany swelling of other body cells.

Symptoms Associated with Hypervolemia
Weight gain

Elevated blood pressure

Edema

Figure 6.5   Hyponatremia

pictures. Although all cases show a depression of plasma sodium concentration (usually below 120 mEq./L.), other symptoms can vary considerably, depending upon history and causative factors. A review of the causes and symptoms of hyponatremia can be found in Figure 6.5.

Hypernatremia

Hypernatremia can be caused by increases of sodium or reductions of water in the body.

CLINICAL CAUSES

Elevated sodium levels can technically be induced by either increasing the intake or decreasing the output of sodium. Clinically, however, hypernatremia is rarely caused by sodium increases except in occasional cases such as saline-induced abortions, near–salt water drownings, and excessive hypertonic sodium intravenous drip.

Most commonly, cases of hypernatremia are associated with depression of body water levels. This depression, in turn, is caused by either decreasing the intake or increasing the output of water. Decreased intake can be found in patients experiencing difficulty in swallowing, impaired thirst, or environmental water deficit.

The most significant manifestations of depressed water levels, however, are found in characteristic cases of excessive water output. Thus *watery* diarrhea, depressed ADH output (diabetes insipidus), excessive perspiration, and pulmonary disorders accompanied by elevated respiratory rate (in which large amounts of water are lost during expiration) could all precipitate hypernatremia.

It is also possible for elevated blood glucose or protein levels to cause the development of hypernatremia. Although, as described earlier in this chapter, these conditions are often accompanied by hypertonic hyponatremia, they can also induce *elevations* in plasma sodium concentration. If the glucose or protein is excreted heavily in the urine, it tends to pull water along with it. To the extent that this happens, water loss will effectively concentrate the electrolytes remain-

ing in the extracellular fluid compartments. There is, unfortunately, no set law or formula available to help determine the effect of hyperglycemia or hyperproteinemia (elevated plasma protein concentration) on any given patient. One can only hope that laboratory values coupled with good patient assessment skills will help to clarify each clinical situation.

SIGNS AND SYMPTOMS

As in the case of hyponatremia, hypernatremia can be accompanied by a variety of clinical symptoms. In all cases of hypernatremia, however, the elevation of plasma sodium concentration (usually to greater than 150 mEq./L.) will predictably cause: (1) thirst, by directly stimulating receptors in the hypothalamus, and (2) fluid shift from the intracellular to the interstitial compartment, as water moves by osmosis to dilute the hypertonic solution bathing the cells.

The resultant cellular dehydration and shrinkage are manifested in a variety of ways. As cerebral cells lose water, symptoms of apprehension, restlessness, and possible coma occur. Dehydration of other body cells results in changes such as dry skin and mucous membranes, dry furrowed tongue, and soft sunken eyeballs.

It is important to realize that in patients experiencing hypernatremia due to sodium gain, symptoms of hypervolemia will commonly be noted. The elevated sodium triggers water reabsorption via the action of ADH on the renal tubules. Hence, indications of weight gain, high blood pressure, edema, and possible circulatory overload are often characteristic.

Most commonly, however, hypernatremia results from water loss. In these instances, one would expect associated symptoms of hypovolemia. Depressed blood pressure, decreased blood flow to the kidneys with possible renal shutdown, and elevations in body temperature are often evident.

HYPERNATREMIA: A SUMMARY

It is clear that the hypernatremic patient may present with a variety of clinical symp-

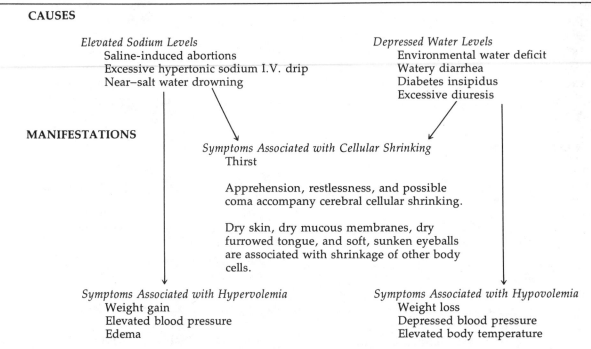

CAUSES

Elevated Sodium Levels
　　　Saline-induced abortions
　　　Excessive hypertonic sodium I.V. drip
　　　Near–salt water drowning

Depressed Water Levels
　　　Environmental water deficit
　　　Watery diarrhea
　　　Diabetes insipidus
　　　Excessive diuresis

MANIFESTATIONS

Symptoms Associated with Cellular Shrinking
　　　Thirst

Apprehension, restlessness, and possible coma accompany cerebral cellular shrinking.

Dry skin, dry mucous membranes, dry furrowed tongue, and soft, sunken eyeballs are associated with shrinkage of other body cells.

Symptoms Associated with Hypervolemia
　　　Weight gain
　　　Elevated blood pressure
　　　Edema

Symptoms Associated with Hypovolemia
　　　Weight loss
　　　Depressed blood pressure
　　　Elevated body temperature

Figure 6.6　Hypernatremia

toms. Although a number of symptoms are characteristic of all cases of elevated sodium concentration, certain aspects of the clinical picture can vary considerably with the cause. A chart summarizing the causes and symptoms of hypernatremia can be found in Figure 6.6.

POTASSIUM IMBALANCES

Potassium, an electrolyte essential to body functioning, poses unique problems with regard to assessment of imbalances. Since the richest stores of potassium are located intracellularly, it is virtually impossible to determine with certainty the status of most potassium ions. All one can do is measure the concentration of the relatively small amount of potassium in the extracellular fluid and use this as an indirect indication of what is happening within the cell membrane. Plasma laboratory values coupled with assessment of the patient's history and clinical picture must be used to evaluate potassium status.

Potassium, in spite of its normally low plasma levels (3.5 to 5.0 mEq./L.), is of critical importance to many major cellular functions. Even a slight deviation from the norm can represent a considerable *percentage* change and is thus potentially life-threatening. In

much the same way that a loss of 5 pounds to a 180-pound man is not nearly as significant as a loss of 5 pounds in a 20-pound infant, so a deviation of 0.5 to 1.0 mEq./L. in potassium can have considerably more physiological impact than would a similar deviation in plasma sodium values.

For our purposes, *hypokalemia* will be defined as a low concentration of potassium in the extracellular fluid, and *hyperkalemia* as an elevated concentration of potassium in the extracellular fluid. Although potassium changes in extracellular fluid are often accompanied by similar alterations in intracellular fluid, it cannot be automatically assumed that the two values will always run in parallel. Just as excess outdoor heat is not necessarily accompanied by higher indoor temperatures, the extracellular and intracellular potassium levels do not consistently change together. Thus, it is conceivable for extracellular potassium to rise at the expense of intracellular stores. This, in fact, does occur at times of cellular trauma, when altered cell membrane permeability allows excessive amounts of potassium to leak out of the cells into interstitial fluid and plasma.

Since it is not possible to effectively measure intracellular fluid composition, the only value of true clinical significance is the measure of extracellular fluid potassium (as reflected in plasma potassium levels). Hence, hypo- and hyperkalemia relate specifically to measurable potassium changes in the extracellular fluid compartment.

Hypokalemia

Hypokalemia is caused primarily by depressed potassium levels in the extracellular fluid.

CLINICAL CAUSES

Depressed potassium levels can be induced either by decreased intake or by increased output of potassium. Decreased intake, although rare, is seen in cases of severe nutritional deficiency accompanying starvation, fasting, and poorly planned dieting. Elevated output is the most common clinical cause of hypokalemia. It often results from *excessive urinary or gastrointestinal losses,* since elevated urinary output tends to wash out potassium, and gastrointestinal contents are rich in potassium.

Specifically, then, conditions causing increased urinary volume will often precipitate hypokalemia. Most diuretics (except those that are potassium-sparing), diabetes insipidus, and a number of renal disorders characterized by excessive output promote potassium loss. Similarly, increased gastrointestinal output, such as is seen in diarrhea, improper use of laxatives or enemas, vomiting, colostomy or ileostomy drainage, and gastric or intestinal suction, can result in hypokalemia.

Another significant factor in regulating extracellular fluid potassium levels is the *output of aldosterone*. This hormone essentially acts upon the nephron to promote the reabsorption of sodium and water as well as the secretion of potassium and hydrogen. Thus, increased aldosterone output (as seen in cases of adrenal cortical tumor and congestive heart failure) facilitates potassium loss. Since steroid drugs mimic the action of aldosterone, excessive use necessitates monitoring for possible side effects of hypokalemia.

Although most cases of hypokalemia are due to excessive urinary or gastrointestinal losses, an alternative mode of depressing extracellular fluid potassium should be mentioned. Since potassium is a positively charged ion, it will often shift from one fluid compart-

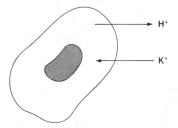

Alkalosis can cause H^+ to shift into interstitial fluid. To maintain electrical neutrality, a positively charged K^+ moves into the intracellular compartment.

Figure 6.7   Alkalosis and potassium balance.

ment to another to compensate for changes in the distribution of another positively charged particle. It is in this way that electrical neutrality is maintained. Thus if sodium (Na^+) or hydrogen (H^+) moves out of intracellular fluid, potassium tends to move into the cell in exchange.

When the body is in a state of *alkalosis,* extracellular hydrogen levels are depressed. In response to this condition, hydrogen tends to move from intracellular into interstitial fluid, attempting to compensate for the existing hydrogen deficit in extracellular fluid. In the process, however, electrical neutrality is compromised, and potassium (K^+) is driven to shift from interstitial into intracellular fluid to maintain ionic balance. In short, alkalosis can trigger a depression in plasma potassium levels through this cellular shift mechanism. This phenomenon is depicted diagrammatically in Figure 6.7.

Facilitating and enhancing these cellular level responses to alkalosis is a similar process occurring simultaneously at the level of the renal tubules. In the nephron, alkalosis affects electrolyte exchanges in the following manner: As normal reabsorption of sodium proceeds in response to aldosterone output, alkalosis renders hydrogen relatively less available for exchange purposes. Thus, a disproportionate amount of potassium must be excreted to balance the retention of positively charged sodium ions. This process, which is illustrated in Figure 6.8, heightens the tendency for alkalosis to be accompanied by hypokalemia.

SIGNS AND SYMPTOMS

As mentioned in Chapter 5, the primary manifestations of potassium imbalance are changes in the neuromuscular irritability

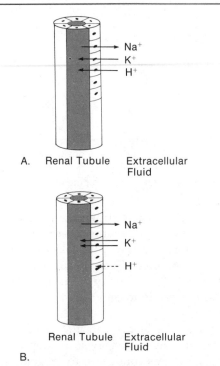

A. Renal Tubule   Extracellular Fluid

B. Renal Tubule   Extracellular Fluid

Figure 6.8 Alkalosis and potassium exchanges in the renal tubule. *A*, Normally, the reabsorption of Na^+ is balanced by elimination of positively charged K^+ and H^+. *B*, During alkalosis, there is relative lack of available H^+. Therefore, proportionately more K^+ than H^+ is eliminated to balance sodium reabsorption.

within the body. More specifically, as the plasma concentration of potassium decreases, muscles will respond less readily to neural stimulation.

Symptoms of hypokalemia thus include:

1. Disturbances in the smooth muscle of the gastrointestinal tract with accompanying abdominal distention, vomiting, and paralytic ileus.

2. Decreases in vascular tone, with associated evolution of hypotension.

3. Disturbances of skeletal muscle as evidenced by flabbiness, weakness, and shallow respirations.

4. Disturbances of the cardiac muscle with possible arrhythmias, rapid weak cardiac rate, heart blockage, and characteristic EKG changes.

Since cardiac changes can be very specific and helpful in the diagnosis of hypokalemia, they warrant further consideration. As potassium concentration falls, the heart becomes less responsive to neural stimulation and repolarization of cardiac muscle is delayed. Associated EKG changes include S-T segment depression and a flattened T wave, as illustrated in Figure 6.9. Hypokalemia is also known to increase the sensitivity of the heart to even low-level doses of digitalis. Hence, patients using digitalis must be carefully monitored with respect to potassium status.

In addition to neuromuscular changes, hypokalemia is also believed to induce a secondary alkalosis. Whereas previously we have discussed the loss of potassium that characteristically accompanies alkalosis, it is significant that hypokalemia can also precipitate or heighten the development of alkalosis. When plasma potassium levels are depleted, the reabsorption of sodium by renal tubule cells must be balanced by excretion of a disproportionately large volume of hydrogen ions.

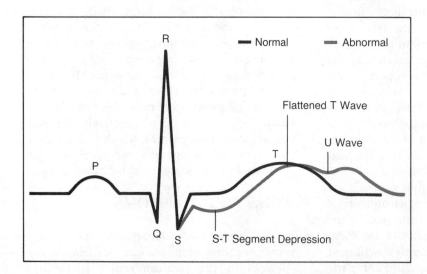

Figure 6.9 EKG changes associated with hypokalemia

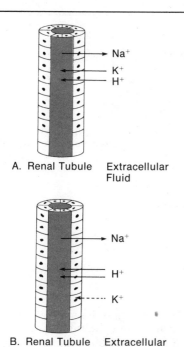

A. Renal Tubule   Extracellular Fluid

B. Renal Tubule   Extracellular Fluid

Figure 6.10 Hypokalemia and acid base balance. *A*, Normally, the reabsorption of Na^+ is balanced by elimination of positively charged K^+ and H^+. *B*, During hypokalemia, there is a relative lack of available K^+. Therefore, proportionately more H^+ than K^+ is eliminated to balance Na^+ reabsorption.

Hence, hydrogen plasma levels will fall, resulting in alkalosis. This phenomenon is illustrated in Figure 6.10. Since the alkalosis thus produced will further precipitate potassium loss, the result is often a spiraling effect that heightens the severity of the hypokalemia.

HYPOKALEMIA: A SUMMARY

Hypokalemia is induced primarily by depressions in extracellular fluid potassium levels. Although changes in water levels in the body affect potassium concentration, they do not seem to be nearly as clinically significant in potassium imbalances as they are in sodium fluctuations.

Depression in extracellular fluid potassium concentration has far-reaching systemic effects. A summary of the primary causes and results of hypokalemia can be found in Table 6.1.

Hyperkalemia

Hyperkalemia is caused primarily by elevated potassium levels in the extracellular fluid.

TABLE 6.1   **Hypokalemia**

Causes of Hypokalemia	Manifestations of Hypokalemia
Nutritional deficit	Altered neuromuscular irritability
Urinary loss	
Excessive use of non–potassium-sparing diuretics	Abdominal distention, paralytic ileus, and vomiting
Excessive diuresis	
Endocrine imbalances (hypersecretion of aldosterone)	Flabbiness and weakness of skeletal muscle
Gastrointestinal loss	Shallow respirations
Diarrhea	Cardiac arrhythmias
Vomiting	Secondary alkalosis
Excessive use of laxatives or enemas	
Gastrointestinal drainage or suction	
Alkalosis	

CLINICAL CAUSES

Elevated potassium levels can be caused by either increased intake or decreased output of potassium. Examples of increased potassium intake include excessive dietary input (often coupled with depressed renal function), elevated I.V. load, and intake of substances such as penicillin G or whole blood, which tend to be high in potassium content.

More commonly, however, hyperkalemia is induced clinically by diminished output. Since the kidneys are the primary route of potassium excretion, renal failure is a frequent cause of hyperkalemia. If potassium cannot be eliminated in the urine, it tends to accumulate in the extracellular fluid.

By altering renal function, decreased aldosterone secretion could similarly induce hyperkalemia. Because aldosterone acts on the renal tubules to promote potassium excretion, lack of aldosterone will result in potassium retention. Hence, individuals with Addison's disease (in which aldosterone output is depressed) or those taking aldosterone-inhibiting drugs (such as Aldactone) should be monitored carefully for signs of hyperkalemia.

Another frequent cause of excess potassium in the extracellular fluid involves the leakage of potassium out of the intracellular compartment into the interstitial fluid. This abnormal shift is seen in cases of cellular trauma accompanied by increased membrane permeability. Common clinical causes include

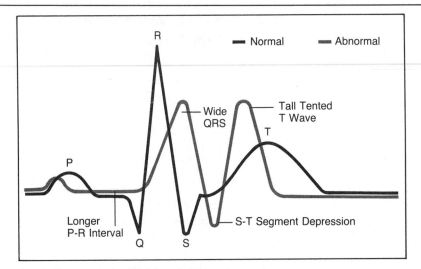

Figure 6.11 EKG changes associated with hyperkalemia.

burns, massive crushing injuries, and severe cellular hypoxia.

Intercompartmental potassium shifts are also induced by acidosis. With elevations in interstitial fluid hydrogen, H^+ ions are driven into the intracellular fluid. In exchange, there is a shift of positively charged potassium ions out of the cells to maintain electrical neutrality. Owing to these shifts, acidosis is almost always accompanied by increases in extracellular fluid potassium.

SIGNS AND SYMPTOMS

As plasma potassium concentration increases, muscles respond more readily to neural stimulation. Simultaneously, however, hyperkalemia causes a *decrease* in the *force* of muscular contraction. As a result of this depressed contractility, clinical manifestations of hyperkalemia are very similar to those associated with hypokalemia. Hence, it can be rather difficult to pinpoint potassium excess symptomatically.

Clinical manifestations of hyperkalemia often depend upon the extent to which potassium is elevated in extracellular fluid. Moderate elevations often cause increases in neuromuscular irritability with associated symptoms of intestinal colic and diarrhea. If hyperkalemia is severe, however, muscular weakness will result causing:

1. Disturbances of skeletal muscle as evidenced by flabbiness, weakness, and shallow respirations.

2. Cardiac muscle disturbances.

Since the specific nature of cardiac changes can prove helpful in supporting a diagnosis of hyperkalemia, some particular alterations are worth elucidating.

As plasma concentration increases, the heart may be affected in two primary ways:

1. Decreasing contractility may cause dilation and flaccidity of cardiac muscle, with an associated depression of cardiac rate. At the extreme, the heart may actually stop pumping while in a state of diastole (at rest).

2. Heightened response to neural stimulation may cause arrhythmias, ultimately culminating in ventricular fibrillation. Some characteristic EKG changes accompanying hyperkalemia can be useful diagnostically. They are presented in Figure 6.11.

TABLE 6.2   **Hyperkalemia**

Causes of Hyperkalemia	Manifestations of Hyperkalemia
Elevated intake of potassium	Altered neuromuscular irritability
Excessive I.V. load	
Penicillin G	Abdominal distention,
Whole blood transfusion	paralytic ileus, and
Depressed output of potassium	vomiting
Renal failure	Flabbiness and weak-
Addison's disease	ness of skeletal muscle
Aldosterone-inhibiting drugs	Shallow respirations
Shift of potassium out of	Cardiac arrhythmias
intracellular compartment	
Acidosis	
Burns	
Crushing injuries	
Cellular hypoxia	

HYPERKALEMIA: A SUMMARY

It can be seen that hyperkalemia is induced in a variety of ways and is symptomatically very similar to hypokalemia. Only EKG changes and serum potassium laboratory values can give some indication of whether an individual is experiencing potassium excess or deficit. A summary of some of the primary causes and results of hyperkalemia can be found in Table 6.2.

CALCIUM IMBALANCES

Calcium, like potassium, is essential to the maintenance of normal neural and muscular irritability. Unlike potassium imbalances, hypo- and hypercalcemia present clinically dissimilar pictures. Hence, one can often distinguish between these two potential calcium imbalances by clinically manifested symptoms.

Throughout the following analysis of calcium imbalances, it is important to keep in mind that only the *ionized* calcium in extracellular fluid can play a physiologically active role. Thus, any calcium bound to plasma proteins or trapped in bone salts does not function significantly as an electrolyte.

Hypocalcemia

Hypocalcemia is caused primarily by the depression of calcium levels in extracellular fluids. This, in turn, can be induced by either decreasing the intake or increasing the output of calcium.

CLINICAL CAUSES

The two primary sources of extracellular fluid calcium are dietary intake and the calcium that can be released from the salts of bone tissue. Thus, hypocalcemia may be induced in one of two ways: (1) by decreasing the ingestion or gastrointestinal absorption of calcium, or (2) by excessive *deposit* of ionized extracellular fluid calcium into bone tissue.

Individuals with nutritionally deficient diets, a milk allergy, or a strong aversion to milk products can develop hypocalcemia. Even with adequate intake, however, hypocalcemia can occur if calcium is not sufficiently absorbed from the gastrointestinal tract. Since the parathyroid hormone is a primary stimulator of gastrointestinal absorption, parathormone deficit is usually accompanied by hypocalcemia.

Assuming adequate calcium intake and normal parathormone levels, however, it is still possible for plasma calcium levels to be depressed. Since vitamin D is also needed to promote gastrointestinal absorption of calcium, hypocalcemia can result from vitamin D deficiency. To serve in its facilitative capacity, vitamin D must first be absorbed from the gastrointestinal tract into the bloodstream. Since it is a fat-soluble vitamin, its absorption is promoted by all secretions and enzymes that normally facilitate lipid digestion. Thus bile (which serves to emulsify fat in the duodenum), and pancreatic lipase (which promotes fat digestion) must both be present in sufficient quantity. Clearly any disease of the liver (which manufactures bile), or the gallbladder (which releases bile), obstruction of biliary ducts, or pancreatic disease can result in reduced vitamin D absorption and secondary hypocalcemia.

Depression of extracellular fluid calcium levels is also evident when excessive amounts of calcium are being withdrawn from plasma and deposited in bone. Once again, since parathormone affects the balance between bone deposit (osteoblastic activity) and bone breakdown (osteoclastic activity), parathyroid output will affect calcium concentration in the extracellular fluid. Deficit of parathormone is known to promote bone deposition. Thus, hyposecretion of this hormone, as seen during accidental surgical removal of the parathyroid glands during a thyroidectomy, is accompanied by hypocalcemia.

Although decreased intake and altered bone metabolism are the two primary causes of calcium deficit, blood levels can also be lowered as a result of increased output. Since the kidneys are the primary route of calcium excretion, increases in urinary calcium output can induce hypocalcemia. Once again, the parathyroid hormone comes into play in regulating the balance between calcium reabsorption and excretion by the nephron. Since parathormone acts to promote calcium retention, depressed hormone levels will be accompanied by increased urinary losses.

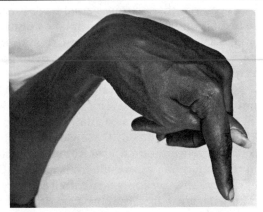

Figure 6.12 Carpopedal spasm, a clinical manifestation of hypocalcemia. (From Guyton, A. C.: Textbook of Medical Physiology, 6th ed. Philadelphia, W. B. Saunders Company, 1981. Used by permission.)

In considering causes of hypocalcemia, it is necessary to examine the effect of hydrogen ion concentration upon blood calcium levels. The concentration of hydrogen ion is known to affect the proportion of ionized calcium in the extracellular fluid. When the concentration of hydrogen ion decreases, as it does during alkalosis, calcium increasingly shifts into a non-ionized form. Since only ionized calcium is physiologically active, this shift produces hypocalcemia by reducing the percentage of functional calcium ions in the plasma.

SIGNS AND SYMPTOMS

A primary result of hypocalcemia is an increase in the permeability and irritability of most neural and muscular tissue. As a result, clinical manifestations of depressed calcium levels largely reflect alterations in neuromuscular performance. Increased irritability of skeletal muscle can result in twitching, carpopedal spasms, tetany, spasms of the larynx, and, in the extreme, epilepsy-like seizures. Smooth muscle irritability, on the other hand, characteristically results in spasms of the blood vessel walls with accompanying numbness and tingling in the fingers.

Characteristic clinical signs of heightened neuromuscular irritability include a positive Trousseau test, as illustrated in Figure 6.12, and Chvostek's sign. In the Trousseau test, a blood pressure cuff is inflated so as to stop circulation to the hand for one to five minutes. If carpopedal spasm results, the test is said to

be positive. Chvostek's sign can be produced by tapping the facial nerve anterior to the ear. If hypocalcemia exists, a momentary twitching of the upper lip and side of the face should result. In both tests, a stimulus is used to induce symptoms in individuals with latent calcium depression.

It is important to note that there is one major exception to the generally excitatory effect of hypocalcemia on neuromuscular tissue. Hypocalcemia is found to decrease cardiac muscle contractility. In extreme cases, arrhythmias and myocardial failure can result from depression of extracellular fluid calcium.

In addition to the organic disorders described, hypocalcemia can also bring about psychoemotional changes. These may be manifested in various ways, including emotional disturbance, irritability, instability, and confusion.

HYPOCALCEMIA: A SUMMARY

Hypocalcemia results from a variety of clinical causes and induces a wide range of symptomatic changes. A review of the causes and results of hypocalcemia can be found in Table 6.3.

Hypercalcemia

Hypercalcemia is caused primarily by an elevation of calcium in the extracellular fluid, which can result from increases in calcium intake or decreases in calcium output.

TABLE 6.3 **Hypocalcemia**

Causes of Hypocalcemia	Manifestations of Hypocalcemia
Decreased ingestion or absorption of calcium	Increased irritability of skeletal muscle
Nutritional deficit	Twitching
Hyposecretion of PTH	Carpopedal spasms
Vitamin D deficiency	Laryngeal spasms
Liver disease	Tetany
Gallbladder disease	Increased irritability of smooth muscle
Pancreatic disease	
Biliary obstruction	Vascular spasms
Excessive deposit of ionized calcium into bone tissue	Numbness and tingling of fingers
Increased elimination of calcium in the urine	
Alkalosis	Decreased irritability of cardiac muscle
	Psychoemotional instability

CLINICAL CAUSES

The two primary means of elevating calcium intake are: (1) increasing the input or gastrointestinal absorption of dietary calcium, or (2) increasing the breakdown of bone and subsequent release of calcium ions into extracellular fluid.

Excessive dietary intake of calcium-rich foods is rarely a cause of hypercalcemia. Occasionally, however, elevated gastrointestinal absorption, as promoted by increased vitamin D or parathormone levels, can produce elevations in serum calcium.

Increasing the release of calcium from bone salts is, perhaps, more clinically common. Elevations of parathormone, prolonged immobilization, and bone cancer all promote osteoblastic activity.

Decreasing the output of calcium, on the other hand, primarily involves alterations in the excretion of calcium by the kidneys. Reabsorption of calcium from the nephron, with subsequent increases in serum calcium levels, is caused mainly by parathormone secretion.

Once again, in examining the causes of calcium imbalance, it is necessary to consider the effect of hydrogen ion concentration on the level of ionized calcium in extracellular fluid. When the concentration of H$^+$ increases, as it does during *acidosis,* increasing proportions of calcium shift into the physiologically active ionized form. Thus, acidosis effectively promotes hypercalcemia by increasing the percentage of functional calcium *ions* in the extracellular fluid.

SIGNS AND SYMPTOMS

As mentioned earlier, hypercalcemia promotes a decrease in the irritability or contractility of most nerve and muscle tissue.

Depression of muscular activity is manifested primarily by decreased tone in the smooth muscle of the gastrointestinal tract. Symptomatically, this can result in abdominal distention, bloating, constipation, nausea, and vomiting.

Alterations in neural function often potentiate some of the gastrointestinal symptoms as well as inducing general lethargy, weakness, and lack of normal reflex response.

Once again, cardiac muscle is an exception to the generally depressant effects of hypercalcemia. Increased concentrations of plasma calcium serve to stimulate the heart, with resulting elevations in cardiac output and blood pressure. If irritability of the heart is excessive, however, arrhythmias can result in diminished pumping capacity with a subsequent fall in blood pressure.

Hypercalcemia induced by increases in parathormone level and osteoclastic activity is usually accompanied by signs of bone pain or softening of bone tissue. As mineral content of the skeleton diminishes, an increased susceptibility to fractures can also be noted.

Regardless of the cause of hypercalcemia, it is important to realize that elevations in blood calcium levels often force abnormal deposits of calcium into soft tissue. A prime target of this pathological classification seems to be the kidneys. Increased incidences of kidney stones, kidney infection, and possible renal failure often result.

HYPERCALCEMIA: A SUMMARY

A wide variety of causes and symptoms may be associated with hypercalcemia. These are summarized in Table 6.4.

SUMMARY

In the previous pages, we have traced the development and results of a number of criti-

TABLE 6.4 **Hypercalcemia**

Causes of Hypercalcemia	Manifestations of Hypercalcemia
Increased intake or absorption of calcium	Decreased neuromuscular irritability
Excessive release of ionized calcium from bone salts	Abdominal distention, constipation, nausea, and vomiting
Hypersecretion of PTH	General lethargy and weakness
Prolonged immobilization	Hyporeflexia
Bone cancer	Increased irritability of cardiac muscle
Decreased renal elimination of calcium	Weakening of bone (if hypercalcemia is associated with osteoclastic activity)
Acidosis	Excessive deposit of calcium into soft tissue
	Kidney stones
	Renal infection

TABLE 6.5   **Systemic Dysfunction Induced by Electrolyte Imbalance**

System	Electrolyte Imbalance	Resulting Systemic Dysfunction	Effect Upon Cellular Equilibrium
CARDIOVASCULAR	Hyperkalemia and hypokalemia	Cardiac arrhythmias	Potential disruption of cellular need for oxygen, nutrients, and elimination
	Hypocalcemia	Decreased irritability of cardiac muscle	
	Hypercalcemia	Increased irritability of cardiac muscle	
RESPIRATORY	Hyperkalemia and hypokalemia	Shallow respirations	Potential disruption of cellular need for oxygen supply and carbon dioxide elimination
	Hypocalcemia	Laryngeal spasms	
GASTROINTESTINAL	Hyponatremia	Nausea and vomiting	Potential disruption of cellular need for nutrients
	Hyperkalemia and hypokalemia }	Abdominal distention; vomiting	
	Hypercalcemia		
RENAL	Hypercalcemia	Renal stones; renal infection	Potential disruption of cellular need for elimination
NEUROMUSCULAR	Hyponatremia	Twitch, hyperirritability, disorientation, coma, weakness	Potential disruption of the integration necessary to support cellular homeostasis
	Hypernatremia	Restlessness, apprehension	
	Hypocalcemia	Twitch, carpopedal spasms, tetany, psychoemotional instability	
	Hypercalcemia	Hyporeflexia, lethargy, weakness	

cal fluid and electrolyte imbalances. Although analysis of acid-base disturbances has been reserved for the following chapter, the effects of isotonic imbalances and alterations in the concentrations of sodium, potassium, and calcium have been discussed.

It is interesting to note the wide variety of systemic changes that result from fluid and electrolyte imbalances discussed thus far. In short, it can be said that disruption of the cellular need for fluid and electrolyte balance can alter the function of a number of organs and structures. The heart, for example, is affected by disturbances in calcium or potassium levels. Malfunction of cardiac muscle can, in turn, initiate a chain of far-reaching pathological problems.

Table 6.5 highlights some of the major systemic disorders that arise from the specific fluid and electrolyte imbalances analyzed in this chapter. It serves to illustrate the extensive downward spiraling physiological changes that can be imposed upon the body as a result of disrupted cellular homeostasis.

STUDY QUESTIONS

1. In each of the following cases, determine whether you would expect an isotonic imbalance to result:
   a. excessive secretion of ADH
   b. hemorrhage
   c. excessive administration of normal (isotonic) saline I.V. fluid
2. Explain why a postoperative patient who is receiving morphine for pain might predictably have depressed plasma sodium levels.
3. Explain why untreated diabetes mellitus might characteristically be associated with hyponatremia.
4. It is 100° F. outside, and you have been playing tennis for two and one-half hours. Why is it *not* a good idea to drink a lot of water?

5. What is responsible for the possible disorientation noted in a hyponatremic or a hypernatremic patient?

6. Identify the sodium imbalance that would predictably accompany each of the following disorders and determine whether you would expect associated symptoms of hypo- or hypervolemia:
   a. diabetes insipidus
   b. vomiting and diarrhea
   c. adrenal cortical tumor
   d. SIADH
   e. excessive administration of a tap water enema

7. Explain why acidosis is characteristically accompanied by: (a) hyperkalemia, and (b) hypercalcemia.

8. Why should a patient on diuretic therapy be monitored for evidence of potassium depletion?

9. Explain why hypokalemia would be a possible complication of colitis (prolonged diarrhea).

10. What would be the effect of (a) steroid therapy and (b) Aldactone therapy upon plasma potassium levels?

11. A patient is admitted to the hospital, after an automobile accident, with massive crushing injuries. Why should he or she be monitored for evidence of hyperkalemia?

12. A patient is hospitalized with extensive hepatic disease. Explain why you should be on the alert for possible (a) hypokalemia, or (2) hypocalcemia.

13. In the course of performing a thyroidectomy, the surgeon accidentally removes the parathyroid glands. What clinical symptoms would predictably result?

14. Why would immobilization or bone cancer promote the development of hypercalcemia?

Suggested Readings

Books

Brooks, S. M.: Basic Facts of Body Water and Ions, 3rd ed. New York, Springer Publishing Company, 1973, pp. 38–45.

Burke, S. R.: The Composition and Function of Body Fluids, 2nd ed. St. Louis, The C. V. Mosby Company, 1976, pp. 34–53.

Luckmann, J., and Sorensen, K. C.: Medical-Surgical Nursing, A Psychophysiologic Approach, 2nd ed. Philadelphia, W. B. Saunders Company, 1980, pp. 171–205.

Maher, J. F., and Bartter, F. C.: Maintenance of dynamic equilibrium of body fluids and electrolytes. In Frohlich, E. D. (ed.): Pathophysiology, Altered Regulatory Mechanisms in Disease, 2nd ed. Philadelphia, J. B. Lippincott Company, 1976, p. 241.

Metheny, N. M., and Snively, W. D.: Nurse's Handbook of Fluid Balance, 3rd ed. Philadelphia, J. B. Lippincott Company, 1979, pp. 64–78.

Reed, G.: Potassium: The chief electrolyte. In Hamilton, H. (ed.): Monitoring Fluids and Electrolytes Precisely. Nursing 79 Books. Horsham, Pa., Intermed Communications, Inc., 1978, p. 79.

Reed, G. M., and Sheppard, V. F.: Regulation of Fluid and Electrolyte Balance: A Programmed Instruction in Clinical Physiology, 2nd ed. Philadelphia, W. B. Saunders Company, 1977, pp. 116–148.

Stroot, V. R., Lee, C. A., and Schaper, C. A.: Fluids and Electrolytes: A Practical Approach, 2nd ed. Philadelphia, F. A. Davis Company, 1977, pp. 49–77.

Thomas, R.: Calcium: The durable electrolyte. In Hamilton, H. (ed.): Monitoring Fluids and Electrolytes Precisely. Nursing 79 Books. Horsham, Pa., Intermed Communications, Inc., 1978, p. 97.

Weldy, N. J.: Body Fluids and Electrolytes—A Programmed Presentation, 3rd ed. St. Louis, The C. V. Mosby Company, 1980, pp. 28–38; 91–117.

Wolfe, L.: Sodium: Controller of fluid volume. In Hamilton, H. (ed.): Monitoring Fluids and Electrolytes Precisely. Nursing 79 Books. Horsham, Pa., Intermed Communications, Inc., 1978, p. 89.

Articles

Aspinall, M. J.: A simplified guide to managing patients with hyponatremia. Nursing 78, *8*:32, 1978.

Bartter, F. C., and Schwartz, W. B.: The syndrome of inappropriate secretion of antidiuretic hormone. Am. J. Med., *42*:790, 1967.

Bay, W. H., and Ferria, T. F.: Hypernatremia and hyponatremia: Disorders of tonicity. Geriatrics, *31*:53, 1976.

Del Bueno, G. J.: Electrolyte imbalance: How to recognize and respond to it. Part 1. RN, *38*:52, 1975.

Khokar, N.: Inappropriate secretion of antidiuretic hormone. Postgrad. Med., *62*:73, 1977.

Narins, G.: A practical approach to managing hyponatremia. Consultant, *19*:25, 1979.

Chapter Outline

chapter 7

Acid-Base Balance and Imbalance

Chapter Objectives

At the completion of this chapter, the student will be able to:

1. Differentiate between acids and bases with respect to chemical nature and behavior.
2. Distinguish between strong acids and bases and weak acids and bases and give examples of each.
3. Differentiate between volatile and nonvolatile acids in the body with respect to (a) origin, and (b) method of elimination.
4. List one volatile and three nonvolatile acids that are present in the body.
5. Identify the primary extracellular fluid base and describe its derivation.
6. Describe the clinical significance of the term *pH.*
7. Distinguish between compensation and correction of an acid-base imbalance.
8. Identify the major regulatory and compensatory mechanisms that function to maintain acid-base balance and describe their modes of action.
9. Trace the functional activity of the bicarbonate buffer system in cases of (a) acidosis, and (b) alkalosis.
10. Define acidosis and describe its clinical manifestations.
11. Differentiate between compensated and uncompensated respiratory and metabolic acidosis with respect to ·causes and characteristic laboratory values.
12. Define alkalosis and describe its clinical manifestations.
13. Differentiate between compensated and uncompensated respiratory and metabolic alkalosis with respect to causes and characteristic laboratory values.

INTRODUCTION

In considering the normal composition of body fluids, it is important to take into account a specific category of electrolytes: acids and bases. In this chapter a general distinction between acids and bases is followed by an analysis of their behavior, function, and regulation in the body. Emphasis is placed upon the complex interactions of the many systems that are essential to the maintenance of acid-base balance.

Since excessive acidity or alkalinity can be so disruptive to all physiological processes, acid-base imbalances will also be discussed. An understanding of acid-base abnormalities can provide a foundation for understanding many pathological mechanisms.

BASIC CONCEPTS

As can be determined by a brief review of Chapters 3 and 5, water is a significant component of living tissue. As we prepare to study acids and bases, it is helpful to take a closer look at the chemical composition of a water molecule. In simple terms, a water molecule consists of one hydrogen atom (H) linked chemically to one hydroxyl group (OH). One water molecule can be drawn as follows: $H-OH$. It can be seen that the chemical bond between the two components is represented by a straight line.

The chemical breakdown of a water molecule involves breaking the bond between H and OH and the simultaneous release of a free H and a free OH into solution. This can be represented chemically as follows: $H-OH \rightarrow$ $H^+ + OH^-$. It is important to note that when the H and the OH are released by this reaction, they each carry an electrical charge. The hydrogen carries one positive charge, the hydroxyl group one negative charge.

It can also be seen how the breakdown of any one water molecule would release one H^+ for every OH^-. It follows, therefore, that the breakdown of 100 water molecules would release 100 hydrogen ions and 100 hydroxyl groups. In short, it can be said that: (1) every time one water molecule is decomposed, it will release one H^+ and one OH^-, or (2) the breakdown of a water molecule releases H^+ and OH^- in equal numbers. It can thus be seen how, in any solution of pure water, the concentration of H^+ would have to equal the concentration of OH^-.

Acids and Bases in General

Acids, by definition, are substances that dissociate to release H^+ into solution. If some acid molecules are placed into pure water, it should be evident that the original equality of H^+ and OH^- would be disrupted. Acid substances added to water will cause the new solution to have a concentration of H^+ greater than the concentration of OH^-. This is illustrated in Figure 7.1.

It is important to realize that not all acid molecules will release their hydrogen with equal ease. The strength with which hydrogen is bonded in an acid molecule will vary with the specific acid. *Strong acids* are substances that release hydrogen readily into solution. These include hydrochloric (H—Cl), nitric (H—NO$_3$), and sulfuric (H$_2$—SO$_4$) acids. *Weak acids,* on the other hand, tend to hold tightly to their hydrogen. Examples include carbonic

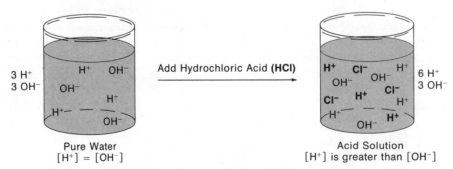

Figure 7.1   The formation of an acid solution.

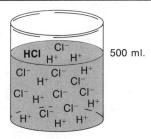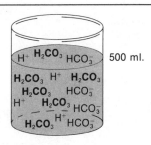

Figure 7.2 The difference between a strong and a weak acid.

Strong Acid:
In this solution of strong acid, nine out of ten acid molecules dissociated to release free H^+.

Weak Acid:
In this solution of weak acid, only four out of ten acid molecules dissociated to release free H^+.

(H_2—CO_3), citric, acetic, lactic, and pyruvic acids.

To clarify the distinction between strong and weak acids, let us imagine two beakers, each containing 500 ml. of pure water. Into beaker A we put 10 molecules of HCl; into beaker B, 10 molecules of H_2CO_3. A look at Figure 7.2 will reveal that the total number of free hydrogen ions released into beaker A by the HCl is 9, whereas the total number of free hydrogen ions released into beaker B by the H_2CO_3 is only 4.

Evidence of characteristic acid properties depends upon the presence of free hydrogen ions. The higher the concentration of hydrogen ions, the stronger the manifestation of acidic properties. Acidic properties include corrosiveness, sour taste, and the ability to turn blue litmus paper pink.

An understanding of the essentials of acidity makes comprehension of base properties (or alkalinity) easier to grasp. Bases, by definition, are substances that either:

1. release free OH^- into solution, or
2. decrease the concentration of free H^+ by trapping it chemically and removing it from solution.

It should be noted that in either case, the result is to render the concentration of OH^- in a solution greater than that of H^+. This is illustrated in Figure 7.3. Note that in beaker A and beaker B, we originally start with 500 ml. of pure water. Beaker A^+ illustrates the result of adding an OH^- donating base to the water. Beaker B^+ illustrates the result of adding a H^+ trapping base to the water. It can be seen that in both cases the equality between hydrogen and hydroxyl, as noted in pure water, is

disrupted. With the addition of a base, the concentration of OH^- in a solution becomes greater than the concentration of H^+.

Potassium hydroxide (KOH) is an example of a base that conforms to definition 1, as stated above. When a molecule of K—OH is put into pure water, it will dissociate as follows: K—OH $\rightarrow$ K^+ + OH^-, thereby increasing the concentration of OH^- in the solution.

Bicarbonate, on the other hand, is an example of a base that conforms to the second definition. When placed into a solution of pure water, the bicarbonate (HCO_3^-) will react with a free H^+ donated by a water molecule as follows:

$$HCO_3^- + \quad H^+ \longrightarrow H_2CO_3$$
from $\qquad$ carbonic acid
water $\qquad$ (a weak acid does not
$\qquad$ release hydrogen readily)

In this way, the concentration of free hydrogen in the water will be reduced, and the relative concentration of free OH^- in the solution will be elevated.

Again, as in the case of acids, base molecules will vary in their chemical capacity to either donate OH^- or trap H^+. Strong bases are those substances that react readily to release OH^- or trap H^+. Weak bases, on the other hand, will have relatively less tendency to release OH^- or attract H^+. Examples of strong bases are sodium hydroxide (NaOH) and potassium hydroxide (KOH). Weak bases include calcium hydroxide ($Ca(OH)_2$), magnesium hydroxide ($Mg(OH)_2$), and bicarbonate (HCO_3^-).

In a manner similar to acids, the display

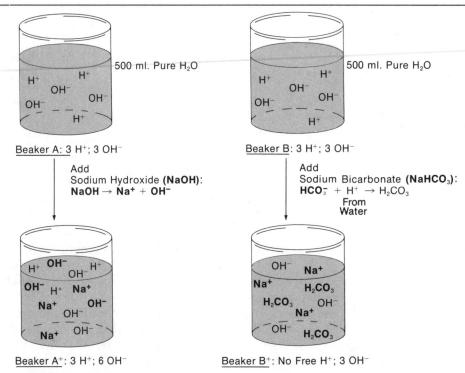

Beaker A: 3 H⁺; 3 OH⁻

Add
Sodium Hydroxide **(NaOH)**:
NaOH → Na⁺ + OH⁻

Beaker B: 3 H⁺; 3 OH⁻

Add
Sodium Bicarbonate **(NaHCO₃)**:
HCO₃⁻ + H⁺ → H₂CO₃
From
Water

Beaker A⁺: 3 H⁺; 6 OH⁻

Beaker B⁺: No Free H⁺; 3 OH⁻

Figure 7.3 The formation of an alkaline solution. When NaOH is added to Beaker A, the release of free OH⁻ causes the formation of an alkaline solution (A⁺). When NaHCO₃ is added to Beaker B, HCO₃⁻ removes free H⁺ from solution, trapping it within a H₂CO₃ molecule. As a result, an alkaline mixture (Beaker B⁺) is generated.

of base, or alkaline, properties will vary with the relative concentration of OH⁻. Typical properties include bitter taste, causticity, and the ability to turn red litmus indicator paper blue.

Although acids and bases can be distinguished from each other on the basis of certain characteristic properties, *pH* measures provide a numerical indication of the relative acidity or alkalinity of a solution. The pH values range from 1, at the acid end of the spectrum, to 14 at the alkaline end. A pH of 7 indicates neutrality. In a solution with a pH of 7, the concentration of H⁺ equals the concentration of OH⁻. The best example is, of course, pure water. As pH values descend from 7 toward 1, they reflect increasing acidity. Con-

versely, as pH values increase from 7 to 14, they reflect increasing alkalinity (see Figure 7.4). Clearly, laboratory slips reporting the pH of blood and urine can be helpful in assessing the acid-base status of the body.

Acids and Bases in the Body

It is perhaps most helpful to view acid-base balance by examining the sources of H⁺ intake and output. The production, behavior, and regulation of hydrogen ions in the body are the primary factors affecting acid-base balance. Although alterations in the concentration of base in extracellular fluid do occur, changes in the hydrogen ion concentration are responsible for most clinical acid-base disruptions.

ACIDS

Acids that are physiologically significant can be classified into two primary groups: (1) *volatile acids*, and (2) *nonvolatile acids*. Al-

pH
Reading

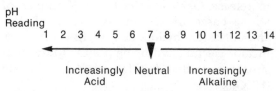

Figure 7.4 pH as a measure of acid-base status.

though both volatile and nonvolatile acids dissociate in water to donate hydrogen ions, they differ in their method of formation and excretion.

Volatile acids are those that can break down to give at least one gaseous (volatile) product. In the body the only substance that qualifies is carbonic acid (H_2CO_3), which, under the proper conditions, will break down to yield water and carbon dioxide gas. The chemical equation for this reaction is as follows: $H_2CO_3 \rightleftharpoons H_2O + CO_2 \uparrow$ (gas).

It should be noted that the arrows in this equation are drawn in both directions. This indicates that the reaction is reversible. In other words, carbonic acid can be formed by the chemical union of water and carbon dioxide. The combination of water with carbon dioxide is, in fact, the primary mechanism for generation of carbonic acid in the body. It thus follows that the quantity of H_2CO_3 in extracellular fluid will be largely affected by extracellular fluid carbon dioxide levels. If carbon dioxide concentration increases, carbonic acid levels will rise; conversely, if carbon dioxide levels fall, carbonic acid levels will decrease.

The concentration of carbon dioxide gas in the extracellular fluid depends upon the balance between two factors: (1) the rate of carbon dioxide production, and (2) the rate of carbon dioxide elimination. The complete metabolism of nutrients via the citric acid cycle is the primary source of carbon dioxide production in the body. This process, which is described in Chapter 2, involves the intracellular oxidation of carbohydrate, protein, or fat particles to yield carbon dioxide, water, and energy. Therefore, any factors affecting the rate of cellular oxidation will indirectly influence the volume of carbon dioxide generated. Some of these factors are summarized in Table 7.1.

Equally important to the status of carbon dioxide in the extracellular fluid is the volume of carbon dioxide excreted. Although the respiratory system is of primary importance in the elimination of carbon dioxide, many other organs and structures are involved. Some of the systems that facilitate carbon dioxide elimination are discussed in Chapter 2. It is important to remember that since the carbon dioxide excreted is derived directly or indirectly from a molecule of carbonic acid, loss of carbon dioxide is functionally equivalent to losing carbonic acid.

All acids in the body except for carbonic acid are classified as *nonvolatile acids*. Nonvolatile acids are a rather diverse category encompassing those acids that do not break down to form gaseous products.

Nonvolatile acids are generated primarily through metabolic processes. The incomplete (anaerobic) metabolism of carbohydrates will generally yield both lactic and pyruvic acid. Alternatively, inability to use carbohydrates metabolically (as is seen in diabetes mellitus or low-carbohydrate diets) will result in elevated utilization of fat and protein molecules. The

TABLE 7.1 **Some Factors Affecting the Rate of Cellular Oxidation**

Factor	Function
Activity levels	Strenuous exercise can considerably increase the generation of energy at the cellular level. Conversely, metabolic rate will decrease during periods of rest or sleep.
Protein intake	Certain amino acids found in proteins are known to directly stimulate cellular metabolic activity.
Age	The rate of cellular oxidation generally declines with age.
Sympathetic neural stimulation	Stimulation by the sympathetic nervous system causes cellular metabolic rate to increase.
Body temperature	Fever triggers an increase in the rate of cellular oxidation.
Endocrine secretions	Thyroid hormone, growth hormone, and the male sex hormone are all known to stimulate cellular metabolism.

metabolic breakdown of these two nutrients causes an increase in the production of acidic ketone bodies.

Nonvolatile acids are excreted primarily by the kidneys. Hence, whereas respiratory failure can lead to an accumulation of volatile carbonic acid, renal failure can result in an increase in nonvolatile acids, such as lactic acid, pyruvic acid, citric acid, uric acid, and so forth.

BASES

In traditional studies of acid-base balance, very little emphasis is placed upon the bases in the body. It is, however, helpful to be aware of the primary base in extracellular fluid as well as its generation and excretion.

The base of greatest clinical significance is *bicarbonate* (HCO_3^-). It may be recalled that bicarbonate is generated primarily by chemical reactions involved with carbon dioxide transport by the blood. In brief, when the carbon dioxide generated by metabolism diffuses from interstitial fluid to plasma, a large percentage enters the red blood cells. Within the erythrocytes, carbon dioxide combines with water to produce carbonic acid, which subsequently dissociates as follows:

$$H_2CO_3 \rightleftharpoons H^+ + HCO_3^-.$$

Most of the bicarbonate thus generated then moves into plasma to be transported throughout the body. The process is illustrated in Figure 2.22 in Chapter 2.

A major pool of bicarbonate is concentrated in the lower gastrointestinal tract. The digestive secretions of the liver and pancreas, which are alkaline, are manufactured by pulling plasma bicarbonate molecules out of circulation and concentrating them in bile and pancreatic juice. When bile and pancreatic juice subsequently enter the gastrointestinal tract at the duodenum, they modify the pH of intestinal contents, as illustrated in Figure 7.5. Although some bicarbonate is thus excreted from the body during defecation, the greatest percentage of base is characteristically eliminated by the kidneys.

pH

As discussed earlier, pH is a measure of the relative acidity or alkalinity of a solution. Hence, it is a convenient diagnostic measure of the acid-base status of the extracellular fluid and certain body secretions. A summary of some body fluids and secretions, and their normal pH range, can be found in Table 7.2.

Most significant for clinical assessment purposes is the pH of extracellular fluid, as reflected by plasma pH. The normal pH range of the blood is 7.35 to 7.45. Even slight deviations from this norm can have serious consequences. If the pH falls below 7.35, the resulting condition is referred to as *acidosis*. If, on the other hand, the pH rises above 7.45, *alkalosis* results.

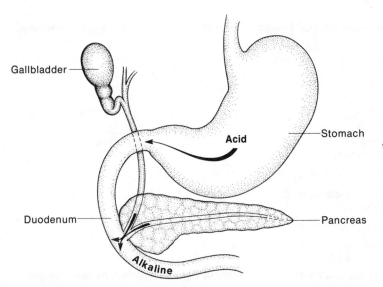

Gallbladder

Acid

Stomach

Duodenum

Pancreas

Alkaline

Figure 7.5 The alkalinizing of gastrointestinal contents.

TABLE 7.2	**The pH of Selected Body Fluids and Secretions**

Fluid	pH
Pure water	7.0
Body fluids	
Blood plasma (arterial)	7.4
Blood plasma (venous)	7.35
Interstitial fluid	7.4
Intracellular fluid	6.5 (average)
Cerebrospinal fluid	7.35–7.45
Body secretions	
Bile	7.0–7.6
Gastric juice	1.2–3.0
Intestinal juice	7.0–8.0
Pancreatic juice	7.5–8.0
Saliva	6.4–7.0
Urine	5–8

Adapted from Cohen, A.: Handbook of Cellular Chemistry. St. Louis, The C. V. Mosby Company, 1975 p. 38.

Regulation of Acids and Bases in the Body

Since the body is a dynamic, nonstable entity, the level of hydrogen ions in the extracellular fluid is in a state of continual flux. In order to prevent accompanying changes in pH, mechanisms exist to compensate for the ongoing increases and decreases in hydrogen ion concentration.

Those processes that function passively, without necessitating the mobilization of a specific organ or system, will be referred to as *regulatory mechanisms*. Included in this category are the effects of dilution and the activity of buffers. Generally helping to blunt the effects of a change in pH, they are only marginally effective in counteracting a major acid-base imbalance.

When a severe or sustained alteration in hydrogen ion concentration occurs, the respiratory or renal system must be activated to re-establish a normal pH. Systemic mobilization, in these cases, comprises what will be referred to as *compensatory mechanisms*, which help to restore acid-base balance.

Although both "regulation" and "compensation" provide a means of re-establishing the pH norm, they are unable to reverse the cause of disequilibrium. Thus, if acidosis develops secondary to pulmonary disease (with associated carbon dioxide retention), dilution, buffers, and the renal system may make adjustments that aid in the restoration of acid-base balance. As a result, plasma pH may return to normal, but the origin of the dysfunction will remain as an ongoing source of stress. True *"correction"* is achieved only when disease of the lung is successfully treated and reversed.

As an aid to understanding this concept, it might be helpful to consider two pots of far too spicy chili. One cook chooses to adjust for the fiery taste by adding rice to mask the problem. The other cook elects to remove the hot peppers that are causing the burning sensation. The first cook is merely compensating for a previous error in judgment. The second cook, on the other hand, is technically correcting the problem by removing the source of the excess.

REGULATORY MECHANISMS

As mentioned earlier, regulatory mechanisms provide ongoing, passive protection against pH fluctuations. Both the effects of dilution and the activity of buffers afford an immediately available means of counteracting alterations in the concentration of hydrogen ions.

DILUTION Dilution is the simplest means of dealing with a hydrogen ion change. As extra hydrogen ions are ingested or generated, the body fluids dilute them. This happens automatically, without any special forces being called into play. As long as the body contains a substantial fluid volume, this fluid will serve to dilute the potency of excessive hydrogen ion input.

BUFFERS Buffers are pairs of chemicals in the body that neutralize the effect of any acid or base that threatens to upset the pH balance. Buffers, which are present in both extracellular and intracellular fluid, contain two components that are closely related structurally:

1. One component serves to neutralize or trap excess hydrogen ion and remove it from solution. It thus functions as a base.

2. The other component serves to donate

a hydrogen ion, which, in turn, traps or neutralizes excess hydroxyl. It thus functions as an acid.

A careful look at the functioning of one buffer pair will facilitate understanding of the buffer mechanism in general. In the body, H_2CO_3 and HCO_3^- serve as a primary buffer pair. It is possible to use a simple rule of thumb to determine which buffer component is more acidic and which is more alkaline: The molecule containing the greater number of hydrogen atoms is the acidic component; the molecule containing the lesser number of hydrogen atoms is the alkaline component. Hence, in the case of the bicarbonate buffer system, H_2CO_3 is the acid, and HCO_3^- is the base.

A second rule of thumb to keep in mind when considering buffer function is that the acid component of the buffer system serves to neutralize excess base in the body; alternatively, the alkaline component neutralizes excess acid.

It thus follows that whenever extra hydrogen ion is being introduced into extracellular fluid, the HCO_3^- component of the bicarbonate buffer system will serve to modify any potential pH change. It does so in the following manner:

$$H^+ \quad + \quad HCO_3^- \quad \longrightarrow \quad H_2CO_3$$

hydrogen from strong acid + bicarbonate from the buffer system → weak acid

It could be asked, "How could this mechanism reduce extracellular fluid acidity if, in fact, it results in the formation of an acid?" The answer lies in the nature of the acid generated. It must be stressed that buffer activity cannot totally remove extra hydrogen ions. Rather, it traps a high percentage of the excess free hydrogen (donated from a stronger acid) into the molecule of a weaker acid. Since carbonic acid does not dissociate too readily, the hydrogens that are part of its structure remain trapped, to a large extent, in molecular form.

It should be noted that as this buffer system responds to excess acidity, one would expect the concentration of HCO_3^- to decrease as H_2CO_3 levels increase. A depression in bicarbonate thus often reflects the existence of acidosis.

Conversely, when excess base (OH^-) is introduced into extracellular fluid, the H_2CO_3 component of the bicarbonate buffer system will respond as follows:

$$OH^- \quad + \quad H_2CO_3 \quad \longrightarrow H_2O \quad + \quad HCO_3^-$$

hydroxyl from strong base + carbonic acid from the buffer system → water + weak base

It should be noted that during this reaction, a strong base (OH^-) is neutralized and trapped into a water molecule, while a weak base (bicarbonate) remains. Alkalosis thus results in the conversion of H_2CO_3 to HCO_3^-, as buffer response progresses. Hence, laboratory assessment of chemical changes associated with alkalosis should reflect decreases in carbonic acid levels and increases in the concentration of bicarbonate.

It is important to realize that there are buffer pairs in the body other than the bicarbonate system described here. They are listed and analyzed with respect to components and primary distribution in Table 7.3.

COMPENSATORY MECHANISMS

Although the pH of the body is kept partially in check by dilution and buffer system activity, these regulatory mechanisms cannot totally adjust for acid-base changes. Effective compensation depends, to a large extent, upon mobilization of the respiratory and renal systems. In both cases, activity is directed toward maintaining normal pH in spite of underlying disease.

RESPIRATORY SYSTEM During times of acid-base excess or deficit, the respiratory

TABLE 7.3 **Buffer Systems in the Body**

Buffer System	Primary Distribution	Acid Component	Alkaline Component
Carbonate	Extracellular fluid	H_2CO_3	HCO_3^-
Phosphate	Intracellular fluid	$H_2PO_4^-$	$HPO_4^=$
Protein	Intracellular fluid	H-Protein	Protein$^-$
Hemoglobin	Red blood cell	H-Hb	Hb$^-$

system can play a significant role in counter-acting fluctuations in hydrogen ion concentration.

As acidosis evolves, compensation can be achieved by increasing the respiratory output of carbon dioxide. In this way, the concentration of H_2CO_3 in extracellular fluid is depressed, and the total pool of hydrogen ions in the body is reduced. Conversely, to compensate for alkalosis, it is necessary to decrease respiratory output of carbon dioxide, thereby retaining CO_2 in the extracellular fluid. The retained carbon dioxide, in turn, combines with water and raises the concentration of carbonic acid.

The mechanism of respiratory compensation is facilitated by neural control, which is sensitive to pH fluctuations. When the concentration of hydrogen ions increases during acidosis, the medulla is directly stimulated to cause an increase in respiratory rate and depth. Conversely, when hydrogen ion levels are depressed during alkalosis, a compensatory decrease in respiratory rate and depth occurs. The responsiveness of respiratory rate to acid-base status is summarized in Figure 7.6.

It is obvious that the respiratory system functions primarily by influencing the concentration of carbonic acid in extracellular fluid. One might well ask, therefore, how respiratory changes can help to modify acidosis or alkalosis caused by excesses or deficits of nonvolatile acids.

The answer lies at the root of acid-base imbalances. Although excess hydrogen ions in the extracellular fluid can be derived from a vast array of acid molecules, compensation can be achieved by removing *any* source of hydrogen ion from the body. It is thus possible to counteract the effects of excess hydrogen ion derived from lactic acid by excreting the

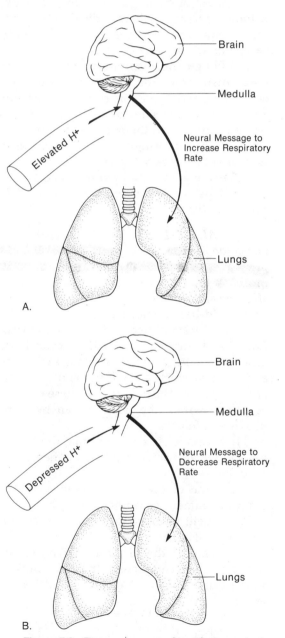

Figure 7.6 Responsiveness of respiratory rate to changes in pH.

hydrogen ion associated with carbonic acid. Conversely, in cases of alkalosis, hydrogen ion depletion (regardless of cause) can be compensated for by the retention of carbon dioxide, with subsequent generation of carbonic acid.

In essence, then, the respiratory system functions to modify pH changes by altering carbonic acid levels in the extracellular fluid. Since acid-base balance depends upon the total *number* of hydrogen ions in the body, without concern for their derivation, respiratory changes can effectively counteract a wide variety of acid-base fluctuations.

Although the respiratory compensation mechanism responds within minutes to a change in hydrogen ion concentration, its ability to compensate for pH deviations is limited. Changes in the rate of respiration are often effective in bringing pH values closer to normal but not totally back to the average 7.35 to 7.45 reading. In the long run, total compensation depends largely upon adequate functioning of the renal system.

RENAL SYSTEM   Although renal compensation is not typically activated until approximately 24 to 48 hours after the onset of a problem, the kidneys are doubtless the most effective and complex mechanism for counteracting acid-base imbalance.

Stated in simplified terms, the presence of excessive hydrogen ion in the extracellular fluid stimulates a series of renal exchanges and chemical reactions within the tubule cells of the nephron. The net result of these internal responses within the nephron can be summarized as follows:

1. Excess H^+ is removed from the tubule cell and secreted actively into the lumen of the nephron.

2. Some of the H^+ that arrives in the nephron lumen combines with ammonia (NH_3) present in urine to be excreted as ammonium (NH_4^+).

3. Some of the H^+ that arrives in the nephron lumen combines with HCO_3^- present in the urine and forms carbonic acid, as follows:

$$H^+ + HCO_3^- \longrightarrow H_2CO_3$$

$$\left[H^+ + \quad \begin{array}{c} H \\ CO_3^- \longrightarrow \quad \end{array} \begin{array}{c} H \\ CO_3 \\ H \end{array} \right]$$

Much of the carbonic acid formed in the preceding reaction then breaks down into H_2O and CO_2, as follows:

$$\begin{array}{c} H \\ \diagdown \\ CO_3 \longrightarrow H\!-\!OH + CO_2 \\ \diagup \\ H \end{array}$$

The originally secreted H^+ can thus be eliminated as part of a water molecule.

4. When H^+ is being secreted into the nephron, a positively charged ion must be reabsorbed to maintain electrical balance. Sodium (Na^+) is the particle most often pulled into the extracellular fluid to compensate for H^+ loss.

5. Finally, accompanying the reabsorbed sodium is a bicarbonate radical, which joins sodium in moving from the nephron into the extracellular fluid. In this way, as acid H^+ levels are being decreased in extracellular fluid, the alkaline bicarbonate levels are being elevated.

The sum total of renal regulatory mechanisms is presented in Figure 7.7.

It can be seen how these activities at the cellular level of the nephron could help to compensate for elevations in hydrogen ion concentrations. As extracellular fluid becomes more acidic, the renal mechanism is mobilized to ward off acidosis by bringing about a loss of acid and an increase in base.

Of course, in cases of alkalosis, this sequence is reversed. There is less hydrogen ion secreted, with more remaining in the extracellular fluid. Increased quantities of bicarbonate and sodium are lost in the urine. Thus, a drastic pH change is minimized by the simultaneous elimination of bicarbonate and retention of hydrogen ions.

FACTORS   AFFECTING   ACID-BASE COMPENSATION   In short, many factors interact to regulate acid-base balance in the body. The primary systems involved in maintaining the normal pH of extracellular fluid are the renal and respiratory systems. It thus follows that disease of any major organ that regulates either nephron function or respiratory activity could affect acid-base balance. A summary of some of the major factors that might indirectly affect acid-base status is presented in Table 7.4.

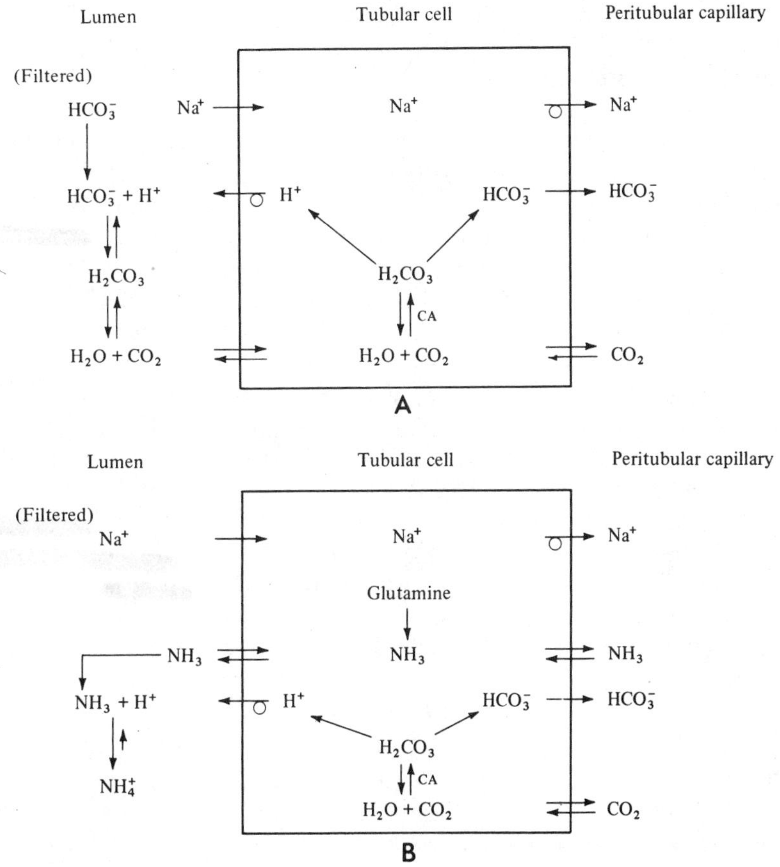

Figure 7.7 Mechanisms for renal excretion of hydrogen and reabsorption of bicarbonate. (A) H^+ eliminated as water (H_2O); (B) H^+ eliminated as ammonium (NH_4^+). (From Rose, B. D.: Clinical Physiology of Acid-Base and Electrolyte Disorders. New York, McGraw-Hill Book Company, 1977. Used by permission.)

ACID-BASE IMBALANCE

The intricacy of the mechanisms that maintain acid-base balance suggests the significance and delicacy of this aspect of homeostasis. In the following pages, many serious imbalances that often develop clinically will be examined.

Before proceeding to a study of pathology, however, it is important to clarify a number of concepts that are central to an understanding of deviations from the acid-base norm:

1. The ideal pH of extracellular fluid is 7.35 to 7.45.

2. When the plasma pH is 7.35 to 7.45,

TABLE 7.4   Some Major Factors that Affect Renal or Respiratory Activity

Functional Activity Affected	Factor	Significance
RESPIRATORY	Cardiovascular status	The diffusion of respiratory gases is dependent upon an adequate alveolar blood supply.
	Neural status	Respiratory rate is regulated by the medulla.
	Skeletomuscular status	Certain muscles control the processes of inspiration and expiration.
RENAL	Cardiovascular status	Renal filtration is dependent upon the maintenance of an adequate glomerular blood pressure.
	Endocrine status	The hormones aldosterone and ADH function in the regulation of urine composition.
	Neural status	The hypothalamus manufactures ADH.

the ratio of H_2CO_3 to HCO_3^- in extracellular fluid is 1:20. This statement is based upon chemical equilibrium considerations and must be accepted as a given.

3. If the normal H_2CO_3/HCO_3^- ratio is altered, the pH of extracellular fluid will change.

4. Conversely, if the pH of extracellular fluid deviates from the norm, one can assume that the ratio between H_2CO_3 and HCO_3^- has changed.

The significance of these points will become apparent as we examine acid-base imbalances in the body. At present, suffice it to say that laboratory information about plasma pH, carbonic acid levels, and HCO_3^- concentration in extracellular fluid is essential to the analysis and diagnosis of acidosis or alkalosis. Although the interpretation of pH laboratory values is fairly straightforward, laboratory data reflecting H_2CO_3 and HCO_3^- levels can be somewhat perplexing.

Laboratory slips, for example, typically report pCO_2 values instead of giving a direct measure of the concentration of H_2CO_3. The pCO_2 value normally ranges from 35 to 50 mm. Hg and is a measure of the pressure exerted by dissolved carbon dioxide in the plasma (technically referred to as *partial pressure*). It is elevated if dissolved CO_2 concentration is high and depressed with decreases in extracellular fluid CO_2. Since dissolved CO_2 gas frequently combines with water in extracellular fluid to form H_2CO_3, elevations or depressions in pCO_2 reflect similar changes in carbonic acid concentration.

It must be remembered, however, that only a small percentage of the CO_2 gas generated by cellular metabolism does dissolve in plasma. By far the largest proportion of CO_2 (approximately 95 per cent) is converted to HCO_3^- in the erythrocytes by a series of reactions described in Chapter 2. The majority of this bicarbonate then diffuses out into plasma, accounting for the high proportion of HCO_3^- in extracellular fluid. Since such a high percentage of CO_2 is normally transported in the form of HCO_3^-, a laboratory measure of *plasma total CO_2 content* (normally 20 to 30 mEq./L.) is actually a very good indicator of HCO_3^- concentration.

Acidosis

Acidosis, in general, is characterized by either an increase of acid or a decrease of base in extracellular fluid. Regardless of the precipitating cause, the cardinal symptoms include the following:

1. A depression in plasma pH.

2. An alteration in the normal 1:20 ratio of H_2CO_3/HCO_3^-. In acidosis, the level of H_2CO_3 may increase while HCO_3^- remains constant. This can result in a new ratio such as 2:20 (1:10). It is also possible to lose excess HCO_3^- while H_2CO_3 stays constant. This might be reflected in an altered ratio such as 1:15.

3. A depression of the central nervous system manifested by possible delirium and coma.

4. Indications of hypercalcemia accompanying the increased ionization of calcium in an acid environment.

5. Indications of hyperkalemia as H^+ shifts into intracellular fluid and potassium ions move into the interstitial compartment to maintain electrical neutrality.

Acidosis is categorized as either *respiratory* or *metabolic*, depending upon the underlying pathophysiology. Respiratory acidosis develops usually as a result of pulmonary disease. It may, however, be associated with any dysfunction characterized by an increase in plasma CO_2 levels. Since the excess carbon dioxide combines with plasma water to form carbonic acid, increases in plasma H_2CO_3 levels are characteristic. Metabolic acidosis, on the other hand, can result from any disorder other than a respiratory one. It is caused by increased levels of an acid other than carbonic acid or by increased output of base.

RESPIRATORY ACIDOSIS: CAUSES

Respiratory acidosis is characterized by an increase in pCO_2, leading to a subsequent elevation in H_2CO_3. It results from any disorder that impairs carbon dioxide output or increases carbon dioxide production. Causes could thus include: (1) disorders resulting in poor diffusion of carbon dioxide from the alveoli into the respiratory tree; (2) disorders resulting in inadequacy of the expiratory process; (3) disorders resulting in depression of respiratory rate or depth; and (4) disorders resulting in the excessive production of carbon dioxide.

Examples of *impaired carbon dioxide diffusion* are commonly seen in patients with COPD (chronic obstructive pulmonary disease). Characteristic obstructive conditions include asthma, bronchitis, and emphysema. The evolution of these disorders will be covered in Unit 3. At this point suffice it to say that alveolar tissue deterioration results in obstruction of the normal carbon dioxide diffusion process.

Inadequacy of the expiratory process can be seen in a variety of clinical situations. Instances of crushed chest trauma, abdominal or thoracic surgery, abdominal binders, blocked airway during choking, and weakness or paralysis of expiratory muscles all tend to impede the depth or efficiency of expiration.

Cases of *depressed respiratory rate or depth* can often be seen accompanying: (1) the use of certain narcotic or sedative drugs, such as morphine; (2) the improper adjustment of an artificial ventilator; and (3) certain central nervous system disorders.

Alternatively, *increases in the production of carbon dioxide* are commonly associated with excessive elevation of metabolic rate. Causes include fever and endocrine imbalances such as hyperthyroidism.

Regardless of the nature of the underlying disease, patients with respiratory acidosis present a rather uniform clinical picture. One can expect to see evidence of depression of the central nervous system, with possible irritability, drowsiness, and hallucinations. There may be an elevation in the rate and depth of respirations (Kussmaul respirations) as the body attempts to compensate for the acidosis. Unfortunately, however, as carbon dioxide accumulates excessively or chronically in the extracellular fluid, it tends to eventually depress the respiratory center of the medulla, resulting in increasingly poor ventilation and shallow respirations. Symptoms of tachycardia and arrhythmia often develop owing to the direct stimulatory effects of increased carbon dioxide upon cardiac activity. Furthermore, if hypercalcemia or hyperkalemia does develop, an entire syndrome of symptoms that relate specifically to these electrolyte disturbances will be precipitated.

RESPIRATORY ACIDOSIS: LABORATORY VALUES

Laboratory values depend, to a large degree, upon whether and to what extent the acidosis is compensated. For this reason, it is worth looking at the mechanisms of compensation for respiratory acidosis and noting how laboratory values can reflect a patient's status.

UNCOMPENSATED RESPIRATORY ACIDOSIS For simplicity's sake, it is better to first consider a *theoretical* picture of totally uncompensated respiratory acidosis. It is important to keep in mind that this case is presented purely for teaching purposes. It would be impossible to observe such a situation clinically.

In the uncompensated state, one would see:

1. A depression of plasma pH below 7.35.

2. An elevation of pCO_2 due to decreased output or excessive production of CO_2.

3. A normal HCO_3^- level, since renal compensation has not yet come into play.

4. A disruption of the normal 1:20 H_2CO_3/HCO_3^- ratio as H_2CO_3 concentration increases while HCO_3^- levels remain unchanged.

COMPENSATED RESPIRATORY ACIDOSIS Since respiratory acidosis is usually caused by a disorder in carbon dioxide expiration, compensation entails utilization of mechanisms other than respiratory ones in attempts to bring the pH back to normal. As a result, it is the *renal system* that is most effective in helping to compensate for respiratory acidosis. Within 24 hours, one can expect to see increased retention of HCO_3^- to balance the elevated H_2CO_3 levels. Thus, laboratory values would reflect an increased pCO_2 accompanied by a significant elevation in HCO_3^-. The

TABLE 7.5   **Respiratory Acidosis: A Comparative Summary of the Uncompensated and the Compensated State**

Type of Respiratory Acidosis	pH	pCO_2	HCO_3^- Concentration	H_2CO_3/HCO_3^- Ratio
Uncompensated	Below 7.35—owing to increases in plasma H_2CO_3	Elevated—owing to insufficient elimination and/or increased production of CO_2	Normal	Elevation of carbonic acid causes ratio to favor carbonic acid (2/20; 3/20, and so forth)
Compensated	7.35–7.45	Elevated—owing to persistence of disease state	Elevated—owing to compensatory renal retention of HCO_3^-	Return to norm of 1/20 as elevation in carbonic acid is balanced by increases in retained HCO_3^-

ideal, of course, is to retain sufficient bicarbonate to bring the carbonic acid–bicarbonate ratio back to 1:20. In reality, the ratio can lie anywhere between the uncompensated theoretical value and the 1:20 norm. Only when the ratio is restored to 1:20 will the pH return to the 7.35 to 7.45 range.

In the totally compensated state, one would see:

1. A pH of 7.35 to 7.45.

2. An elevation of pCO_2 above 40 mm. Hg, indicating continued respiratory dysfunction.

3. An elevation of HCO_3^- above 30 mEq./L., indicating compensatory renal retention of bicarbonate.

4. An acidic urine with increased levels of NH_4^+, indicating renal compensatory elimination of excess H^+.

5. A restoration of the 1:20 ratio between H_2CO_3 and HCO_3^-.

Some primary distinctions between compensated and uncompensated respiratory acidosis are presented in Table 7.5.

METABOLIC ACIDOSIS: CAUSES

Metabolic acidosis can be caused by a variety of clinical disorders. Elevations in the concentration of nonvolatile acids can be caused by an increased intake of acidic substances, such as salicylic acid or boric acid. More commonly, however, acid levels increase as a result of altered metabolic patterns.

Anoxia, or hypoxia, for example, will result in the initiation of *anaerobic metabolism*, which, in turn, causes the accumulation of *lactic acid* (see Chapter 2). Hence, any disorders that reduce the supply of cellular oxygen will induce the development of metabolic acidosis. Examples include cardiac arrest or failure, occlusion of blood vessels, depressed inspiration, decreased diffusion of oxygen into the pulmonary capillaries, anemia, and decreases in environmental oxygen levels.

Alternatively, any disorders that inhibit the ability of the body to use carbohydrates effectively promote the mobilization of fats and proteins for energy generation. As described in Chapter 2, fat and protein mobilization is accompanied by increased generation of intermediary acidic *ketone bodies*. Hence, acidosis develops. This type of metabolic disorder may occur in the untreated diabetic (whose lack of insulin renders him or her unable to utilize carbohydrates), individuals on low-carbohydrate diets, and individuals subjected to general nutritional starvation.

Even in cases characterized by normal metabolic patterns, nonvolatile acids can accumulate if excretory routes are blocked. Hence, metabolic acidosis will inevitably accompany cases of renal failure.

It can be seen that metabolic acidosis is commonly caused by disorders that promote increases of nonvolatile acids in the extracellular fluid. Metabolic acidosis can also result from *excessive loss of base bicarbonate.* Clinically, this type of loss is most often associated with increased output of lower gastrointestinal contents. Since pancreatic and small intestinal secretions tend to be alkaline by nature, prolonged diarrhea, lower gastrointestinal drainage, or vomiting of intestinal contents can precipitate metabolic acidosis.

Many of the symptoms accompanying metabolic acidosis mirror those of respiratory acidosis. They thus include indications of central nervous system depression, Kussmaul respirations, and possible hyperkalemia or hypercalcemia with accompany cardiac irritability and neuromuscular changes.

METABOLIC ACIDOSIS: LABORATORY VALUES

Once again, in considering the laboratory values of the patient with metabolic acidosis, it is helpful to compare the compensated and the uncompensated states.

UNCOMPENSATED METABOLIC ACIDOSIS It must be remembered that one cannot expect to see a clinical case of totally uncompensated metabolic acidosis. Nevertheless, examination of theoretical laboratory values can be useful in elucidating the underlying mechanisms of compensation. As metabolic acidosis first evolves, one would expect to see:

1. A pH of less than 7.35.
2. A pCO_2 within normal limits, since respiratory compensation has not yet come into play.
3. A depression of HCO_3^- levels caused by (a) increased clinical loss of base bicarbonate, or (b) conversion of buffer bicarbonate to carbonic acid as excess nonvolatile acids are neutralized.
4. A disruption in the normal 1:20 H_2CO_3/HCO_3^- ratio as HCO_3^- concentration decreases.

COMPENSATED METABOLIC ACIDOSIS It is significant to note that in cases of metabolic acidosis, compensation is effected primarily by the respiratory system. Thus, the laboratory values in cases of totally compensated metabolic acidosis reflect excess output of carbon dioxide as follows:

1. A pH of 7.35 to 7.45.
2. A depression of HCO_3^- concentration, indicating ongoing dysfunction.
3. A depression of pCO_2, indicating compensatory respiratory response to acidosis.
4. A restoration of the 1:20 ratio between H_2CO_3 and HCO_3^-.

Some major differences between compensated and uncompensated metabolic acidosis are summarized in Table 7.6.

TABLE 7.6 Metabolic Acidosis: A Comparative Summary of the Uncompensated and the Compensated States

Type of Metabolic Acidosis	pH	pCO_2	HCO_3^- Concentration	H_2CO_3/HCO_3 Ratio
Uncompensated	Below 7.35—owing to decreases in plasma HCO_3^-	Normal	Depressed—owing to clinical loss of HCO_3^-, or conversion of buffer HCO_3^- into carbonic acid (as excess nonvolatile acids are neutralized)	Decreases in bicarbonate causes ratio to favor H_2CO_3 (1/15; 1/10, and so forth)
Compensated	7.35–7.45	Depressed—owing to compensatory respiratory elimination of CO_2 (H_2CO_3)	Depressed—owing to persistence of causative disorders	Return to norm of 1/20 as decreases in HCO_3^- are balanced by compensatory elimination of CO_2 (H_2CO_3)

TABLE 7.7 Respiratory and Metabolic Acidosis: A Comparative Summary

Type of Acidosis	Origin of Acidosis	Primary Characteristics	Primary Compensation Mechanism
Respiratory	Excessive generation or retention of plasma carbon dioxide	↑ pCO_2 ↑ HCO_3^- (with compensation)	Renal retention of bicarbonate
Metabolic	Elevation in plasma levels of nonvolatile acids or decrease of base in extracellular fluid, or both	↓ HCO_3^- ↓ pCO_2 (with compensation)	Respiratory elimination of carbon dioxide; renal retention of bicarbonate

ACIDOSIS: A SUMMARY

There are several similarities between respiratory and metabolic acidosis. Both conditions share many signs and symptoms, although causes, compensations, and laboratory values differ. A comparative summary of respiratory and metabolic acidosis is presented in Table 7.7.

In reviewing the changes associated with hydrogen excess, it is significant to note that a wide range of systemic dysfunction can be precipitated by acidosis. Some of the major organs and structures characteristically affected are shown in Figure 7.8.

Alkalosis

Alkalosis, is a condition generally characterized by a decrease of acid or an increase of base in the extracellular fluid. Regardless of cause, some primary symptoms include:

1. An elevation in plasma pH.
2. An alteration in the normal 1:20 ratio of H_2CO_3/HCO_3^-. In alkalosis, the level of H_2CO_3 may decrease while that of HCO_3^- remains constant. This results in a new ratio such as 0.5:20 (1:40). Conversely, it is also possible for the base to increase while acid levels remain unchanged. The altered ratio would then move in the direction of 1:30 or 1:40.

3. An excitation of the central nervous system reflected by hyperirritability, disorientation, and heightened reflex responses.
4. Possible symptoms of hypocalcemia, as alkalosis causes decreased ionization of extracellular fluid calcium.
5. Possible hypokalemia, as kidneys retain H^+ (to compensate for alkalosis) and excrete positively charged K^+ ions in the urine (in an attempt to maintain electrical neutrality).

As in the case of acidosis, alkalosis is categorized as either *respiratory* or *metabolic*, depending upon underlying causes. Respiratory alkalosis, for example, is precipitated by any clinical disorder that promotes increases in carbon dioxide output. As a result of eliminating excessive CO_2, the level of H_2CO_3 in the extracellular fluid falls, thereby inducing alkalosis. Metabolic alkalosis, on the other hand, is characterized by an excessive loss of any acid, other than H_2CO_3, or by an elevation of base in the extracellular fluid.

RESPIRATORY ALKALOSIS: CAUSES

Respiratory alkalosis is caused most often by a pathological state that promotes an increase in respiratory rate and depth. Clinical causes of such elevations vary widely, and in-

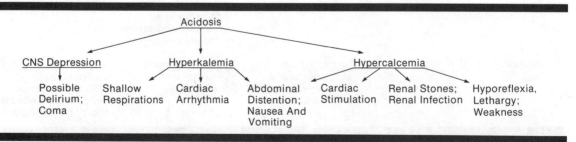

Figure 7.8 Clinical manifestations of acidosis.

clude:

1. Elevated temperature (fever). It is predicted that respiratory rate will increase approximately 10 respirations per minute for every 1° F. increase in temperature.

2. Hypoxia at high altitudes. Depressed oxygen levels will stimulate the medulla directly to initiate a compensatory increase in respiratory rate.

3. A poorly adjusted mechanical ventilator, promoting excessive output of carbon dioxide.

4. Anxiety and tension. It has been noted that anxiety and tension will often lead to subconscious episodes of deep sighing or hyperventilation, which cause excessive carbon dioxide output.

5. Pain, which is often accompanied by hyperventilation.

6. Central nervous system trauma. In certain cases, CNS disorders may be accompanied by hyperventilation.

7. Drugs. Some drugs, such as aspirin, if taken in excess, often cause hyperventilation.

Typical symptoms of respiratory alkalosis include those listed previously. Characteristically noted are the numb tingling fingers, carpopedal spasms, cardiac arrhythmias, and tetany that often accompany hypocalcemia.

RESPIRATORY ALKALOSIS: LABORATORY VALUES

As with cases of acid-base imbalance, it is helpful to contrast the laboratory values of the theoretically uncompensated patient with those of the compensated individual.

UNCOMPENSATED RESPIRATORY ALKALOSIS In theoretical cases of uncompensated respiratory alkalosis, one would expect to see:

1. A pH greater than 7.45.

2. Depression in pCO_2 values due to excessive elimination of carbon dioxide.

3. Normal HCO_3^- levels, since renal compensation has not yet taken effect.

4. Disruption in the normal 1:20 H_2CO_3/HCO_3^- ratio as H_2CO_3 decreases while HCO_3^- remains constant.

COMPENSATED RESPIRATORY ALKALOSIS In cases of respiratory alkalosis, the primary compensation mechanism is renal. Once compensation is complete, one can expect to see:

1. A pH within the normal limits of 7.35 to 7.45.

2. A depression in pCO_2, indicating an ongoing expiratory disorder.

3. Depressed HCO_3^- levels, as the kidneys compensate for alkalosis by eliminating bicarbonate.

4. A return of the H_2CO_3/HCO_3^- ratio to a norm of 1:20.

Some primary distinctions between compensated and uncompensated respiratory alkalosis are summarized in Table 7.8.

TABLE 7.8 **Respiratory Alkalosis: A Comparative Summary of the Uncompensated and the Compensated States**

Type of Respiratory Alkalosis	pH	pCO$_2$	HCO$_3^-$ Concentration	H$_2$CO$_3$/HCO$_3^-$ Ratio
Uncompensated	Above 7.45—owing to decreases in plasma H$_2$CO$_3$	Depressed—owing to excessive elimination of CO$_2$ (H$_2$CO$_3$)	Normal	Depression of CO$_2$ (H$_2$CO$_3$) causes ratio to favor HCO$_3^-$ (0.5/20→1/40; 0.2/20→1/100)
Compensated	7.35–7.45	Depressed—owing to persistence of disease state	Depressed—owing to elimination of HCO$_3^-$	Return to norm of 1/20 as depression in H$_2$CO$_3$ is balanced by compensatory elimination of HCO$_3^-$

TABLE 7.9   **Metabolic Alkalosis: A Comparative Summary of the Uncompensated and the Compensated States**

Type of Metabolic Alkalosis	pH	pCO$_2$	HCO$_3^-$ Concentration	H$_2$CO$_3$/HCO$_3^-$ Ratio
Uncompensated	Above 7.35–owing to increases in plasma HCO$_3^-$	Normal	Elevated–owing to clinical retention of HCO$_3^-$, or conversion of buffer H$_2$CO$_3$ into HCO$_3^-$ (as excess plasma bases are neutralized)	Increases in bicarbonate cause ratio to favor HCO$_3$ (1/30; 1/40, and so forth)
Compensated	7.35–7.45	Elevated–owing to compensatory respiratory retention of CO$_2$ (H$_2$CO$_3$)	Elevated–owing to persistence of disease state	Return to norm of 1/20 as increases in HCO$_3^-$ are balanced by compensatory retention of CO$_2$ (H$_2$CO$_3$)

TABLE 7.10   **Respiratory and Metabolic Alkalosis: A Comparative Summary**

Type of Alkalosis	Origin of Alkalosis	Primary Characteristics	Primary Compensation Mechanism
Respiratory	Excessive elimination of plasma carbon dioxide	↓ pCO$_2$ ↓ HCO$_3^-$ (with compensation)	Renal retention of hydrogen ions and elimination of bicarbonate
Metabolic	Depletion of nonvolatile acids or increases of base in extracellular fluid, or both	↑ HCO$_3^-$ ↑ pCO$_2$ (with compensation)	Respiratory retention of carbon dioxide Renal elimination of bicarbonate and retention of hydrogen ions

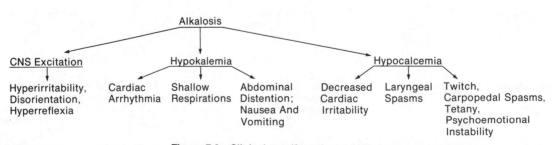

Figure 7.9 Clinical manifestations of alkalosis.

METABOLIC ALKALOSIS: CAUSES

Metabolic alkalosis, as described earlier, is characterized either by excessively high levels of base or by depressed concentrations of acid in the extracellular fluid. Cases of excessively high base levels are seen clinically in patients who ingest chronically high doses of alkaline medication (such as antacids). Acid loss, however, is a more common cause of metabolic alkalosis. Excessive output of gastric content associated with vomiting, gastric lavage, or gastric suction results in alkalosis.

Symptoms of metabolic alkalosis are often similar to those of respiratory alkalosis. In addition, as the respiratory system attempts to compensate for the acid-base imbalance, a depression in respiratory rate, with possible cyanosis and decreased thoracic movements, is likely to be noted.

METABOLIC ALKALOSIS: LABORATORY VALUES

As one contrasts the laboratory values for compensated and uncompensated metabolic alkalosis, the underlying mechanisms of this acid-base disturbance become clear.

UNCOMPENSATED METABOLIC ALKALOSIS In the theoretically uncompensated state, one could expect to see:

1. A pH of greater than 7.45.
2. An elevated bicarbonate level caused by: (a) the combination of any excess base (other than HCO_3^-) with H_2CO_3 to form bicarbonate, or (b) the retention of negatively charged HCO_3^- to compensate for any loss of Cl^- through the upper gastrointestinal tract.
3. Normal pCO_2 levels, since respiratory compensation has not been activated.

4. An alteration in the normal 1:20 H_2CO_3/HCO_3^- ratio as bicarbonate levels increase while carbonic acid concentrations remain unchanged.

COMPENSATED METABOLIC ALKALOSIS Once respiratory compensation has been initiated, one would expect to see a move toward normal laboratory values. The kidneys, however, must also support compensation if equilibrium conditions are to be fully re-established. In the completely compensated state, one would see:

1. A pH of 7.35 to 7.45.
2. An elevation in HCO_3^- level, indicating continued dysfunction.
3. An elevation in pCO_2 as the respiratory system compensates by retaining carbon dioxide.
4. Alkaline urine, as urinary output of HCO_3^- increases, and elimination of H^+ (NH_4^+) decreases.
5. A return of the H_2CO_3/HCO_3^- ratio to 1:20.

A comparative summary of compensated and uncompensated metabolic alkalosis can be found in Table 7.9.

ALKALOSIS: A SUMMARY

In retrospect, it can be seen that there are a number of similarities and quite a few differences between metabolic and respiratory alkalosis. A brief comparative summary of these two imbalances can be found in Table 7.10.

It is important to keep in mind that alkalosis, like acidosis, can precipitate dysfunction in a variety of organs and structures and, in this way, initiate far-reaching physiological dysfunction. A summary of some of the systems affected by alkalosis is presented in Figure 7.9.

STUDY QUESTIONS

1. Given a test tube of each of the following acids (in equivalent concentrations), determine which tubes would have the lowest pH and which the highest.

pyruvic acid
nitric acid (HNO_3)
hydrochloric acid (HCl)
citric acid
sulfuric acid (H_2SO_4)
lactic acid
carbonic acid (H_2CO_3)

2. Identify the normal mode of elimination for each of the following:
   a. lactic acid
   b. carbonic acid
   c. bicarbonate
   d. uric acid

3. Under which of the following circumstances would plasma pCO_2 predictably increase?
   a. renal failure
   b. respiratory obstruction
   c. hyperventilation
   d. hyperthyroidism
   e. starvation

4. What chemical formula defines the relationship between pCO_2 and carbonic acid in the plasma?

5. Under which of the following circumstances would nonvolatile acids predictably accumulate in the extracellular fluid?
   a. untreated diabetes mellitus
   b. anemia
   c. extensive diarrhea
   d. gastric vomiting
   e. respiratory depression
   f. renal failure

6. Explain the derivation of bicarbonate in the plasma.

7. Determine whether a patient is in a state of acidosis, alkalosis, or acid-base balance when the plasma pH is:
   a. 7.1
   b. 6.9
   c. 7.8
   d. 7.4

8. Describe one way to *correct* for respiratory acidosis that develops secondary to bacterial pneumonia.

9. In each of the following cases, determine whether the H_2CO_3 or HCO_3^- component of the buffer system would be active in attempting to normalize plasma pH:
   a. prolonged starvation
   b. renal failure
   c. excessive intake of alkaline medication

10. Within 48 hours after the onset of metabolic acidosis, would you expect the following laboratory values to be elevated or depressed? Why?
    a. plasma HCO_3^-
    b. urinary NH_4^+
    c. pCO_2
    d. urinary pH

11. Within 48 hours after the onset of respiratory alkalosis, would you expect the laboratory values (listed in question 10) to be elevated or depressed? Why?

12. A patient is in a state of respiratory failure. Describe the regulatory and compensatory mechanisms that would be functional in attempting to restore acid-base equilibrium.

13. You are caring for a patient who is in a state of compensated metabolic alkalosis. What would be the ratio between bicarbonate and carbonic acid in his or her extracellular fluid?

Suggested Readings

Books

Burgess, A.: The Nurses' Guide to Fluid and Electrolyte Balance, 2nd ed. New York, McGraw-Hill Book Company, 1979, pp. 77–86; 205–215.

Burke, S. R.: The Composition and Function of Body Fluids, 2nd ed. St. Louis, The C. V. Mosby Company, 1976, pp. 56–83.

Davenport, H. W.: The ABC of Acid-Base Chemistry, 6th ed. Chicago, University of Chicago Press, 1974.

Guyton, A. C.: Textbook of Medical Physiology, 5th ed. Philadelphia, W. B. Saunders Company, 1976, pp. 485–500.

Hills, A. G.: Acid-Base Balance. Baltimore, The Williams & Wilkins Company, 1973.

Jones, D. A., Dunbar, C. F., and Jirovec, M. M.: Medical-Surgical Nursing, A Conceptual Approach. New York, McGraw-Hill Book Company, 1978, pp. 464–470.

Lee, C.: Acid base imbalance: How to recognize it. *In* Hamilton, H. (ed.): Monitoring Fluids and Electrolytes Precisely. Nursing 79 Books. Horsham, Pa., Intermed Communications, Inc., 1978, p. 67.

Lennon, E. J.: Body buffering mechanisms. *In* Frolich, E. D. (ed.): Pathophysiology, Altered Regulatory Mechanisms in Disease, 2nd ed. Philadelphia, J. B. Lippincott Company, 1976, p. 287.

Luckmann, J., and Sorensen, K. C.: Medical-Surgical Nursing, A Psychophysiologic Approach, 2nd ed. Philadelphia, W. B. Saunders Company, 1980, pp. 182–198.

Masoro, E. J., and Siegel, P. D.: Acid-Base Regulation: Its Physiology, Pathophysiology, and the Interpretation of Blood-Gas Analysis, 2nd ed. Philadelphia, W. B. Saunders Company, 1977.

Metheny, N. M., and Snively, W. D.: Nurse's Handbook of Fluid Balance, 3rd ed. Philadelphia, J. B. Lippincott Company, 1979, pp. 85–96.

Pflanzer, R. G., and Tanner, G. A.: Acid-base regulation. In Selkurt, E. E. (ed.): Basic Physiology for the Health Sciences, Boston, Little, Brown & Company, 1975, p. 519.

Reed, G. M., and Sheppard, V. F.: Regulation of Fluid and Electrolyte Balance: A Programmed Instruction in Clinical Physiology, 2nd ed. Philadelphia, W. B. Saunders Company, 1977, pp. 157–216.

Robinson, J. R.: Fundamentals of Acid-Base Regulation, 4th ed. Philadelphia, J. B. Lippincott Company, 1972.

Stroot, V. R., Lee, C. A., and Schaper, C. A.: Fluids and Electrolytes: A Practical Approach, 2nd ed. Philadelphia, F. A. Davis Company, 1977, pp. 83–111.

Weldy, N. J.: Body Fluids and Electrolytes — A Programmed Presentation, 3rd ed. St. Louis, The C. V. Mosby Company, 1980, pp. 39–68.

Woodbury, J. W.: Body acid-base state and its regulation. In Ruch, T. C., and Patton, H. D. (eds.): Physiology and Biophysics. Vol II. Philadelphia, W. B. Saunders Company, 1974.

Articles

Cohen, S.: Metabolic acid-base disorders. Part 1: Chemistry and physiology. Programmed instruction. Am. J. Nurs., 77:(PI insert), 1977.

Cohen, S.: Metabolic acid-base disorders. Part 2: Physiological abnormalities and nursing actions. Programmed instruction. Am. J. Nurs., 78:(PI p. 1), 1978.

Cohen, S.: Metabolic acid-base disorders. Part 3: Clinical and laboratory findings. Am. J. Nurs., 78:(PI p. 1), 1978.

Lee, C. A., Stroot, V. R., and Schaper, C. A.: What to do when acid-base problems hang in the balance. Nursing 75, 5:32, 1975.

Sharer, J. E.: Reviewing acid-base balance. Am. J. Nurs., 75:980, 1975.

Sieger, P.: The physiologic approach to acid-base balance. MCNA, 57:863, 1973.

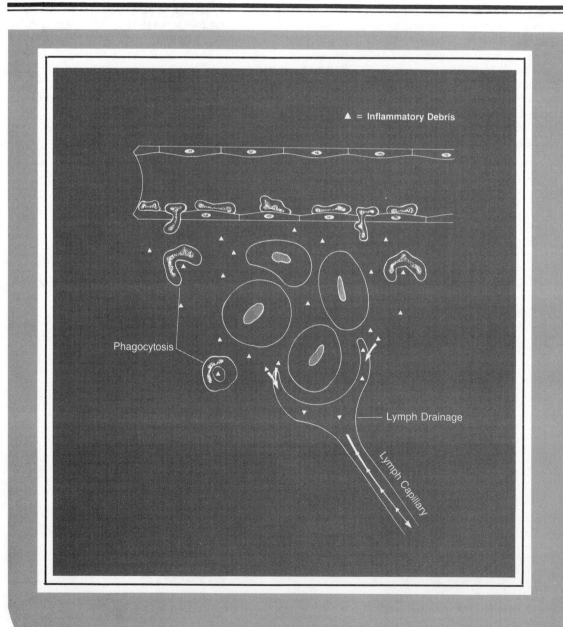

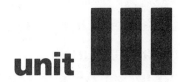

The Evolution of Disease in Some Critical Systems

Throughout earlier chapters, it was shown that many systems in the body work jointly to service the basic cellular survival needs. Conversely, maintenance of the cell is essential to the support of systemic health. To the extent that stress initiates cellular dysfunction, organs and systems in the body can eventually be affected. In a chain-reaction fashion, disorders that significantly alter the status of the cell frequently precipitate further dysfunction.

An understanding of systemic disorders requires a working knowledge of the underlying processes whereby individual cells of the body respond to stress. Only in this way can one acquire a deep-seated appreciation for the intricacies of pathophysiology. Toward this end, an overview of cellular level response patterns to stress (such as inflammation, hypertrophy, and hypersensitivity) is followed by specific examination of disease in five major systems: cardiovascular, respiratory, gastrointestinal, renal, and nervous. Diseases of metabolic, endocrine, and hematopoietic origin will not be treated separately in this Unit. Instead, they are integrated into chapters where they fit most appropriately.

Although disorders are classified systemically for the sake of clarity, it is important to remember that pathophysiology is, in reality, a dynamic and ongoing process that defies arbitrary categorization. In much the same way that one domino in a carefully balanced standing row can initiate the fall of many neighboring pieces, so disease originating at one point can eventually affect a variety of secondary organs. In essence, the complex realities of pathological states pose a truly challenging and changing puzzle for the clinician to solve.

Chapter Outline

INTRODUCTION

SOURCES OF STRESS

NONADAPTIVE CELLULAR RESPONSES TO STRESS

ADAPTIVE CELLULAR RESPONSES TO STRESS
Changes in the Structural Characteristics of the Cell
HYPERTROPHY
HYPERPLASIA
The Inflammation and Repair Response
MAJOR COMPONENTS OF THE INFLAMMATORY MECHANISM
Vascular Changes
Phagocytic Activity
THE CLINICAL MANIFESTATIONS OF INFLAMMATION
Local Effects of Inflammation
Serous Exudate
Fibrinous Exudate
Purulent-Suppurative Exudate
Hemorrhagic Exudate
Systemic Effects of Inflammation
THE RESOLUTION OF INFLAMMATION
Regeneration
Scar Formation
The Resolution of Inflammation: An Illustrative Example
NONADAPTIVE INFLAMMATION
Inappropriate Target
Secondary Dysfunction
SUPPRESSION OF THE INFLAMMATORY RESPONSE
Natural Suppression
Deficiency of Blood Supply
Inadequate Migration of Phagocytic Cells
Insufficient Function of Phagocytic Cells
Inadequate Support of the Inflammatory Mechanism by the Immune System
Artificially Induced Suppression
THE INFLAMMATION AND REPAIR RESPONSE: A SUMMARY
The Immune Response
IMMUNE CELLS
T-Lymphocytes
B-Lymphocytes
FACILITATORS OF THE IMMUNE RESPONSE
NONADAPTIVE IMMUNE RESPONSES
Immediate or Anaphylactic Type Hypersensitivity
Cytotoxic Type Hypersensitivity
Immune Complex–Mediated Hypersensitivity
Cell-Mediated Hypersensitivity
Adaptive Cellular Responses to Stress: A Summary
NEOPLASMS
Benign Growths
Malignant Growths
BEHAVIORAL CHARACTERISTICS
CELLULAR CHARACTERISTICS
CELLULAR RESPONSES TO STRESS: A SUMMARY

142

chapter **8**

Cellular Responses to Stress

Chapter Objectives

At the completion of this chapter, the student will be able to:

1. Define stress and list five major sources of cellular stress.
2. Define necrosis and identify two major cellular changes that often precede necrosis.
3. Differentiate between coagulation, liquefaction, and caseous necrosis.
4. Identify and describe two diagnostic tools that may be utilized to confirm the existence of necrosis.
5. List three adaptive cellular responses to stress.
6. Distinguish between hyperplasia and hypertrophy.
7. Describe the inflammatory process with respect to vascular changes, phagocytic activity, clinical manifestations, and resolution.
8. Define nonadaptive inflammation and give some clinical examples of this phenomenon.
9. Describe two major mechanisms whereby the inflammatory response may be suppressed.
10. Differentiate between nonspecific and specific immunity.
11. Describe specific immunity with respect to: (a) functional activity of T-lymphocytes and B-lymphocytes, (b) facilitation of the immune response, and (c) the phenomenon of nonadaptive immunity.
12. Define the term *neoplasm* and distinguish between benign and malignant growths.

INTRODUCTION

In the healthy body, individual cells are surrounded by fluid of ideal volume and composition. All major systems contribute to the maintenance of equilibrium, and homeostasis prevails. Unfortunately, however, many external and internal stress factors can act to alter the optimal cellular environment. When this happens, a chain of reactive response is initiated. In some cases, the response mechanism is *nonadaptive* (degenerative) and culminates in the death of the cells. In others, the response pattern results in adjustments that help to combat or compensate for the impinging stress or trauma. These changes are referred to as *adaptive* and are functional in the restoration of health.

In this chapter, a brief introduction to some sources of stress is followed by an analysis of certain nonadaptive and adaptive cellular responses. It is important to realize that, in the clinical setting, disruption of homeostasis is often followed by both degenerative and adaptive changes. If the adaptive reactions are dominant, cellular equilibrium is restored; if not, cellular death results. This concept is illustrated in Figure 8.1.

In the study of disease processes, neoplasms stand apart as the black sheep of pathophysiology. Defying all attempts at definitive

classification, they await solutions to problems about the nature of abnormal cellular growth. Do tumors start growing as an adaptive response to an irritant, which subsequently becomes a nonadaptive response? Are they nonfunctional from their inception? Until such questions can be answered, tumors cannot really be categorized as adaptive or nonadaptive with any degree of certainty. Accordingly, they are discussed in a separate section at the end of the chapter.

It is important to keep in mind that throughout this chapter we are dealing primarily with *cellular level* phenomena. Although the response patterns described may ultimately affect larger organs and systems throughout the body, they occur primarily at the micro- level. Because the body is a summation of its parts, these cellular responses to stress frequently have widespread systemic ramifications. In fact, one cannot understand organic disease without comprehending the processes initiated at the cellular level.

SOURCES OF STRESS

For our purposes, stress is defined as any change or stimulus causing the disruption of cellular homeostasis. Sources of stress can thus include:

1. *mechanical injury* — defined as injury resulting from the application of force or pressure. Examples include fractures, abrasions, contusions, and lacerations.

2. *injury caused by a physical agent* — commonly caused by abnormal environmental conditions (such as excessive fluctuations in heat, cold, or atmospheric pressure) and exposure to electricity or ionizing radiation.

3. *injury caused by a chemical agent* — due to excessive intake of or exposure to toxic chemicals such as drugs, alcohol, and poisons.

4. *injury caused by physiological deficit* — characterized by insufficient supply of certain critical substances such as oxygen or glucose.

5. *infection* — defined as invasion by a parasitic organism that depends upon its host for survival. It is significant to realize that only some microbes cause disease. They are referred to as pathogens. Other microorganisms

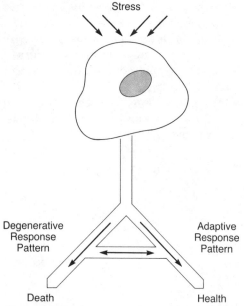

Figure 8.1 Cellular response patterns to stress.

can exist within their host without causing infection.

Although not listed here, congenital or developmental abnormalities may also cause structural and functional changes. Many birth defects, however, do not technically affect cellular homeostasis. Mental retardation, color blindness, clubfoot, and cleft lip, for example, do not lead to physiological disharmony. Congenital disorders will be treated in this text only to the extent that they disrupt the servicing of cellular needs. As such, they can be classified in the above-listed categories according to the specific stress that they induce.

Sickle cell anemia, for example, is a hereditary enzyme disorder that results in the formation of abnormal hemoglobin. Since deficiency in oxygen transport leads to cellular hypoxia, sickle cell anemia is an example of a disease that induces stress through "physiological deficit."

NONADAPTIVE CELLULAR RESPONSES TO STRESS

Under certain circumstances, stress can engender a series of nonadaptive cellular changes that are degenerative in nature. This nonfunctional response pattern is characterized by:

1. *accumulation of water within the cells.* Cells appear cloudy and swollen under the microscope. This change is believed to be due to a failure in the cellular metabolic mechanism and is accompanied by a decrease in the formation of ATP. Loss of available ATP results in an energy deficit, which, in turn, causes failure of the energy-driven sodium-potassium membrane pump. The subsequent loss of selective permeability is believed to cause excessive influx of sodium and water into the intracellular fluid compartment.

2. *accumulation of neutral fat in the cells.* Fat globules deposit abnormally in the cytoplasm and coalesce, pushing the nucleus off to the side. This change occurs commonly in diseased liver cells and is often associated with alcoholism.

Although these changes are reversible, continued or acute stress can bring cells to a point of no return. When this occurs, degenerative changes lead to cellular death.

Cellular death can be defined as the cessation of cellular function or reproduction or both. When a cell dies, the citric acid cycle ceases to operate, but anaerobic glycolysis may continue for a short period of time. As a result, lactic acid is produced, and the pH of adjacent interstitial and intracellular fluid declines.

Cellular death is often accompanied by characteristic structural changes collectively referred to as *necrosis*. Necrosis is commonly caused by anoxia, but it can also be induced by mechanical injury or infection. Stored cellular enzymes are released, promoting a process of cellular self-digestion called *autolysis*. The characteristic microscopic appearance of necrotic cells varies and can be indicative of the cause of death. Some typical patterns include:

1. *coagulation necrosis* — characterized by a firm cytoplasm resembling cooked egg white. It commonly accompanies anoxic injury.

2. *liquefaction necrosis* — frequently resulting from rapid cytoplasmic destruction. It is characterized by liquefied cellular breakdown products and often accompanies suppurative (pus-producing) bacterial infections.

3. *caseous necrosis* — manifested by the formation of cheese-like cellular debris. It follows in the wake of certain infections such as tuberculosis.

The necrotic process is often accompanied by a phenomenon referred to as pathological calcification. For unknown reasons, injured or necrotic tissue that is not immediately digested or removed attracts abnormal deposits of calcium salts. Occasionally, these calcified areas can be visualized on x-rays. In certain cases, therefore, soft tissue calcium deposits may indicate undiagnosed necrosis.

To confirm the presence of necrosis, however, it is helpful to use one of two major diagnostic procedures: microscopic examination or chemical analysis.

1. *Microscopic examination.* Microscopic examination of suspect tissue should reveal the presence of characteristic nuclear changes. With the onset of necrosis, the nucleus normally becomes extremely dense-staining. It is

subsequently either digested or broken into small fragments. All these alterations can be detected under the microscope and help to indicate the extent of necrotic damage.

2. *Chemical analysis.* As necrosis progresses, a number of cellular enzymes often diffuse into the extracellular fluid. Following severe soft tissue injury, for example, there is frequently a detectable elevation in the plasma levels of SGOT (serum glutamic oxaloacetic transaminase), LDH (lactic dehydrogenase), and CPK (creatine phosphokinase). Since the presence of these enzymes can be confirmed by chemical analysis, any significant increase in their concentration reflects the existence of deep-seated necrosis.

In summary, it can be said that stress frequently initiates a chain of nonadaptive cellular responses. Early metabolic abnormalities can terminate in cellular death and necrosis depending on the severity and duration of the causative trauma. It must be remembered, however, that the effect of any cellular level change upon the total organism will depend largely upon the number and type of cells involved. The loss of a small number of cardiac muscle cells, for example, would be more physiologically significant than the death and necrosis of a much larger quantity of connective or epithelial cells.

ADAPTIVE CELLULAR RESPONSES TO STRESS

Fortunately, the cells do not always react to stress in a nonadaptive manner. In many cases response patterns promote compensation for disruptions in equilibrium. The most common adaptive mechanisms include: (1) changes in the structural characteristics of the cell, (2) the inflammation and repair response, and (3) the immune response.

Changes in the Structural Characteristics of the Cell

Most cells in the body manifest the ability to accommodate to changing environmental demands by structural adaptation. In much the same way that we would put on a slicker before going out into a storm, or take off

weight before running in a marathon, the cells can adjust appropriately to changing needs. Two primary adaptive mechanisms available to the cell are *hypertrophy* and *hyperplasia.*

HYPERTROPHY

Hypertrophy can be defined as an increase in the *size* of individual cells. This alteration occurs primarily in response to increased work demands. It is characteristically seen in heavily exercised skeletal muscle; hence, the bulging biceps of the weight lifter.

Cellular enlargement can also occur in response to the need for increased productivity in the vital organs. Typical examples of this phenomenon can be found in the heart and the kidney.

In the case of the renal system, hypertrophy of one kidney often occurs in response to disease or surgical removal of its mate. Cellular enlargement can cause the remaining healthy kidney to increase in size by as much as 100 per cent. In this way, the continued functioning of the renal system is facilitated.

Under certain circumstances, the myocardium will also show evidence of adaptive hypertrophy. To the extent that the muscle of the heart must increase productivity to maintain normal output, cellular enlargement results. In cases of arterial hypertension, for example, the muscle of the left ventricle must work harder to eject blood against a resistive force. Subsequent enlargement of left ventricular cells serves an adaptive purpose unless it proceeds to excess. When this happens, organic functional capacity declines. In much the same way that an excessively overgrown skeletal muscle may lose strength and flexibility, so myocardial hypertrophy beyond a critical point will trigger physiological dysfunction.

HYPERPLASIA

Hyperplasia is defined as an increase in the *number* of individual cells. This change may or may not be accompanied by hypertrophy.

Hyperplasia can be induced by a number of stimuli and under a variety of circumstances. It is commonly seen in the liver, as a response to the loss of hepatic cells through disease or surgery. It is also noted on surface skin (in the form of a protective callus) as an adaptive response to increased mechanical stress.

In considering hypertrophy and hyperplasia, it is important to realize that both these response mechanisms are reversible. Removal of the initially stressful stimulus is often followed by a return to normal growth patterns.

The Inflammation and Repair Response

Inflammation is an inherently adaptive, protective response that can be directed against a variety of stressful stimuli. Although typically accompanied by symptoms of redness, warmth, and pain, it is not by nature a pathological process. It is, perhaps, helpful to regard the characteristic discomfort of inflammation as an unfortunate but necessary auxiliary phenomenon. In much the same way that penicillin, while preventing the development of rheumatic fever, can induce diarrhea, inflammation imposes a penalty upon those who reap its adaptive benefits.

Since the inflammatory process is so essential to the maintenance of health, it is discussed at some length in the following pages. An initial look at the mechanism of inflammation is followed by an analysis of its clinical manifestations and resolution.

Although the inflammatory response is normally beneficial, there are instances in which it functions nonadaptively. These exception conditions, and the means whereby the inflammatory response can be suppressed, are noted at the conclusion of this section.

MAJOR COMPONENTS OF THE INFLAMMATORY MECHANISM

The inflammatory process is actually a series of physiological responses to cellular injury. The ultimate goal of the process is to re-establish equilibrium and pave the way for the repair of damaged tissue. It is typically induced by factors such as infection, ischemia, and necrosis, and it can range in intensity from acute to subacute to chronic. Regardless of differences, however, the basic response pattern consists of two major components: (1) *vascular changes*, and (2) *phagocytic activity*.

VASCULAR CHANGES When stress or trauma disrupts cellular equilibrium, certain chemicals are released at the site of injury. Primary among these are histamine, which is active initially, followed by serotonin and bradykinin. In promoting increased transport of fluid to the damaged area, they act by simultaneously (1) stimulating localized vasodilation of arterioles, precapillary sphincters, and venules, and (2) triggering increased permeability of capillaries and venules.

These vascular changes, illustrated in Figure 8.2, cause the appearance of typical inflammatory symptoms. Vasodilation, for ex-

A. INCREASE IN CAPILLARY PERMEABILITY

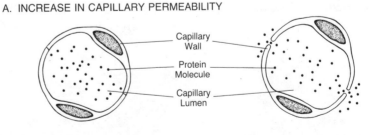

Figure 8.2 The vascular changes associated with inflammation.

B. VASODILATION

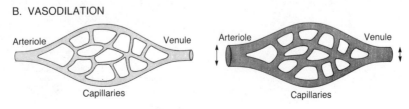

TABLE 8.1 **Clinical Manifestations of Inflammation**

Clinical Symptom	Underlying Causative Mechanism
Redness	Vascular dilation promotes an increased flow of blood to the inflamed site.
Warmth	Vascular dilation promotes the transport of blood to the area of inflammation. Since the temperature of plasma is elevated by the heat of cellular metabolism, warmth is associated with an increase in blood flow.
Edema	An increase in vascular permeability causes fluid and protein to shift from the plasma into the interstitial compartment.
Pain	Fluid pressure associated with the development of edema is believed to be largely responsible for stimulating nerve endings and causing the subsequent transmission of pain impulses from the site of inflammation to the central nervous system.

ample, results in *warmth* and *redness* as a larger volume of blood is brought to the site of injury. Capillary permeability changes, on the other hand, allow for leakage of excessive amounts of fluid and protein out of the vascular tree into the interstitial fluid. This flux is accompanied by characteristic signs of localized *edema, swelling,* and *pain.* The development of clinically evident vascular changes is summarized in Table 8.1.

PHAGOCYTIC ACTIVITY The alterations in diameter and permeability of blood vessels noted during inflammation facilitate the transport of specialized "clean-up" cells into the area of tissue injury. "Clean-up" cells are derived from the blood and are designed to phagocytize, or digest and destroy, foreign protein, necrotic tissue, and bacteria. They are of two primary types:

1. *Neutrophils.* These are white blood cells (WBC's) with many-lobed nuclei and cytoplasm of granular appearance. They arrive at the site of inflammation within 30 to 60 minutes to initiate phagocytic activity. Also called *polymorphonuclear neutrophils, PMN's,* or *polys* (because of their distinctive nuclear appearance), these cells contain many tiny membrane-enclosed enzyme packages called lysozymes. It is, in fact, the intracellular enzymes that digest foreign material at the inflammatory site.

2. *Monocytes.* These are white blood cells with large nonlobed nuclei and nongranular cytoplasm. A number of these cells are found in tissue spaces and are immediately available to encircle and "wall off" foreign particles. Having previously wandered out of plasma to become "fixed" within the interstitial compartment, these monocytes, specifically referred to as *histiocytes,* function to prevent the spread of infection. Additional monocytes normally appear within four to five hours of the initial injury and are referred to as *macrophages,* as they move out of the blood vessel directly into the inflamed tissue. Although late arrivers, they seem to be able to survive longer than neutrophils and under adverse conditions. They are thus particularly effective

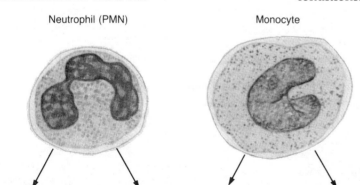

Neutrophil (PMN)   Monocyte

57–67% of Total Leukocytes | Primary Phagocyte during Initial Inflammatory Reaction | 3–7% of Total Leukocytes | Primary Phagocyte in Chronic Inflammation

Figure 8.3 Some differences between neutrophils and monocytes. (Blood cell enlargements reprinted with permission from Jacob, S., Francone, C., and Lossow, W.: Structure and Function in Man. Philadelphia, W. B. Saunders Company, 1978.)

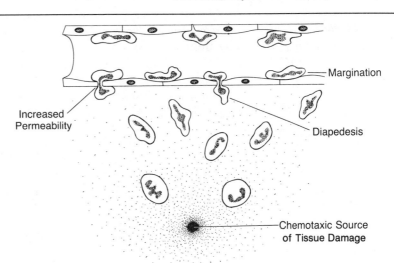

Figure 8.4 Movement of white blood cells by the process of chemotaxis toward an area of tissue damage.

in sustaining phagocytosis at the site of long-term injury.

Some structural and functional differences between neutrophils and monocytes are summarized in Figure 8.3.

Despite the differences between these two types of phagocytic cells, they share many functional similarities. In order to be effective, both neutrophils and monocytes must move out of the vascular system directly into the area of tissue injury. Proceeding in a sequential and directed manner, monocytes and neutrophils prepare for exit from the plasma compartment by flattening themselves against the walls of blood vessels. This phenomenon, called *margination,* is preparatory to the squeezing of these phagocytic cells through blood vessel pores out into the interstitial fluid. Moving in an ameboid fashion by a process called *diapedesis,* they are attracted toward the site of injury by chemical signals emanating from the traumatized area. This responsiveness to chemical stimuli is referred to as *chemotaxis.* The intricate and ordered mechanisms whereby phagocytic blood cells escape from the plasma compartment are illustrated in Figure 8.4.

Ultimately, the goal of phagocytosis is to destroy toxic and foreign substances at the site of inflammation. Toward this end, monocytes and neutrophils are aided by antibodies and other chemicals that are released by immuno-active cells. The immune mechanism and its relationship to the inflammatory response will be discussed later in this chapter.

THE CLINICAL MANIFESTATIONS OF INFLAMMATION

In the clinical setting, evidence of inflammation is usually easy to detect. In addition to the obvious localized changes, there are more subtle systemic effects that often compound the patient's discomfort. A careful look at both local and systemic effects will enhance understanding of the inflammatory process.

LOCAL EFFECTS OF INFLAMMATION At the site of tissue trauma, the inflammatory response generates redness, warmth, swelling, and pain. As mentioned earlier, these symptoms arise as reflections of underlying vascular changes. They are accounted for by the increase in blood flow and vascular permeability at the inflammatory site.

More specifically, it is helpful to look at the nature of the fluid that leaks from capillaries and venules into the interstitial compartment. This fluid, called *exudate*, can vary considerably in composition and often reflects the type of stress that induced its formation. The primary types of inflammatory exudate include: (1) *serous,* (2) *fibrinous,* (3) *purulent-suppurative,* and (4) *hemorrhagic.*

Serous Exudate Serous exudate is composed primarily of plasma fluid and plasma proteins. The fluid is clear and watery, similar to the material that would drain from a ruptured blister. It occurs in cases in which there is only a mild increase in vascular permeability and frequently accumulates in the pleural or peritoneal body cavities at times of cellular stress.

Fibrinous Exudate Fibrinous exudate is similar in composition to serous exudate. It does, however, contain higher concentrations of the protein fibrinogen and the fibrin strands that are derived from this protein. Frequently found on the moist surfaces of inflamed organs, such as the heart and lungs, it coats these structures with a sticky, shaggy, often restrictive deposit.

Purulent-Suppurative Exudate A purulent exudate contains high concentrations of neutrophils and most often accompanies bacterial infection. When the neutrophils accumulate and die, they release potent enzymes, which proceed to digest adjacent tissue. The resulting combination of fluid, dead and live neutrophils, liquefied tissue, and (often) bacteria is called *pus*.

Hemorrhagic Exudate Hemorrhagic exudate contains high concentrations of red blood cells. It usually accompanies severe vascular damage and reflects the leakage of whole blood out of the vascular tree.

SYSTEMIC EFFECTS OF INFLAMMATION Normally the localized manifestations of inflammation are accompanied by a variety of more generalized systemic symptoms. These include fever, increased production of white blood cells (leukocytosis), and vague feelings of generalized discomfort variously manifested as malaise, loss of appetite (anorexia), and weakness.

The mechanisms linking systemic symptoms to cellular level inflammatory activity have not been totally elucidated. In many instances, however, it has been found that chemicals released at the site of tissue injury help to promote systemic changes.

Fever, for example, is believed to be triggered by low molecular weight proteins called *pyrogens* that are released from the inflamma-

tory site directly into the bloodstream. These pyrogens, in turn, stimulate the hypothalamus of the brain to generate an elevation in body temperature. Sweat production decreases, and surface vasoconstriction increases. Metabolic heat is thereby denied its normal escape route, and fever subsequently develops.

Leukocytosis is similarly induced by chemicals released at the inflammatory site. These chemicals, which have not as yet been clearly identified, directly stimulate bone marrow to increase the production and release of neutrophils. The subsequent development of leukocytosis can be confirmed by standard laboratory blood tests.

THE RESOLUTION OF INFLAMMATION

Ultimately, the goal of the inflammatory process is to promote a return to cellular equilibrium. More specifically, vascular changes and phagocytic activity are directed at paving the way for the repair or replacement of damaged tissue.

To the extent that the inflammatory mechanism does its job, the stage is set for subsequent healing. In other words, before the healing process can occur, the inflammatory response must provide a relatively clean environment, free from bacteria, toxins, and other irritating factors. Normally, repair is further facilitated by the removal of inflammatory debris and exudate through the lymph vessels. The readying of traumatized tissue for repair is illustrated in Figure 8.5.

The healing process, unfortunately, is not always characterized by a total return to normal. Repair is initiated in one of two ways. Through the process of *regeneration*, damaged tissue is replaced with cells identical to the original. As a result, there is no significant loss of functional capacity. In certain instances, however, healing occurs through a process of *scar formation*. When injured tissue is replaced with connective tissue filler (called a scar), a considerable decline in functional capacity may be noted.

REGENERATION Tissues vary considerably in their ability to regenerate. Structures

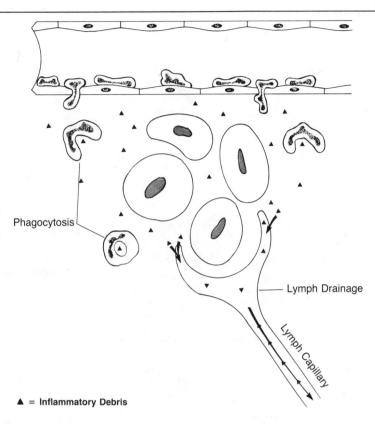

Figure 8.5 Clean-up at the site of inflammation. Note the removal of inflammatory debris via phagocytosis and lymph drainage.

Phagocytosis

Lymph Drainage

Lymph Capillary

▲ = Inflammatory Debris

containing a large proportion of epithelial cells, such as surface skin, the lining of the gastrointestinal tract, the vaginal lining, and the endometrial lining, regenerate readily. Muscle tissue and most neural tissue, on the other hand, regenerate poorly, if at all. Thus, myocardium damaged by an infarction and brain cells destroyed by inadequate blood supply are likely to remain forever nonfunctional. In attempting to predict the extent to which activity can be restored after disease, it is helpful to know specifically what types of tissue have been most affected by injury or disease.

SCAR FORMATION Whenever a connective tissue scar replaces damaged cells, one can expect some degree of functional deficit to result. This type of repair is seen commonly in cases of extensive or chronic liver damage. When such damage culminates in cirrhosis, the replacement of diseased liver cells with fibrous filler produces a relatively crippled organ. In these instances, the "healed" struc-

ture is repaired only in a limited physical sense. Functional and physiological capacity remain significantly diminished.

THE RESOLUTION OF INFLAMMATION: AN ILLUSTRATIVE EXAMPLE In considering the relationship between inflammation and healing, it is helpful to use a study of skin puncture as an illustrative model. Such a model is presented diagrammatically in Figure 8.6.

It can be seen that penetration of the skin is typically followed by an acute inflammatory response. Vascular changes and phagocytic activity facilitate clean-up and pave the way for the repair process. Healing is often initiated approximately one to three days following the injury and is manifested by an increase in blood supply and fibroblast cells at the site. Fibroblast cells function specifically in the deposit of a collagen protein filler into the injured area. This filler, called granulation tissue, becomes increasingly dense with time, eventually culminating in the formation of a

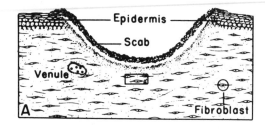

Initial skin penetration followed by formation of dried blood scab

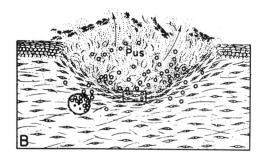

Inflammatory response and clean-up

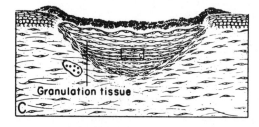

Deposit of granulation filler tissue

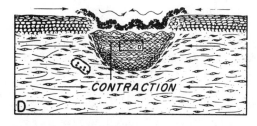

Growth of epithelium over the surface of the wound

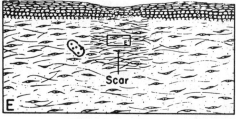

Healing with residual scar formation

Figure 8.6   The healing of a superficial skin wound. (from Majno, G.: The Healing Hand: Man and Wound in the Ancient World. Cambridge, Harvard University Press, 1974. Used by permission.)

scar. As can be seen in the pictorial summary, surface skin is ultimately reconstructed as epithelial cells grow to cover the underlying granulation tissue in the dermis.

NONADAPTIVE INFLAMMATION

Although essentially a beneficial process, inflammation can at times act nonadaptively to produce harmful results. In much the same way that a bullet may miss its target, the inflammatory reaction is occasionally misdirected. Most typically, nonadaptive inflammation is noted when: (1) the target of the inflammatory response is inappropriate, or (2) the inflammatory response induces secondary dysfunction in a critical organ.

INAPPROPRIATE TARGET The success of inflammation depends largely upon the phagocytosis and enzymatic digestion of foreign or harmful material. To the extent that these processes are abnormally directed against healthy, normal tissue, inflammation becomes a pathological reaction. Unfortunately, this inappropriate cellular destruction is not uncommon. It provides the impetus for the development of. many disease conditions including gout, silicosis, rheumatic fever, acute poststreptococcal glomerulonephritis, and many forms of arthritis.

The vascular component of the inflammatory response is also responsible for some aspects of nonadaptive inflammation. Most commonly in these cases, allergic or hypersensitivity reactions trigger the inflammatory mechanism. Subsequent increases in capillary-venule permeability promote the loss of fluid from the plasma compartment. At the extreme, this reaction is referred to as anaphylactic shock.

Whether inappropriate inflammation is phagocytic or vascular in nature, the underlying disorder is tied closely to related immune mechanisms. As immunity is discussed later in this chapter, its intimate relationship with the inflammatory response will become increasingly apparent.

SECONDARY DYSFUNCTION Even in cases in which the inflammatory response is directed appropriately against bacteria or necrotic cells, secondary dysfunction of critical organs may at times be generated. Most typical are instances of the accumulation of normal inflammatory exudate that interferes with organic functional activity. The alveoli of the lungs, for example, will support only marginal gas exchange when filled with inflammatory fluid. Thus, at the very site where phagocytes are struggling to normalize the cellular environment, fallout is occurring that interferes with the restoration of equilibrium.

SUPPRESSION OF THE INFLAMMATORY RESPONSE

In the clinical setting, suppression of the inflammatory response is associated with one of two primary mechanisms:

1. *Natural suppression* is noted in cases in which a physiological deficit or abnormality interferes with some aspect of the inflammatory mechanism. In these instances, loss of the inflammatory response results in greater susceptibility of infection and less potential for healing. Natural suppression is thus considered to be an inherently pathological phenomenon.

2. *Artificially induced suppression* is associated with a medical attempt to depress inflammation in cases in which the inflammatory response is nonadaptive (as discussed earlier). Under these circumstances the benefits derived from suppression are considered to outweigh the associated decline in resistance and repair.

NATURAL SUPPRESSION When inflammation is suppressed naturally, the causative factor usually falls into one of four major categories: (1) deficiency of blood supply, (2) inadequate migration of phagocytic cells, (3) insufficient function of phagocytic cells, and (4) inadequate support of the inflammatory mechanism by the immune system.

Deficiency of Blood Supply A deficiency of blood supply to the inflammatory site could occur in a wide variety of clinical conditions that induce ischemia. Examples include the atherosclerosis accompanying diabetes mellitus, the obstruction of blood flow caused by emboli or thrombi, and the hardening of arteries characteristic of old age. Regardless of the circumstances, the vascular component of the inflammatory mechanism will be suppressed as blood flow declines.

Inadequate Migration of Phagocytic Cells   The migration of phagocytic cells out of the plasma compartment into the area of tissue trauma is a significant aspect of the inflammatory mechanism. When the number of phagocytic cells is decreased or the mechanisms of migration are impeded, the inflammatory response will suffer. Decline in the quantity of phagocytic cells is often induced by malignancies or toxic drug activity at the sites of white blood cell production (the bone marrow or lymph nodes or both). Interference with diapedesis or chemotaxis, on the other hand, is

frequently evident in certain metabolic disorders such as diabetes mellitus, malnutrition, and acute alcoholism.

Insufficient Function of Phagocytic Cells   At times, the ability of phagocytes to ingest and destroy foreign or toxic material is inhibited. In cases of hypersecretion of steroid hormones, for example, a decrease is noted in the release of enzymes from the neutrophils. This phenomenon explains, in part, the increased susceptibility to infection manifested in patients with Cushing's disease.

Inadequate Support of the Inflammatory Mechanism by the Immune System   As mentioned earlier, the function of phagocytes is normally facilitated by the release of chemicals

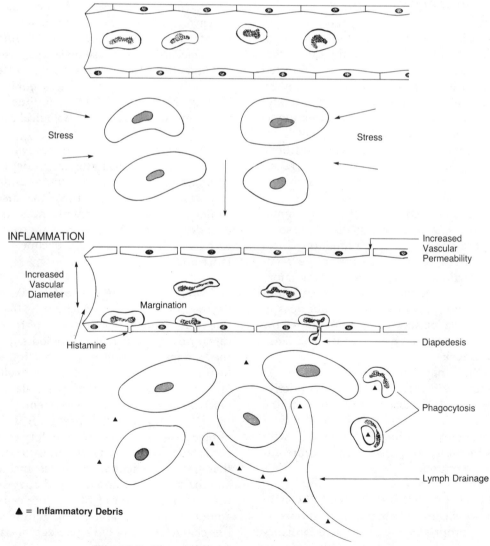

Figure 8.7   Some major aspects of the inflammatory response.

by immunoactive cells at the inflammatory site. To the extent that the immune mechanism is suppressed or deficient, the inflammatory response is rendered less effective.

ARTIFICIALLY INDUCED SUPPRESSION In cases in which disease is associated with nonadaptive inflammation, it is often desirable to medically suppress the inflammatory mechanism. Drugs typically used to produce the desired changes include aspirin and aspirin-like compounds and steroids such as cortisone and prednisone. Aspirin is believed to act by inhibiting the production of hormones involved in the inflammatory response, while steroids suppress both the vascular and the phagocytic components of the inflammatory mechanism. The use of anti-inflammatory drugs can provide much relief to those suffering from disorders associated with nonfunctional inflammation. Unfortunately, however, predictable side effects include increased susceptibility to infection and reduced healing capacity. It becomes evident that patients on such therapy must be monitored carefully for signs of secondary disease.

THE INFLAMMATION AND REPAIR RESPONSE: A SUMMARY

In review, it can be said that inflammation is inherently a beneficial and adaptive process. Although it is typically associated with pain and discomfort, the protection it affords far outweighs any negative side effects.

In the clinical setting, it is sometimes difficult to reconcile the positive aspects of inflammation with the ugly reality of a swollen, hot, pus-filled wound awaiting treatment. One must, however, constantly guard against the temptation to throw out the baby with the bath water. It should always be remembered that the inflammatory process is a necessary precursor to healing. A brief unifying summary of some of the major aspects of inflammation can be found in Figure 8.7.

The Immune Response

Immunity, like inflammation, is an inherently protective and adaptive mechanism

that functions to inactivate potentially toxic substances within the body. Mobilized by the presence of a foreign body (called an *antigen*), the immune response can generally be described as either nonspecific or specific.

Nonspecific immunity is mediated by any factor that provides nonselective opposition to the invasion of foreign substances. Operating without distinction against most potentially harmful agents, it encompasses a wide variety of devices including intact skin and mucous membranes, phagocytic activity of white blood cells, and chemically based resistance of certain body secretions. It is significant to note that the inflammatory mechanism is also considered to be an example of this type of immune response (see Table 8.2). Operating in a nonselective manner, inflammation func-

TABLE 8.2 **Nonspecific Immunity**

Mechanism	Examples
Mechanical barrier	*Intact skin; intact mucous membranes. Mucus* and *cilia* associated with certain membranes also help to trap foreign materials.
Enzymatic activity	*Lysozyme* enzyme associated with skin and mucous membranes helps to combat infection; *gastric pepsin* and *HCl* serve to inactivate certain antigens that enter through the gastrointestinal tract.
Inflammation	The inflammatory mechanism acts nonselectively against a variety of foreign substances.
Interferon	Interferon is a chemical released by certain cells in response to viral infection. Interferon is believed to act by triggering the production of antiviral protein by other cells in the body, thus inhibiting the further reproduction of pathogenic viruses.
Reticuloendothelial activity	Some phagocytic cells are found fixed in specific tissues such as the lymph nodes, spleen, bone marrow, and liver. Described as reticuloendothelial cells, they help to filter foreign substances from the bloodstream.
High acidity	Acidity, as noted in the stomach and vagina, serves to inhibit the growth of microbes.

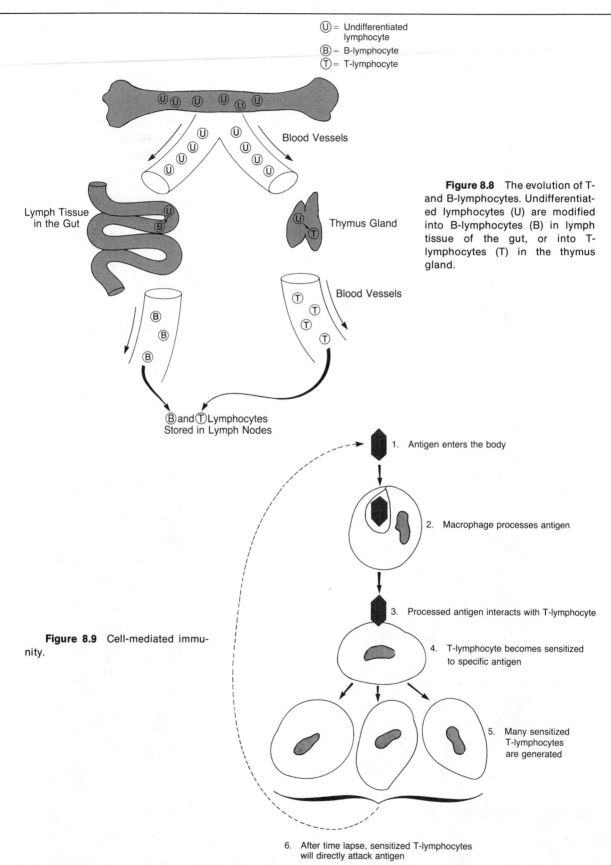

Ⓤ = Undifferentiated lymphocyte
Ⓑ = B-lymphocyte
Ⓣ = T-lymphocyte

Blood Vessels

Lymph Tissue in the Gut

Thymus Gland

Blood Vessels

Ⓑ and Ⓣ Lymphocytes Stored in Lymph Nodes

Figure 8.8 The evolution of T- and B-lymphocytes. Undifferentiated lymphocytes (U) are modified into B-lymphocytes (B) in lymph tissue of the gut, or into T-lymphocytes (T) in the thymus gland.

Figure 8.9 Cell-mediated immunity.

1. Antigen enters the body

2. Macrophage processes antigen

3. Processed antigen interacts with T-lymphocyte

4. T-lymphocyte becomes sensitized to specific antigen

5. Many sensitized T-lymphocytes are generated

6. After time lapse, sensitized T-lymphocytes will directly attack antigen

tions to support the mission of nonspecific immunity.

Specific immunity provides an additional and very discriminatory means of protection. The agents of this response pattern are programmed to act against only one particular type of antigen, to recognize this antigen, and to remember it if it is introduced into the body more than once.

To ensure this type of selectivity, the specific immune process must be quite complex. The following pages are devoted to elucidating the major aspects of specific immunity. Primary emphasis is placed upon (1) immune cells, (2) facilitators of the immune response, and (3) nonadaptive immunity.

IMMUNE CELLS

Immune cells, the primary mediators of specific immunity, are of two distinct types: *T-lymphocytes* and *B-lymphocytes*. Although they both originate embryonically as stem cells in the yolk sac and fetal liver, they are processed differentially to become two functionally independent entities.

At the time of birth, all lymphocytes are manufactured primarily by the bone marrow. Discrimination occurs as those cells destined to become T-lymphocytes are transported to the thymus gland for processing and subsequently stored in lymphoid tissue, such as lymph nodes, spleen, and bone marrow. B-lymphocytes, on the other hand, are processed directly by the bone marrow or in gut-related lymph tissue and are then released to be stored in lymph nodes adjacent to the T-lymphocytes. The comparative evolution of T- and B-lymphocytes is summarized in Figure 8.8.

T-LYMPHOCYTES With the introduction of an antigen into the body, the functional distinction between T- and B-lymphocytes can be clarified. Upon contact with the antigen, T-cells become specifically sensitized and undergo reproduction to generate a number of similarly sensitized T-cells.

Within approximately 48 hours, these sensitized T-cells are ready to assume a defensive role. Attaching directly to their specific antigen, they proceed to release enzymes that promote antigenic destruction. This process,

depicted in Figure 8.9, is described as *cell-mediated immunity (CMI)*. It is, in general, responsible for: (1) the killing of harmful microbes that live in intracellular fluid, (2) the rejection of transplanted organs, and (3) the ongoing defense mechanism believed to combat the establishment of cancer cells.

Since sensitized T-lymphocytes can survive for long periods within the vascular system, they are available to act against any subsequent entry of the same antigen. T-cells thus serve the immune process with a "memory" component, thereby extending protection far beyond the time of initial exposure to the foreign substance.

B-LYMPHOCYTES Unlike T-cells, B-lymphocytes respond to the presence of an antigen by cellular transformation. They change into *plasma cells*, which subsequently produce chemicals called *antibodies*. These antibodies, in turn, are released into the blood to inactivate the invading antigen. This process, described as *humoral (blood-related) immunity*, is illustrated in Figure 8.10. It is particularly functional in protecting the body against a wide variety of bacterial infections but is also responsible for the generation of many nonadaptive immune responses, as described later in this chapter.

Following exposure to an antigen, some sensitized B-lymphocytes remain in the blood for an extended period of time. They thus provide a memory pool that enables rapid regeneration of antigen-specific plasma cells and antibodies upon re-exposure to the foreign substance.

Ultimately, the immune function of B-cells is linked to antibody activity. Each antibody, also called an *immunoglobulin (Ig)*, is designed to inactivate a specific antigen. It accomplishes its purpose in a variety of ways, including:

1. *precipitation* — rendering a soluble antigen insoluble.

2. *agglutination* — causing antigen particles or cells to clump together.

3. *opsonization* — coating an antigenic particle so as to render it more attractive to phagocytes.

4. *neutralization* — inactivating the harmful chemicals (toxins) released by pathogenic microorganisms.

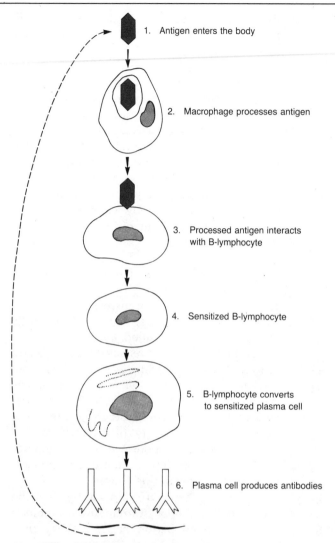

1. Antigen enters the body

2. Macrophage processes antigen

3. Processed antigen interacts with B-lymphocyte

4. Sensitized B-lymphocyte

5. B-lymphocyte converts to sensitized plasma cell

6. Plasma cell produces antibodies

7. Antibodies help to specifically destroy antigen

Figure 8.10   Humoral immunity.

FACILITATORS OF THE IMMUNE RESPONSE

Although lymphocytes function quite effectively in protecting the body against foreign substances, the immune response can be heightened or enhanced in a number of ways.

T-lymphocytes, for example, will respond most effectively to antigens pretreated by macrophages. Macrophages, it will be remembered, are large phagocytic cells, derived from monocytes, that escape from the vascular tree to service the inflammatory process.

B-lymphocyte activity, on the other hand, is potentiated by a number of factors, includ-ing *macrophage activity, opsonization,* and *complement activity.*

Opsonization involves the coating of an antigen with a specific form of antibody designated as *immunoglobulin G (IgG)*. This process enhances macrophage activity by rendering the antigen more attractive and "tasty" to the phagocytic cell.

Complement is the name given to a series of enzyme proteins in the blood. If these proteins attach to an antigen-antibody complex, an *immune complex* is formed. The activation of complement by an antigen-antibody complex may occur in localized extracellular spaces or on select cellular membranes. In the latter case, cellular destruction, or lysis, will result. In extracellular fluid, antigen-antibody complexes associated with complement will promote degeneration to the extent that they trigger inflammatory breakdown of body tissue. Specific examples of immune-complex disorders will be cited in the following section.

NONADAPTIVE IMMUNE RESPONSES

Thus far, immunity has been treated as an essentially adaptive and protective mechanism. Whenever the immune response is directed against foreign substances for the purpose of rendering them inactive, the results are beneficial. As in the case of inflammation, however, there are instances in which the immune process is directed against inherently harmless substances or against normal body tissue. When this happens, of course, cellular disequilibrium occurs and disease results.

Nonadaptive immune responses, also called *hypersensitivity reactions*, are classified into four major groups: (1) immediate or anaphylactic type hypersensitivity, (2) cytotoxic type hypersensitivity, (3) immune complex–mediated hypersensitivity, and (4) cell-mediated hypersensitivity.

IMMEDIATE OR ANAPHYLACTIC TYPE HYPERSENSITIVITY Anaphylactic type hypersensitivity is usually seen in individuals with allergies. It is a particular form of the immune response in which the immune mechanism is directed against materials that are not inherently harmful. In cases of immediate hypersensitivity, substances as innocuous as pollen, dog hair, or milk can trigger an immunity-mediated reaction.

Typically, initial exposure to the allergy-inducing agent (called an *allergen*) results in the production of a specific form of antibody described as *immunoglobulin E (IgE)*. These antibodies, as they accumulate, tend to coat *mast cells*, which are dispersed throughout the body and contain high concentrations of vasodilator chemicals such as *histamine*.

Once antibodies have been formed, the introduction of the allergen is followed by an allergen-antibody interaction. The allergen combines with IgE antibodies that are waiting in readiness on the mast cell membranes. Their interaction leads to mast cell rupture. Histamine is thereby released, followed by evidence of symptomatic clinical changes.

To better understand the allergic reaction, it is helpful to review the functional activity of histamine. In brief, histamine triggers physiological change by promoting vasodilation and increases in capillary-venule permeability. On the local level, the results are redness, warmth, and swelling. These symptoms are characteristic of the typical allergic wheal that can often be noted on the skin.

If the response occurs in the respiratory tree, it is frequently accompanied by bronchiolar smooth muscle constriction. Resulting airway obstruction, compounded by fluid accumulation in the alveoli, is a characteristic manifestation of a classic allergic-asthmatic attack.

If permeability changes are widespread and generalized, they cause a massive flux of fluid out of the plasma compartment into the interstitial compartment. The resulting rapid drop in blood volume and blood pressure is potentially life-threatening. At this extreme, the allergic response pattern is referred to as *anaphylaxis,* or *anaphylactic shock.*

The major physiological changes underlying the development of immediate type hypersensitivity are illustrated in Figure 8.11. The significance of histamine as a primary mediator of the allergic response is clear. In fact, drugs that counteract the activity of histamine (*antihistaminic agents*) are frequently used to alleviate allergy symptoms.

CYTOTOXIC TYPE HYPERSENSITIVITY This response is initiated when complement attaches to antigen-antibody complexes that already exist on cellular surfaces. The result is destruction of the cell involved. Since this phenomenon is frequently associated with red blood cells, it commonly induces hemolytic anemia. It is noted in cases of transfusion reactions and erythroblastosis fetalis. The underlying mechanism is illustrated in Figure 8.12.

IMMUNE COMPLEX–MEDIATED HYPERSENSITIVITY This response pattern is triggered by the attachment of complement to

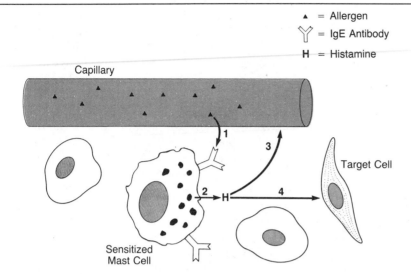

▲ = Allergen

Y = IgE Antibody

H = Histamine

Figure 8.11 The evolution of immediate or anaphylactic hypersensitivity. 1. IgE antibody generated in response to the presence of a specific allergen attaches to a mast cell. 2. Histamine is released when additional allergen is introduced and reacts with the IgE antibody on the sensitized mast cell. 3. Histamine causes vascular dilation and increases in capillary permeability. 4. Histamine may also cause smooth muscle constriction in the bronchioles.

antigen-antibody complexes circulating in plasma or localized in extracellular tissue spaces. Common sites of immune complex reactions are the capillaries of skin, kidneys, heart, or joints. Subsequent destruction of healthy tissue in the area is caused by inflammatory phagocytosis with secondary release of lysosomal enzymes.

This mechanism is central to the development of such disorders as acute poststreptococcal glomerulonephritis, rheumatic fever, and serum sickness as well as the Arthus reaction. Major aspects of this type of hypersensitivity are summarized in Figure 8.13.

CELL-MEDIATED HYPERSENSITIVITY This type of hypersensitivity results when the activity of normally adaptive T-lymphocytes is directed against a harmless substance. The most common example of this phenomenon is the graft rejection reaction, in which new tissue introduced into the body for medical reasons is attacked and destroyed as antigenic.

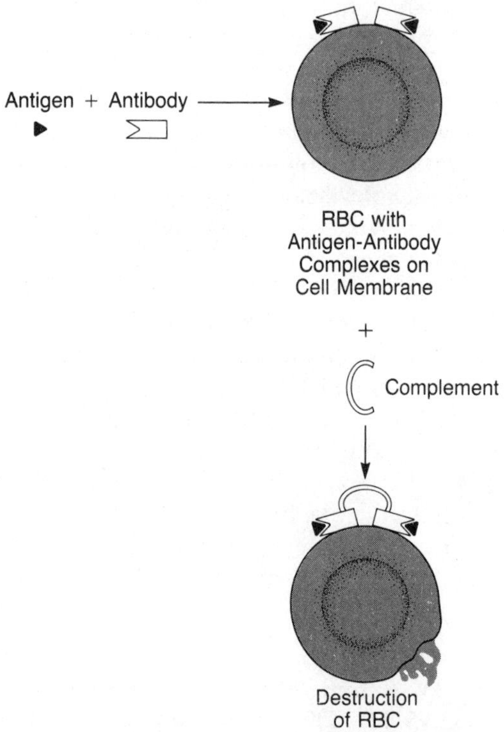

Antigen + Antibody

▶   ⊐

RBC with Antigen-Antibody Complexes on Cell Membrane

+

C Complement

Destruction of RBC

Figure 8.12 Cytotoxic type hypersensitivity.

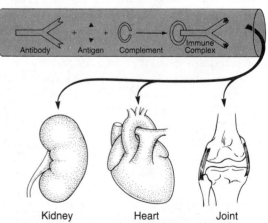

Antibody   Antigen   Complement   Immune Complex

Kidney   Heart   Joint

Figure 8.13 Complement-mediated hypersensitivity. When complement interacts with antigen and antibody, immune complexes form that may trigger the destruction of healthy tissue in the kidneys, heart, and joints.

Adaptive Cellular Responses To Stress: A Summary

This chapter has described the primary mechanisms of adaptive cellular responses to stress. They include changes in the structural characteristics of the cell, the inflammation and repair response, and the immune response. In most cases, they are processes initiated at *the cellular level* that are directed toward eliminating stress and promoting a return to homeostasis. Under certain circumstances, however, these normally adaptive mechanisms can result in inappropriate pathological responses.

In considering adaptive response patterns, it is significant to note that stress or disequilibrium can invoke *systemic* as well as cellular adaptive mechanisms. In these cases, reflex compensations are mediated at the macro- instead of the micro- level. Hypoxia, for example, will trigger reflex increases in respiratory and cardiac rates. These systemic changes compensate for insufficient cellular oxygenation and promote the re-establishment of homeostasis. Some examples of similar mechanisms and their mode of action are presented in Table 8.3.

TABLE 8.3 **Some Systemic Adaptations to Stress**

Source of Stress	Mechanism of Restoring Equilibrium
Low blood pressure	Increase in cardiac rate Arterial vasoconstriction Renal retention of fluid
Acidosis	Increase in respiratory rate Renal secretion of hydrogen, and reabsorption of bicarbonate
Hypercapnia	Increase in respiratory rate Localized vasodilation
Temperature elevation	Increased sweat production Superficial vascular dilation
Physical exercise	Increase in cardiac rate Increase in respiratory rate Dilation of blood vessels servicing skeletal muscles Increased sweat production

NEOPLASMS

As mentioned earlier, neoplasms, or "new tissue," are a particularly diffuse and unresolved area for investigation. The term *neoplasm*, often used interchangeably with *tumor*, refers to an area of inappropriate and excessive cellular growth. Most commonly, neoplasms are categorized as either *benign* (theoretically harmless) or *malignant* (cancerous).

Benign Growths

Benign growths can take a variety of forms, depending upon the location and type of tissue involved. Although theoretically harmless, they will cause physiological disruption if they exert pressure on a critical structure. A benign brain tumor, for example, can cause serious dysfunction if pressure induces a neural disorder at a vital site.

Fortunately, benign growths are not inherently disruptive. Characteristically developing in a well-localized and encapsulated manner, they usually can be successfully removed surgically. Once excised, benign tumors seldom recur.

Malignant Growths

Unlike benign growths, malignancies, or cancers, are pathological in nature. Although varied in form and location, they generally can be identified by certain unique behavioral and cellular characteristics.

BEHAVIORAL CHARACTERISTICS

In general, malignant growths are more invasive than benign neoplasms. Whereas normal cells stop growing when they come into contact with nearby tissue, cancer cells fail to exhibit this *contact inhibition*. The invasiveness of malignancies is also believed to be enhanced by the production of enzymes that dissolve intercellular cement in surrounding tissues.

In addition to this tendency to invade locally, cancerous growths commonly spread to other more distant sites in the body. This phenomenon, called *metastasis*, is frequently initiated by the lymph system, blood vessels, or physical displacement within a body cavity. A cancer cell that originates in the stomach, for example, could be carried to the liver or lungs in either blood or lymph vessels. Alternatively, it could dislodge from its site of origin and be pulled downward by gravity to "land" on another organ in the abdominopelvic cavity.

Metastasis is generally facilitated by the relative lack of cohesion and increased motility characteristic of cancer cells. A deficit in calcium and increase in surface negative charges noted in malignant cells seems to be responsible for decreased intercellular bonding. As a result, cancer cells may be shed rather easily from the surface of a tumor. Once released from extracellular fluid and spaces, the characteristic mobility of malignant cells enables them to migrate throughout the body.

Unfortunately, the surgical removal of a malignancy carries with it no guarantee of permanent recovery. The tendency of excised malignancies to recur adds to the aura of mystery and fear that surrounds the diagnosis of cancer.

CELLULAR CHARACTERISTICS

The diagnosis of cancer is often confirmed by a biopsy, or microscopic examination of a small sample of the tissue in question. Cancer cells typically exhibit characteristic structural changes, which include:

1. irregularity in the size, shape, and arrangement of the cells, as illustrated in Figure 8.14.

2. abnormal increase in the size of the nucleus and the nucleolus of the cells, as illustrated in Figure 8.15.

3. decrease in structural specialization of the cells. The tendency of malignant cells to

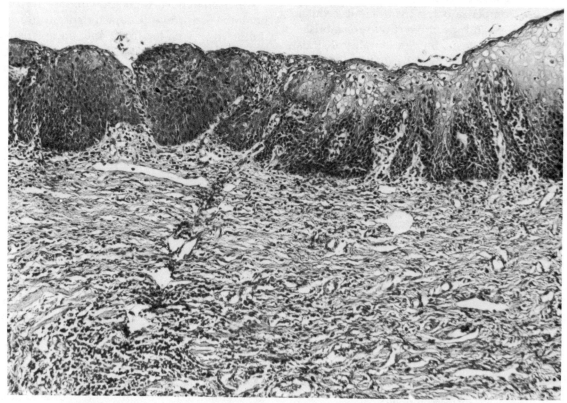

Figure 8.14 Irregularity in the size, shape, and arrangement of cells as seen in dysplasia of the cervical mucosa. The normal epithelium is seen at the right. Note the gradual conversion into the dysplastic epithelium at the left. The dysplastic cells are smaller and more crowded together, and there is loss of the orderly maturation of the cell layers. (From Robbins, S. L., and Angell, M.: Basic Pathology. Philadelphia, W. B. Saunders Company, 1976.)

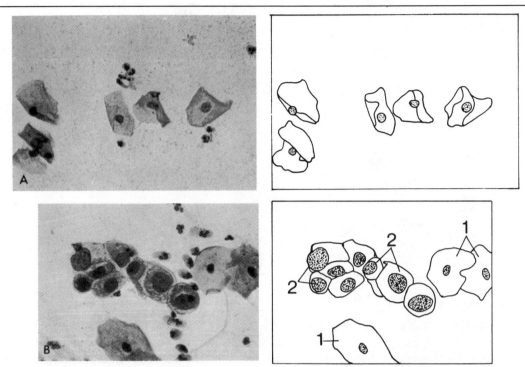

Figure 8.15   Abnormal nuclear characteristics. *A*, Photomicrograph and drawing of normal cells with nuclei of normal size. *B*, Photomicrograph and drawing of abnormal nuclear characteristics in carcinoma. *1*. Normal cells of the intermediate cell layer (in this case of the ectocervix of an adult premenopausal woman). *2*. Severely dysplasic cells with large nuclei having an abnormally large amount of chromatin material (hyperchromasia) and with prominent nuclear membranes. (From Schneider M. L., and Staemmler. H: Gynecologic Cytopathology. A Color Atlas of Differential Diagnosis, Philadelphia, W. B. Saunders Company, 1977. Used by permission.)

lose certain characteristic structural components, such as cilia or glandular elements, is accompanied by increased generalization of functional capacity. The entire phenomenon is referred to as *anaplasia*.

Accompanying these microscopic structural changes are alterations in cellular metabolic patterns. Malignant cells seem progressively unable to carry out normal aerobic metabolism and increasingly revert to glycolysis for energy generation. As a result, lactic acid accumulates and clinical manifestations of metabolic acidosis may occur. Simultaneously, the selective hoarding of plasma amino acids by the malignant cells gives the cancerous tissue a competitive growth advantage. Malignancies thus thrive at the expense of other cells and are often referred to as nitrogen traps.

As cancer develops, an initial inflammatory response is frequently mounted against the malignant growth. Vasodilation and increased vascular permeability are accompa-

nied by localized accumulation of fluids and phagocytes. With progressive establishment of the malignancy, however, blood supply to the cancerous tissue decreases. The associated lack of oxygen and nutrient supply often causes necrosis, hemorrhage, and infection within the core of the tumor.

Ultimately, the complex cellular level changes spawned by malignancy are manifested symptomatically in a variety of ways. Typically, weight loss, pain, disfigurement, and fever accompany the invasion and establishment of malignant neoplasms.

CELLULAR RESPONSES TO STRESS: A SUMMARY

Stress, as defined in this chapter, is considered to be any stimulus that precipitates cellular disequilibrium. We have considered alternative cellular response patterns to disruptions in homeostasis. Degenerative, or

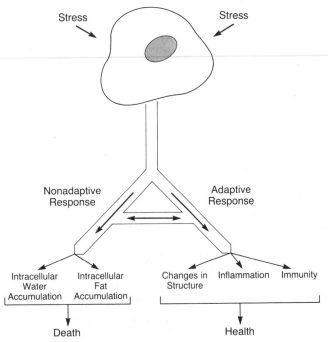

Figure 8.16 Cellular responses to stress.

nonadaptive, responses are those that do not facilitate a return to equilibrium. They include specific metabolic alterations and necrosis. Adaptive cellular response patterns, on the other hand, are generally beneficial and promote the restoration of health. They include certain changes in the structural characteris- tics of the cell, the inflammation and repair response, and the immune responses. Even inherently adaptive mechanisms, however, can engender disorders under certain circum- stances. A comparison of adaptive and non- adaptive cellular response patterns to stress is shown in Figure 8.16.

STUDY QUESTIONS

1. In each of the following cases, identify the source of cellular stress:
   a. drug overdose
   b. pneumonia
   c. prolonged malnutrition
   d. overexposure to radiation
   e. crushing injury
   f. severe anemia
   g. frostbite
   h. alcoholism

2. Define necrosis.

3. Explain why, after a massive heart at- tack, there is a characteristic increase in plasma levels of SGOT, LDH, and CPK.

4. In response to stress, muscle tissue will typically undergo hypertrophy but not hyperplasia. Why?

5. Explain the mechanisms responsible for the following manifestations of inflam- mation:

   a. swelling
   b. pain
   c. fever
   d. redness
   e. warmth
   f. leukocytosis

6. In each of the following cases, indicate whether repair is most likely to occur by regeneration or scar formation:
   a. surface skin abrasion
   b. cirrhosis of the liver
   c. damage to cerebral neurons second- ary to a stroke
   d. replacement of the uterine lining after menstruation
   e. damage to the myocardium second- ary to ischemia

7. List three examples of nonadaptive in- flammation.

8. In each of the following cases, describe why the inflammatory response might be suppressed:

a. acute alcoholism
b. drug toxicity
c. diabetes mellitus
d. Cushing's disease
e. atherosclerosis
f. excessive intake of aspirin

9. Describe the differences between T-lymphocytes and B-lymphocytes.

10. What is the function of complement in the immune process?

11. Identify the type of hypersensitivity reaction associated with each of the following disorders:
    a. serum sickness
    b. hemolytic anemia
    c. graft rejection
    d. hay fever
    e. acute poststreptococcal glomerulonephritis
    f. anaphylactic reaction to penicillin

12. Why is a benign tissue growth not necessarily harmless?

13. You are caring for a patient with possible uterine cancer. The terms *metastasis* and *anaplasia* appear on a pathology laboratory slip. Define these terms and explain their significance.

Suggested Readings

Books

Anderson, W. A. D., and Scotti, T. M.: Synopsis of Pathology, 10th ed. St. Louis, The C. V. Mosby Company, 1980, pp. 22–93, 240–276.

Bellanti, J. A.: Immunology II, 2nd ed. Philadelphia, W. B. Saunders Company, 1978.

Blue, J. A.: Anaphylaxis and serum sickness. *In* Conn, H. F. (ed.): Current Therapy. Philadelphia, W. B. Saunders Company, 1979.

Cameron, R.: Inflammation and repair. *In* Robbins, S. L.: Pathology. Philadelphia, W. B. Saunders Company, 1967.

Guyton, A. C.: Textbook of Medical Physiology, 5th ed. Philadelphia, W. B. Saunders Company, 1976, pp. 67–86.

Holborow, E. J.: An ABC of Modern Immunology, 3rd ed. Boston, Little, Brown & Company, 1977.

Jones, D. A., Dunbar, C. F., and Jirovec, M. M.: Medical-Surgical Nursing, A Conceptual Approach. New York, McGraw-Hill Book Company, 1978, pp. 123–127; 281–289; 303–416.

Kent, T. H., Hart, M. N., and Shires, T. K.: Introduction to Human Disease. New York, Appleton-Century-Crofts, 1979, pp. 24–55; 443–451.

Luckmann, J., and Sorensen, K. C.: Medical-Surgical Nursing, A Psychophysiologic Approach, 2nd ed. Philadelphia, W. B. Saunders Company, 1980, pp. 98–168; 430–443.

McCluskey, R. T., and Cohen, S. (eds.): Mechanisms of Cell-Mediated Immunity. New York, John Wiley & Sons, 1974.

Meyer, E. A.: Microorganisms and Human Disease. New York, Appleton-Century-Crofts, 1974, pp. 60–69.

Movat, H. Z. (ed.): Inflammation, Immunity, and Hypersensitivity, 2nd ed. New York, Harper & Row, 1979.

Phair, J. P.: Assessment of the inflammatory and immune response. *In* Youmans, G. P., Paterson, P. Y., and Sommers, H. M.: The Biological and Clinical Basis of Infectious Diseases, 2nd ed. Philadelphia, W. B. Saunders Company, 1980, p. 163.

Purtillo, D. T.: A Survey of Human Diseases. Menlo Park, Addison-Wesley Publishing Company, 1978, pp. 74–128; 157–172.

Robbins, S. L., and Cotran, R. S.: Pathologic Basis of Disease, 2nd ed. Philadelphia, W. B. Saunders Company, 1979, pp. 12–103: 141–166; 262–278.

Roitt, I.: Essential Immunology, 3rd ed. Oxford, Blackwell Scientific Publishing, 1977.

Tucker, E. S., and Nakamura, R. M.: Dynamics of immune response, immunocompetence, immunodeficiency, and tumor immunology. *In* Sodeman, W. A., and Sodeman, T. M. (eds.): Pathologic Physiology, Mechanisms of Disease, 6th ed. Philadelphia, W. B. Saunders Company, 1979, p. 110.

Articles and Monographs

Auld, M. E., et al.: Wound healing. Nursing 72, 2:36, 1972.

Glasser, R.: How the body works against itself — autoimmune diseases. Nursing 77, 7:38, 1977.

Jerne, N. K.: The immune system. Sci. Am., 229:52, 1973.

Mayer, M. M.: The complement system. Sci. Am., 229:54, 1973.

Nysanther, J., et al.: The immune system: its development and functions. Am. J. Nurs., 76:1614, 1976.

Raff, M. C.: T and B lymphocytes and immune responses. Nature, 242:19, 1973.

Ryan, G. B., and Majno, G.: Inflammation. Kalamazoo, Upjohn Company, 1977.

Scarpelli, D. G., and Trump, B. F.: Cell Injury. Kalamazoo, Upjohn Company, 1971.

Chapter Outline

166

chapter 9

Cardiovascular Pathology

Chapter Objectives

At the completion of this chapter, the student will be able to:

1. Distinguish between arteries, arterioles, capillaries, venules, and veins with respect to basic structure and function.
2. Identify two major causes of vascular disease and the mechanism whereby they induce physiological disruption.
3. Define hypertension and describe its development and clinical manifestations.
4. Describe the basic cardiac structure and trace normal blood flow through the heart.
5. Describe the cardiac cycle and its relationship to (a) the conduction system and (b) the electrocardiogram.
6. Define cardiac output and describe the significance of stroke volume and cardiac rate in determining output.
7. Describe myocardial blood supply.
8. Differentiate between direct and indirect cardiac stress.
9. Distinguish between four major sources of direct cardiac stress with respect to cause and development.
10. Differentiate between three major sources of indirect cardiac stress with respect to causative factors and development.
11. Describe the way in which cardiac muscle compensates for stress.
12. Define congestive heart failure and describe the causes and development of this disorder.
13. Differentiate between left-sided and right-sided heart failure.
14. Define shock and describe its primary causes, development, and clinical manifestations.
15. Describe the way in which cardiovascular disease may disrupt the servicing of cellular needs.

INTRODUCTION

If not for the cardiovascular system, the cells of the body would be permanently isolated within a sea of stagnant interstitial fluid. In the ongoing struggle for cellular survival, plasma plays a crucial role. Continually circulating through the capillaries, it delivers oxygen and nutrients to the cells, provides an exit route for metabolic wastes, and helps maintain the fluid-electrolyte and acid-base balance.

In facilitating the transport of plasma throughout the body, the cardiovascular system lies at the crossroads of homeostasis. Consisting of a cardiac pump and vascular pipelines, the system is designed to support and maintain a fluid environment compatible with cellular health.

Cardiovascular disease develops when structural or functional abnormalities affect the heart or the blood vessels or both. The results are frequently devastating, accounting for four out of every ten deaths in the United States.

Cardiovascular disorders are classified in this chapter as either vascular disease, or cardiac disease. In each case, a brief review of normal structure and function is followed by an analysis of dysfunction. The intimate functional relationship that exists between the heart and the blood vessels is illustrated by the phenomenon of shock, which is discussed at the end of the chapter.

THE BLOOD VESSELS: A BRIEF REVIEW OF NORMAL STRUCTURE AND FUNCTION

To maintain homeostasis, the blood vessels and the heart must work together to provide a continuous pipeline for the servicing of cellular needs. Normally, they transport blood from the left heart to metabolizing cells, and then back to the right heart, in a continuous closed circuit. The routing of blood through arteries, arterioles, capillaries, venules, and veins is illustrated in Figure 9.1.

Although all vessels are responsible for the transport of oxygen, nutrients, and metabolic wastes, they do differ from each other

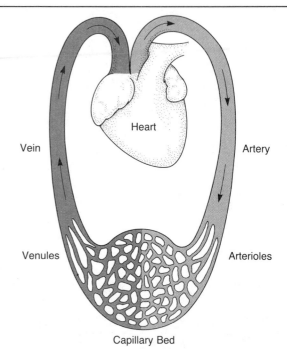

Figure 9.1 The routing of blood through the vascular pipelines.

both structurally and functionally. Arteries, for example, are designed to receive freshly oxygenated blood and transport it to the capillaries that directly service cells. To facilitate the reception of blood as it is ejected, under fairly high pressure, from the left ventricle, arterial walls are relatively thick and elastic. They are composed of three major coats of tissue: an outer layer of connective tissue, a middle layer of primarily smooth muscle, and an inner layer of specialized epithelium, called endothelium. Their structure is illustrated in Figure 9.2. The arterial walls stretch to accommodate the entrance of blood during systole, then recoil during diastole to propel fluid along. Their inherent elasticity thus plays an important role in the maintenance of circulation.

Arterioles receive blood from arteries. They are, in fact, structurally derived from arteries, with a similar configuration but much thinner walls. It is primarily the smooth muscle in the walls of arterioles that function to regulate the flow of blood from arteries into capillaries (see Figure 9.3). While constriction causes blood to be retained in the arteries, dilation causes a decrease in arterial blood volume and an increase in capillary blood

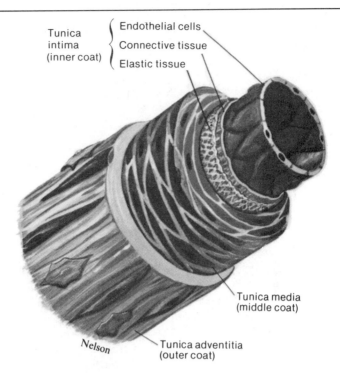

Tunica intima (inner coat)
{
Endothelial cells
Connective tissue
Elastic tissue

Tunica media (middle coat)

Nelson

Tunica adventitia (outer coat)

Figure 9.2 The wall of an artery. (From Hole, J. W.: Human Anatomy and Physiology. Dubuque, Wm. C. Brown Company, 1978. Used by permission.)

flow. Because of their strategic location, arterioles play a significant role in the generation of *peripheral resistance* by posing opposition to the flow of arterial blood through the vascular system.

Capillaries, also called the *microcirculation*, are very small vessels constructed from a continuation of the endothelial tissue that lines arteries and arterioles. With connective and muscle layers peeled away, these epithelial cells remain essentially naked and facilitate exchange between plasma and interstitial fluid. Capillary structure is illustrated in Figure 9.4.

As blood moves from capillaries into venules, it is low in oxygen and high in metabolic wastes. The pressure exerted against vascular walls diminishes relative to increasing dis-

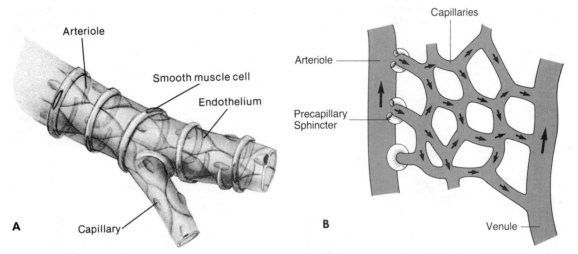

Figure 9.3 *A,* The structure of an arteriole. Note the smooth muscle cells in the wall of the vessel and the endothelial lining. (From Hole, J. W.: Human Anatomy and Physiology. Dubuque, Wm. C. Brown Company, 1978. Used by permission.) *B,* The routing of blood through arterioles into capillaries. Note the location of precapillary sphincter muscles, which serve to regulate the flow of blood through the capillaries.

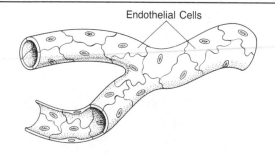

Endothelial Cells

VASCULAR PATHOLOGY

For blood vessels to adequately service cellular needs, circulation cannot be obstructed or altered to any significant extent. When the flow of blood is disrupted by an abnormality originating in the blood vessels, a vascular disorder is present. Common causative mechanisms include (1) obstruction of blood flow through the vascular lumen, and (2) inappropriate contraction or relaxation of smooth muscle in the vascular walls.

The factors that initiate vascular disease are discussed in the following pages. A conceptual integration of vascular pathophysiology is presented in a study of hypertension, which provides a model for the merging of diverse pathological phenomena into a single clinical entity.

tance from the pumping source. The walls of venules, although similar to those of arterioles, are thus considerably thinner, with less elastic tissue.

When blood moves into veins to be transported back to the heart, the majority of circulation is occurring against the force of gravity. Therefore, internal valves exist to prevent the backflow of blood as it makes its way "uphill" toward the thoracic cavity. Venous return is also facilitated by the contraction of skeletal muscle that surrounds veins. A "milking" effect is thereby initiated as normal physical activity promotes the incremental transport of plasma back toward the right side of the heart. The structure of veins is illustrated in Figure 9.5.

It is important to remember that veins are very distensible and can thus stretch to accommodate a disproportionately large volume of blood. The constriction of smooth muscle within the walls of the veins reduces venous capacity and propels blood more rapidly toward the right atrium. In this way, venous return is increased.

Obstruction of Blood Flow Through the Vascular Lumen

Whenever obstruction occurs in the lumen of a vessel, blood flow is slowed or impeded. Ensuing physiological changes vary in nature and depend upon the location and extent of the occlusion.

ARTERIAL OBSTRUCTION

The most common clinical cause of vascular obstruction is a degenerative disorder called *arteriosclerosis*. Arteriosclerosis is a general term for any disorder characterized by hardening and thickening of the arterial walls.

If degenerative vascular changes are ac-

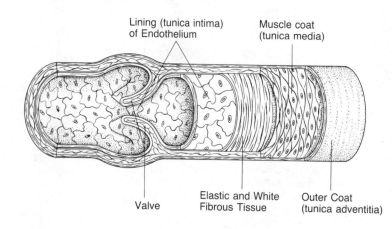

Lining (tunica intima) of Endothelium

Muscle coat (tunica media)

Valve

Elastic and White Fibrous Tissue

Outer Coat (tunica adventitia)

Figure 9.5 The structure of the vein.

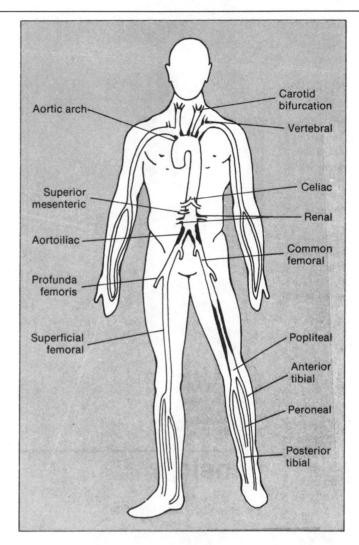

Figure 9.6 Major sites of peripheral arteriosclerotic occlusive disease. (From Royster, et al.: Postgrad. Med., *62*:154, 1977. Used by permission.)

companied by the deposit of fatty plaques within the arterial lumens, the condition is referred to as *atherosclerosis*. As the most common cause of disease and death in the elderly, its development merits further study.

Although it is possible to identify the structural changes accompanying atherosclerosis, definitive causes have not yet been established. Contributory risk factors include obesity, cigarette smoking, high-cholesterol diets, and high blood pressure.

When degenerative vascular changes occur, they usually develop gradually and progressively, typically affecting the major large arteries in the body (see Figure 9.6). As early as the age of ten, fatty streaks can be noted in the lumen of the aorta. These streaks consist of subendothelial accumulations of smooth mus-

cle–like tissue surrounded by fat cells. With the passage of time, these streaks develop into similarly composed larger structures called *fibrous plaques*. Finally, with the addition of elastic fibers and mucopolysaccharides, the plaques are transformed into degenerative sites called *complicated lesions*, or *atheromatous plaques*. Attracting calcium deposits, these lesions harden and obstruct the flow of blood through the vascular lumen. The development of atherosclerosis is illustrated in Figure 9.7.

With vascular narrowing and obstruction comes the danger of blood clot, or *thrombus*, formation. As plasma flows increasingly slowly through a restricted opening, platelets tend to catch and rupture on the atherosclerotic plaques. This, in turn, initiates the clotting process. Subsequent thrombus formation will,

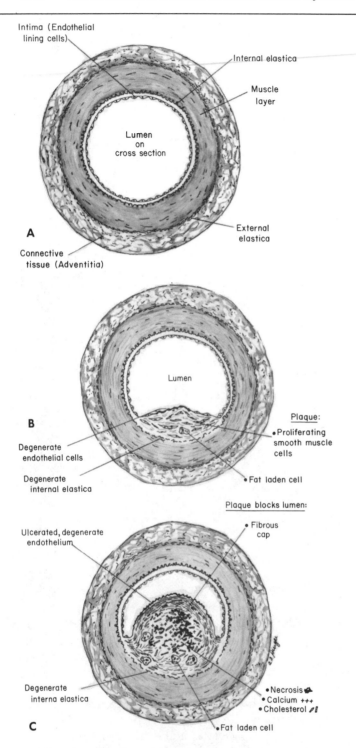

Intima (Endothelial lining cells)

Internal elastica

Muscle layer

Lumen on cross section

External elastica

A

Connective tissue (Adventitia)

Lumen

B

Plaque:

• Proliferating smooth muscle cells

Degenerate endothelial cells

Degenerate internal elastica

• Fat laden cell

Plaque blocks lumen:

• Fibrous cap

Ulcerated, degenerate endothelium

Degenerate interna elastica

• Necrosis
• Calcium +++
• Cholesterol

C

• Fat laden cell

Figure 9.7 The evolution of atherosclerosis. Note the progressive degeneration and plaque formation illustrated in *A* through *C*. (From Purtilo, D. T.: Survey of Human Disease. Reading, Mass., Addison-Wesley Publishing Company, 1978. Used by permission.

Illustration continued on opposite page

of course, occlude the already narrowed vascular opening.

The clots generated in this manner can, unfortunately, also cause damage at a point distant from their site of formation. If a portion of a blood clot breaks away, it can cause obstruction wherever it lodges in the vascular system. Such a moving clot, which is called an *embolus,* precipitates severe physiological dysfunction if it chooses to "land" in the myocardial, pulmonary, or cerebral circulatory pathway.

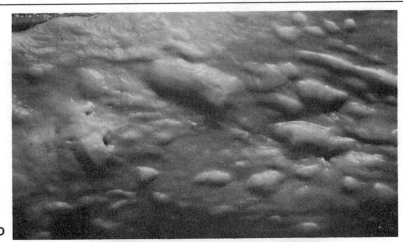

D

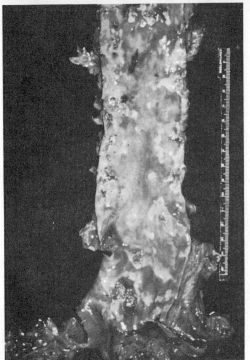

E

Figure 9.7 *Continued. D,* A close-up of atherosclerotic plaques within the lumen of the aorta. (From Benditt, E. P.: The origin of atherosclerosis. Sci. Am., *236*:74, 1977. Used by permission.) *E,* Extensive atherosclerotic lesions. (From Robbins, L. S., and Cotran, R. S.: Pathologic Basis of Disease. Philadelphia, W. B. Saunders Company, 1979. Used by permission.)

Symptoms of atherosclerosis are varied and depend largely upon the degree and location of vascular occlusion. Early indications of disease include the absence of a palpable pulse, coolness, and cyanosis in the areas that are deprived of adequate circulation.

As cellular hypoxia develops, anaerobic metabolism causes the accumulation of lactic acid, generating pain impulses. Initially, pain in the lower limbs is associated with exercise but is relieved by rest. This phenomenon is referred to as *intermittent claudication.*

In more advanced stages of vascular degeneration, pain is no longer dependent upon physical exertion and is frequently noted in the toes, heel, or metatarsophalangeal joints of the foot. In the extreme case, ischemia in these areas will result in cellular death and necrosis, with tissue ulceration and gangrene.

To the extent that blood supply to vital organs is occluded by atherosclerotic deposits, major disruptions in homeostasis can occur. Blockage of the coronary arteries feeding the heart, for example, (referred to as arteriosclerotic heart disease, or *ASHD*) can result in severe myocardial tissue damage. Accompanying physiological changes will be discussed later in this chapter. In a similar fashion, the

TABLE 9–1.   **Clinical Manifestations of Atherosclerosis**

Manifestations	Causative Mechanism
Intermittent claudication: exercise-induced pain in the lower limbs, which is relieved by rest	Hypoxia and accumulation of metabolic wastes associated with muscle ischemia
Shiny, thin skin Thick, opaque nails Loss of hair Cool extremities Pallor/cyanosis of skin Decrease or absence of peripheral pulse	Decrease of blood supply to the periphery
Mental confusion Monocular blindness Dizziness Motor instability Occasional loss of consciousness	Cerebral hypoxia, secondary to arterial occlusion
Angina pectoris	Transient myocardial ischemia
Myocardial infarction	Myocardial necrosis, secondary to occlusion of the coronary arteries
Abnormal ECG's	Disruption of the cardiac conduction system, secondary to ischemia
Renal failure	Disruption of functional activity in the nephron, secondary to renal ischemia

occlusion of renal arteries, feeding the kidneys, or carotid arteries, feeding the brain, can cause renal or cerebral dysfunction. A brief summary of some systemic clinical manifestations of atherosclerosis is presented in Table 9.1.

VENOUS OBSTRUCTION

Although clot formation most commonly occurs in the arteries, thrombi can also develop in the veins. Most often, this occurs in cases of *thrombophlebitis,* or inflammation of the venous wall. The development of thrombophlebitis is facilitated by a number of factors, including:

1. *venous stasis* (pooling of blood in the venous vessels). This can occur in individuals with varicose veins, a condition in which vessels are characteristically dilated and valves are nonfunctional. It is also noted following periods of prolonged immobility, when skeletal muscles are not functioning to promote venous return.

2. *injury to the venous endothelial lining.* This disorder often results from intravenous injections, fractures, and dislocations.

3. *hypercoagulability of blood* (blood excessively prone to clotting). This phenomenon, characterized by elevated platelet counts, can occur secondary to cancer, long-term use of oral contraceptives, and certain hematopoietic disorders.

Because of the general pattern of venous blood flow, obstruction in the veins does not usually lead to extensive functional changes. This is due largely to the fact that venous return is characterized by simultaneous flow through superficial and deep vessels. If occlusion or stasis occurs in superficial veins, blood may be shunted through communicating vessels into deep veins. In this way, an alternate circulatory pathway is provided (see Figure 9.8). If, however, obstruction develops in deep vessels, return to the heart can be significantly slowed. Under these conditions, blood pressure will increase in the capillaries feeding the occluded veins. The resulting flux of fluid from plasma into the interstitial compartment will cause edema, tenderness, and pain.

Although thrombus formation in a vein does not typically result in ischemia, tissue hypoxia can result if an embolus derived of a

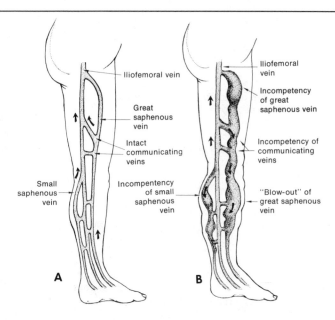

Figure 9.8 *A,* Healthy venous circulation. Note that blood ascends in both superficial and deep veins and can pass from superficial to deep veins via the communicating veins. *B,* The effect of varicosities upon venous circulation. Note that blood cannot ascend via incompetent superficial veins and thus must return to the heart via the deeper vessels. (From Abramson, D. I.: Vascular Disorders of the Extremities, 2nd ed. New York, Harper & Row, 1974. Used by permission.)

venous clot lodges in an arterial vessel. This phenomenon is a frequent complication of thrombophlebitis, and extreme care must be taken to prevent or minimize the generation of pulmonary, myocardial, or cerebral emboli. Patients with a venous clot are thus often treated with anticoagulant drugs and instructed to rest the affected limb until the thrombus is sufficiently dissipated.

Inappropriate Vascular Constriction or Dilation

Although obstruction is a common cause of vascular disease, blood flow through the vessels can also be impeded by excessive narrowing or widening of the vascular walls. Contraction and relaxation of the smooth muscle in arteries, arterioles, venules, and veins are normally adaptive in nature and contribute to the maintenance of optimal circulation. When alterations are extreme or inappropriate, however, disorders can result. In the following pages, a distinction is made between the causes and manifestations of nonadaptive vascular constriction and dilation.

INAPPROPRIATE VASCULAR CONSTRICTION

Inappropriate vascular constriction is most often induced by nonadaptive neural or chemical stimulation of the smooth muscle in the vascular walls.

In general, nerve-induced vasoconstriction is triggered by impulses originating in the vasoconstrictor center of the medulla. Transmitted to the vascular walls by fibers of the sympathetic nervous system, they govern smooth muscle contraction. An inappropriate increase in vasoconstrictor impulses is frequently noted at times of tension or anxiety. Certain tumors in the brain can also cause excessive vasoconstriction.

Chemically induced contraction, on the other hand, is most commonly caused by norepinephrine and angiotensin. Epinephrine also functions in vasoconstriction but acts selectively upon superficial blood vessels, while causing dilation of vessels that supply the brain, heart, and skeletal muscles.

Epinephrine and norepinephrine are secreted and released by the medulla (internal tissue) of the adrenal glands. Although output of these chemicals is normally controlled by the hypothalamus of the brain, clinical excesses most often result from adrenal medullary tumors (*pheochromocytomas*). This condition is often life-threatening if not corrected surgically.

Angiotensin formation is normally triggered by the release of renin from the nephrons of the kidney. The renin-angiotensin mechanism has been previously described in Chapter 5, and is summarized diagrammatically in Figure 9.9. In short, it can be said that

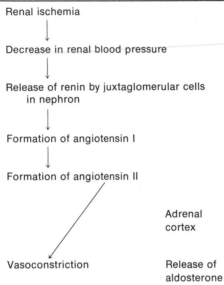

Renal ischemia

↓

Decrease in renal blood pressure

↓

Release of renin by juxtaglomerular cells in nephron

↓

Formation of angiotensin I

↓

Formation of angiotensin II

Adrenal cortex

Vasoconstriction   Release of aldosterone

Figure 9.9   The renin-angiotensin mechanism

as renal ischemia promotes the output of renin, vasoconstriction results from the effects of angiotensin upon the smooth muscle in vascular walls.

Regardless of the cause of vasoconstriction, associated physiological changes include:

1. an increase in arterial blood pressure, as peripheral resistance increases and fluid accumulates excessively within narrowed arterial lumens.

2. an increase in venous return and cardiac output, as narrowing of the veins promotes a more rapid return of blood to the right side of the heart.

3. a decrease in capillary blood pressure and the servicing of cellular needs, as the volume of blood entering the microcirculation is compromised.

INAPPROPRIATE VASCULAR DILATION

Most often, inappropriate vascular dilation is induced by parasympathetic neural stimulation or massive systemic release of histamine. Vasodilation may also be caused by chemical agents such as bradykinin, muscle metabolites, acetylcholine, and bacterial toxins.

Regardless of the cause of vascular dilation, characteristic clinical manifestations include:

1. a decrease in arterial blood pressure, as peripheral resistance decreases and fluid presses with less force upon dilated arterial walls.

2. a decrease in venous return and cardiac output, as dilation promotes venous stasis.

3. an increase in capillary blood pressure and fluid flux into the interstitial compartment as blood accumulates in the microcirculation.

Causes of Vascular Pathology: A Summary

In review, it can be said that vascular disease, as defined in this text, evolves secondary to obstruction or inappropriate constriction or dilation of the blood vessels.

The clinical manifestations of obstruction vary with the location and extent of the blockage. Whether occlusion originates in the arteries or veins, however, physiological disruption will ensue only to the extent that cellular blood supply is compromised. Thus, during the early stages of atherosclerosis, or in minor cases of nonembolizing thrombophlebitis, homeostasis can frequently be maintained.

Similarly, in disorders characterized by excessive contraction or relaxation of the smooth muscle in vascular walls, only extreme or prolonged alterations lead to cellular disequilibrium. A comparative summary of the causes and manifestations of vascular disorders can be found in Table 9.2.

Hypertension: A Study in Vascular Pathology

Hypertension is a clinical phenomenon characterized by an elevation in arterial blood pressure. When arterial blood pressure is measured clinically, two numbers are recorded, as follows: 120/80. The first number (120), which reflects the pressure exerted against the arterial walls when the ventricles are in systole, is referred to as *systolic blood pressure*. The second number (80) is a measure of *diastolic blood pressure*, or the force exerted against arterial walls when the ventricles are in diastole. The difference between systolic and diastolic blood pressure is designated as *pulse pressure*. In our example, pulse pressure

TABLE 9–2.   **Vascular Pathology**

Pathological Mechanism	Causative Clinical Disorders	Manifestations

Obstruction of blood flow through arterial lumen	Atherosclerosis
	Thrombi
	Emboli
		In area affected by circulatory deficit:
		    coolness
		    pain
		    ulceration and gangrene
		    organic dysfunction (typically renal, myocardial, and/or cerebral)

Obstruction of blood flow through venous lumen	Thrombophlebitis secondary to:
	    venous stasis
	    injury to venous endothelium
	    hypercoagulability of blood
		Edema, tenderness, and pain in affected area

Inappropriate vascular constriction	Tension; anxiety Pheochromocytoma Renal ischemia	Increased arterial blood pressure Possible cellular ischemia
Inappropriate vascular dilation	Anaphylactic shock Septic shock	Decreased arterial blood pressure Decreased venous return and cardiac output

would be equal to 120 mm. Hg minus 80 mm. Hg, or 40 mm. Hg.

Hypertension is defined by the American Heart Association as a persistent, sustained condition in which the systolic pressure is greater than 140 mm. Hg, and the diastolic pressure is greater than 90 mm. Hg. Often associated with phenomena that: (1) decrease the distensibility of the arterial wall, (2) increase peripheral resistance, or (3) cause hypervolemia, hypertension is described as *primary* or *essential* when a specific causative disorder cannot be identified. Less frequently (approximately 10 per cent of the time), high blood pressure may be associated with a particular organic disorder, and is described as *secondary hypertension*. Regardless of precipitating factors, hypertension poses a major threat to the health of many Americans. An understanding of its development and manifestations enables integration of many clinical aspects of vascular disease.

DEVELOPMENT OF HYPERTENSION

When blood is ejected from the ventricles of the heart into the large arteries, disten-sibility of the vascular walls normally militates against an excessive increase in systolic pressure. During ventricular relaxation, on the other hand, elastic recoil of the arteries helps to propel blood through the vascular tree. In this way, a sudden drop in diastolic pressure is avoided.

If hardening of the major arteries should occur, a condition described as *benign arteriosclerotic hypertension* may result. Characterized by an increase in systolic blood pressure and a decrease in diastolic pressure, this form of hypertension is considered to be a relatively harmless manifestation of vascular disease.

When high blood pressure is associated with an increase in peripheral resistance, however, the resulting condition is a potentially serious threat to physiological equilibrium. Most often caused by widespread constriction of arterioles throughout the body, this condition is characterized by retention of fluid within the arterial vessels (see Figure 9.10). An increase in both systolic and diastolic pressures will predictably occur.

Most often in cases of hypertension associated with arteriolar vasoconstriction an exact causative mechanism cannot be identified.

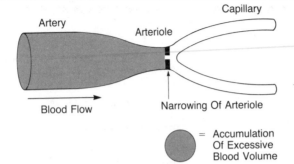

Figure 9.10 The effect of narrowing of the arterioles upon blood pressure in the arteries.

Frequently, however, renal mechanisms may be implicated in one of two ways:

1. Vasoconstriction triggered by neural or endocrine disorders of unknown origin may promote secondary release of renin from is-chemic kidneys. Subsequent formation of angiotensin II will cause additional vasoconstriction and release of aldosterone. Resulting retention of sodium and water aggravates the hypertensive condition.

2. Renal disease of unknown origin may cause abnormal increases in the secretion of renin. Secondary formation of angiotensin II will cause changes, as described earlier.

Although essential hypertension is the most common clinical form of high blood pressure, secondary hypertension is also a significantly pathological entity. Often associated with renal or endocrine dysfunction (see Table 9.3), high blood pressure can also be induced by select vascular occlusion. In cases of coarctation of the aorta, for example, constriction of the aorta is characteristically

TABLE 9–3. **Causes of Secondary Hypertension***

Cause	Etiology	Symptoms	Physical Findings
Coarctation of aorta	Constriction of portion of aorta causes elevated blood pressure proximal to obstruction	Absence of femoral pulses; decreased blood pressure in legs as compared with arms; weight loss	X-ray shows notching of ribs; intercostal bruits on auscultation
Pheochromocytoma	Adrenal medullary tumor causes excess secretion of catecholamines	Half of all patients have sudden attacks of severe headache with palpitation; hypermetabolic state; excessive sweating; meat intolerance; flushed, anxious appearance	Elevated basal metabolic rate (BMR); elevated fasting blood sugar; excess excretion of catecholamines in urine
Primary aldosteronism	Functioning adenoma of adrenal cortex	Moderate elevation of blood pressure; muscular weakness; polyurea; nocturia; polydipsia; tetany; pares-thesias; headache	Dilute alkaline urine, persistently low serum K$^+$ levels
Cushing's syndrome	Excess glucocorticosteroids excreted from adrenal cortex; cause may be an adrenocortical adenoma (or carcinoma) or adreno-cortical hyperplasia	Mild hypertension; moon facies; "buffalo" hump on back; edema; hirsutism	Excretion of large amounts of 17-hydroxycorticoids and 17-ketosteroids in urine
Renovascular hypertension	Narrowing of renal artery due to atherosclerosis, fibrosis of wall or renal artery, or trauma to renal area	Hypertension; fluid retention with edema	Difference in length of kidneys; delayed appearance of dye from one kidney during intravenous pyelogram (IVP); decreased urine and Na$^+$ output
Parenchymal disease (acute and chronic glomerulonephritis)	Allergic response to infection in body (usually streptococcal), causing in-flammatory changes in glomeruli	Hypertension; sodium and water retension; edema; oliguria; orthopnea; dyspnea; pulmonary edema; uremic odor	Cardiac enlargement; evidence of myocardial failure of ECG, elevated nonprotein nitrogen (NPN)

*From Luckmann, J., and Sorensen, K. C.: Medical-Surgical Nursing: A Psychophysiologic Approach. Philadelphia, W. B. Saunders Company, 1980. Used by permission.

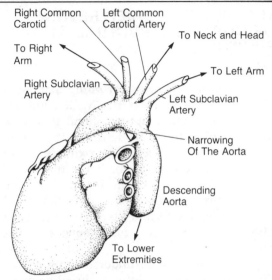

Right Common Carotid

Left Common Carotid Artery

To Neck and Head

To Right Arm

To Left Arm

Right Subclavian Artery

Left Subclavian Artery

Narrowing Of The Aorta

Descending Aorta

To Lower Extremities

Figure 9.11 Coarctation of the aorta.

noted at a point beyond the exit of the left subclavian artery (see Figure 9.11). This phenomenon causes an increase of blood pressure in vessels proximal to the obstruction (such as those servicing the right and left arms) and a decrease of blood pressure in the lower extremities. Fortunately, coarctation of the aorta is a disorder that can be corrected surgically.

Regardless of the nature of hypertension, elevations in blood pressure are considerably exacerbated by the existence of hypervolemia. Whenever plasma volume is elevated, the quantity of fluid pushing against the arterial walls will be increased. For this reason, hypertensive patients are frequently treated with diuretics to reduce extracellular fluid volume. In cases in which fluid is retained excessively (such as in Cushing's disease, primary aldosteronism, or SIADH), increases in blood pressure are characteristic.

CLINICAL MANIFESTATIONS OF HYPERTENSION

Regardless of cause, hypertension, once established, can initiate a series of very disruptive physiological changes. Increased fluid pressure against the vascular walls causes further degenerative changes. Large vessels harden and narrow; smaller vessels show indications of constriction and damaged linings. The result is further aggravation of the hypertensive condition and depletion of the blood supply to many vital organs (See Table 9.4).

TABLE 9–4. **Some Manifestations of Essential Hypertension***

Symptoms	Base of Symptoms
Blood pressure persistently elevated above 140/90	Arterioles are constricted, causing abnormal resistance to blood flow
Anginal pain	Insufficient blood flow through coronary arteries to the myocardium
Intermittent claudication†	Decrease in blood supply to the legs
Retinal hemorrhages and exudates	Damage to arterioles that supply the retina
Severe occipital headaches associated with nausea and vomiting, drowsiness, giddiness, anxiety, and mental impairment	Vessel damage within the brain
Polyuria; nocturia; diminished ability of kidneys to concentrate urine; protein and RBC's in urine	Arteriolar nephrosclerosis (hardening of arterioles within the kidney)
Dyspnea upon exertion	Left-sided heart failure
Edema of the extremities	Right-sided heart failure

*From Luckmann, J., and Sorensen, K. C.: Medical-Surgical Nursing: A Psychophysiologic Approach. Philadelphia, W. B. Saunders Company, 1980. Used by permission.
†Intermittent claudication is a severe pain that develops in the calf muscles when a patient walks and subsides at rest; this is a symptom of peripheral vascular disease.

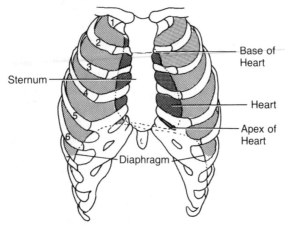

Figure 9.12 The location of the heart.

THE HEART: A BRIEF REVIEW OF NORMAL STRUCTURE AND FUNCTION

The heart is a muscular pump that ejects blood into the vascular tree with sufficient pressure to promote optimal circulation. It is located within the thoracic cavity in an area called the *mediastinum;* approximately two thirds of its mass lies to the left of the body's midline. As illustrated in Figure 9.12, the heart is surrounded laterally by the lungs and extends from the second rib to the level of the fifth intercostal space, just above the diaphragm.

To facilitate better understanding of cardiac activity, it is helpful to briefly review some basic aspects of normal anatomy and physiology, as follows: (1) cardiac structure, (2) the flow of blood through the heart, (3) the cardiac cycle, (4) cardiac output, and (5) myocardial blood supply.

Cardiac Structure

Internally, the heart is divided into four chambers: a right and a left atrium, and a right and a left ventricle. The atria are superior, small chambers that are separated from each other by a thin interatrial partition called a

Symptoms reflect the extent and location of vascular degeneration. The structures most sensitive to impeded circulation are the *heart, brain, and kidneys.* Twenty-five to 35 per cent of hypertensive patients die of congestive heart failure induced by myocardial ischemia and the indirect stress imposed by hypertension. Another 15 per cent succumb to cerebrovascular accidents (strokes) caused by damage to blood vessels feeding the brain. An additional 20 per cent of hypertensive patients fall victim to renal failure precipitated by degenerative changes in the blood vessels supplying the nephrons.

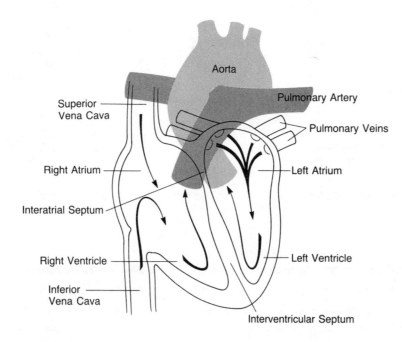

Figure 9.13 The basic structure of the heart.

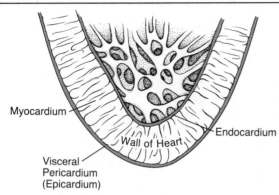

Figure 9.14   The wall of the heart.

Myocardium

Endocardium

Wall of Heart

Visceral Pericardium (Epicardium)

septum. They serve as receptacles for blood and contract to promote optimal filling of the larger, inferior, ventricular chambers. The ventricles are also isolated from one another by a thick muscular wall called the interventricular septum. They pump blood either to the lungs (from the right side) or into the systemic arterial tree (from the left side). This general structure is illustrated in Figure 9.13.

Although the wall of the heart consists primarily of muscle tissue (*myocardium*), it is covered and lined by thin membranes called the *epicardium* (or *visceral pericardium*) and *endocardium,* respectively (see Figure 9.14). While epicardium is found exclusively on the surface of cardiac muscle, endocardium ex-

tends from the chambers of the heart to line all blood vessels in the body. It thereby provides an uninterrupted, smooth surface for interface with circulating blood.

To supplement the protection afforded by epicardium and endocardium, the heart is encased within a sac of tough, fibrous *parietal pericardium*. As illustrated in Figure 9.15, the narrow pericardial cavity that exists between visceral and parietal pericardium normally contains a clear, watery, serous fluid. This fluid, secreted by the pericardial membranes, functions in both lubrication and shock absorption.

The Flow of Blood Through the Heart

In general, the heart is designed to propel blood into two major circulatory pathways. While the right ventricle is expelling deoxygenated blood into the pulmonary blood vessels (where diffusion of respiratory gases can occur), the left heart is simultaneously pumping freshly oxygenated arterial blood into the systemic circulation.

Ideally, a drop of blood should move in a fixed route from the time it enters the right atrium until it is ejected from the left ventricle. As illustrated in Figure 9.16, blood normally

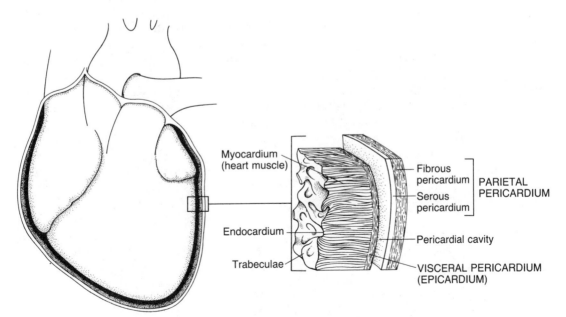

Myocardium (heart muscle)

Fibrous pericardium

PARIETAL PERICARDIUM

Serous pericardium

Endocardium

Pericardial cavity

Trabeculae

VISCERAL PERICARDIUM (EPICARDIUM)

Figure 9.15   The pericardial cavity.

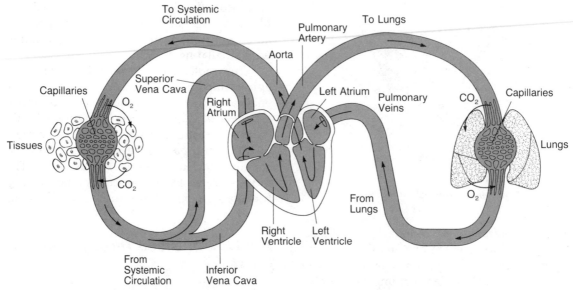

Figure 9.16 The flow of blood through the heart.

travels through the heart in the following way: right atrium → right ventricle → pulmonary arteries → lungs → pulmonary veins → left atrium → left ventricle → aorta.

The valves of the heart ensure the transport of blood through this carefully prescribed pathway. When ventricular *systole* (contraction) occurs, valves between the atria and the ventricles snap shut to prevent blood from flowing backward into the atria. These valves (specifically designated as atrioventricular, or cuspid valves) are fashioned from three leaflets of tissue on the right side (the *tricuspid valve*) and two on the left (the *bicuspid, or mitral, valve*).

Alternately, during ventricular *diastole* (relaxation), semilunar valves at the base of the pulmonary artery (*pulmonic valve*) and aorta (*aortic valve*) function to prevent reflux of blood from these major vessels back into the ventricles. The location and function of the four major valves in the heart are summarized in Figure 9.17.

The Cardiac Cycle

While cardiac valves facilitate the effective circulation of blood through the heart, the cardiac pump must alternately contract and relax in a rhythmic fashion, if output is to be maintained. Normally, atrial systole is followed by ventricular systole. A period of total rest, or diastole, precedes the initiation of any subsequent contractions. This pattern, referred to as the *cardiac cycle*, repeats itself inexorably, approximately 70 to 80 times a minute, throughout the life of the individual.

As illustrated in Figure 9.18, any given cardiac cycle lasts approximately 0.8 second and consists of 0.1 second of atrial systole, 0.3 second of ventricular systole, and 0.4 second of cardiac diastole. This intricately orchestrated time sequence is designed to facilitate optimal filling and emptying of the chambers of the heart. Any deviation from these norms can, therefore, lead to a decrease in cardiac output.

Because the valves of the heart normally close and open in response to fluctuating intraventricular pressures, it is possible to predict their status at any given point in the cardiac cycle. As illustrated in Figure 9.19, the atrioventricular valves typically snap shut during ventricular systole, while the semilunar valves close during cardiac diastole.

Figure 9.17 *A*, The valves of the heart. *B*, A frontal section of the heart showing location of cardiac valves. *C*, A view of the heart from above showing location of cardiac valves. (From Jacob, S. W., Francone, C. A., and Lossow, W. J.: Structure and Function in Man, 4th ed. Philadelphia, W. B. Saunders Company, 1978. Used by permission.)

Valves of the Heart

Valve		Location	Function
Cuspid valves	Tricuspid	Between right atrium and right ventricle	Prevents the backflow of blood from right ventricle to right atrium during systole
	Bicuspid (mitral)	Between left atrium and left ventricle	Prevents the backflow of blood from left ventricle to left atrium during systole
Semilunar valves	Pulmonary semilunar	At the base of the pulmonary artery	Prevents the backflow of blood from pulmonary artery to right ventricle during diastole
	Aortic semilunar	At the base of the aorta	Prevents the backflow of blood from aorta to left ventricle during diastole

A

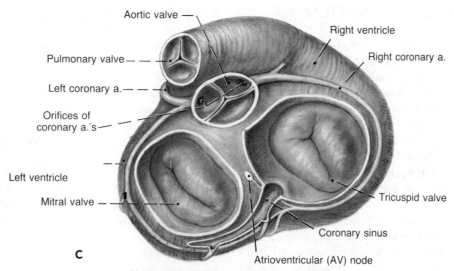

B

C

Figure 9.17 *See legend on opposite page*

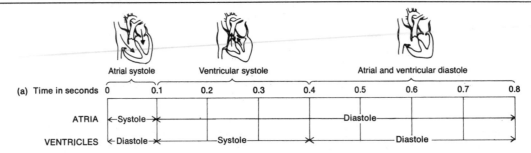

(a) Time in seconds

Figure 9.18 The cardiac cycle. (From Tortora, G. J., and Anagnostakos, N. P.: Principles of Anatomy and Physiology, 2nd ed. New York, Harper & Row, 1978. Used by permission.)

By applying a stethoscope to the wall of the chest, it is possible to hear heart sounds that reflect specific aspects of valvular activity. Normally, a long, low *lub* sound is followed by a shorter, higher *dup*, and then by a pause. While the *lub* sound is caused by turbulence due to the closure of the cuspid valves, the *dup* is associated with the snapping shut of the semilunar valves. If a valvular disorder exists, abnormal sounds called *murmurs* may be detectable.

In order to fully understand the nature of the cardiac cycle, it is helpful to clarify specific ways in which rhythmic contraction is (1) regulated and (2) visualized diagnostically. Therefore, the structure and function of the conduction system and the significance of the electrocardiogram print-out will be described.

THE CONDUCTION SYSTEM

Cardiac muscle, like skeletal muscle, is composed of striated fibrous cells that shorten to produce muscular contraction. In the case of the myocardium, however, fibers are organized into two discrete networks of interconnecting cells — one in the atrial walls and the other in the ventricular walls. Impulses originating at any point in a given network (called a *syncytium*) will normally spread rapidly and uniformly, causing each muscle mass to contract as a unit.

Because of the functional separation between the two myocardial syncytiums, a mechanism must exist to coordinate atrial and ventricular contractions. Ultimately, these contractions are integrated by the *conduction system* of the heart. Fashioned from modified cardiac muscle tissue, the conduction system consists of four major components:

1. *The sinoatrial (SA) node.* This node of tissue is located in the posterior wall of the right atrium, adjacent to the point at which the superior vena cava enters the heart. It discharges impulses at a rate of approximately 72 to 80 times a minute, and it will maintain this inherent beat whether it is inside the heart or excised from it. Normally, the SA node is responsible for determining the rate of contraction for all cardiac muscle and is thus referred to as the cardiac pacemaker.

2. *The atrioventricular (AV) node.* This node of tissue sits on top of the interventricular septum. It receives impulses from the SA node and transmits them to ventricular muscle via the bundle of His. If excised from the heart, the AV node will generate impulses at a rate of 40 to 50 times a minute. Under normal circumstances, however, its discharge rate is determined by the rhythm of the pacemaker.

3. *The bundle of His.* This bundle of conducting fibers extends through the interventricular septum, ultimately dividing into a right and a left bundle branch. These fibers transmit impulses from the AV node to the ventricular walls.

4. *The Purkinje fibers.* These fibers run within the ventricular wall. They receive impulses from the bundle branches and transmit them rapidly and uniformly through the ventricles, thereby triggering contraction.

The entire conduction system is illustrated in Figure 9.20.

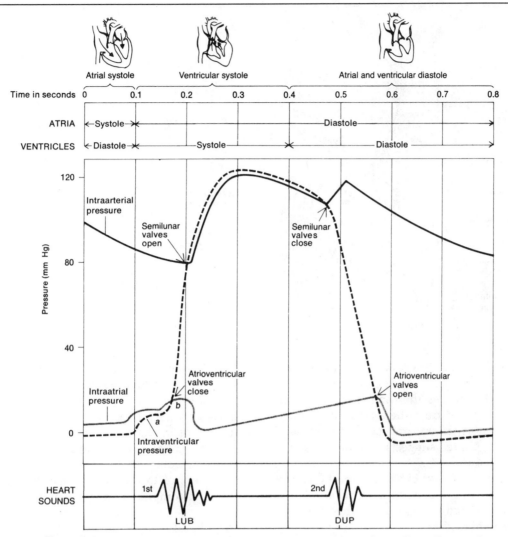

Figure 9.19 The opening and closure of valves during the cardiac cycle. (From Tortora, G. J., and Anagnostakos, N. P.: Principles of Anatomy and Physiology, 2nd ed. New York, Harper & Row, 1978. Used by permission.)

THE ELECTROCARDIOGRAM

The conduction system functions to initiate and sustain the normal cardiac cycle. If a pathologic condition develops, however, serious arrhythmias may result. In these cases, diagnosis is greatly aided by the electrocardiograph apparatus, which provides the clinician with a print-out that reflects myocardial activity.

The normal *electrocardiogram (ECG)* strip records the electrical changes in cardiac muscle during systole and diastole. As illustrated in Figure 9.21, it consists of three basic subunits. The *P wave* indicates atrial contraction; the *QRS complex*, ventricular contraction; and the *T wave*, ventricular recovery following systole. The appearance of these waves and complexes can provide relevant information to the clinician about the status of the heart.

In examining the ECG strip, it is important to be aware of the length and position of certain specified intervals that normally exist between the waves and complexes of any given cardiac cycle.

The *P-R interval*, for example, is illustrat-

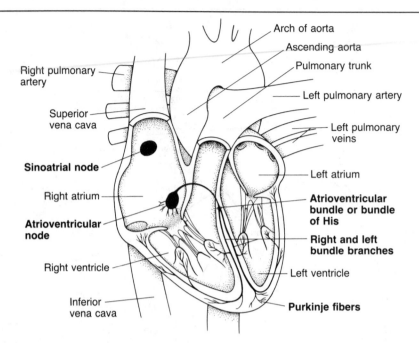

Figure 9.20 The conduction system of the heart.

ed in Figure 9.22. It extends from the beginning of the P wave to the beginning of the Q wave and indicates the time it takes for impulses to spread from the atria to the ventricles. Any delay in transmisison, or increase in the interval, often suggests organic damage to the AV node.

The *S-T segment* extends from the end of the S wave to the beginning of the T wave. It may be elevated or depressed when myocardial ischemia exists.

The measurement of quantitative deviations from the norm is simplified by the type of paper that ECG tracings are printed on. As illustrated in Figure 9.23, uniform little squares provide a horizontal measure of time elapsed as well as a vertical measure of the strength or intensity of a wave.

By providing a noninvasive way of assessing cardiac activity, the ECG offers a major service to the health care practitioner. Although comprehensive interpretation of the

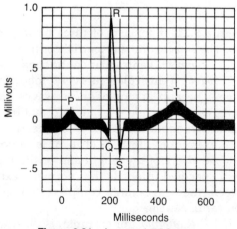

Figure 9.21 A normal ECG strip.

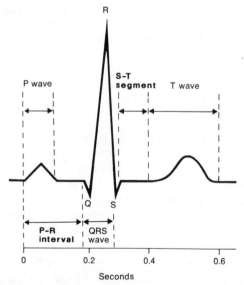

Figure 9.22 Some major components of a normal ECG strip.

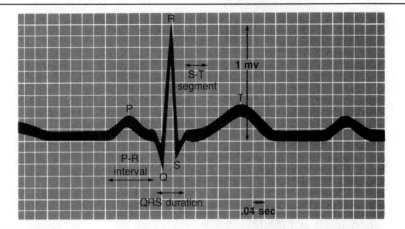

Figure 9.23 The basic ECG complex.

print-outs must be left to the experts, it is nevertheless helpful to be generally familiar with some basic ECG norms. These are presented, in tabular form, in Figure 9.24.

Cardiac Output

Ultimately, the cardiac cycle facilitates the ejection of optimal quantities of blood into the pulmonary and systemic circulations. *Cardiac output*, defined as the quantity of blood ejected by each ventricle per minute, normally

equals around 5 liters. Varying as a function of cardiac rate and *stroke volume* (the amount of blood ejected from each ventricle per beat), cardiac output can be determined as follows:

cardiac output = cardiac rate × stroke volume
   5040 ml.   72/minute   70 ml.

Although a cardiac output of 5 liters is usually sufficient to service cellular needs during periods of rest and relaxation, it does not represent the maximal pumping capacity of

WAVES OF EXCITATION SEEN IN A TYPICAL ELECTROCARDIOGRAM

Wave	Meaning and Significance	Time Period	Abnormalities
P Wave	Signifies depolarization and contraction of the atria	0.08 sec.	Abnormal or absent P waves imply that another area of the heart muscle is acting as pacemaker in place of SA node
PR Interval	Section from beginning of P wave to beginning of QRS complex; signifies time it takes impulse to pass from atria to ventricles	Average time = 0.16 sec. Usually less than 0.20 sec.	Prolonged PR interval: Impulse being conducted more slowly than normal through AV node *Shortened PR interval:* impulse being conducted over a shortened abnormal route from atria to ventricles
QRS Complex	Depolarization and contraction of ventricles	0.06– 0.12 sec.	Prolonged QRS complex signifies abnormal conduction or delay of conduction through the ventricles
ST Segment	Period following completion of depolarization of ventricles and preceding repolarization of ventricles	0.12 sec.	*Elevation* or *depression* of ST segment indicates ischemia or infarction of the heart muscle
T Wave	Repolarization of ventricles following contraction	0.16 sec.	*Inverted* T wave: implies ischemia or infarction of heart muscle

Figure 9.24 Some characteristic features of a typical electrocardiogram. (From Luckmann, J., and Sorensen, K. C.: Medical-Surgical Nursing: A Psychophysiologic Approach, 2nd ed. Philadelphia, W. B. Saunders Company, 1980. Used by permission.)

the heart. Considerable *cardiac reserve* does exist, which allows output to increase to as much as 12 to 13 liters during times of stress or physical exertion. Clearly, it is alterations in cardiac rate or stroke volume or both that are primarily responsible for this variability in cardiac output.

STROKE VOLUME

Stroke volume is defined as the amount of blood ejected with each ventricular contraction. Normally, ventricles fill during relaxation to an *end diastolic volume (EDV)* of approximately 100 ml. of blood. Contraction typically forces about two thirds of this volume (or 70 ml.) into arterial blood vessels; thus leaving approximately 30 ml. in the ventricles at the end of systole (referred to as the *end systolic volume,* or *ESV*). As illustrated in Figure 9.25, any variation in either EDV or ESV can cause considerable fluctuation in stroke volume (SV).

While EDV is largely affected by cardiac rate and venous return (both of which will be discussed subsequently), ESV and SV are in-

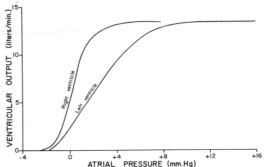

Figure 9.26 Approximate normal right and left ventricular output curves for the human heart (as extrapolated from data obtained in dogs). (From Guyton, A. C.: Textbook of Medical Physiology, 6th ed. Philadelphia, W. B. Saunders Company, 1981. Used by permission.)

fluenced by three major factors: (1) preload, (2) contractility, and (3) afterload.

PRELOAD Preload refers to the stretch of myocardial muscle initiated by the return of venous blood to the heart. Since, according to *Frank-Starling's law*, the force of contraction will increase as a result of muscular fiber stretch, this mechanism provides a means of intrinsically adapting to varying levels of venous return. As increasing quantities of blood enter the atria (and subsequently the ventricles), an associated rise in intra-atrial and intraventricular pressures should cause an increase in cardiac output (see Figure 9.26).

CONTRACTILITY Contractility is defined as alterations in the strength of cardiac muscle contraction caused by factors other than preload stretch. Contractility is typically increased by exposure to calcium, norepinephrine, or epinephrine and stimulation by the sympathetic nervous system. Acidosis, hypocalcemia, hyperkalemia, and parasympathetic neural stimulation, on the other hand, all tend to decrease the force of myocardial contraction.

AFTERLOAD Afterload can be defined as the amount of force that must be generated during systole to eject blood into the arterial vessels. Varying primarily as a function of arterial blood pressure and ventricular radius, afterload explains why myocardial work must increase under certain conditions, if stroke volume is to be maintained (see Figure 9.27).

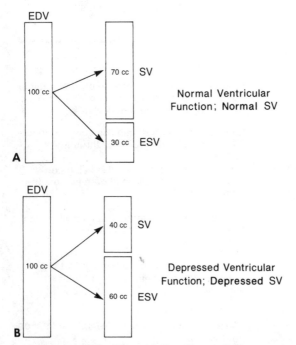

Figure 9.25 The relationship between end-diastolic volume (EDV), stroke volume (SV), and end-systolic volume (ESV), under normal circumstances *(A)*, and in cases of depressed ventricular function *(B)*.

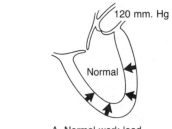

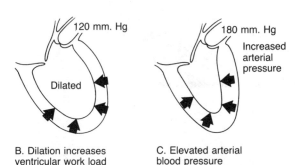

A. Normal work load

B. Dilation increases ventricular work load

C. Elevated arterial blood pressure increases work load

Figure 9.27 Myocardial work as a function of arterial blood pressure and ventricular diameter. Note that work must increase in cases in which ventricles are dilated, as in (B), or arterial blood pressure is elevated, as in (C).

If rising arterial blood pressure poses resistance to the exit of blood from the heart, for example, the cardiac muscle will have to exert greater effort to sustain output. Likewise, if ventricular muscle dilates, the pumping work of the heart is increased.

Ultimately, stroke volume will remain within normal limits only if the heart is able to continuously respond to varying degrees of afterload stress. To the extent that disease depresses the functional adaptability of cardiac muscle, output will decrease.

CARDIAC RATE

Under normal circumstances, the impetus for cardiac contraction originates in the SA node. Although the rate dictated by this node is usually stable within a narrow range, it can be modified by a number of external influences.

Decreases in cardiac rate, for example, may be caused by increased parasympathetic neural stimulation, decreased sympathetic neural stimulation, hyperkalemia, or depressed body temperatures.

Cardiac acceleration, on the other hand, is frequently triggered by decreases in arterial blood pressure, decreases in pO_2, elevations in pCO_2, exercise, or alarm. In these cases, mobilization of the sympathetic nervous system is responsible for cardiac stimulation (see Figure 9.28).

Elevations in cardiac rate may also be caused by chemical agents, such as epinephrine, norepinephrine, and thyroxine. If disease causes hypersecretion of these hormones, tachycardia and palpitation will predictably result.

Although increases in cardiac rate cause blood to be ejected more frequently from the heart, cardiac output will not always rise accordingly. In cases in which acceleration is excessive, for example, a decrease in diastolic filling time will ultimately cause EDV to fall. Under these circumstances, the volume of blood that can be ejected from the heart per beat will decline, and cardiac output may subsequently be compromised.

Myocardial Blood Supply

In order for cardiac muscle to function optimally, it must receive an adequate supply of oxygen and nutrients. Normally, blood is transported to myocardial cells by the *coronary arteries*. As illustrated in Figure 9.29, these vessels originate immediately above the aortic semilunar valve and branch to service specific segments of the heart, as follows:

1. The *right coronary artery* supplies the right atrium, the right ventricle, and part of the posterior wall of the left ventricle.

2. The *left circumflex artery* supplies the left atrium and the lateral and posterior walls of the left ventricle.

3. The *left anterior interventricular artery* supplies the anterior left ventricle.

After supplying cellular needs, blood initially passes into the *cardiac veins*, which parallel the route taken by major coronary arteries. Subsequent transport into an enlarged vessel called the *coronary sinus* is followed by delivery of blood back into the right atrium of the heart.

Since cardiac muscle is extremely sensitive to oxygen or nutrient deprivation, the maintenance of adequate myocardial circula-

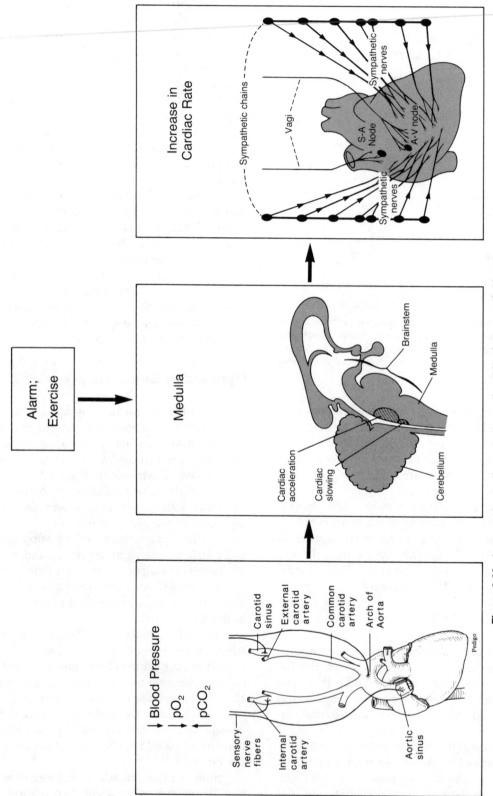

Figure 9.28   Increase in cardiac rate as mediated by the sympathetic nervous system.

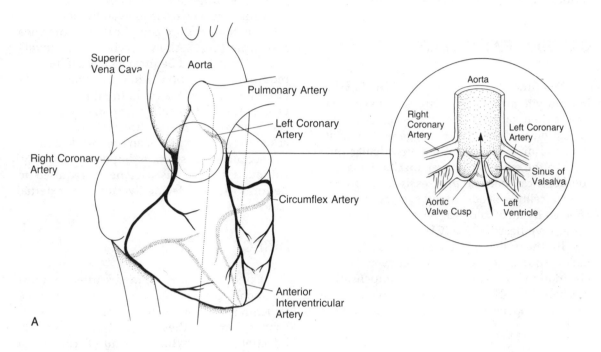

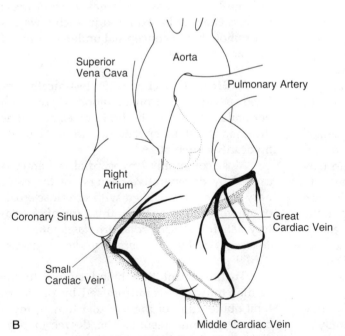

Figure 9.29 Myocardial circulation. *A,* The transport of freshly oxygenated arterial blood to the myocardium via coronary arteries. *B,* The return of venous blood from the myocardial cells to the right atrium via cardiac veins.

tion is of primary physiological significance. If blood flow to the myocardium is disrupted, serious functional disequilibrium will result.

CARDIAC PATHOLOGY

The functional significance of the heart is its ability to propel blood through the vascular tree. When cardiac muscle is stressed, compensation mechanisms are triggered that facilitate the maintenance of left ventricular output. To the extent that these mechanisms fail, the heart can become progressively unable to service cellular needs. Many systems are then affected by a pathological syndrome known as congestive heart failure (CHF).

In the following pages, an analysis of major sources of stress is followed by an elucidation of myocardial compensation mechanisms. The evolution of nonadaptive cardiac compensation is clarified by a study of CHF.

Sources of Cardiac Stress

Cardiac muscle is said to be stressed when circumstances force the heart to work harder in order to maintain output. Adaptation to changing environmental demands is not necessarily a pathological phenomenon. Fluctuations in cardiac activity can be noted throughout any normal day and reflect parallel alterations in need. Physical exertion or increased metabolic rate, for example, normally trigger adaptive elevations in cardiac output.

When stress is induced by a pathological cause, however, the demands placed upon the heart muscle are more sustained and extensive. The purpose of this chapter is to elucidate the major sources of pathological stress. Toward this end, causative factors are categorized as follows:

1. *Direct stress* — characterized by disorders that alter the heart either structurally or functionally in such a way as to reduce pumping effectiveness.

2. *Indirect stress* — characterized by a disorder external to the heart that increases the workload of the heart indirectly.

This conceptual distinction between direct and indirect stress can be further clari-

fied by considering the case of John Doe, physical laborer. One could theoretically impose stress upon John by demanding that he carry his normal workload even though he has a 103° F. temperature complicated by diarrhea and vomiting. Alternatively, a relatively healthy John could be incapacitated if he were required to function while carrying a 200-pound weight on his back. In either case, Mr. Doe is destined to suffer. The first hypothetical situation imposes direct stress: John is asked to work in spite of an organic disease. In the second case, stress is imposed indirectly. Although free of disease, he is required to perform under decidedly adverse external conditions.

DIRECT STRESS

Direct stress, as defined earlier, is most commonly caused by disorders that alter the structural or functional nature of the heart. Primary among these are: (1) ischemia, (2) infection, (3) arrhythmias, and (4) congenital defects. In the following pages, each of these phenomena will be explored in such a way as to promote better conceptual understanding of cardiac pathology.

ISCHEMIA Ischemia is technically defined as the reduction of blood supply to a particular area in the body. In cases of cardiac disease, it refers specifically to inadequate myocardial circulation.

Most commonly, myocardial ischemia is caused by degenerative changes in the coronary arteries. Associated with arteriosclerosis or atherosclerosis or both, this type of circulatory deficit is described as *arteriosclerotic heart disease (ASHD)* or *coronary heart disease (CHD)*.

To the extent that blood supply to the cardiac muscle is compromised by partial or total obliteration of the vascular lumen, myocardial ischemia results. The degree of physiological disruption that ensues depends largely upon the location and extent of circulatory deficit. As illustrated in Figure 9.30, any obstruction at point X in the coronary arteries would lead to more extensive damage than would a similar occlusion at point Y.

Since degeneration of the coronary arte-

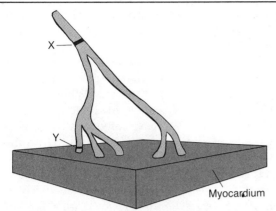

Figure 9.30 Occlusion of coronary arteries. Note that considerably more ischemia would result if an obstruction developed in a larger coronary artery (X), as opposed to a smaller vessel (Y).

ries often develops progressively, over an extended period of time, specific clinical expressions of disease may vary considerably. Under the best of circumstances, vascular disorders may be minimal and disease asymptomatic. At the other extreme, critical dysfunction may lead to sudden death. Some specific causes and manifestations of CHD will be discussed in the following pages.

Causes of Ischemia Myocardial ischemia is most directly triggered by either *spastic constriction* or *occlusion* of diseased coronary arteries. In either case, the narrowing of the vascular lumen will deprive cardiac muscle of adequate blood supply.

SPASTIC CONSTRICTION Spastic constriction of the coronary arteries is a reversible phenomenon often associated with the early stages of ASHD. Most often, spastic vasoconstriction is triggered by exposure to wind or cold, excessive intake of caffeine or nicotine, anxiety, or physical exertion. Patients with CHD can thus modify their activities and

habits so as to minimize ischemic stress. Often warned against exposure to frigid, windy conditions or involvement in anxiety-producing situations, they are also encouraged to avoid the use of coffee and tea and to refrain from smoking cigarettes.

OCCLUSION Occlusion of coronary arteries is characteristically a progressive and irreversible phenomenon that is associated with the later stages of ASHD. As blood flow is impeded by degenerative vascular changes, there is more opportunity for platelets to catch and rupture on the rough edges of fatty plaques. Clotting subsequently occurs, and a small clot, or *thrombus*, begins to develop. To the extent that the thrombus increases in size, it can eventually cause total obstruction of a coronary artery. Early thrombus formation is illustrated in Figure 9.31.

Manifestations of Ischemia Whenever myocardial ischemia exists, the volume of blood available to service cardiac cellular needs is diminished. The muscle of the heart must generate energy anaerobically, and lactic acid is produced by the myocardium. It is believed that the localized accumulation of this acid is irritating to nerve endings in the area, causing cardiac pain. Chest pain and decreased cardiac capacity are, in fact, noted in most cases of myocardial oxygen deficit.

Myocardial ischemia will also trigger a number of cellular level and systemic responses that more specifically reflect the degree of circulatory deprivation. In the clinical setting, several different expressions of ischemia can be cited, as summarized in Table 9.5. While *angina* is characterized by temporary and reversible ischemia, *infarction* is associated with more sustained and extensive oxygen deprivation. A study of these two disease

Figure 9.31 Early thrombus formation within an atherosclerotic vessel: a schematic presentation.

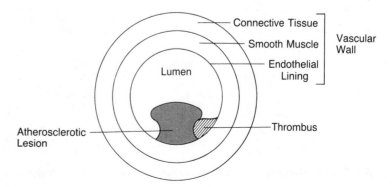

TABLE 9–5 **Clinical Expressions of Myocardial Ischemia***

Clinical Expression	Mechanism
1. Angina pectoris	1. Transient, localized myocardial ischemia
2. Acute myocardial infarction	2. Arterial occlusion
3. Intermediate coronary syndrome (unstable angina)	3. Prolonged myocardial ischemia, with or without myocardial necrosis
4. Heart failure, acute and chronic arrhythmias, conduction disturbances, abnormal ECG	4. Gradual fibrosis of myocardium or conduction system; may result from (2) or (3) also
5. Sudden death	5. Any of the above, plus ventricular arrhythmia, or Stokes-Adams attacks

*From Krupp, M. A., and Chatton, M. J. (eds.): Current Medical Diagnosis and Therapy. Los Altos, CA: Lange Medical Publications, 1978. Used by permission.

states is helpful in clarifying the pathogenesis of myocardial ischemia.

ANGINA If ischemia is short-lived and is due to a temporary spastic constriction of coronary arteries, the resulting disorder is referred to as *angina pectoris.*

Anginal pain is characteristically of brief duration (from 3 to 15 or 20 minutes) and can be rapidly alleviated by the administration of vasodilator drugs, such as nitroglycerin. Since the effects are reversible with the elimination of stress, tissue is not permanently damaged.

In cases of advanced vascular disease,

manifestations of angina may become more frequent and intense as well as less predictable. This phenomenon, described as *crescendo angina* or *intermittent coronary syndrome,* often culminates in a true infarction.

MYOCARDIAL INFARCTION When myocardial ischemia is severe or prolonged (over 35 to 40 minutes), associated cardiac pain is usually of sudden onset and extended duration (see Table 9.6). The cardiac tissue that is deprived of oxygen and glucose will die and undergo necrotic changes. Since necrosis induced by ischemia is called an *infarction* (or *infarct*), the death of myocardial cells caused by coronary arterial occlusion is referred to as a *myocardial infarction (MI).*

Unfortunately, the cellular damage of myocardial infarction is not reversible. Necrosis can be diminished, however, if accessory (or *collateral*) vessels are present to transport blood around the vascular blockage. These accessory vessels do not suddenly appear in response to an immediate need. Instead, they develop over a period of time as a result of sustained demands upon cardiac output. A regular and well-planned exercise program, for example, is likely to encourage good collateral circulation— hence, the value of jogging, biking, swimming, or other aerobic activity.

To the extent that collateral vessels can function to effectively bypass an occlusion, cellular health is maintained (see Figure 9.32). If, on the other hand, collateral circulation is insufficent, myocardial necrosis will result.

TABLE 9.6 **Characteristics of Cardiac Pain**

	Onset and Length of Pain	Location	Quality and Severity	Signs and Symptoms	Initiating Factors
Angina	Can begin slowly or suddenly; pain often lasts no more than 15 minutes and rarely more than 30 minutes.	Pain is in the substernal or anterior chest; diffuse and radiating to neck, back, arms, jaw, and sometimes upper abdomen or fingers.	Pressure of low to medium intensity; attacks follow the same pattern; pain is deep-seated: tight and constricting.	Labored breathing, profuse sweating, nausea, feeling of need to urinate, belching, apprehension.	Stress, physical exercise, eating, urination or bowel movement, cold or hot or humid weather.
Myocardial infarction	Begins suddenly; pain lasts 1/2–2 hours; soreness lasts 1–3 days.	Pain is substernal, along the midline, or along the anterior of the chest. Pain radiates down the arms to the neck, back, or jaw.	Intense pressure; deep-seated: stabbing or crushing type of pain.	Apprehension, nausea, labored breathing, profuse sweating, a galloping heart sound.	Physical or emotional stress; also occurs at rest.

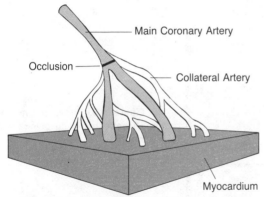

Main Coronary Artery

Occlusion

Collateral Artery

Myocardium

Figure 9.32 Collateral circulation to the myocardium. Main coronary artery is shaded. Collateral vessels are shown in white. Note that obstruction in a main coronary artery could be bypassed if sufficient collateral circulation existed.

The existence of a full-blown myocardial infarction is often confirmed in one of two ways. Clinical symptoms of pain, shock, depressed urinary output, nausea, vomiting, low-grade fever, and extreme anxiety (see Table 9.7) are characteristically accompanied by:

1. Elevation in the plasma levels of certain intracellular enzymes. These enzymes, released from the myocardium during necrosis, include SGOT, LDH, and CPK. Although not conclusive evidence of cardiac disease, they are nevertheless extremely useful diagnostic tools when combined with other evaluative procedures (see Figure 9.33).

2. Changes in the normal electrocardio-

TABLE 9–7. **Symptoms Associated with a Myocardial Infarction***

Symptoms	Bases of Symptoms
Pain: Crushing, severe, prolonged, unrelieved by rest or nitroglycerin, often radiating to one or both arms, the neck, and back.	Complete stoppage of blood suppy to myocardium caused by thrombotic occlusion evidently causes accumulation of unoxidized metabolites within ischemic part of myocardium; this affects the nerve endings.
Shock: Systolic blood pressure below 80 mm. Hg, gray facial color, lethargy, cold diaphoresis, peripheral cyanosis, tachycardia or bradycardia, weak pulse.	In some cases, shock caused primarily by the severe pain; in others, by a severe reduction in cardiac output and by inadequate tissue perfusion resulting in tissue hypoxia.
Oliguria: Urine flow of less than 20 ml./hr. as measured by indwelling Foley catheter.	Inadequate urine flow indicates renal hypoxia owing to inadequate tissue perfusion resulting from shock.
Low-grade fever: Temperature rises within 24 hours and lasts 3 to 7 days; usually 37.5 to 39.5°C. (100 to 103°F), accompanied by leukocytosis, elevated sedimentation rate, LDH, and SGOT.	Fever and elevated white counts result from destruction of myocardial tissue and the ensuing inflammatory process; fever drops when fibroblasts begin to replace leukocytes and scar tissue starts to form.
Apprehension, great fear of death, restlessness.	The severe pain of heart attack is terrifying; also, most lay people are aware of the heart's importance and the significance of a heart attack; restlessness results from shock and pain.
"Indigestion," "gas pains around the heart," nausea and vomiting.	Patients may prefer to believe that their pain is caused by "gas" or "indigestion" rather than by heart disease; nausea and vomiting may result from severe pain or from vagovagal reflexes conducted from the area of damaged myocardium to the gastrointestinal tract.
Acute pulmonary edema: Sense of suffocation, dyspnea, orthopnea, gurgling; bubbling respirations.	In some cases, the left ventricle becomes severely crippled in pumping action owing to infarction; severe pulmonary congestion results, accompanied by low cardiac output and shock.

*From Luckmann, J., and Sorensen, K. C.: Medical-Surgical Nursing: A Psychophysiologic Approach. Philadelphia, W. B. Saunders Company, 1980. Used by permission.

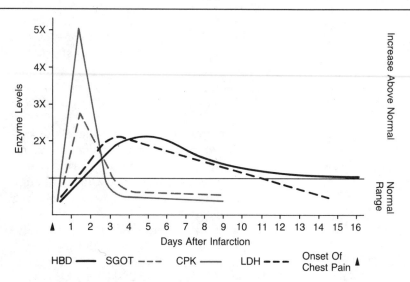

Figure 9.33 How serum enzyme levels change in myocardial infarction.

graph (ECG) readings. As illustrated in Figure 9.34, a wide deep Q wave, S-T segment elevation, or T wave inversion are all indicative of myocardial infarction.

Subsequent to cellular death and necrosis, the healing process begins. Inflammatory clean-up is followed by repair at the site of ischemia. In the case of the myocardium, removal of necrotic cells begins about the second or third day post infarction. Fibrous scar formation is initiated by about the third week, and repair is normally complete at the con-

clusion of the sixth week. Unfortunately, however, the new tissue is not nearly as functional as the original. When connective tissue filler replaces myocardial cells, the effective capacity of the organ declines.

Following an MI, a reduction in the contractility and pumping capacity of the heart muscle is usually noted. Ischemic damage can cause abnormal patterns of contraction (as illustrated in Figure 9.35), with associated decrease in cardiac output. Potential complications such as cardiac arrhythmias, congestive heart failure, pulmonary edema, pulmonary embolism, rupture of the heart, and acute heart failure may further alter the clinical picture and seriously compromise physiological equilibrium.

INFECTION Infection triggers cardiac disorders whenever pathogenic microorganisms invade or affect the heart. The pericardium, myocardium, or endocardium may be affected by the infectious process, with resulting variability in associated clinical symptoms. In the following pages, a closer look is taken at the development and manifestations of infection in the three primary cardiac tissues. Ultimately, rheumatic fever is studied as a disease entity that pathologically affects all major cardiac components.

Pericardial Infection Pericarditis is an inflammation of the visceral or parietal pericardium, or both, which often occurs second-

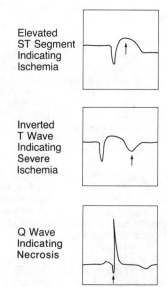

Figure 9.34 Some ECG changes associated with a myocardial infarction.

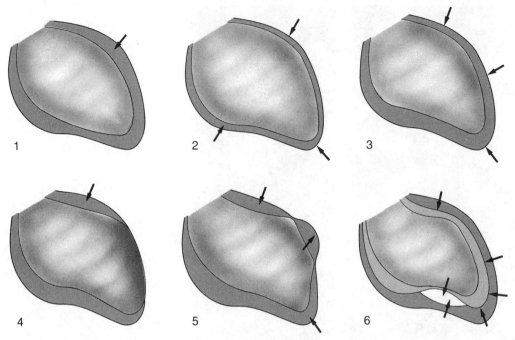

Figure 9.35 Some abnormal patterns of cardiac contraction.
  1. Uniform contraction of a normal heart. If damaged by a myocardial infarction (MI), abnormal contraction patterns may develop.
  2. A *hypokinetic* contraction is weak but uniform.
  3. *Asyneresis* is a localized hypokinetic contraction.
  4. *Akinesis* refers to a contraction failure in a portion of the ventricular wall.
  5. *Dyskenesis* is a bulging of a portion of the ventricular wall during systole.
  6. *Asynchrony* refers to a failure in the sequencing and coordination of contraction.

ary to infections elsewhere in the body. Common causative agents include staphylococcus, pneumococcus, streptococcus, meningococcus, and certain viruses, but pericarditis may also be associated with myocardial infarction, systemic lupus erythematosus, rheumatic fever, chest trauma, and neoplasms.

Although pericarditis may take a number of forms, it is generally described as acute or chronic. Acute pericarditis is typically associated with the growth of pericardial adhesions (acute fibrinous pericarditis), or with an exudate that accumulates in the pericardial sac (acute pericarditis with effusion). Chronic pericarditis, on the other hand, develops secondary to acute disease and is characterized by fibrous calcification of the visceral pericardium. In all cases, cardiac restriction may occur, with a resulting decrease in functional contractility. The phenomenon of restrictive defects will be discussed subsequently in this chapter as an example of indirect cardiac stress.

Regardless of the exact nature of pericarditis, associated manifestations often include chest pain, pericardial frictional rub (detectable with a stethoscope), dyspnea, fever, leukocytosis, chills, and tachycardia.

Myocardial Infection. Myocarditis, or inflammation of the myocardium, frequently occurs secondary to infections such as acute pericarditis, acute endocarditis, diphtheria, influenza, poliomyelitis, measles, mumps, toxoplasmosis, trichinosis, and, most significantly, rheumatic fever. The illness is usually of sudden onset and is characterized by the appearance of isolated pockets of inflamed and necrotic myocardial cells. Symptoms are often varied and include fever, malaise, anorexia, fatigue, leukocytosis, and chest pain. Ultimately diagnosed on the basis of ventricular enlargement, myocarditis may cause acute heart failure and sudden death in cases in which disease is sufficiently extensive.

Endocardial Infection Endocarditis, or inflammation of the lining and the valves of

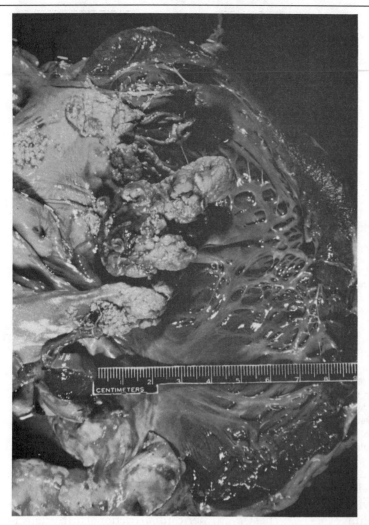

Figure 9.36 Infective bacterial endocarditis of the mitral valve. (From Robbins, S. L., and Cotran, R. S.: Pathologic Basis of Disease, 2nd ed. Philadelphia, W. B. Saunders Company, 1979. Used by permission.)

the heart, generally arises secondary to acute infection elsewhere in the body or in cases of pre-existing cardiac disease.

The acute form of bacterial endocarditis (*ABE*) is usually caused by highly pathogenic microorganisms such as *Staphylococcus aureus*, and, less frequently, by pneumococci, beta-hemolytic streptococci, or gonococci. Subacute bacterial endocarditis (*SBE*), on the other hand, is a chronic, smoldering infection typically caused by *Streptococcus viridans. S. faecalis* or *Staphylococcus aureus* may be causative agents. In either case, the condition is characterized by vegetative growths on the leaflets of cardiac valves (see Figure 9.36). Laden with pathogenic microbes, these lesions may cause dysfunction in a variety of ways: (1) spread of infectious organisms from the valves to other structures in the heart; (2)

spread of infectious microbes, via the bloodstream, to organs such as the spleen, kidney, and brain; (3) release of small vegetative particles into the bloodstream (as emboli), causing secondary ischemia and infarction in a number of critical structures; and (4) functional valvular disruption.

Whereas infection is associated with generalized manifestations of fever, chills, fatigue, and anorexia, emboli may cause a range of symptoms that vary with the site of ischemia (see Table 9.8). Thus, while tenderness, enlargement, and upper abdominal pain are reflections of splenic infarction, blood in the urine is a characteristic result of renal ischemia.

Since valves of the heart normally facilitate optimal circulation of blood through the cardiac chambers, functional valvular disrup-

TABLE 9.8 **Rheumatic Fever: Manifestations of Organic Dysfunction Secondary to the Discharge of Emboli from Diseased Heart Valves**

Site of Ischemia	Clinical Manifestations
Pulmonary	Dyspnea, cough, expectoration of blood, pleuritic pain
Splenic	Splenic tenderness and enlargement; pain in the upper abdomen
Renal	Flank pain; blood in the urine; possible renal failure
Cerebral	Inability to speak; paralysis of one side of the body; sudden onset of visual problems
Extremities	Pain; necrosis; gangrene

tion may alter both the distribution and the flow of blood through the heart. Most commonly, such disruption affects either the mitral or the aortic valve, resulting in a narrowing or insufficient closure of valvular components.

Stenosis refers to a condition in which the valve hardens and narrows, impeding the free forward flow of blood. As a result, blood tends to accumulate behind the obstruction. Thus, a stenosed mitral valve causes increased retention of blood in the left atrium. This concept is visualized in Figure 9.37.

Valvular *regurgitation* (or *incompetence*) refers to a condition in which the valves do not snap shut effectively. An abnormal reflux of blood results. With aortic incompetence, for example, blood will leak out of the aorta back into the left ventricle during diastole. This phenomenon is illustrated in Figure 9.38.

Regardless of the specific nature of valvular dysfunction, it can be seen that circulation of blood through the heart is disrupted. Pumping effectiveness will subsequently decline to the extent that a particular cardiac chamber is stressed by abnormal accumula-

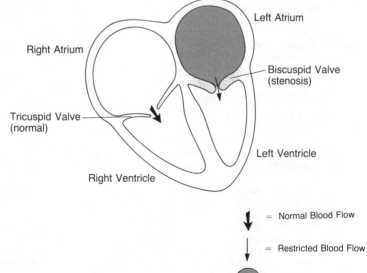

Figure 9.37 Stenosis of the mitral valve: a schematic presentation.

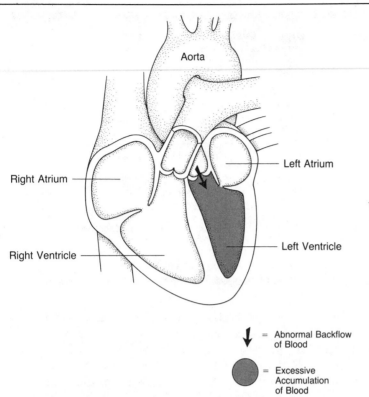

Figure 9.38 Aortic valve incompetence: a schematic presentation.

TABLE 9.9 **Valvular Disease and Associated Cardiac Stress**

When This Valvular Disorder Exists	Excessive Accumulation of Blood May Be Noted in the
Stenosis of the tricuspid valve	Right atrium
Incompetence of the tricuspid valve	Right atrium
Stenosis of the bicuspid valve	Left atrium
Incompetence of the bicuspid valve	Left atrium
Stenosis of the pulmonic valve	Right ventricle
Incompetence of the pulmonic valve	Right ventricle
Stenosis of the aortic valve	Left ventricle
Incompetence of the aortic valve	Left ventricle

TABLE 9.10 **Effects of Rheumatic Fever upon the Myocardium, Endocardium, and Pericardium***

Condition	Characteristic Lesion	Factors in Causation of Lesion	Significance of Patho-physiological Involvement
Rheumatic myocarditis	Aschoff bodies, minute nodules, usually found in connective tissue around small arteries in myo-cardium	Formed by leukocytes that mass in inflamed tissues	Nodules may eventually become fibrotic; damage from fibrosis may eventually damage arter-ies in myocardium; myocarditis may cause a temporary loss in contractile power of the heart; permanent damage rarely results
Rheumatic endocarditis	Tiny *vegetations* resem-bling little beads form along line of closure of valve flaps	Probably result from in-flammation, ulceration, and erosion of valve flaps	Inflammatory damage of valves results in *permanent* severe heart disease
Pericarditis	Nonspecific lesions	Result from a diffuse, non-specific fibrinous or sero-fibrinous inflammatory reaction	May cause pericardial friction rub; usually no serious sequelae

*From Luckmann, J., and Sorensen, K. C.: Medical-Surgical Nursing: A Psychophysiologic Approach. Philadelphia, W. B. Saunders Company, 1980. Used by permission.

tions of blood. A summary of the stress patterns induced by major valvular disorders can be found in Table 9.9.

Rheumatic Fever Rheumatic fever is a systemic inflammatory disorder characterized by joint pain, fever, and cardiac dysfunction. Although the exact causative mechanism remains unknown, pathogenesis is believed to be associated with an immune complex–mediated hypersensitivity response to group A beta-hemolytic streptococcus. Characteristically, an acute streptococcal infection (such as sore throat or tonsillitis) is followed by the delayed formation of immune complexes between noneradicated streptococci, streptococcal antibody, and complement. Within two to three weeks after onset of the initial infection, immune complexes deposit in joints and small myocardial blood vessels, causing subsequent tissue destruction. Joints become tender and swollen. Systemic edema is noted, and large nodules frequently form under the skin. Most significantly, all tissues of the heart may be affected by rheumatic fever (a phenomenon referred to as *pancarditis*). While damage to the myocardium and pericardium is usually reversible, endocarditis often causes permanent valvular dysfunction, as noted in Table 9.10.

ARRHYTHMIAS Arrhythmias can be defined as alterations in the rate or the rhythm or both of cardiac contraction. Induced by a variety of factors including myocardial ischemia, electrolyte imbalances, and neural-endocrine disturbances, arrhythmias may trigger stress by decreasing pumping effectiveness.

In general, it can be said that cardiac output may be compromised by any disorders that *excessively* slow down or speed up the rate of myocardial contraction. In considering this type of disorder, it is important to stress the interdependency of the four cardiac chambers. Although the volume of blood ejected into the systemic circulation depends directly upon left ventricular output, this critical chamber must be adequately serviced by both the right side of the heart and the left atrium, if physiological needs are to be met.

Patterns of arrhythmia can vary considerably with respect to causative factors, site of origin, and clinical manifestations. In the subsequent pages, disorders are classified according to whether they arise (1) in the SA node, (2) in the atria, (3) in the AV node, or (4) in the ventricles.

Disorders Arising in the SA Node These disturbances are primarily due to alterations

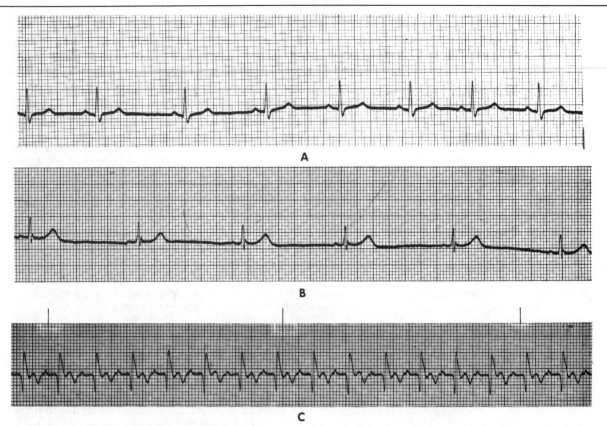

Figure 9.39 *A*, Normal sinus rhythm: Note normal upright P waves preceding each QRS complex. Cardiac rate is 60 to 100 beats per minute. *B*, Sinus bradycardia: Strip appears similar to normal sinus rhythm, but cardiac rate is slower than 60 beats per minute. *C*, Sinus tachycardia: Note rapid cardiac rate of 100 to 160 beats per minute. (From Phillips, R., and Feeney, M. K.: The Cardiac Rhythms, 2nd ed. Philadelphia, W. B. Saunders Company, 1980. Used by permission.)

in neural or chemical stimulation of the SA node. Most often, they trigger accelerations (sinus tachycardia) or depressions (sinus bradycardia) in the rate of contraction. The rhythm usually remains normal, except in relatively rare cases in which the cardiac rate is keyed to respiratory activity — increasing with inspirations and decreasing with expirations. Most often, SA node disorders are of minor clinical significance, since they do not typically alter the functional capacity of the heart. Some examples of ECG's that reflect this condition can be found in Figure 9.39.

Disorders Arising in the Atria These disturbances occur when a focal center in the atrial muscle begins to discharge impulses at an abnormal rate or rhythm. Often originating in an area of fibrotic postinfarction scarring, the pathologically discharging site takes over the function of the SA node and dictates a new pattern of cardiac contraction. Because the source of these disorders lies in the atrium, ECG's are typically characterized by an absent or abnormal P wave. Examples of atrial arrhythmias include:

1. *Premature atrial contractions (PAC's).* Frequently noted in patients with a history of rheumatic heart disease, these disorders are characterized by extra atrial contractions, which discharge regularly or sporadically before a normal cardiac cycle. A typical ECG strip is presented in Figure 9.40.

2. *Extremely rapid discharge of atrial impulses.* Examples of these arrhythmias include paroxysmal atrial tachycarida (160 to 240 beats per minute), atrial flutter (250 to 400 beats per minute), and atrial fibrillation (over 400 beats per minute). As rate increases excessively, a decline in atrial pumping capacity will be noted. In much the same way that a fluttering

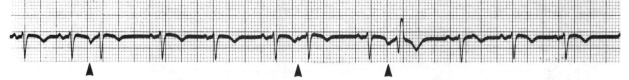

Figure 9.40 Premature atrial contraction (PAC). Arrows indicate premature waves. (From Phillips, R., and Feeney, M. K.: The Cardiac Rhythms, 2nd ed. Philadelphia, W. B. Saunders Company, 1980. Used by permission.)

set of bellows cannot eject large volumes of air, so a rapidly contracting cardiac chamber will neither fill nor empty sufficiently for optimal effectiveness.

3. *Atrial-ventricular block.* As the rate of atrial discharge increases, the AV node cannot respond to every arriving impulse. In many instances, the node will respond to every second (2:1 block), third (3:1 block), or fourth (4:1 block) atrial beat. When atrial contraction climbs excessively high, however, as it does during fibrillation, ventricular discharge can become extremely irregular. In these cases a classic block pattern is no longer evident. ECG strips illustrating the phenomenon of atrial-ventricular block are presented in Figure 9.41.

Disorders Arising in the AV Node These disturbances characteristically accompany organic disease of the AV node. Often induced by myocardial infarction, rheumatic fever, or degeneration of conduction tissue due to age, they can also be caused by excessive intake of drugs such as digitalis or quinidine.

Arrhythmias originating in the AV node are commonly associated with a syndrome of

heart block. In these disorders, impulses are not transmitted normally from the atria, through the AV node, and into the ventricles. Manifestations vary in severity, and are categorized as follows:

1. *First-degree block* — in which there is a slight delay in impulse conduction to the AV node, but the cardiac cycle remains essentially normal. These blocks are characterized by a prolonged P-R interval, as illustrated in Figure 9.42.

2. *Second-Degree Block* — in which ventricular contraction does not always follow an atrial discharge. Conduction will characteristically occur from the SA node through the atria, but the ventricles frequently respond to only two out of three (3:2 ratio) or three out of four (4:3 ratio) impulses.

This type of block is more specifically described as Mobitz type I or Mobitz type II depending upon the nature of the underlying disorder. In type I disorders, the diseased AV node becomes increasingly fatigued with the transmission of each successive impulse. The resulting delay in conduction is reflected by progressive lengthening of the P-R interval,

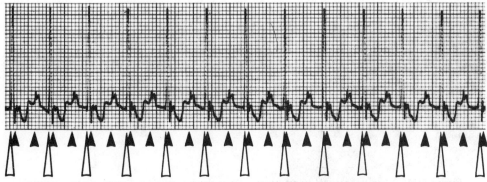

Figure 9.41 Atrial ventricular block associated with atrial tachycardia. Black arrows indicate P waves. White arrows indicate QRS complexes. Note that there are two atrial beats for every one ventricular contraction in this strip. (From Phillips, R., and Feeney, M. K.: The Cardiac Rhythms, 2nd ed. Philadelphia, W. B. Saunders Company, 1980. Used by permission.)

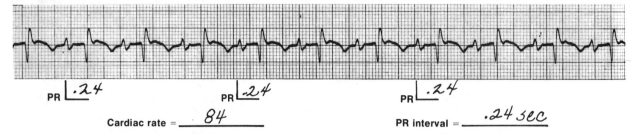

PR L.24   PR L.24   PR L.24

Cardiac rate = _____84_____   PR interval = _____.24 sec_____

Figure 9.42 First-degree AV heart block. Note that PR interval is greater than 0.20 second. (From Phillips, R., and Feeney, M. K.: The Cardiac Rhythms, 2nd ed. Philadelphia, W. B. Saunders Company, 1980. Used by permission.)

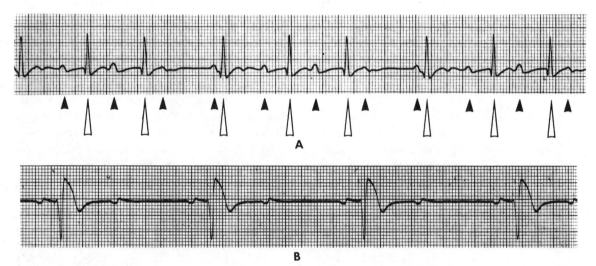

Figure 9.43 Second-degree AV heart block. *A,* Mobitz type I (Wenckebach). Black arrows indicate P waves. White arrows indicate QRS complexes. *B,* Mobitz type II. (From Phillips, R., and Feeney, M. K.: The Cardiac Rhythms, 2nd ed. Philadelphia, W. B. Saunders Company, 1980. Used by permission.)

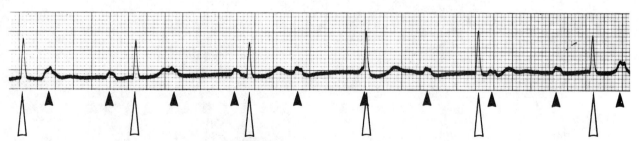

Figure 9.44 Third-degree AV heart block. Black arrows indicate P waves. White arrows indicate QRS complexes. Note that the atria and ventricles are completely dissociated and beat independently of one another. (From Phillips, R., and Feeney, M. K.: The Cardiac Rhythms, 2nd ed. Philadelphia, W. B. Saunders Company, 1980. Used by permission.)

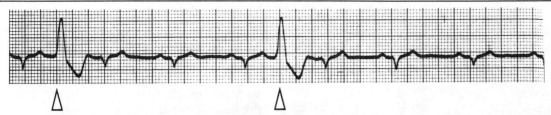

Figure 9.45 Premature ventricular contractions (PVC's) (indicated by white arrows). (From Phillips, R. E., and Feeney, M. K.: The Cardiac Rhythms, 2nd ed. Philadelphia, W. B. Saunders Company, 1980. Used by permission.)

ultimately terminating in a dropped ventricular beat. Subsequent nodal recovery allows for a cyclical repetition of the type I pattern. In type II arrhythmias, on the other hand, the P-R interval remains relatively constant, and QRS complexes are skipped rather abruptly, without any forewarning. One ventricular beat may sequentially follow every two (2:1), three (3:1), or four (4:1) atrial discharges, or the ventricles may contract at irregular and fluctuating intervals during the cardiac cycle. Illustrative ECG strips are presented in Figure 9.43.

3. *Third-degree block* — in which all impulses from the atria are blocked from passing into the ventricles. In these cases, the atria may be contracting at a normal SA node rhythm, while the ventricles are discharging impulses at the depressed rate dictated by the bundle of His or bundle branches (30 to 40 times a minute). A typical ECG strip is presented in Figure 9.44.

Disorders Arising in the Ventricles These disturbances arise when a focal center in the ventricular muscle itself begins to abnormally discharge impulses. Typically brought on by severe myocardial ischemia, they result in an abnormal pattern of ventricular contraction. Manifestations include:

1. *Premature ventricular contractions (PVC's)* — in which ventricular contractions sporadically discharge out of normal sequence. A characteristic ECG strip is illustrated in Figure 9.45.

2. *Ventricular tachycardia* — in which the ventricular contraction rate can rise to 140 to 250 per minute. Actually reflecting a run of consecutive PVC's, this disorder can be extremely serious, as cardiac output declines with elevations in ventricular rate.

3. *Ventricular fibrillation* — evidenced by an extremely rapid and abnormal pattern of ventricular contraction. Since left ventricular output is effectively reduced to almost nothing, death will result unless fibrillation can be reversed.

Cardiac Arrhythmias: A Summary Many cardiac arrhythmias induce stress by causing one or more chambers of the heart to work harder in order to maintain output. If the precipitating disorder is chronic or sustained, myocardial compensation responses predictably occur. If, on the other hand, the arrhythmia is severe or acute, all systems in the body may be affected by rapid reversals in cellular equilibrium. A tabular summary of major patterns of cardiac and systemic stress induced by arrhythmias is presented in Figure 9.46.

CONGENITAL DEFECTS   Abnormal fetal development of the heart, or of the major

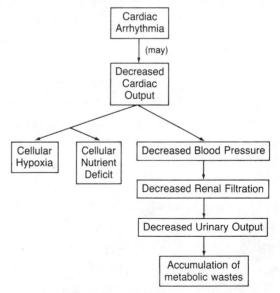

Figure 9.46 Cellular disequilibrium triggered by cardiac arrhythmias.

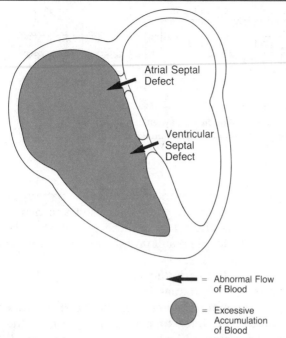

Figure 9.47 Septal defects: a schematic presentation.

vessels entering and leaving the heart, can also stress the cardiac muscle.

Primary examples of congenital cardiac structural abnormalties are disorders referred to as *septal defects*. A baby born with an atrial septal defect, for example, has a hole in the septum between the right and the left atrium.

A ventricular septal defect, on the other hand, is characterized by a hole in the septum between the right and the left ventricle. Since systolic pressure is usually greater within the left cardiac chambers, blood typically flows back through the septum into the right side of the heart. Described as a left-right shunt, this phenomenon does not typically interfere with oxygenation in the alveoli. It does, however, impose a strain upon the right cardiac chambers as excessive volumes of blood leak from the left side of the heart into the right. The stress imposed by septal defects is illustrated in Figure 9.47.

Occurring more commonly than a septal defect is a congenital heart disease referred to as the *tetralogy of Fallot*. Characterized by four structural abnormalities, it results in poorly oxygenated blood (manifested by cyanosis or a "blue baby" appearance) and excessive right ventricular strain. The specific causative defects are illustrated in Figure 9.48.

SOURCES OF DIRECT STRESS: A SUMMARY   In the previous pages, the major sources of direct cardiac stress have been elucidated. It was shown how ischemia, infection, arrhythmias, and congenital defects contribute to cardiac disorders by directly altering the structure or function of the heart. Although each of these four factors is unique

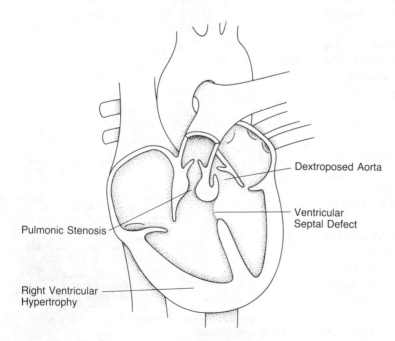

Figure 9.48 The tetralogy of Fallot.

TABLE 9.11 **Sources of Direct Cardiac Stress**

Sources of Stress	Causative Factors	Clinical Manifestations
Ischemia	Atherosclerosis Thrombi Emboli	Angina Myocardial infarct

Infection	Invasion by pathogenic
	  microbes such as:
	    Beta-hemolytic streptococci
	    Streptococcus viridans
	    Staphylococcus aureus
	    Treponema pallidum
		Rheumatic fever
		Myocarditis
		Pericarditis
		Endocarditis

Arrhythmias	Myocardial ischemia Fluid and electrolyte imbalance Neural disorders Endocrine disorders	Atrial fibrillation AV block First-, second-, or third-degree heart block PVC's Ventricular fibrillation
Congenital defects	Genetic defects Developmental defects	Septal defects Tetralogy of Fallot

with respect to pathogenesis and clinical manifestations, they all force cardiac muscle to work harder in order to maintain normal output. A comparative summary of the major sources of direct stress is presented in Table 9.11.

INDIRECT STRESS

Sources of indirect stress, as defined earlier, also impose an increase in cardiac workload. They are, however, derived of disorders external to the heart and commonly originate with: (1) volume imbalances, (2) restrictive defects, or (3) vascular disease.

VOLUME IMBALANCES Volume imbalances are characterized by an excess or deficit of total body fluid. At either extreme, deviations from the norm are inevitably mirrored by alterations in plasma volume.

When the volume of blood falls, the heart has to work harder to maintain normal output. Clinically, this phenomenon is noted most frequently in cases in which the amount of blood returning to the right heart is depressed owing to hemorrhage, severe dehydration, or excessive pooling of blood in the venous vessels. A more thorough elucidation of the causes and evolution of fluid deficit can be found in Chapter 3.

Alternatively, elevations in plasma volume force the heart to work harder to eject larger quantities of blood. At the extreme, this situation terminates in "circulatory overload," a clinical condition marked by severe cardiac stress. Elevations in fluid levels are frequently caused by increasing fluid intake or decreasing output or both. Causative disorders range from endocrine imbalances to renal failure and are detailed in Chapter 3.

RESTRICTIVE DEFECTS When external pressure is exerted upon the heart in such a way as to obstruct cardiac filling, a restrictive defect is said to exist. Caused most frequently by inflammation of the pericardial membranes, restrictive defects commonly develop in one of two primary ways: (1) The generation of excess fluid can overload the pericardial sac, thereby preventing normal cardiac filling; or (2) a thickening and calcification of the epicardium can restrict normal cardiac activity.

Pericarditis, or the inflammation of pericardial membranes, is induced by a variety of disorders, including infections, myocardial infarctions, hypersensitivity reactions, neo-

---

TABLE 9.12 **Some Causes of Pericarditis**

Infection
  A. Bacterial
    1. Meningococcus
    2. Gonococcus
    3. Streptococcus
    4. Staphylococcus
    5. *Mycobacterium tuberculosis*
  B. Viral
    1. Coxsackie virus type B
    2. Echovirus type A
    3. Mumps virus
  C. Fungal
    1. Histoplasmosis
    2. Actinomycosis
    3. Nocardiosis

Myocardial infarction

Chest trauma

Connective tissue disorders
  A. Acute rheumatic fever (in children)
  B. Rheumatoid arthritis
  C. Systemic lupus erythematosus (SLE)

Drug allergies
  A. Penicillin
  B. Diphenylhydantoin
  C. Hydralazine
  D. Procainamide

Metabolic disorders
  A. Uremia
  B. Hypothyroidism

Physical or chemical agents
  A. Radiation
  B. Asbestosis

---

plasms, and trauma. A list of major causative factors can be found in Table 9.12.

When disease is of rapid onset, acute pericarditis results. In these cases, *pericardial effusion*, or the accumulation of excess fluid in the pericardial space, is characteristically noted. Chronic pericarditis, on the other hand, evolves more slowly and is commonly accompanied by constrictive fibrosis of the visceral pericardium.

Regardless of the pattern of development, restrictive defects engendered by pericarditis can precipitate critical alterations in cellular equilibrium. To the extent that compression impedes filling, end diastolic volume will decline, and cardiac output will be compromised. Often a decrease in pumping effectiveness will aggravate myocardial stress by reducing blood supply to the heart muscle itself. As myocardial ischemia develops, an ominous downward spiral is initiated. This clinical syndrome, referred to as *cardiac tamponade*, is the most feared complication of restrictive defects (see Figure 9.49).

VASCULAR PATHOLOGY Vascular pathology, as defined in this text, is characterized by an inability of the blood vessels to adequately service cellular needs. Disorders are most commonly caused by obstruction or inappropriate constriction-dilation of vascular walls.

The mechanisms whereby vascular disorders can induce myocardial stress are twofold: The heart is forced to work harder if and when (1) venous return is depressed, or (2) resistance to cardiac output is increased.

Decreased Venous Return When return of blood to the right side of the heart is impeded, cardiac muscle is stressed. In the face of declining input, the heart is forced to work harder to maintain an adequate output.

Assuming normal plasma volume, depression of venous return is most commonly caused by vascular dilation. As the lumens of blood vessels enlarge, plasma is propelled through the vascular tree more slowly. Blood often pools in distended veins, and the heart is forced to contend with an ever-diminishing venous return.

Resistance to Cardiac Output When arterial blood pressure rises, the left ventricle must work increasingly hard to eject blood against the resistance posed by fluid pressure in the arteries.

Assuming normal plasma volume, elevations in arterial pressure are caused most commonly by occlusion, hardening, or constriction of the vascular walls. The pathogenesis of cardiac stress secondary to elevated arterial blood pressure is illustrated in Figure 9.27C.

SOURCES OF CARDIAC STRESS: A SUMMARY

In brief review, cardiac stress is induced by any factor that forces the heart to work harder in order to maintain output. Sources of stress are classified as *direct* or *indirect* accord-

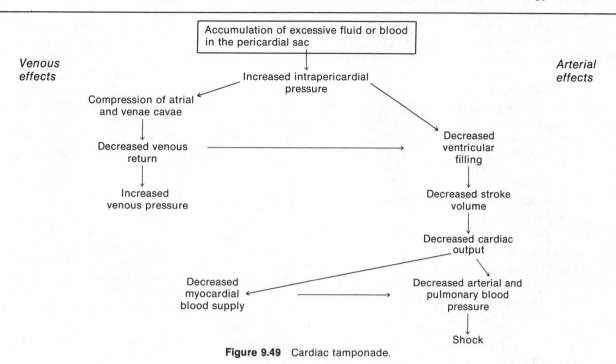

Figure 9.49   Cardiac tamponade.

TABLE 9.13   **Sources of Cardiac Stress**

Type of Stress	Sources of Stress	Causative Factors
DIRECT	Ischemia	Atherosclerosis Thrombi Emboli
	Infection	Invasion by pathogens: Beta-hemolytic streptococcus *Streptococcus viridans* *Staphylococcus aureus* *Treponema pallidum*
	Arrhythmias	Myocardial ischemia Fluid and electrolyte imbalance Neural disorders Endocrine disorders
	Congenital defects	Genetic defects Developmental defects
INDIRECT	Volume imbalances	Hemorrhage Dehydration Endocrine disorders Renal failure
	Restrictive defects	Pericarditis Pericardial effusion
	Vascular disease	Venous stasis Hypertension

ing to whether the disturbance originates in the heart or external to cardiac muscle.

Direct stress is triggered most commonly by ischemia, infection, arrhythmias, or congenital defects. Indirect stress, on the other hand, is usually derived from volume imbalances, restrictive defects, or vascular disorders. A tabular comparative summary of the major sources of cardiac stress is presented in Table 9.13.

Myocardial Compensation for Stress

Cardiac muscle, when stressed, will usually respond adaptively in an attempt to maintain normal output. To facilitate compensation, three primary mechanisms can normally be activated: (1) dilatation, (2) hypertrophy, and (3) tachycardia.

DILATATION

Whenever stress leads to the accumulation of an excessive volume of blood in a chamber of the heart, cardiac muscle fibers characteristically respond by dilating, or increasing in length. Potential causes of excess volume accumulation are detailed in Table 9.14.

Regardless of the initiating factor, dilatation is adaptive on two counts. As cardiac muscle stretches, increasing volumes of blood can be accommodated in the stressed chamber. Furthermore, in accordance with Frank-Starling's law, the dilated fibers will contract more forcefully than normal myocardial tissue.

Unfortunately, however, dilatation is adaptive and beneficial only up to a point. If tissue is stretched excessively, compensation value is lost as contraction force actually declines.

HYPERTROPHY

Whenever cardiac muscle is forced to work harder to maintain output, the response of myocardial muscle fibers is to hypertrophy, or increase in diameter. This change is accompanied by a thickening of the cardiac walls and an increase in the size and weight of the heart.

Like dilatation, hypertrophy facilitates an increase in myocardial pumping effectiveness. As cardiac muscle enlarges, however, its need for oxygen and nutrients increases accordingly. To the extent that myocardial blood supply cannot support escalating cellular needs, the force of cardiac contraction soon takes a downward plunge.

TACHYCARDIA

In the face of declining output, the rate of cardiac contraction often accelerates. This increase is governed by the nervous system in

TABLE 9.14   **The Accumulation of Excessive Volumes of Blood Within the Cardiac Chambers**

Causative Factors	Pathological Mechanisms
Hypertension	An increase in arterial blood pressure poses resistance to the ejection of blood from the left heart.
Left-to-right shunt	A left-to-right shunt (often associated with septal defects) is characterized by an abnormal flux of blood from left to right cardiac chambers.
Valvular disease	Valvular stenosis or incompetence causes excessive accumulation of blood in certain cardiac chambers, as detailed in Figure 9.25.
Hypervolemia	In cases of extracellular fluid excess, venous return to the right side of the heart will characteristically be elevated.
Pulmonary disease	Constriction of the blood vessels servicing the lungs (associated with pulmonary disease) poses resistance to the ejection of blood from the right heart.

reflex response to decreases in the pressure of blood against vascular or cardiac walls.

When blood pressure falls, for example, specialized nerve endings (pressoreceptors), located in the aortic arch, carotid sinus, venae cavae, and right atrium, send neural messages to the medulla. The medulla, in turn, transmits excitatory impuses to the SA node via sympathetic nerves, causing cardiac rate to increase. Although inherently adaptive, tachycardia is effective only up to a point. As rate increases excessively, pumping effectiveness declines and output decreases.

Congestive Heart Failure: A Study in Nonadaptative Myocardial Compensation

In spite of the arsenal of compensatory mechanisms at its command, the heart is often unable to maintain cardiac output in the presence of prolonged stress. This functional inability is described as *congestive heart failure (CHF)* when it develops slowly and is characterized by (1) sustained stress that triggers the activation of the three cardiac compensation mechanisms: dilatation, hypertrophy, and tachycardia; (2) overcompensation to the point of ineffectiveness, also described as *decompensation*; and (3) depressed cardiac output.

In the following pages, a brief look at the causes of congestive heart failure is followed by an overview of its pathogenesis. A subsequent distinction between the clinical manifestations of left-sided and right-sided failure will further clarify the complexity of this physiologically disruptive.disorder.

CAUSES OF CONGESTIVE HEART FAILURE

Congestive heart failure is a slowly developing condition that results from chronic long-term exposure to physiological stress. In reality, all causes of direct or indirect stress can eventually terminate in CHF. To the extent that compensation mechanisms succeed in maintaining cardiac output, equilibrium can be sustained. Failure is caused by the onset of decompensation and characterized by the disruption of cellular homeostasis. Some primary causes of congestive heart failure are summarized in Figure 9.50.

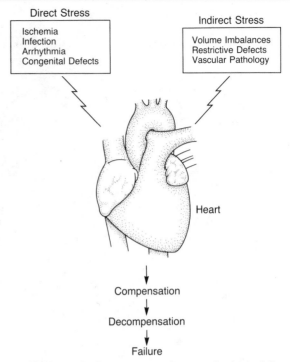

Figure 9.50 Some causes of congestive heart failure.

DEVELOPMENT OF CONGESTIVE HEART FAILURE

Characteristically, the congestive heart failure syndrome begins with the failure of one chamber and progresses to involve other chambers of the heart. In elucidating the mechanisms of this disorder, it is helpful to trace the pathogenesis of CHF initiated secondary to a left ventricular myocardial infarction.

As healing of the necrotic cardiac muscle proceeds, functional myocardium is replaced with fibrous scar tissue. Since this connective tissue filler lacks the capacity to actively contract, the "repaired" ventricle is rendered less effective as a pump. Dilatation, hypertrophy, and tachycardia are initiated to compensate for decreased efficiency. Unfortunately, however, these mechanisms proceed to excess, and decompensation results.

With the onset of decompensation, the left ventricle performs even less efficiently than it did initially. Left ventricular output declines, and blood accumulates in the chamber, unable to be ejected. This *congestion* poses a resistance to the outflow of blood from

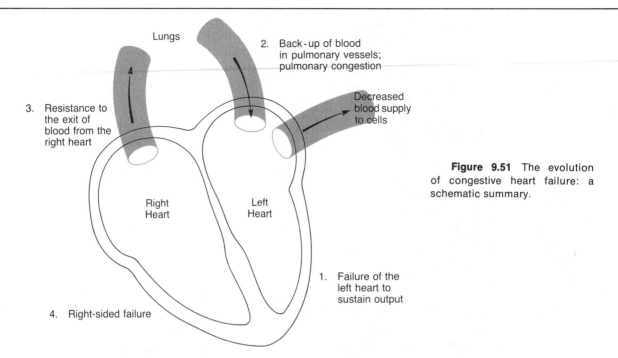

Lungs

2. Back-up of blood in pulmonary vessels; pulmonary congestion

Decreased blood supply to cells

3. Resistance to the exit of blood from the right heart

Right Heart

Left Heart

1. Failure of the left heart to sustain output

4. Right-sided failure

Figure 9.51 The evolution of congestive heart failure: a schematic summary.

the left atrium. Unrelieved, it will lead to left atrial compensation, decompensation, and eventual failure.

When the left atrium fails, congestion poses resistance to the entry of blood from the pulmonary veins. As blood backs up and pools in the pulmonary vascular tree, increased capillary pressure causes a shift of fluid into the alveolar spaces (*pulmonary edema*). Symptoms of respiratory stress appear, and resistance is posed to the exit of blood from the right side of the heart. Right ventricular and, subsequently, right atrial failure typically develop secondary to pulmonary congestion. The pathogenesis of congestive heart failure is summarized in Figure 9.51.

A DISTINCTION BETWEEN LEFT-SIDED AND RIGHT-SIDED FAILURE

The functional significance of the heart lies in its ability to propel blood through the vascular tree. To fully understand the distinctions between left and right failure, it is important to remember that the heart actually consists of two functional units that work together to service cellular needs: the *right heart* and the *left heart*. Separated by a muscular wall called the septum, these units function

interdependently but are serviced by their own networks of entry and exit vessels.

The right heart receives blood low in oxygen from the venous system and pumps it to the lungs through the pulmonary arteries. Oxygenated blood, cleansed of carbon dioxide wastes, subsequently returns to the left heart via the pulmonary veins. Pumped into the arterial tree by the left ventricle, it ultimately serves to support cellular survival needs.

In the following pages, the clinical manifestations of right-sided and left-sided failure are described. It is interesting to note that symptoms typically arise in direct response to alterations in the input or output or both. Since supply and exit routes for the right and left side of the heart differ, each disorder is characterized by a unique pathological pattern.

It is important to remember, however, that left- and right-sided failure are not normally isolated phenomena. Because left-sided failure often leads to right-sided failure, and vice versa, the patient with congestive heart failure most frequently shows evidence of both left- and right-sided disease.

LEFT-SIDED FAILURE Left-sided failure is a disorder specifically initiated by stress to the left heart. Most commonly, it is induced by (1) factors posing resistance to the ejection of blood from the left ventricle, such as arterial hypertension or aortic stenosis; (2) ischemia of the left myocardium; or (3) restrictive disorders, such as pericarditis.

The characteristic symptoms of left-sided failure reflect, for the most part, either pulmonary congestion or decreased left ventricular output.

As a result of *pulmonary congestion*, respiratory disorders develop. Excess fluid in the blood vessels and tissue spaces of the lungs cause difficulty in breathing (*dyspnea*), which is aggravated by the prone position. When an individual lies down, the return of venous blood to the heart is accelerated, thereby promoting further fluid congestion. Sporadic shortness of breath at night (*paroxysmal nocturnal dyspnea*) is, thus, an early sign of left-sided failure. Other respiratory symptoms often include coughing (as pulmonary edema causes irritation of the alveoli and respiratory passages) and, occasionally, wheezing.

As a result of *decreasing left ventricular output*, the ability to service cellular needs declines. Many critical organs suffer functional incapacity as a result. Evolving *cerebral hypoxia*, for example, is accompanied by symptoms of restlessness and irritability. Similarly, as skeletal muscles are deprived of adequate circulation, evidence of fatigue and muscular weakness can be noted.

Most damaging, perhaps, is the effect of decreased cardiac output upon the renal system. As blood flow through the renal arteries falls, the renin-angiotensin mechanism is called into play. Aldosterone is subsequently released and promotes the reabsorption of sodium and water from the nephron. Ultimately, hypervolemia develops, with associated increases in plasma volume. Unfortunately, this elevation in fluid levels further aggravates the congestion characteristic of left heart failure.

The primary clinical manifestations of left heart failure are summarized in Table 9.15. It is important to remember, however, that left heart failure is rarely seen in its pure form. Most often it is accompanied by reflections of right failure that typically occur secondary to pulmonary congestion.

RIGHT-SIDED FAILURE Right-sided failure is a dysfunction that can be precipitated by a number of factors, including:

1. Disorders that pose resistance to the ejection of blood from the right ventricle, such as stenosis of the pulmonic valve or pulmonary congestion. Pulmonary congestion, in turn, can occur secondary to left-sided failure or be caused directly by respiratory disease. When right heart failure is specifically linked to elevated pulmonary blood pressure, the resulting condition is technically referred to as *cor pulmonale*. Causative factors in cor pulmonale are discussed in Chapter 10.

2. Ischemia of the right myocardium.

3. Restrictive cardiac disorders, such as pericarditis.

Regardless of the initiating factors, the symptoms of right-sided failure primarily reflect venous congestion. Since the right heart

TABLE 9.15   Clinical Manifestations of Left-Sided Heart Failure

Clinical Manifestation	Causative Mechanism
Dyspnea, coughing, wheezing	Failure to eject sufficient quantities of blood from the left heart causes pulmonary congestion.
Restlessness; irritability	Cerebral hypoxia secondary to declining cardiac output.
Fatigue; muscular weakness	Declining cardiac output causes secondary deficit in the supply of oxygen and nutrients to skeletal muscle.
Hypervolemia	Declining cardiac output triggers the release of aldosterone via the renin-angiotensin mechanism. Renal retention of sodium and water results.

cannot adequately eject blood, there is a back-up of fluid in the veins, and return to the right atrium is subsequently depressed. Distention of the neck veins is often an early indication of right-sided failure.

As venous congestion progresses, resistance is posed to the flow of blood out of arteries and capillaries. A resulting increase in capillary blood pressure promotes fluid flux into the interstitial compartment.

In the abdominopelvic cavity, edema is prominent in hepatic tissue. If congestion in the liver is chronic, long-standing, and severe, depressed circulation can lead to hepatic anoxia and subsequent necrosis. The resulting condition, referred to as *cardiac cirrhosis,* is accompanied by hepatic malfunction, jaundice, and ascites (the shift of fluid into the peritoneal cavity). Congestion of other organs in the gastrointestinal tract can further aggravate symptoms of bloat, nausea, and loss of appetite.

The general pattern of depressed circulation affects the extremities of the body as well. In the hands and feet, return of blood to the heart is characteristically sluggish because of the effects of gravity. With venous congestion, circulation through these peripheral areas is significantly affected. Circulatory stagnation and increases in capillary blood pressure promote anoxia and edema. Bluish nail beds and puffy ankles and fingers are frequently noted.

In summary, it can be said that accumula-tion of blood in the right side of the heart sets the stage for the development of venous congestion. Primary clinical manifestations of right-sided failure are presented in Table 9.16.

LEFT-SIDED AND RIGHT-SIDED FAIL-URE: A SUMMARY   Congestive heart failure must be regarded as a total syndrome, involving components of both left- and right-sided failure. One could thus expect the patient with chronic heart failure to show indications of pulmonary congestion, decreased left ventricular output, and venous congestion. As circulation is progressively compromised, cellular malnutrition evolves, accompanied by symptoms of tissue wasting and weight loss. At the extreme, the syndrome can terminate in shock and death.

SHOCK: A UNIFYING MODEL OF CARDIOVASCULAR PATHOLOGY

Shock is a pathological process characterized by inadequate circulation to body tissues. As an area of study, it facilitates integration, correlation, and application of many physiological concepts elucidated throughout this chapter. An understanding of the causes, evolution, and manifestations of shock serves to clarify the multisystemic consequences of cardiovascular pathology.

TABLE 9.16   **Clinical Manifestations of Right-Sided Heart Failure**

Clinical Manifestation	Causative Mechanism
Distention of neck veins	Accumulation of blood in the right side of the heart poses resistance to venous return.
Liver enlargement; jaundice; abdominal pain	Venous congestion within the liver can lead to enlargement, pain, secondary hepatic necrosis, and jaundice.
Bloat, anorexia; nausea	Venous congestion within the gastrointestinal tract causes these symptoms to develop.
Edema of lower extremities	Sluggish circulation, secondary to venous congestion, decreases the return of blood from the extremities. Compensatory renal vasoconstriction often aggravates edema by promoting the retention of sodium and water.
Coolness and cyanosis of extremities	Sluggish circulation, secondary to venous congestion, reduces peripheral blood flow.

TABLE 9.17 **The Primary Classifications of Shock**

Type of Shock	Definition	Causative Pathological Condition
Hematogenic	Decrease in blood volume	Hemorrhage Burns Excessive gastrointestinal losses (vomiting, diarrhea) Excessive diaphoresis Excessive diuresis
Cardiogenic	Decrease in cardiac pumping capacity	Myocardial infarction Cardiac arrhythmias Valvular disease Pericarditis Congestive heart failure
Neurogenic	Excessive vasodilation induced by neural stimulation	Cerebral disease Spinal anesthetic reaction Insulin shock
Vasogenic	Excessive vasodilation induced by chemical agents	Anaphylactic shock Septic shock

Causes of Shock

In general, shock can be classified as *hematogenic, cardiogenic,* or *neurogenic-vasogenic,* depending upon the causative factors.

Hematogenic shock, for example, is induced by a depression in blood volume. As such, losses of whole blood (hemorrhage), or extracellular fluid depletion accompanying burns, excessive urinary output, diarrhea, vomiting, and so forth, can trigger hematogenic shock.

Cardiogenic shock, on the other hand, is caused by factors that stress the heart by forcing it to work harder in order to maintain output. Thus, all sources of direct and indirect stress, as elucidated earlier in the chapter, could theoretically trigger cardiogenic shock.

Neurogenic-vasogenic shock is a disorder specifically caused by inappropriate vascular dilation. If the dilation is due to neural stimuli (as in cases of insulin reaction, spinal anesthesia, or brain damage), it is termed neurogenic. If, however, it is due to chemical agents acting directly upon the smooth muscle of vascular walls (as in cases of anaphylaxis or dilation induced by bacterial toxins), it is called vasogenic. A comparative summary of the pri-

mary types of shock is presented in Table 9.17.

Development of Shock

Regardless of initiating factors, shock evolves in a characteristic and progressive manner. In general, pathological changes proceed through four major stages, as follows:

1. *Initial Stage* — circulation is only marginally depressed. Deviations from the norm are not of sufficient magnitude to cause dysfunction.

2. *Compensatory stage* — circulation is more severely depressed. Compensation mechanisms are activated to maintain blood pressure and promote blood supply to vital organs.

3. *Progressive stage* — compensation mechanisms fail to maintain adequate circulation. Lack of blood supply to vital organs precipitates serious physiological disequilibrium.

4. *Irreversible stage* — conditions deteriorate rapidly, terminating in death.

As shock develops, the inability to adequately service cellular needs triggers compensatory mechanisms. Typically, the maintenance of left ventricular output and arterial blood pressure is supported by an increase in cardiac rate and vasoconstriction. Activation of the sympathetic nervous system and release of epinephrine and norepinephrine from the adrenal medulla are primarily responsible for these adaptive responses.

Shock is further compensated for by the release of renin from ischemic nephrons, the release of ADH from the posterior pituitary gland, and the release of ACTH (adrenocorticotropic hormone) from the anterior pituitary.

ADH, as discussed earier, stimulates the reabsorption of water from renal tubules. It thereby serves to elevate plasma volume and promote an increase in arterial blood pressure. ACTH, on the other hand, stimulates the

secretion of mineralocorticoids (such as aldosterone) and glucocorticoids from the cortex, or outer layer, of the adrenal glands. While aldosterone potentiates the activity of ADH by promoting retention of sodium and water, the glucocorticoids function to provide fuel for metabolically deprived cells. By mobilizing fats and proteins to be used in the generation of much-needed glucose (gluconeogenesis), these hormones sustain cellular metabolism in the face of depleted carbohydrate reserves. A tabular summary of the compensatory mechanisms associated with shock can be found in Figure 9.52.

Although initially beneficial, these compensatory mechanisms can, with time, become nonadaptive. For example, when the rate of cardiac contraction increases excessive-

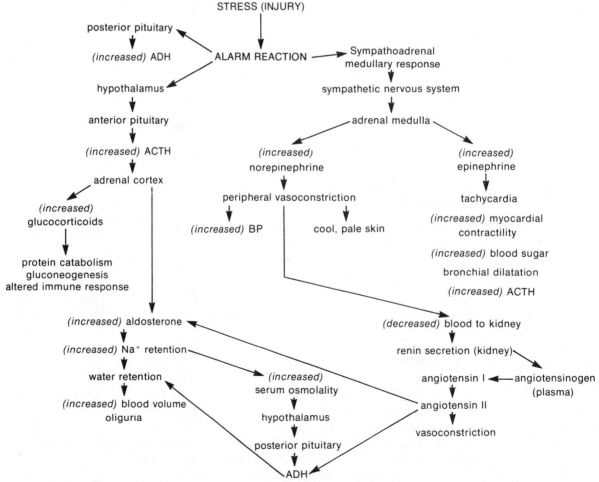

Figure 9.52 Compensatory mechanisms associated with shock. (From Marcinek, M. B.: Am. J. Nurs., 77:1809, 1977. Used by permission.)

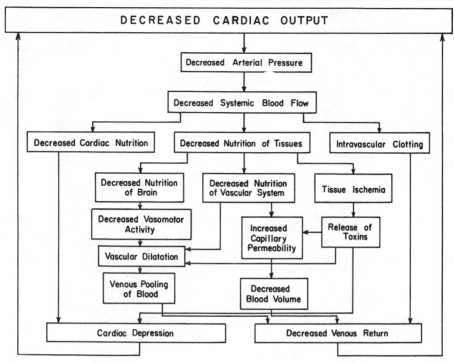

Figure 9.53 Some mechanisms that lead to the progression of shock. (From Guyton, A. C.: Textbook of Medical Physiology, 6th ed. Philadelphia, W. B. Saunders Company, 1981. Used by permission.)

ly, pumping effectiveness eventually declines. Even vasoconstriction can ultimately aggravate the shock syndrome. With sustained narrowing of the arterioles, arterial blood pressure is often maintained at the expense of capillary blood supply. Under these circumstances, a seemingly normal blood pressure reading can mask considerable cellular ischemia. The characteristic release of histamine by hypoxic tissue cells will, moreover, further complicate the phenomenon of nonadaptive compensation. As histamine triggers dilation of the precapillary sphincters, large volumes of blood pool in the microcirculation. Simultaneous increases in capillary permeability cause fluid to shift from plasma into the interstitial compartment. Venous return is thereby depleted, and arterial blood pressure falls as a consequence. When compensation mechanisms thus fail to provide for the maintenance of cellular equilibrium, the "progressive" stage of shock is said to be reached. A summary of some primary factors contributing to the evolution of shock can be found in Figure 9.53.

Manifestations of Shock

Although it can be seen that shock is typically initiated by disorders that trigger cardiovascular dysfunction, all systems eventually suffer from the effects of depressed circulation. Characteristic symptoms of weak rapid pulse, pallor, and falling blood pressure are thus accompanied by critical alterations in metabolism, pulmonary function, renal function, gastrointestinal function, and neural function. A survey of some primary manifestations of the shock syndrome is presented in the following pages.

METABOLISM DURING SHOCK

With the onset of shock, cellular oxygen supply is compromised, and anaerobic metabolism (glycolysis) is initiated. Although generating little energy, this metabolic pathway does produce significant amounts of lactic acid, ultimately resulting in metabolic acidosis. At the extreme, acidosis will directly trigger vasodilation, thereby initiating a drop in blood pressure, which aggravates the general depression of circulatory capacity.

If the ischemia accompanying shock is not corrected, metabolic and structural degeneration will ultimately culminate in cellular death and necrosis. Clinical symptoms will increasingly reflect cellular level changes to the extent that critical organs such as the heart, lungs, kidneys, and brain are victimized by these metabolic derangements.

PULMONARY FUNCTION DURING SHOCK

Pulmonary disorders often arise in the early stages of shock. At the extreme, dysfunction culminates in adult respiratory distress syndrome (ARDS) or shock lung. Sluggish circulation and ischemia characteristically promote the development of pulmonary vascular thrombi and pulmonary edema. As small vessels become plugged with blood cells, degenerative changes trigger the destruction of both capillary and alveolar tissue. Resulting depression of pulmonary diffusion is reflected by decreasing oxygen and increasing carbon dioxide levels in circulating plasma. Although these alterations in blood gas concentrations trigger a reflex stimulation of respiratory rate, compensation is not always effective or complete. Most often, the hypoxia and metabolic and respiratory acidosis generated by pulmonary dysfunction potentiate the escalating physiological disequilibrium characteristic of the shock syndrome.

RENAL FUNCTION DURING SHOCK

In order to function adequately in the elimination of wastes and the maintenance of fluid and electrolyte balance, the nephrons of the kidneys must receive an adequate supply of blood. The formation of urine is, in fact, initially dependent upon the filtration of fluid out of the plasma into the Bowman's capsule of the nephron.

As shock progresses, compensation mechanisms promote vasoconstriction of the afferent arterioles feeding blood into Bowman's capsule. Consequently, the rate and efficiency of urine formation declines, and nitrogenous wastes begin to accumulate in the plasma. Unfortunately, if renal ischemia is prolonged, death and necrosis of the nephrons ensue. With extensive tissue degeneration, damage becomes irreversible, and renal failure results.

GASTROINTESTINAL FUNCTION DURING SHOCK

The compensatory vasoconstriction initiated during shock is particularly effective in narrowing the blood vessels serving the liver and intestines. Resulting ischemic damage is frequently considerable. Necrosis of the intestinal mucosa is characteristically accompanied by the release of bacteria from the gastrointestinal tract into the bloodstream. The deleterious effects of toxins released by these microorganisms is potentiated by the degeneration of hepatic cells that normally function in detoxification. To the extent that the liver is unable to destroy harmful bacterial toxins, these foreign chemicals will aggravate the shock syndrome by directly triggering systemic vasodilation.

More recently, the ischemic pancreas has been implicated in the evolution of progressive shock. Believed by some researchers to function in the generation of myocardial depressant factor (MDF), this gland could play an indirect role in triggering the decreases in cardiac contractility that are frequently associated with hypovolemic or vasogenic-neurogenic shock.

NEURAL FUNCTION DURING SHOCK

Neural tissue is extremely sensitive to lack of oxygen and glucose supply. The brain, in fact, is protected from the effects of ischemia by a mechanism that facilitates vasodilation of cerebral blood vessels when the medulla is initiating vasoconstriction in most other areas of the body. As shock progresses, however, this protective dilation is often unable to maintain adequate cerebral circulation. With oxygen deprivation come symptoms of confusion, agitation, and restlessness, possibly accompanied by drowsiness and stupor.

TABLE 9.18   **Clinical Manifestations Associated with the Earlier Stages of Shock**

Clinical Manifestations	Causative Mechanism
Restlessness; apprehension	Cerebral hypoxia secondary to declining cardiac output
Hyperventilation	Increase in respiratory rate induced by anxiety or stress
Rapid pulse	Increase in cardiac rate as compensatory response to decreasing blood pressure
Pallor	Compensatory vasoconstriction of blood vessels servicing the skin

Shock: A Summary

In review, it can be said that shock is a physiological state characterized by circulatory depression. Homeostasis is disrupted as all four cellular life needs are compromised. The systemic effects are widespread and reflected by a broad range of symptoms. A summary of some major clinical manifestations of early shock can be found in Table 9.18.

As the shock syndrome progresses sequentially, advancing circulatory disruption will ultimately culminate in irreversible cellular damage and death. An overview of some primary symptoms associated with later shock is presented in Table 9.19.

CARDIOVASCULAR PATHOLOGY: DISRUPTION OF CELLULAR NEEDS

Since the cardiovascular system is so critical in providing for cellular needs, dis-

TABLE 9.19   **Clinical Manifestations Associated with the Later Stages of Shock**

Clinical Manifestation	Causative Mechanism
Metabolic acidosis	Decrease in cellular oxidation associated with circulatory failure
Hyperventilation	Compensatory response to development of metabolic acidosis
Rapid, weak, thready pulse; may culminate in cardiac arrest	Compensatory response to progressively decreasing blood pressure
Oliguria, possibly terminating in anuria	Decrease in renal blood flow
Apathy; may be followed by coma	Advancing cerebral hypoxia
Dyspnea; hypoxia	Pulmonary edema and decrease in pulmonary compliance characteristically associated with later stages of shock
Decreasing blood pressure	Failure of compensatory mechanism to maintain circulation. Vasodilation triggered by: (1) accumulation of cellular metabolic wastes, and (2) release of toxins into bloodstream by ischemic gastrointestinal tract

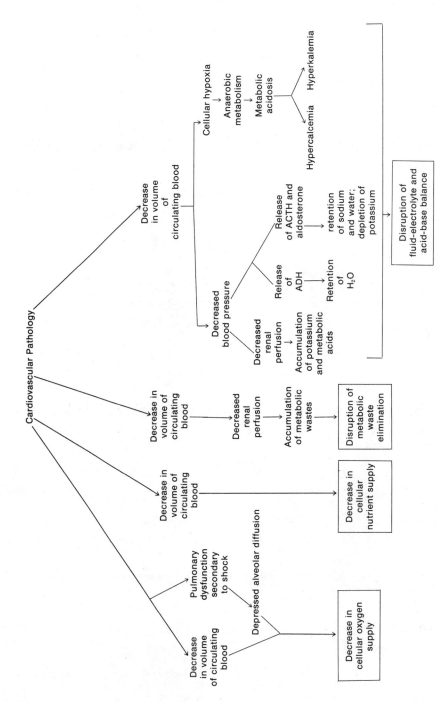

Figure 9.54 Cardiovascular pathology: disruption of homeostasis.

orders of the heart or blood vessels or both will trigger severe disruption of homeostasis, as follows:

1. *The cellular need for oxygen.* Oxygen is normally carried to the cells by the blood. Any interference with the pumping or transport of plasma will compromise the cellular oxygen supply.

2. *The cellular need for nutrients.* Absorbed nutrients are normally carried from the gastrointestinal tract to metabolizing cells through the blood. Once again, a functional cardiovascular system is needed to facilitate this transport.

3. *The cellular need for elimination.* Metabolic wastes are carried from the cells to organs of elimination by the blood. Cardiovascular disease can thus trigger physiological disruption by promoting the retention of potentially toxic chemicals.

4. *The cellular need for fluid-electrolyte and acid-base balance.* The maintenance of fluid-electrolyte and acid-base balance is controlled by extremely intricate mechanisms, as discussed in Chapters 6 and 7. Support for these mechanisms is derived from the cardiovascular system. Hormones regulating fluid and electrolyte levels are transported through the blood to target organs. Buffers compensating for acid-base imbalance are an integral part of plasma. Ultimately, cardiovascular disorders can interfere with the maintenance of fluid-electrolyte and acid-base balance in a variety of ways. Some of the mechanisms whereby cardiovascular disease can trigger cellular disequilibrium are summarized in Figure 9.54.

STUDY QUESTIONS

1. Describe the evolution of atherosclerosis.

2. Mrs. Coombs is diagnosed as suffering from atherosclerosis. List three predictable symptoms and explain their derivation.

3. Mrs. Rafael has been taking birth control pills for 15 years. She is admitted to the hospital with a tentative diagnosis of pulmonary embolism. Explain how such a condition could develop.

4. Why do anxiety and tension often cause an increase in blood pressure?

5. A patient in hematogenic (hemorrhagic) shock is given a vasoconstrictor drug. How would the administration of this drug affect cellular blood supply?

6. Explain why the rapid release of histamine during an allergic reaction would cause blood pressure to fall.

7. Explain why hypertension is often associated with renal disease.

8. Briefly identify, define, or describe the following:
   a. the structure that separates the right ventricle from the left ventricle
   b. the endocardium
   c. the tough, fibrous sac that encases the heart
   d. aortic valve
   e. the valve that prevents reflux of blood from the right ventricle into the right atrium during systole
   f. the normal pattern of the cardiac cycle
   g. abnormal heart sounds associated with valvular pathology
   h. the SA node
   i. the component of the electrocardiogram reflecting ventricular systole
   j. the P-R interval
   k. the volume of blood within the ventricles at the end of diastole (approximately 100 ml.)
   l. end systolic volume
   m. the stretch of myocardial muscle initiated by the return of venous blood to the heart.
   n. afterload
   o. cardiac output
   p. vessels that transport blood to the myocardial muscle

9. Assuming all other factors are constant, predict and explain the effect of the following upon cardiac output:
   a. hyperkalemia
   b. hypothermia

c. physical activity

d. hypocalcemia

10. Diagnostic testing reveals occlusion of the following coronary vessels. In each case, identify the portion of the myocardium that will most likely suffer from ischemia:
    a. left anterior descending artery
    b. right coronary artery
    c. left circumflex artery

11. Determine whether the following are examples of direct or indirect cardiac stress:
    a. rheumatic fever
    b. hemorrhage
    c. angina pectoris
    d. Cushing's disease
    e. myocarditis
    f. ventricular tachycardia
    g. myocardial infarction
    h. pericardial effusion
    i. tetralogy of Fallot
    j. hypertension
    k. anaphylactic shock
    l. SIADH

12. Which of the following may characteristically *result* from myocardial ischemia?
    a. hypertension
    b. arrhythmias
    c. chest pain
    d. elevation of plasma SGOT levels
    e. myocarditis

13. A patient is admitted to the hospital with severe chest pain. Indicate what tests will predictably be run to confirm a tentative diagnosis of myocardial infarction, and why.

14. Why does endocarditis often cause secondary systemic disease?

15. Differentiate between valvular stenosis and regurgitation.

16. In each of the following cases, identify the cardiac chamber in which excessive blood is most likely to accumulate:
    a. aortic stenosis
    b. mitral incompetence
    c. incompetence of the pulmonic valve

17. David Storrow, age 7, is brought to the pediatrician complaining of tiredness and loss of appetite. He has intermittent periods of fever and diffuse joint pain. Several weeks previously he had a streptococcal sore throat that was diagnosed and treated, but penicillin was discontinued after initial symptoms abated. What disease condition do you expect?

18. Explain why a baby with a ventricular septal defect would not typically show signs of cyanosis.

19. Determine whether the following phenomena would most likely cause a (1) decrease in venous return, or (2) resistance to cardiac output:
    a. hemorrhage
    b. hypertension
    c. vascular dilation
    d. aortic stenosis

20. List the three primary myocardial compensation mechanisms.

21. Mr. Boles is admitted to the hospital with pulmonary congestion secondary to emphysema. Describe how and why right-sided heart failure might develop.

22. Mrs. Taylor is showing signs of left-sided heart failure after a left ventricular myocardial infarction. List some predictable clinical manifestations.

23. In each of the following cases, determine whether shock would be classified as hematogenic, cardiogenic, neurogenic, or vasogenic.
    a. insulin reaction
    b. cardiac tamponade
    c. extensive burns
    d. hemorrhage
    e. anaphylactic reaction to penicillin
    f. severe myocardial infarction
    g. ventricular fibrillation

24. Explain briefly the mechanism responsible for each of the following shock symptoms:
    a. falling blood pressure
    b. weak, rapid pulse
    c. pallor
    d. pulmonary edema
    e. depressed urinary output
    f. confusion, agitation, and restlessness

Suggested Readings

Books

Abboud, F. M.: Shock. *In* Beeson, P. B., McDermott, W., and Wyngaarden, J. B. (eds.): Cecil

Textbook of Medicine, 15 ed. Philadelphia, W. B. Saunders Company, 1979, p. 1107.

Abel, F. L.: Functional characteristics of the heart. *In* Selkurt, E. E. (ed.): Basic Physiology for the Health Sciences. Boston, Little, Brown & Company, 1975, p. 349.

Abel, F. L.: The peripheral circulation. *In* Selkurt, E. E. (ed.): Basic Physiology for the Health Sciences. Boston, Little, Brown & Company, 1975, p. 375.

Anderson, W. A. D., and Scotti, T. M.: Synopsis of Pathology, 10th ed. St. Louis, The C. V. Mosby Company, 1980, pp. 279–382.

Berry, M. A.: Normal structure and function of the cardiovascular system. *In* Hudak, C. M., Lohr, T. S., and Gallo, B. M.: Critical Care Nursing, 2nd ed. Philadelphia, J. B. Lippincott Company, 1977, p. 73.

Bowers, S. A.: Cardiac complications: Often catastrophic. *In* Hamilton, H. (ed.): Combatting Cardiovascular Diseases Skillfully. Nursing 78 Books. Horsham, Pa., Intermed Communications, Inc., 1978, p. 103.

Brammell, H. L.: Pathophysiology of heart failure. *In* Hudak, C. M., Lohr, T. S., and Gallo, B. M.: Critical Care Nursing, 2nd ed. Philadelphia, J. B. Lippincott Company, 1977, p. 87.

Cannon, C. W.: Coronary artery disease: Stages of progression. *In* Hamilton, H. (ed.): Combatting Cardiovascular Diseases Skillfully. Nursing 78 Books. Horsham, Pa., Intermed Communications, Inc., 1978, p. 75.

Canobbio, M. M.: Inflammatory heart disease: Four most common. *In* Hamilton, H. (ed.): Combatting Cardiovascular Diseases Skillfully. Nursing 78 Books. Horsham, Pa., Intermed Communications, Inc., 1978, p. 115.

Clark, M. F.: Disturbances in the blood-pumping mechanism. *In* Jones, D. A., Dunbar, C. F., and Jirovec, M. M.: Medical-Surgical Nursing, A Conceptual Approach. New York, McGraw-Hill Book Company, 1978, p. 813.

Coffman, J. D.: Diseases of the peripheral vessels. *In* Beeson, P. B., McDermott, W., and Wyngaarden, J. B. (eds.): Cecil Textbook of Medicine, 15th ed. Philadelphia, W. B. Saunders Company, 1979. p. 1299.

Cromwell, R. L., et al.: Acute Myocardial Infarction: Reaction and Recovery. St. Louis, The C. V. Mosby Company, 1977.

Dodge, H. T., and Kennedy, J. W.: Cardiac output, cardiac performance, hypertrophy, dilatation, valvular disease, ischemic heart disease, and pericardial disease. *In* Sodeman, W. A., and Sodeman, T. M. (eds.): Pathologic Physiology, Mechanisms of Disease, 6th ed. Philadelphia, W. B. Saunders Company, 1979, p. 271.

Dollery, C. T.: Arterial hypertension. *In* Beeson, P. B., McDermott, W., and Wyngaarden, J. B. (eds.): Cecil Textbook of Medicine, 15th ed. Philadelphia, W. B. Saunders Company, 1979, p. 1199.

Fairbairn, J. F., II: Peripheral Vascular Diseases, 4th ed. Philadelphia, W. B. Saunders Company, 1972.

Fishman, A. P.: Heart failure. *In* Beeson, P. B., McDermott, W., and Wyngaarden, J. B. (eds.): Cecil Textbook of Medicine, 15th ed. Philadelphia, W. B. Saunders Company, 1979, p. 1080.

Guyton, A. C.: Textbook of Medical Physiology, 5th ed. Philadelphia, W. B. Saunders Company, 1976, pp. 160–196; 222–309; 320–369.

Hershey, S. G. (ed.): Shock. International Anesthesiology Clinics. Vol. 2, No. 2. Boston, Little, Brown & Company, 1964.

Hole, J. W.: Human Anatomy and Physiology. Dubuque, Wm. C. Brown Company, 1978, pp. 572–618.

Holm, K. M.: Blood vessel disruption. *In* Jones, D. A., Dunbar, C. F., and Jirovec, M. M.: Medical-Surgical Nursing, A Conceptual Approach. New York, McGraw-Hill Book Company, 1978, p. 981.

Hume, M.: Massive thrombophlebitis of the lower extremities. *In* Conn, H. F. (ed.): Current Therapy 1978. Philadelphia, W. B. Saunders Company, 1978.

Hurst, J. W. (ed.): The Heart, Arteries, and Veins. New York, McGraw-Hill Book Company, 1978.

Isacson, L. M., and Schultz, K. J.: Congestive failure: Severe cardiac impairment. *In* Hamilton, H. (ed.): Combatting Cardiovascular Diseases Skillfully. Nursing 78 Books. Horsham, Pa., Intermed Communications, Inc., 1978, p. 93.

Julian, D. G.: Angina pectoris. *In* Beeson, P. B., McDermott, W., and Wyngaarden, J. B. (eds.): Cecil Textbook of Medicine, 15th ed. Philadelphia, W. B. Saunders Company, 1979, p. 1223.

Julian, D. G.: Myocardial infarction. *In* Beeson, P. B., McDermott, W., and Wyngaarden, J. B. (eds.): Cecil Textbook of Medicine, 15th ed. Philadelphia, W. B. Saunders Company, 1979, p. 1229.

Kent, T. H., Hart, M. N., and Shires, T. K.: Introduction to Human Diseases. New York, Appleton-Century-Crofts, 1979, pp. 74–104.

Kim, M. J.: Disturbances in blood pressure. *In* Jones, D. A., Dunbar, C. F., and Jirovec, M. M.: Medical-Surgical Nursing, A Conceptual Approach. New York, McGraw-Hill Book Company, 1978, p. 933.

Levy, R. I.: Prevalence and epidemiology of cardiovascular disease. *In* Beeson, P. B., McDermott, W., and Wyngaarden, J. B. (eds.): Cecil Textbook of Medicine, 15th ed. Philadelphia, W. B. Saunders Company, 1979, p. 1059.

Luckmann, J., and Sorensen, K. C.: Medical-Surgical Nursing, A Psychophysiologic Approach, 2nd ed. Philadelphia, W. B. Saunders Company, 1980, pp. 229–285; 757–892; 1085–1138.

Maloney, R. J.: Hypertension: Risk factor in atherosclerosis. *In* Hamilton, H. (ed.): Combatting Cardiovascular Diseases Skillfully. Nursing 78 Books. Horsham, Pa., Intermed Communications, Inc., 1978, p. 67.

Manzi, C. C.: Acute myocardial infarction: Severe ASHD. *In* Hamilton, H. (ed.): Combatting Cardiovascular Diseases Skillfully. Nursing 78 Books. Horsham, Pa., Intermed Communications, Inc., 1978, p. 83.

McFarland, M. B.: Conduction disturbances as a cause of pump failure. *In* Jones, D. A., Dunbar, C. F., and Jirovec, M. M.: Medical-Surgical Nursing, A Conceptual Approach. New York, McGraw-Hill Book Company, 1978, p. 841.

Murphy, K., and Stahler, K.: Cardiac babies: Know six common anomalies. *In* Hamilton, H. (ed.): Combatting Cardiovascular Diseases Skillfully. Nursing 78 Books. Horsham, Pa., Intermed Communications, Inc., 1978, p. 23.

Purtillo, D. T.: A Survey of Human Diseases. Menlo Park, Addison-Wesley Publishing Company, 1978, pp. 259–283.

Ream, I.: Peripheral vascular lesions: Cause of leg pain. *In* Hamilton, H. (ed.): Combatting Cardiovascular Diseases Skillfully. Nursing 78 Books. Horsham, Pa., Intermed Communications, Inc., 1978, p. 155.

Robbins, S. L., and Cotran, R. S.: Pathologic Basis of Disease, 2nd ed. Philadelphia, W. B. Saunders Company, 1979, pp. 593–709.

Ross, J.: Acquired valvular heart disease. *In* Beeson, P. B., McDermott, W., and Wyngaarden, J. B. (eds.): Cecil Textbook of Medicine, 15th ed. Philadelphia, W. B. Saunders Company, 1979, p. 1174.

Sherry, S.: Thrombophlebitis and phlebothrombosis. *In* Beeson, P. B., McDermott, W., and Wyngaarden, J. B. (eds.): Cecil Textbook of Medicine, 15th ed. Philadelphia, W. B. Saunders Company, 1979, p. 1124.

Shires, G. T., et al.: Shock. Philadelphia, W. B. Saunders Company, 1973.

Storlie, F. J.: Structural defects of the heart. *In* Jones, D. A., Dunbar, C. F., and Jirovec, M. M.: Medical-Surgical Nursing, A Conceptual Approach. New York, McGraw-Hill Book Company, 1978, p. 899.

Strong, A. B.: Diagnostic tests: Invasive and noninvasive. *In* Hamilton, H. (ed.): Combatting Cardiovascular Diseases Skillfully. Nursing 78 Books. Horsham, Pa., Intermed Communications, Inc., 1978, p. 55.

Swan, H. J. C., and Parmley, W. W.: Congestive heart failure. *In* Sodeman, W. A., and Sodeman, T. M. (eds.): Pathologic Physiology, Mechanisms of Disease, 6th ed. Philadelphia, W. B. Saunders Company, 1979, p. 313.

Tarazi, R. C., and Gifford, R. W.: Systemic arterial pressure. *In* Sodeman, W. A., and Sodeman, T. M. (eds.): Pathologic Physiology, Mechanisms of Disease, 6th ed. Philadelphia, W. B. Saunders Company, 1979, p. 198.

Tortora, G. J., and Anagnostakos, N. P.: Principles of Anatomy and Physiology, 2nd ed. San Francisco, Canfield Press, 1978, pp. 441–493.

VanMeter, M., and Lavine, P. G.: Reading EKG's Correctly, 2nd ed. Horsham, Pa., Intermed Communications, Inc., 1975.

Walter, J. B.: An Introduction to the Principles of Disease. Philadelphia, W. B. Saunders Company, 1977, pp. 428–466.

Weber, M. A., and Laragh, J. H.: Hypertension. *In* Conn, H. F. (ed.): Current Therapy 1978. Philadelphia, W. B. Saunders Company, 1978.

Whalen, R. E.: Disorders of the pericardium. *In* Beeson, P. B., McDermott, W., and Wyngaarden, J. B. (eds.): Cecil Textbook of Medicine, 15th ed. Philadelphia, W. B. Saunders Company, 1979, p. 1268.

Wolf, P. S., et al.: Assessment skills for the nurse: cardiovascular system. *In* Hudak, C. M., Lohr, T. S., and Gallo, B. N.: Critical Care Nursing, 2nd ed. Philadelphia, J. B. Lippincott Company, 1977, p. 141.

Wolinsky, H.: Atherosclerosis. *In* Beeson, P. B., McDermott, W., and Wyngaarden, J. B. (eds.): Cecil Textbook of Medicine, 15th ed. Philadelphia, W. B. Saunders Company, 1979, p. 1218.

Articles

Barnes, R. W.: Axioms on acute arterial occlusion of an extremity. Hosp. Med., *14*:34, 1978.

Baron, H. C.: Chronic arterial insufficiency of the lower limbs. Hosp. Med., *14*:33, 1978.

Burch, G. E.: Axioms on myocardial infarction. Hosp. Med., *14*:8, 1978.

CHF diagnosis and treatment today. Emergency Med., *11*:109, 1979.

Chandler, J. G.: The physiology and treatment of shock. RN, *34*:42, 1971.

Ciuca, R.: Cor pulmonale. Nursing 78, *8*:46, 1978.

Cobey, J., and Cobey, J. H.: Chronic leg ulcers. Am. J. Nurs., *74*:258, 1974.

Denny, M. P.: Septic shock. J. Emergency Nurs., *3*:19, 1977.

Fagin-Dubin, L.: Atherosclerosis: a major cause of peripheral vascular disease. Nurs. Clin. North Am., *12*:101, 1977.

Friedman, S. A.: Guide to diagnosis of peripheral arterial disease. Hosp. Med., *15*:87, 1979.

Gould, L., et al.: Pericardial effusion as an early complication of acute myocardial infarction. Am. Fam. Physician, *19*:197, 1979.

Henry, J. P.: Understanding the early pathophysiology of essential hypertension. Geriatrics, *31*:59, 1976.

Hollander, G., and Lichstein, E.: Guide to evaluation of ischemic heart disease. Hosp. Med., *16*:46, 1979.

Juergens, J. L.: Venous thromboembolism. Cardiovasc. Clin., *3*:234, 1971.

Katz, F. H.: Primary hypertension. Hosp. Med., *13*:26, 1977.

Kennedy, J.: Myocardial infarction in coronary artery disease. Cardiovasc. Nurs., *12*:23, 1976.

Keys, A.: Atherosclerosis, coronary heart disease — the global picture. Atherosclerosis, *22*:149, 1975.

Mayer, G. G., et al.: Arrhythmias and cardiac output. Am. J. Nurs., *72*:1597, 1972.

McNeal, G. J.: Tracing arrhythmias. Am. J. Nurs., *79*:98, 1979.

Mechanisms of edema in myocardial failure. Hosp. Med., *12*:79, 1976.

Miller, K. M.: Assessing peripheral perfusion. Am. J. Nurs., *8*:1673, 1978.

Parmley, W. W.: Axioms on congestive heart failure. Hosp. Med., *13*:44, 1977.

Ream, I.: Counseling patients with leg pain. A review of peripheral vascular disease. Nursing 77, *7*:54, 1977.

Robinson, P. H.: Pericarditis. Med. Times, *107*:73, 1979.

Sacksteder, S., et al.: Common congenital cardiac defects. Am. J. Nurs., *78*:264, 1978.

Sochocky, S.: Axioms on cor pulmonale. Hosp. Med., *12*:7, 1976.

Spodick, D. H.: Acute pericarditis and pericardial effusion: Guide to diagnosis and management. Hosp. Med., *15*:72, 1979.

Stude, C.: Cardiogenic shock. Am. J. Nurs., *74*:1636, 1974.

Wilson, R. F., and Wilson, J. A.: Pathophysiology, diagnosis and treatment of shock. J. Emergency Nursing, *3*:11, 1977.

Chapter Outline

chapter 10

Respiratory Pathology

Chapter Objectives

At the completion of this chapter, the student will be able to:

1. Describe the processes of pulmonary inflation, ventilation, and diffusion.
2. Define ventilation pathology and identify two major causative mechanisms.
3. Give five examples of ventilation disorders of neurological origin.
4. List two primary types of disorders that increase the "work of ventilation."
5. Differentiate between restrictive and obstructive pathology with respect to the nature of dysfunction and causative factors.
6. Define diffusion pathology and identify four major causative mechanisms.
7. Describe the significance of alveolar perfusion and ventilation-perfusion imbalances with respect to diffusion.
8. Describe the way in which the respiratory membrane may affect pulmonary diffusion.
9. Identify ten major disorders that may cause diffusion disorders, and describe the pathogenesis of dysfunction.
10. Differentiate between respiratory insufficiency and respiratory failure.
11. Trace the development of respiratory failure.
12. List and define four major pulmonary volumes and four major pulmonary capacities and describe their significance.
13. Define the term *alveolar ventilation* and describe its clinical relevance.
14. Identity and describe arterial blood gas values and elucidate their diagnostic significance.

INTRODUCTION

The respiratory system consists of a series of organs that function to promote the exchange of gases between the atmosphere and plasma. Through the processes of *ventilation* (the transport of gases between the atmosphere and the alveoli of the lungs) and *diffusion* (the exchange of gases between the alveoli and the pulmonary capillaries), respiratory structures work to support homeostasis. By providing an interface between the internal and external environments, the respiratory system helps to service all basic cellular needs, as follows:

1. *Oxygen.* Oxygen derived from inspired air normally diffuses from the alveoli into pulmonary capillaries, thence to be transported by the blood to all cells of the body.

2. *Nutrient utilization.* Cellular metabolism is maintained to the extent that oxygen is available to support aerobic catabolism.

3. *Elimination.* Carbon dioxide generated by cellular metabolism normally diffuses from pulmonary capillaries into alveoli and is subsequently eliminated by expiration.

4. *Acid-base balance.* Carbon dioxide, by reacting chemically with water in the blood, affects the plasma levels of carbonic acid, thereby influencing acid-base balance.

Respiratory disorders occur when structural or functional changes alter the processes of ventilation or diffusion. In this chapter, a basic review of normal respiratory physiology lays the groundwork for the later study of ventilation and diffusion abnormalities. Since such dysfunction often culminates in respiratory insufficiency or failure, it is important to understand the pathogenesis and manifestations of this pathological syndrome.

RESPIRATORY PHYSIOLOGY: A REVIEW

Assuming a functional cardiovascular system and normal transport of gases through the bloodsteam, the distribution and elimination of respiratory gases are dependent largely upon the respiratory system. The components of the system must function together to support cellular homeostasis. To facilitate a better understanding of pathology, it is essential to review some of the complexities of normal respiratory physiology.

The lungs are composed of a large amount of elastic tissue. As such, they exhibit a natural tendency to recoil or collapse. During fetal development, in fact, the lungs are actually filled with fluid, deflated and unable to perform any work. It is not until birth that pulmonary fluid is expelled or absorbed, and lung expansion begins. For functional capacity to be maintained, pulmonary tissue must remain inflated throughout the life of the individual. Some major factors that counteract recoil and promote inflation will be discussed in the following pages.

The optimally functional lung is designed to service cellular needs by participating in both ventilation and diffusion. Because these two processes are the basis of respiratory activity, their mechanisms will also be clarified in this introductory review.

Pulmonary Inflation

In the human body, inflation of the collapsed fetal lung is initiated at birth and is maintained primarily through the combined effects of *negative intrapleural pressure* and *surfactant production*.

As the baby is delivered from the birth canal, pulmonary fluid is replaced by air and activation of the respiratory center causes chest expansion. Inherent pulmonary recoil is counteracted, in part, by complex changes that cause the pressure in the thoracic cavity surrounding the lungs to be *less* than the pressure within the lungs. As gases attempt to move from the area of greater pressure (within the lungs) to the area of lesser pressure (surrounding the lungs), pulmonary tissue expands. The evolution of negative intrapleural pressure, as illustrated in Figure 10.1, is essential to the initiation and maintenance of pulmonary inflation.

Further facilitating postnatal pulmonary expansion is the secretion of a special substance, called surfactant, into the alveoli. By

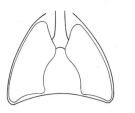   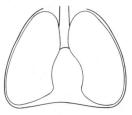

Prenatal Thoracic Cavity   Postnatal Thoracic Cavity

Figure 10.1 Pulmonary inflation at birth.

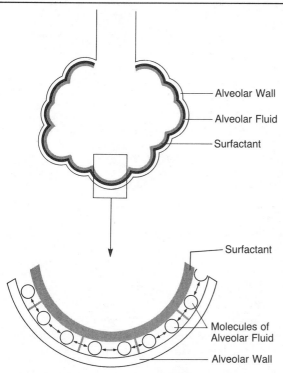

Alveolar Wall

Alveolar Fluid

Surfactant

Surfactant

Molecules of
Alveolar Fluid

Alveolar Wall

Figure 10.2 The function of surfactant. Note that surfactant works to decrease the intermolecular attraction in alveolar fluid.

decreasing *surface tension,* or the intermolecular attraction exhibited between molecules of fluid lining the alveoli, surfactant acts to stabilize the lungs and prevent alveolar collapse. Occasionally, however, premature babies are born with inadequate surfactant. The resulting pathological condition, referred to as *infant respiratory distress syndrome (hyaline membrane disease),* is characterized by inadequate pulmonary inflation, the formation of a fibrinous hyaline membrane over the cells lining the alveoli, and acute respiratory distress. The way in which surfactant functions to counteract pulmonary collapse is depicted in Figure 10.2.

Assuming normal inflation of the lungs at birth, collapse of pulmonary tissue can be induced by a variety of disorders. When such disorders lead to "imperfect lung expansion," the resulting condition is generally referred to as *atelectasis.* Causative factors include restrictive and obstructive conditions, which will be examined later in this chapter.

Ventilation

Ventilation is defined as the movement of gases between the atmosphere and the alveoli of the lungs. As such, it involves the inspiration of air through the respiratory passages into the terminal air sacs, and the expiration of air containing metabolic wastes up through the respiratory tree into the environment. To appreciate the intricacies of the inspiration-expiration process, it is necessary to look more closely at three major aspects of ventilation: (1) the mechanics of ventilation, (2) the work of ventilation, and (3) the rate of ventilation.

THE MECHANICS OF VENTILATION

In general, the mechanics of ventilation involve alternately enlarging and compressing the thoracic cavity and the lungs. In accordance with natural laws governing the behavior of gases, pressure within the lungs decreases as thoracic and pulmonary volumes increase. Air subsequently flows from where it is under greater pressure (in the atmosphere) to where it is under lesser pressure (in the alveoli), resulting in inspiration. Alternately, as thoracic and pulmonary volumes decrease, rising pressure forces gases out of the lungs into the atmosphere, causing expiration. An illustrative summary of the processes governing inspiration and expiration is presented in Figure 10.3.

Normally, ventilation is regulated by control centers in the medulla and the pons. Inspiration is initiated by neural impulses that stimulate contraction of the muscles of inspiration, such as the diaphragm and external intercostals. Shortening of these muscles increases the anterior-posterior and inferior-superior dimensions of the thoracic cavity, thereby facilitating inspiration. Expiration, on the other hand, is an essentially passive process. Induced by decreases in thoracic volume as the diaphragm relaxes and elastic tissue in the lungs and chest cavity recoils, normal expiration requires no expenditure of energy. During forced expiration however, a few muscles may be recruited to help generate thoracic pressure increases. Abdominal muscles, for example, function to pull the ribs down while simultaneously pushing gastrointestinal organs up into the thoracic cavity. Compression is further facilitated by contraction of the internal intercostals, which pull the upper ribs backward, thereby lowering the chest cage. The mechanics of inspiration and expiration are illustrated in Figure 10.4.

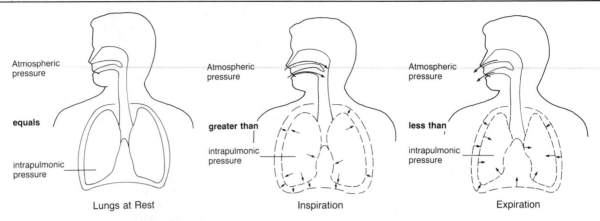

Figure 10.3   A schematic summary of inspiration and expiration.

THE WORK OF VENTILATION

Under normal circumstances, the ventilation process is executed with relative ease, encountering only a marginal amount of resistance. During quiet breathing, for example, the muscular work required to support ventilation constitutes only 2 to 3 per cent of total energy output. As respiratory dysfunction develops, however, as much as 30 per cent of metabolic output must be utilized just to facilitate inspiration and expiration. Energy is thus drained from other processes, and multisystemic dysfunction can result.

The "work of ventilation" is specifically directed at counteracting (1) resistance posed by pulmonary and thoracic recoil, (2) resistance posed by friction within the airways,

and (3) resistance posed by inherent viscosity of the lungs and chest cage. Since the demands of inspiration and expiration can differ considerably, it is helpful to evaluate each process independently. Only in this way is it possible to isolate the complex threads that are woven into the intricate pattern of respiratory pathology.

RESISTANCE TO INSPIRATION To facilitate the intake of air, elastic tissue of the lungs and thorax must expand in response to volume and pressure changes. The extent to which the lungs and thorax can enlarge during ventilation is referred to as *compliance*. Expressed numerically as the change in pulmonary volume generated by each unit increase

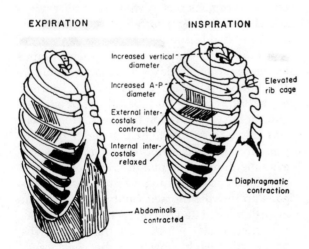

Figure 10.4   The mechanics of ventilation. (From Guyton, A. C.: Textbook of Medical Physiology, 6th ed. Philadelphia, W. B. Saunders Company, 1981. Used by permission.)

TABLE 10.1 Disorders That Cause Resistance to Expiration

Type of Disorder	Examples
Obstructive	Chronic obstructive pulmonary disease (COPD) Bronchiectasis Cystic fibrosis Lung cancer
Infectious	Pneumonia Tuberculosis
Inflammatory	Pneumoconioses

in inter-alveolar pressure, compliance specifically reflects the amount of energy required to counteract pulmonary and thoracic elastic recoil. Any factor that reduces compliance will predictably increase the "work of ventilation." Causative disorders are varied in nature ranging from fibrous degenerative changes in pulmonary tissue to structural deformities of the thoracic cage. Regardless of the underlying disorder, however, declining expansibility will force inspiratory muscles to work harder in attempts to overcome tissue resistance.

Airway obstruction can also pose an impediment to the inspiratory process. Frequently caused by excessive accumulation of bronchial or alveolar fluid, by constriction of the bronchioles, or by neoplasms, the resistance generated will also tax the muscles of respiration and ultimately increase the "work of ventilation."

RESISTANCE TO EXPIRATION As mentioned earlier, expiration is largely a passive process facilitated by the elastic recoil of pulmonary and thoracic tissue. In the event that elasticity is reduced, expiratory muscles must work harder to produce pulmonary compression, and the "work of ventilation" is consequently increased. Some causative disorders are listed in Table 10.1.

Since the ultimate goal of expiration is to eliminate gaseous wastes by transporting them from the alveoli into the atmosphere, it stands to reason that airway obstruction can also pose resistance to the expiratory process.

The degree of resulting dysfunction will, of course, depend upon the nature, extent, and location of the obstruction.

THE RATE OF VENTILATION

To facilitate the optimal intake and output of air, the rate, depth, and rhythm of inspiration and expiration must be carefully regulated. Any change in the pattern of ventilation is normally adaptive in nature and designed to promote cellular homeostasis. The respiratory system is particularly responsive to alterations in plasma concentration of oxygen, carbon dioxide, and hydrogen ions.

As carbon dioxide and hydrogen levels rise, or oxygen level falls, for example, a reflex increase in respiratory rate and depth is initiated. Referred to as *hyperventilation*, this response functions to bring carbon dioxide, carbonic acid (hydrogen ions), and oxygen levels back toward normal. Conversely, if carbon dioxide and hydrogen ion concentrations decline, reflex *hypoventilation* occurs. Respiratory rate and depth are depressed to enable the retention of carbon dioxide and the build-up of carbonic acid. The responsiveness of respiratory rate to blood gas and acid levels is summarized in Figure 10.5.

The mechanism that supports this respiratory response pattern is based primarily upon sensitivity of the medulla to chemical changes in plasma. As carbon dioxide and hydrogen ions accumulate in the body they trigger the initiation of hyperventilation by the medulla. Unfortunately, however, extensive or chronic elevation of carbon dioxide has been found to eventually desensitize the medulla. When this occurs, the respiratory center does not respond normally to changing blood chemistry, and respiratory depression ensues.

Hypoventilation, on the other hand, is normally initiated by the medulla in direct response to decreases in carbon dioxide and hydrogen ion concentrations. Neural impulses are sent less frequently to the muscles of respiration, causing retention of carbon dioxide and hydrogen ions.

It is significant, but surprising, to note that respiratory rate is *not* particularly responsive to changes in plasma oxygen levels. Con-

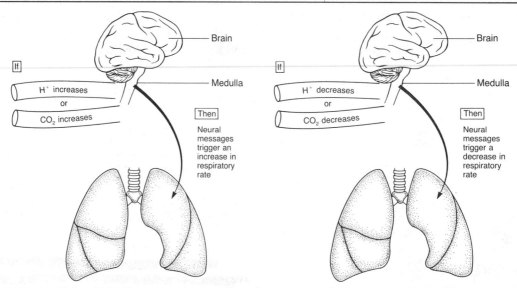

Figure 10.5 The responsiveness of respiratory rate to fluctuations in pH and CO_2.

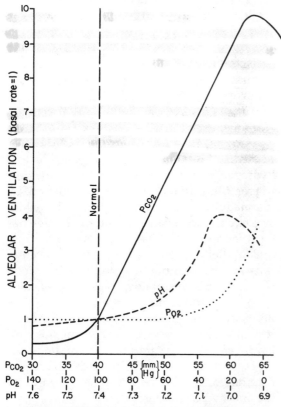

Figure 10.6 The relative impact of pCO_2, pH and pO_2 upon respiratory rate. (From Guyton, A. C. Textbook of Medical Physiology, 6th ed. Philadelphia, W. B. Saunders Company, 1981. Used by permission.)

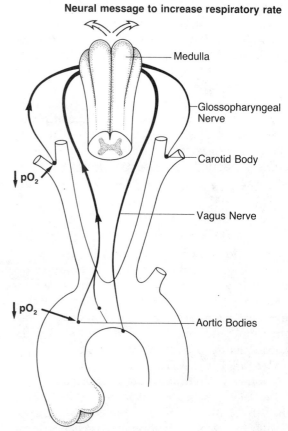

Figure 10.7 The mechanism whereby hypoxemia can trigger an increase in respiratory rate.

trary to expectation, the body can tolerate rather extensive depressions in pO_2 before cellular oxygen supply is compromised. In fact, alveolar ventilation can decrease by approximately one half and still adequately support cellular metabolism. This is true primarily because the body normally inspires considerably more oxygen than is needed by the cells, thereby providing a margin of safety. The relative responsiveness of respiratory rate to changes in pCO_2, pH, and pO_2 is summarized in Figure 10.6.

Under certain circumstances, however, oxygen deprivation can significantly stimulate respiratory rate. In these cases, declining oxygen concentration initiates increases in ventilation primarily by stimulating chemoreceptors in the aortic arch and carotid bodies. Neural messages are sent to the medulla, which, in turn, triggers respiratory changes. The mechanism is illustrated in Figure 10.7.

Oxygen-induced stimulation is characteristically noted in high-altitude, low-oxygen environments. As respiratory rate increases, carbon dioxide and hydrogen ion concentrations decrease. The resulting decline in pCO_2 and increase in pH would normally depress the rate of respiration, thereby modifying the stimulatory effect of low pO_2. In cases of environmentally reduced oxygen levels, however, the medulla adapts, with time, to altered carbon dioxide and hydrogen concentrations. Within about a week, the influence of declining pO_2 takes precedence, and respiratory rate may increase considerably.

Oxygen levels also function to significantly affect ventilation rate in cases of long-term pulmonary disease characterized by restricted diffusion. In these instances, pO_2 is chronically depressed while pCO_2 and hydrogen ion concentrations are elevated. It has been discovered that when carbon dioxide and hydrogen ions are increased over prolonged periods of time, the medulla adapts and become unresponsive to their influence. In the resulting condition, described as *CO2 narcosis*, elevations in carbon dioxide and hydrogen ions no longer serve as primary respiratory stimulants. Rather, it is depressed pO_2 that becomes the major impetus to respiration. Under these circumstances, alleviation of hypoxia can actually precipitate respiratory arrest. The clini-

cian is thus cautioned to monitor carefully the administration of oxygen to any patients suffering from chronic respiratory distress.

VENTILATION: A SUMMARY

Ventilation is the process whereby gases are continually transported between the atmosphere and the alveoli of the lungs. While inspiration is initiated by increases in pulmonary and thoracic volumes, expiration is facilitated by compression.

Under normal circumstances, only minimal resistance is posed to the intake or output of air during respiration. To the extent that resistance factors are increased with disease, inspiratory and expiratory muscles must work harder just to maintain the status quo.

The effectiveness of ventilation is also influenced by the rate and rhythm of inspiration and expiration. Primarily regulated and controlled by the respiratory centers in the brainstem, activity is particularly responsive to alterations in plasma levels of carbon dioxide and hydrogen ions.

Diffusion

To support homeostasis, ventilation must be coupled with adequate diffusion of gases between the alveoli and the pulmonary capillaries. The diffusion process has been described previously in Chapter 2. In brief, it involves the movement of oxygen from alveoli into pulmonary capillaries and the passage of carbon dioxide from pulmonary capillaries into alveoli. Each respiratory gas moves independently, according to the laws of diffusion, from the area where it is under *greater* pressure to the area where it is under *lesser* pressure. The normal exchange is illustrated diagrammatically in Figure 10.8.

If diffusion is disrupted, the cellular needs for oxygen and waste elimination may be compromised. Most commonly, *hypoxemia* (depression of pO_2) and *hypercapnia* (elevation of pCO_2) will result. In the evaluation of alveolar gas exchange, several factors that support diffusion must be taken into account. These include:

1. *Ventilation of the alveoli.* Alveolar ventilation can be defined as the movement of

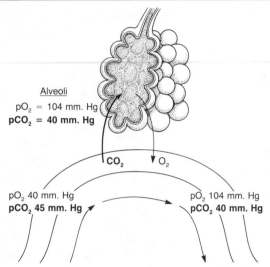

Alveoli
pO_2 = 104 mm. Hg
pCO_2 = 40 mm. Hg

CO_2 O_2

pO_2 40 mm. Hg
pCO_2 45 mm. Hg

pO_2 104 mm. Hg
pCO_2 40 mm. Hg

Figure 10.8 Diffusion of oxygen and carbon dioxide between the alveoli and the pulmonary capillary.

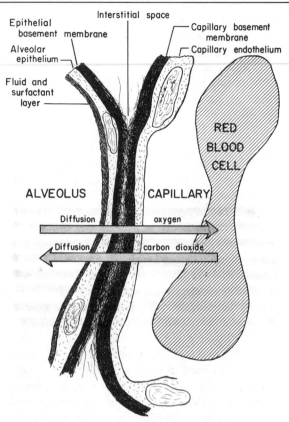

Figure 10.9 Ultrastructure of the respiratory membrane. (From Guyton, A. C.: Textbook of Medical Physiology, 6th ed. Philadelphia, W. B. Saunders Company, 1981. Used by permission.)

gases between the alveoli and the rest of the respiratory tree. Although inspiration and expiration may appear to be adequate, it is important to estimate the extent to which gases are actually entering and leaving the tiny air sacs hidden deep within the lungs.

2. *Perfusion of the alveoli.* To facilitate diffusion, the alveoli must be provided with an adequate volume of pulmonary blood. The degree to which blood circulates through the alveolar wall is referred to as alveolar perfusion.

3. *Ventilation-perfusion ratio.* The ventilation-perfusion ratio is a measure of the balance between alveolar ventilation and perfusion. Ideally, ventilation and perfusion are relatively matched. To the extent that ventilation-perfusion imbalances occur, gas exchange may be disrupted.

4. *Integrity of the "respiratory membrane."* The respiratory membrane is actually a composite structure through which gases must pass in their movement between alveolus and pulmonary capillary. It consists of the alveolar membrane, the pulmonary capillary wall, and the narrow interstitial space between the two. The "respiratory membrane," illustrated in Figure 10.9, is extremely thin (0.2 to 0.5 microns) and freely permeable to carbon dioxide and oxygen. Presenting a total surface area of approximately 70 square meters, its structure greatly facilitates gas exchange.

VENTILATION PATHOLOGY

The ventilation process is the essential first step in respiratory function. Any disruption of the ventilation mechanism can, of course, interfere with both the intake and the output of air. A pathological state is generally induced in one of two major ways:

1. Alteration of the normal respiratory rate or rhythm. Causative disorders usually have a neurological origin.

2. Increases in the "work of ventilation." These dysfunctions are usually classified as *restrictive* or *obstructive*, according to the nature and result of characteristic changes.

Disorders of Neural Origin

The central nervous system normally directs respiratory activity by regulating the rate and rhythm of inspiratory and expiratory muscular contraction. As a result, neural disorders can often precipitate changes in ventilation.

Respiratory depression, for example, is typically caused by many disorders of neurological origin. *Cerebral edema* resulting from a concussion will frequently inactivate neurons of the respiratory centers and thus depress respiratory rate. Alternatively, tumors exerting pressure on the medulla can cause nerve damage and deactivation of the respiratory center. Disease conditions such as poliomyelitis, Guillain-Barré syndrome, or myasthenia gravis depress the ventilation process by affecting neurons that normally stimulate the muscles of respiration. Perhaps the most common cause of respiratory depression, however, is an overdose of *anesthetics or narcotics*. These chemical agents act directly upon the medulla to reduce the rate of respiration. In excessive amounts, they can cause respiratory arrest or death.

Alternatively, respiratory rate can be increased by factors that stimulate ventilation activity. Caffeine, Benzedrine, and theophylline, for example, are chemical agents that directly excite the respiratory center. Thyroxine, epinephrine, norepinephrine, and growth hormone, on the other hand, are hormones that activate the respiratory center indirectly by promoting cellular metabolism. Subsequent increases in carbon dioxide production provide the impetus for respiratory changes.

Disorders That Increase the "Work of Ventilation"

Disorders that increase the work of ventilation are generally classified as either *restrictive* or *obstructive*. Restrictive disorders are characterized by a decrease in compliance of the lungs or thorax or both. Obstructive disorders, on the other hand, are caused by factors that pose resistance to the free movement of gases through the respiratory tree.

RESTRICTIVE PULMONARY DISORDERS

Restrictive disorders are induced clinically in three primary ways. They generally accompany (1) abnormalities in the size, shape, or expansibility of the chest cage; (2) changes in the pressure dynamics within the thoracic cavity; or (3) fibrous degeneration of pulmonary tissue.

ABNORMALITIES OF THE CHEST CAGE The chest cage is a bell-shaped cavity that accommodates both the heart and the major organs of respiration. Any alteration in the size, shape, or expansibility of the thorax can interfere with the generation of volume and pressure changes essential to normal ventilation.

Structural deformities such as *scoliosis* and *kyphosis*, for example, are characterized by lateral and hunchback curvature of the spine, respectively. Illustrated in Figure 10.10, these disorders frequently increase the work of ventilation by abnormally compressing the lungs. Respiratory restriction can also be imposed by traumatic damage to the chest cage, as evidenced in cases of crushing injuries or rib fractures.

Decreases in the volume of the thorax can also be caused by pressure of abdominal origin. Distention of gastrointestinal organs, abdominal binders, or abdominal pain will restrict the downward movement of the diaphragm that normally accompanies inspiration. Ventilation patterns are thereby altered, and respiratory effectiveness declines.

CHANGES IN THORACIC PRESSURE DYNAMICS Normally, the surface of the lungs is covered with a thin, serous membrane called *visceral pleura;* the thoracic cavity is lined with a similar membrane, described as the *parietal pleura*. The relationship between these two membranes is clarified by picturing a drawer that is to be filled with two boxes. If one takes some paper and lines the drawer, then wraps each box and places it in the drawer, the drawer lining can be likened to parietal pleura, and the box wrapping to visceral pleura. This concept is illustrated in Figure 10.11.

The narrow *pleural space* existing between visceral and parietal pleura usually contains a small volume of lubricating *pleural fluid*. This fluid functions to reduce friction between the lungs and the thoracic walls during ventilation. If pleural fluid accumulates excessively, however, compression can reduce

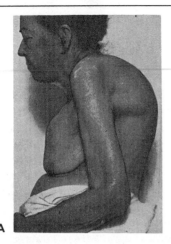

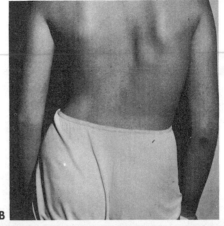

Figure 10.10 Kyphosis *(A)* and scoliosis *(B and C)* are structural deformities that can interfere with ventilation. (From Delp, M. H., and Manning, R. T.: Major's Physical Diagnosis, 9th ed. Philadelphia, W. B. Saunders Company, 1981. Used by permission.)

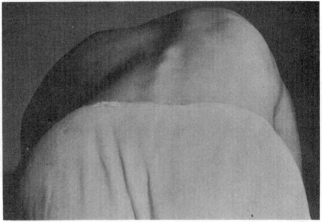

effective respiratory capacity, resulting in dysfunction.

In considering the pleural space, it is important to remember that the pressure within the pleural cavity *(intrapleural gas pressure)* must always remain less than gas pressure within the lungs *(intrapulmonic pressure)* if

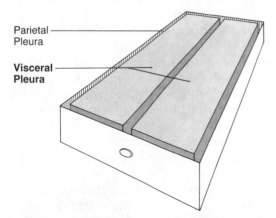

Figure 10.11 The pleural membranes: a conceptual illustration.

Parietal Pleura

Visceral Pleura

pulmonary inflation is to be sustained. If negative pressure is not maintained, partial or total collapse of the lungs can ensue.

In the following pages, a closer look is taken at disorders that characteristically cause increases in (1) intrapleural gas pressure, or (2) pleural fluid pressure.

Regardless of causative mechanism, pulmonary compression may ultimately result in *atelectasis*. In these cases, resistance to pulmonary expansion culminates in the collapse of lung tissue.

Increases in Intrapleural Gas Pressure Normally, the thoracic cavity is an airtight structure. Negative pressure within this cavity can be supported only to the extent that a closed seal is maintained. If a communicating opening should occur between the pleural space and an area of higher pressure, gases would rush in to equalize the pressure differences. Any disorder that increases intrapleural gas pressure will therefore cause varying degrees of pulmonary compression.

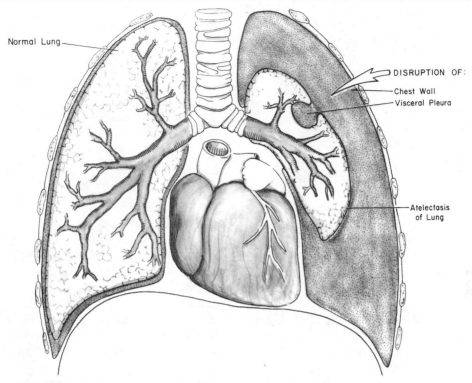

Normal Lung

DISRUPTION OF:
Chest Wall
Visceral Pleura

Atelectasis
of Lung

Figure 10.12 Pneumothorax (increase in gas pressure within the pleural cavity) can be caused by disruption of either the chest wall or the visceral pleura. Atelectasis (collapse) of the lung results. (From Purtilo, A.: Survey of Human Diseases, p. 292. Copyright 1978 by Addison-Wesley Publishing Company. Used by permission.)

A primary cause of elevated intrapleural pressure is a condition referred to as *pneumothorax*. Pneumothorax is a disorder characterized by an abnormal increase of air pressure in the pleural space. As illustrated in Figure 10.12, pressure elevation usually occurs secondary to the development of an opening between (1) the pleural space and the respiratory tree, or (2) the pleural space and the atmosphere.

Most commonly, leaks out of the respiratory tree arise from a ruptured bronchus or alveolus. This type of defect can accompany degenerative changes associated with emphysema, pneumonia, or neoplasms.

Communication between the pleural space and the atmosphere, on the other hand, is usually induced by penetration of the thoracic cavity. Knife wounds, gunshot wounds, and compound rib fractures all disrupt the airtight seal of the chest cage and allow equalization with atmospheric pressure.

Increases in Pleural Fluid Pressure Although increasing intrapleural gas pressure is a common cause of pulmonary restriction, compression of the lungs can also be induced

by an elevation in the volume and pressure of pleural fluid.

Pleural fluid is believed to be derived from capillaries lying under the highly permeable pleural membranes. To the extent that fluid shifts excessively out of pulmonary or thoracic blood vessels into the interstitial compartment, it can subsequently pass with relative ease into the pleural space (see Figure 10.13). If the lymph system cannot adequately drain accumulating pleural fluid, a condition described as *pleural effusion* results. Most often, pleural effusion develops in one of two primary ways: (1) increased blood pressure or decreased colloid osmotic pressure in pulmonary capillaries promote the flux of fluid out of plasma into interstitial and pleural spaces; or (2) inflammation of pleural membranes causes increased permeability of associated capillaries, with excessive flux of protein-rich fluid into the interstitial and pleural spaces.

The fluid accumulating secondary to blood pressure or colloid osmotic pressure changes is called a *transudate*. It is usually associated with the pulmonary vascular con-

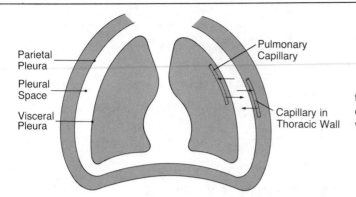

Figure 10.13 The generation of pleural fluid. Note that pleural fluid can be derived from capillaries located on the surface of the lung or within the thoracic wall.

gestion characteristic of left heart failure. Transudate can also be produced when *hypoproteinemia* (decreased plasma protein levels) causes depression in capillary colloid osmotic pressure, with subsequent accumulation of fluid in the interstitial and pleural spaces. A more detailed examination of the clinical disorders that precipitate fluid pressure imbalances can be found in Chapter 4.

When fluid build-up in the pleural space is caused by increases in capillary permeability, the excess is referred to as an *exudate*. Because of increased porosity of the capillary walls, fluid leaking under these circumstances contains a disproportionately high concentration of large protein molecules. This condition often accompanies inflammation or malignancy of the pleura.

FIBROUS DEGENERATION OF PULMONARY TISSUE Although decreased compliance of the lungs and thorax can be caused by alterations in chest cage volume or elevations in external pressures, restriction is frequently induced by degenerative changes in pulmonary tissue itself.

When respiratory disease is characterized by *fibrosis*, or the generation of excessive amounts of fibrous connective tissue, pulmonary elasticity declines. Resulting decreases in expansability and recoil causes the lung to function less effectively in both inspiration and expiration.

Common causes of pulmonary fibrosis include *obstructive disorders* (such as bronchiectasis), *infectious diseases* (such as pneumonia and tuberculosis), and *inflammatory responses* (such as pneumoconioses). Since the evolu-

tion of obstructive disorders will be discussed subsequently in this chapter, emphasis, at this point, will be placed on the pathogenesis of infectious and inflammatory conditions.

Infectious Diseases When pathogenic microorganisms invade pulmonary tissue, considerable disruption of alveolar ventilation and diffusion may result. In order to establish themselves within the lungs, however, infectious agents must effectively overpower a number of defensive barriers. Designed to filter, remove, or inactivate foreign substances within the respiratory tract, these protective mechanisms include:

1. Nasal hairs — hairs within the nasal cavity that function to filter foreign particles out of inhaled air.

2. Nasal turbinates — plates of bone within the nasal cavity that obstruct the transport of foreign particles into the lower respiratory tract.

3. Mucus — secretion produced by epithelial cells lining the respiratory tract; contains the enzyme lysozyme, which functions to break down bacterial cell walls.

4. Mucociliatory escalator — combined action of mucus and cilia within the respiratory tract; serves to sweep foreign particles toward the pharynx, where swallowing or expectoration may occur.

5. Alveolar macrophages — phagocytic cells within the alveoli that function to ingest and destroy invading microorganisms.

6. Cough reflex — forceful expiration triggered by the presence of foreign particles or irritants within the respiratory tract.

To the extent that any of these mechanisms is disrupted or obliterated, it becomes easier for pulmonary infection to set in. Some factors that increase susceptibility to respiratory infection are listed in Table 10.2.

Of the pulmonary infectious diseases, pneumonia and tuberculosis are among the most common. Although tuberculosis may lead to the development of pneumonia, these two conditions differ sufficiently in pathogenesis and clinical manifestations to warrant separate consideration.

PNEUMONIA Pneumonia, which can be defined as an inflammation of pulmonary tissue, is commonly caused by bacterial or viral infection. Some major types of pneumonia are elucidated in Table 10.3.

To better understand this illness, it is helpful to trace the pathogenesis of a classic case of pneumonia caused by the invasion of pneumococcal bacteria.

Initially, the pneumococci are carried to the alveoli in droplets of mucus or saliva. Their arrival sets off a typical inflammatory response, as described in Chapter 8. Increasing capillary dilation and permeability cause fluid and white blood cells to fill the interstitial spaces and alveoli. Fibrin strands also accumulate with the initiation of the healing or repair process. Resulting alveolar congestion, or *consolidation,* is reflected in symptoms

of pain, coughing, and depressed pO_2 (to the extent that alveolar gas diffusion is impaired). Normally, symptoms abate by the seventh to eleventh day as pathogenic microbes are destroyed and pulmonary tissue returns to normal.

It is important to remember that the extent to which inflammatory and immune mechanisms can successfully combat pulmonary disease depends largely upon factors such as virulence of the causative agent, general health, and age. In the event that microorganisms are not inactivated, death and necrosis of tissue can ensue. Mortality in these cases can rise to more than 70 per cent.

TUBERCULOSIS Tuberculosis is a disease caused by a rod-shaped bacterium, *Mycobacterium tuberculosis.* As with pneumonia, these microorganisms commonly enter the respiratory tract by inhalation. Once established on the alveolar surface, they induce characteristic reactions in pulmonary tissue.

Initially, an acute inflammatory response occurs, causing leakage of fluids, white blood cells, and macrophages into the interstitial spaces. This exudate then drains into lymph vessels and is carried to lymph nodes located toward the center of the chest.

Within the lymph nodes, an immune re-

TABLE 10.2 **Factors that Increase Susceptibility to Pulmonary Infection**

Defense Barrier	Factor Interfering with Barrier	Disruptive Mechanism
Mucus secretion	Dehydration	Fluid deficit ⟶ production of scant and viscous mucus
	Inspiration of dry air	Production of viscous mucus
	Anesthetics	Depress mucus production
Ciliary action	Cigarette smoking/atmospheric pollution	Depresses ciliary activity
	Chronic bronchitis	Overproduction of mucus ⟶ ineffective ciliary activity
	Anesthetics	Depress ciliary activity
Alveolar macrophage	Inspiration of silica or asbestos particles	Damages or destroys macrophages
Cough reflex	Pain	Reduces forcefulness of expiration
	Sedatives and narcotics	Inhibit the cough reflex

TABLE 10.3 **Some Major Types of Pneumonia**

Type of Pneumonia	Causative Agent	Characteristics
Bacterial pneumonia	May be caused by a variety of bacterial agents, including:	Generally characterized by a suppurative exudate within the alveoli. Specific pathological changes vary with the causative agent.
	Pneumococcus *(Streptococcus pneumoniae)*	Most common cause of bacterial pneumonia.
	Klebsiella	Extremely destructive. More common in males. Often associated with alcoholism or chronic bronchopulmonary disease.
	Staphylococcus	Causes extensive damage. Lung abscesses are frequent complications.
	Mycobacterium tuberculosis	Associated with characteristics of tuberculosis, such as the formation of granulomas, and subsequent necrosis.
Mycoplasmal pneumonia	Mycoplasma are similar to bacteria but are smaller and contain no cell wall. The species *Mycoplasma pneumoniae* has been identified as a cause of pneumonia.	Highly contagious form of pneumonia. Characterized by edema between the alveoli but lack of intra-alveolar exudate. Responds to antibiotics.
Viral pneumonia	Types A and B influenza virus are common causative agents. The chickenpox virus may also cause pneumonia.	Primarily associated with mild form of disease. Similar in characteristics to mycoplasmal pneumonia but may pave the way for the invasion of secondary bacterial infection. Not treatable with antibiotics.

sponse is prompted by sensitized T lymphocytes (see Chapter 8). The tubercular bacteria are walled off by lymphocyte, macrophage, and fibroblast activity, forming small localized lesions called *granulomas*. Necrosis often develops deep within these granulomas, resulting in the formation of a cheesy or liquid material. In the case of liquefaction necrosis, drainage can leave cavities or spaces at the site of the lesion. If liquefied necrotic material drains into the respiratory tree, it will be expelled as highly infectious sputum.

With time, granulomas are rendered increasingly fibrous and hard as they become the site of connective scar tissue formation and calcium deposition. The appearance of calcified spots in lung x-rays, in fact, commonly reflects tubercular disease. The evolution of tuberculosis is illustrated in Figure 10.14.

To the extent that tubercular bacilli are effectively localized within granulomas, the disease can remain essentially asymptomatic for long periods of time. Inside the lesions, however, bacteria remain active and can cause damage if they spread, via blood or lymph vessels, to other areas of the lung or to nonrespiratory tissue, such as the brain, kidneys, or joints.

Most often, cases of clinical tuberculosis represent *secondary*, or *reinfection*, tuberculosis. In these instances, individuals who have already been exposed to the tubercular pathogen will have developed granulomas. When resistance is lowered, the tubercular bacillus escapes from its walled-off site to cause further pulmonary damage. It is at this point that clinical symptoms most commonly appear. Very often nonspecific, they include fatigue,

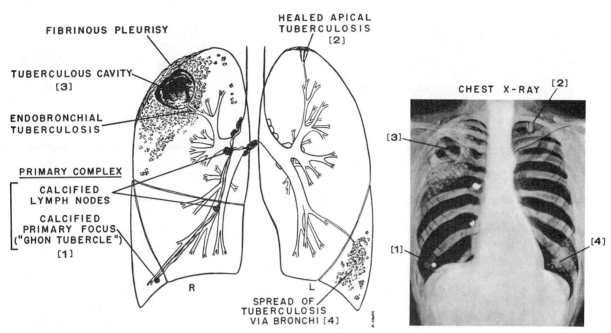

FIBRINOUS PLEURISY

TUBERCULOUS CAVITY
[3]

ENDOBRONCHIAL
TUBERCULOSIS

PRIMARY COMPLEX

CALCIFIED
LYMPH NODES

CALCIFIED
PRIMARY FOCUS
("GHON TUBERCLE")
[1]

HEALED APICAL
TUBERCULOSIS
[2]

SPREAD OF
TUBERCULOSIS
VIA BRONCHI [4]

R   L

CHEST X-RAY   [2]

[3]

[1]

[4]

Figure 10.14   The evolution of tuberculosis. (From Introduction to Lung Disease, 6th ed. New York, American Lung Association, 1975. Used by permission.)

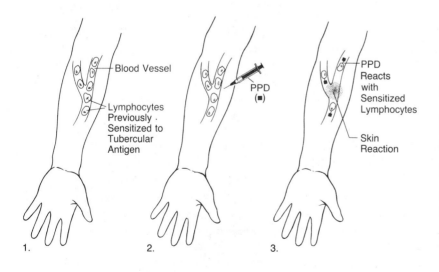

Blood Vessel

Lymphocytes
Previously .
Sensitized to
Tubercular
Antigen

PPD
(∎)

PPD
Reacts
with
Sensitized
Lymphocytes

Skin
Reaction

1.   2.   3.

Figure 10.15   The tuberculin skin test.

1. In person previously exposed to tubercular antigen, lymphocytes become sensitized.

2. PPD (a form of tubercular antigen) is injected.

3. A localized skin reaction is noted as PPD reacts with sensitized lymphocytes.

tiredness, irritability, low-grade fever, anorexia, and weight loss as well as cough, dyspnea, and possible rales.

Because invasion by the tubercular bacillus does not usually precipitate immediately obvious clinical symptoms, it is helpful to have a means of identifying individuals who are carrying dormant bacteria. Such a tool is provided by the tuberculin skin test. Following exposure to the tubercular pathogen, specifically sensitized T lymphocytes are generat-ed within three to ten weeks. After this time, introduction of the tubercular antigen, in the form of an injected purified protein derivative *(PPD)*, causes a hypersensitivity skin reaction at the site of application. This characteristic inflammatory response, which is caused primarily by previously sensitized T lymphocytes, is particularly helpful in identifying individuals who have been exposed to tuberculosis. The tuberculin skin test is presented diagrammatically in Figure 10.15.

TABLE 10.4   **Physical and Chemical Irritants: Working Classification of their Pulmonary Effects***

Category of Agents	Effect on Lung	Agent	Circumstances of Exposure, Including Occupation(s) or Industry at Risk
Inorganic dusts	1. Pneumoconiosis (noncollagenous)	Carbon, tin, iron, coal, graphite	Mining, welding
	2. Acute silicolipoproteinosis	Free silica (uncombined SiO_2)	Tunneling, sandblasting: exposure to high doses of fine particles
	3. Pneumoconiosis (collagenous)		
	a. Nodular	Free silica	Hardrock mining of any sort; quarrying, stonecutting and dressing; foundry, pottery, and enamel workers
	b. Diffuse	Asbestos (all fiber types)	Asbestos mining, milling and manufacturing; insulating
		Fume and other fine silica	Sandblasting
		Beryllium	Fluorescent light and space industry
	c. Complicated	An altered response to usually nonfibrogenic dust	Coal miners (progressive massive fibrosis)
	4. Neoplasia (lung)	Asbestos (all fiber types)	Mining and industrial exposures
		Radioactive dusts	Mining operations
		Metal mining	Hematite, chrome
		Metal refining	Nickel, chrome
	5. Neoplasia (pleura)	Asbestos (excluding anthophyllite)	Industrial exposure more at risk than mining exposures
	6. Chronic bronchitis	All dusts, given a high enough dose	Probably all types of exposure
Organic dusts	1. Asthma-like reactions	Enzymes of *B. subtilis*	Manufacture of detergents
		Western red cedar dust	Wood workers
	2. Late-onset airflow obstruction (eventually irreversible)	Cotton, hemp, flax, and jute	Processing of vegetable fiber, especially carding of cotton
	3. Hypersensitivity pneumonitis	Fungal spores, especially *M. faeni*	Haymaking, grain handling, mushroom cultivating, sugar cane picking or processing the residue
	4. Chronic bronchitis	Organic material (nonspecific)	Grain handling
	5. Chronic interstitial pneumonia	Vaporized mineral oil	Smoking blackfat tobacco (Guyana); certain industrial exposures
Chemicals, including fumes and vapors	1. Acute pulmonary edema	Oxides of nitrogen	Silo filling, fire fighting
		Phosgene	Fire fighting
		Certain insecticides, e.g., paraquat	Accidental ingestion
	2. Asthma-like reactions	Complex platinum salts	Platinum refining
		Aluminum solder flux	
		Toluene di-isocyanate (TDI)	Manufacture of polyurethane plastic
	3. Acute bronchitis	TDI (in heavier doses)	Manufacture of polyurethane plastic
		SO_2	Pulp and paper mills
		NH_3	Refrigeration industry
		Vanadium	
	4. Chronic bronchitis	All the aforementioned agents in lower dose	As above
	5. Pneumonitis	Cadmium, Hg, Mn	
Radiation	1. Pneumonitis	X-radiation	Medical treatment
	2. Neoplasia	Radioactive dusts	Uranium and other mining

*From Beeson, P. B., McDermott, W., and Wyngaarden, J. (eds.): Cecil Textbook of Medicine, 15th ed. Philadelphia, W. B. Saunders Company, 1978. Used by permission.

TABLE 10.5   **Restrictive Pulmonary Diseases**

Type of Disorder	Examples
Abnormalities in the size, shape, or expansibility of the chest cage	Scoliosis Kyphosis Abdominal distention Abdominal pain Flail chest
Changes in the pressure dynamics within the thoracic cavity	Pneumothorax Pleural effusion
Fibrous degeneration of pulmonary tissue	COPD Bronchiectasis Pneumonia Tuberculosis Pneumoconioses

Inflammatory Responses   Pulmonary inflammatory diseases are frequently characterized by the formation of fibrous connective tissue. *Pneumoconioses*, or disorders triggered by the inhalation of respiratory irritants, commonly initiate such fibrous tissue formation.

Pneumoconioses are usually grouped according to causative agent. *Silicosis*, for example, is induced by the continued inhalation of small silicon dioxide particles that are often derived from sandstone blasting or quartz and granite polishing. *Asbestosis* is caused by the inhalation of fine asbestos fibers, and *anthracosis* (black lung disease) is precipitated by the chronic inhalation of coal dust. A tabular summary of some primary pulmonary irritants and their effect upon the lung can be found in Table 10.4.

Regardless of the source of irritation, the resulting inflammatory response will lead to generation of excessive fibrous connective tissue. Subsequent reduction of pulmonary elasticity results in decreased compliance and increased "work of ventilation."

RESTRICTIVE PULMONARY DISORDERS: A SUMMARY   The work of ventilation is generally increased by any disorder that restricts the normal expansion or recoil of pulmonary tissue. This type of dysfunction originates with disorders characterized by (1) abnormalities in the size, shape, or expansibility of the chest cage; (2) changes in the pressure dynamics within the thoracic cavity; or (3) fibrous degeneration of pulmonary tissue.

In the preceding pages, specific clinical examples of each type of disorder have been presented. A summary of restrictive pulmonary diseases is presented in Table 10.5.

It is significant to note that alterations in the size, shape, or pressure dynamics of the thoracic cavity will primarily increase the work of inspiration. By reducing compliance, these disorders specifically tax the muscles of inspiration. Changes in pulmonary tissue, on the other hand, will stress both the inspiratory and the expiratory processes. As inherent pulmonary elasticity declines, muscles must work harder to facilitate normal intake and output of gases.

As we continue to explore the pathogenesis of respiratory dysfunction, note that many "restrictive" diseases can also cause obstruction or diffusion disorders. Since many varied aspects of respiratory dysfunction are often manifested simultaneously, overlap is frequently the rule rather than the exception.

OBSTRUCTIVE PULMONARY DISORDERS

Obstructive disorders, as defined earlier, are caused by any factors posing resistance to the normal transport of air through the respiratory tree. Characteristically, they arise from blockage or constriction of the passageways carrying gases between the atmosphere and the alveoli. In either case, such disorders will trigger an increase in the "work of ventilation."

The most common clinical manifestations of obstruction are found in individuals with chronic bronchitis, emphysema, or asthma. These three disorders, considered together, constitute a pathological syndrome referred to as *chronic obstructive pulmonary disease (COPD)*. In the following pages, a discussion of the pathogenesis of COPD will be followed by a brief description of other obstructive diseases.

CHRONIC OBSTRUCTIVE PULMONARY DISEASE

Chronic obstructive pulmonary disease is typically caused by long-term resistance to air flow. Characteristically, resistance is greater during expiration than during inspiration. This is true because respiratory passageways normally enlarge during inspiration as pulmonary tissue expands to facilitate the intake of air. During expiration, compression occurs, often restricting the diameter of the airway. In the healthy lung, this compression poses no significant problem. When obstructive disease is present, however, expiration can be considerably impeded.

Further complicating the clinical picture in obstructive disorders is the potential for alveolar collapse, or atelectasis. To the extent that occlusion in an airway prevents the adequate filling of pulmonary air sacs, the gas already present in the alveoli will be slowly absorbed into the bloodstream. Under these conditions, the alveoli will subsequently collapse, thereby accelerating the development of pulmonary dysfunction.

Chronic Bronchitis Chronic bronchitis is a disorder most commonly induced by cigarette smoking or severe air pollution. Tissue irritation leads to hypertrophy of the mucus-producing cells in the bronchi, with a consequent rise in mucus production. Increased secretions, in turn, stimulate the cough reflex, causing progressive damage to the smaller bronchioles and increased susceptibility to respiratory infection.

It is the accumulation of mucous secretions and the swelling of tissue lining the bronchi that most specifically obstruct air passage during the evolution of chronic bronchitis (see Figure 10.16). A large number of alveoli are inadequately ventilated, causing disruption of diffusion, with subsequent depression of pO_2 and elevation of pCO_2.

In many cases of respiratory dysfunction, reflex hyperventilation could help to compensate for abnormal blood gas values. In the individual with chronic bronchitis, however, the medulla becomes relatively insensitive to sustained hypercapnia. Simultaneously, the peripheral chemoreceptors in the aortic arch and carotid body respond only marginally to developing hypoxia. As a result, compensatory hyperventilation does not characteristically occur. Because insufficient oxygenation of hemoglobin often causes cyanosis, patients with chronic bronchitis are frequently referred to as *blue bloaters.*

Further complicating the clinical picture is the evolution of pulmonary vasoconstriction secondary to depressions in pO_2. Subsequent increases in pulmonary blood pressure cause resistance to the output of blood from the right ventricle. As a result, *cor pulmonale* (or right-sided heart failure) is characteristically associated with chronic bronchitis.

Emphysema Although emphysema is technically identified as a discrete obstructive

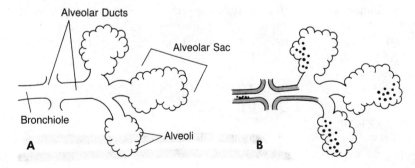

Figure 10.16 Bronchitis. *A,* Normal bronchiole and alveoli. *B,* Bronchiole and alveoli during bronchitis. Note thickening of walls in respiratory passageways and increase in secretions (indicated by black dots).

Alveolar Ducts

Alveolar Sac

Bronchiole

Alveoli

A

B

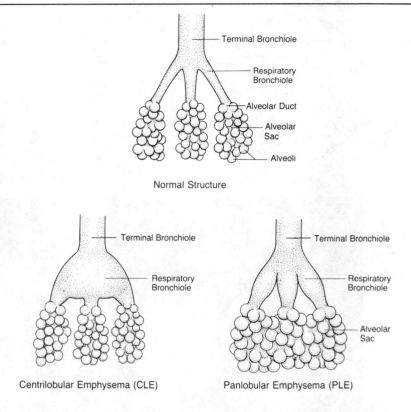

Figure 10.17 The effect of centrilobular emphysema and panlobular emphysema upon the respiratory tract. Note that in CLE the respiratory bronchioles merge, while the more distal alveolar ducts and sacs remain unaffected. In PLE, on the other hand, all segments of the respiratory tree distal to the respiratory bronchiole are distended.

disease, 60 per cent of emphysemic patients present with associated symptoms of bronchitis. Although chronic bronchitis may frequently trigger the onset of emphysema, the disorder can also develop without a history of previous obstructive disease. Predisposing factors include long-term inhalation of cigarette smoke or other pulmonary irritants as well as genetically determined deficiency of alpha-1-antitrypsin (A1AT) enzyme.

In spite of the fact that A1AT deficiency is noted in only a limited number of COPD patients, study of this defect has been helpful in elucidating some potential mechanisms of emphysema. It was determined, for example, that emphysema developed in individuals with A1AT deficiency because of excessive digestion of pulmonary tissue by protein-destructive leukocytic enzymes. Since A1AT normally suppresses the proteolytic activity of white blood cell enzymes, individuals with A1AT deficit are high-risk candidates for the development of primary pulmonary disease.

Regardless of the specific cause of dysfunction, emphysema is generally characterized by inflammatory swelling and narrowing of bronchioles. Most commonly, the respiratory bronchioles in the upper segments of the lung are selectively involved, causing the formation of large coalescing air spaces as the walls of individual bronchioles disintegrate. Referred to as *centrilobular emphysema (CLE)*, this form of disease does not usually affect the more distal alveolar ducts or alveolar sacs. In cases of *panlobular emphysema (PLE)*, on the other hand, all segments of the respiratory tree distal to the terminal bronchiole are usually involved. Degeneration and distention of the respiratory bronchioles, alveolar ducts, and alveolar sacs result. Some of the distinctions between CLE and PLE are illustrated in Figure 10.17.

In all forms of emphysema, obstruction commonly causes trapping of air in the alveoli during expiration. Large air spaces, or cysts, are formed as alveolar walls break down and many individual alveoli coalesce into a single unit. These changes are illustrated in Figure 10.18.

The patient with emphysema is particularly stressed during expiration. The extra effort expended in attempting to exhale adequate quantities of air meets with very little success. In time, the lungs become chronic-

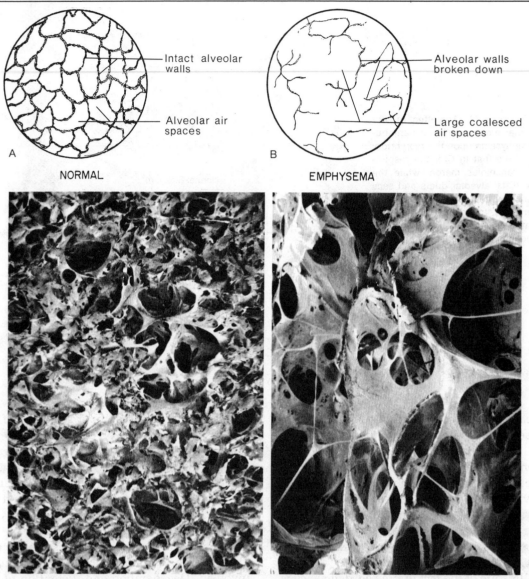

Figure 10.18 Contrast between the normal lung *(A)* and the emphysematous lung *(B)*. (From Guyton, A. C.: Textbook of Medical Physiology, 6th ed. Philadelphia, W. B. Saunders Company, 1981. Used by permission.)

ally overinflated, and the entire configuration of the chest cavity is altered to take on a barrel shape, as illustrated in Figure 10.19.

In cases in which emphysema is not preceded by chronic bronchitis, changes in the plasma concentration of oxygen and carbon dioxide are not typically noted. Although alveolar destruction could theoretically interfere with pulmonary diffusion, simultaneous breakdown of the capillaries that serve the degenerating alveoli helps to minimize the development of any ventilation-perfusion imbalance. To the extent that marginal hypox-

emia or hypercapnia does develop, compensatory hyperventilation usually serves to bring arterial blood gases back within normal limits. Because patients with primary emphysema do not typically become hypoxic or cyanotic, they are referred to as *pink puffers.*

Frequently, however, as disease progresses an individual with emphysema may develop secondary chronic bronchitis. In these cases, oxygen levels decrease, carbon dioxide accumulates, and respiratory acidosis occurs.

Asthma Asthma, unlike bronchitis or

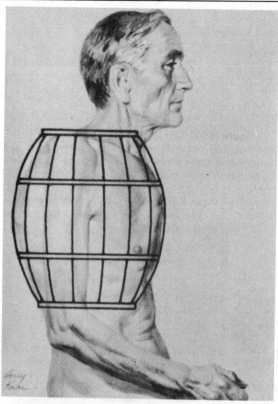

Figure 10.19 The barrel chest of emphysema. (From Knoll Pharmaceutical Company. Used by permission.)

emphysema, is an obstructive disorder characterized primarily by spastic constriction of the respiratory airways. Often accompanied by tissue swelling and elevated mucus secretion (as illustrated in Figure 10.20), this dysfunction is frequently triggered by hypersensitivity allergic responses to pollens or food. Asthmatic attacks, however, can also be induced by a large number of nonspecific factors, such as emotional upset or exercise.

As is the case in emphysema, the primary effects of obstruction are seen during expiration. The output of air is seriously restricted, and characteristic wheezing sounds are generated as the patient attempts to expire air through constricted passageways.

Although the effects of bronchospasm are largely reversible, chronic and sustained asthmatic attacks can cause smooth muscle hypertrophy and permanent narrowing of the respiratory tract. In these cases, clinical manifestations may become very similar to those of emphysema.

Chronic Obstructive Pulmonary Disease:

A Summary   As can be seen, the COPD Syndrome is of considerable significance in the evolution of respiratory disease. Characterized by obstruction, disorders increase the "work of ventilation" and commonly trigger diffusion problems. The significance of resulting alterations in pO_2 and pCO_2 levels will be discussed later in this chapter.

In evaluating chronic obstructive pulmonary disease, it is important to realize that, in reality, one rarely encounters a "pure" case of emphysema, bronchitis, or asthma. Often, patients present with some combination of these disorders, thus complicating the clinical picture. The potential effects of COPD overlap are summarized in Figure 10.21.

OTHER OBSTRUCTIVE PULMONARY DISORDERS   Although COPD is the classic obstructive syndrome, other diseases can also result in the restriction of air flow through the respiratory tree. Among these are a genetic disorder called *cystic fibrosis* and a pulmonary

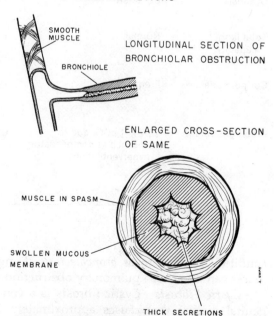

BRONCHIOLE OBSTRUCTED
ON EXPIRATION BY:

1. MUSCLE SPASM
2. SWELLING OF MUCOSA
3. THICK SECRETIONS

SMOOTH MUSCLE

BRONCHIOLE

LONGITUDINAL SECTION OF BRONCHIOLAR OBSTRUCTION

ENLARGED CROSS-SECTION OF SAME

MUSCLE IN SPASM

SWOLLEN MUCOUS MEMBRANE

THICK SECRETIONS

Figure 10.20 Pathophysiological changes in bronchial asthma. (From Introduction to Lung Disease, 6th ed. New York, American Lung Association, 1975. Used by permission.)

A

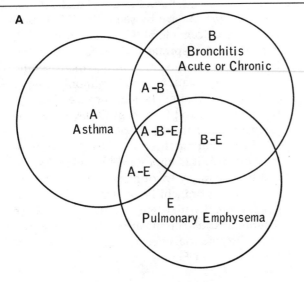

Figure 10.21 COPD. *A*, The rings illustrate the overlap that may occur between asthma, bronchitis, and emphysema. Each disease entity may occur alone or in combination with other COPD disorders. (From Tomashefski, J. F., and Pratt, P. C: Pulmonary emphysema. Med. Clin. North Am., *51*:269, 1967. Used by permission.) *B*, Chronic obstructive pulmonary diseases: a comparative summary.

B

	Chronic Bronchitis ("Blue Bloater")	Emphysema ("Pink Puffer")	Asthma
Causative factors	Cigarette smoking Severe air pollution	Cigarette smoking Severe air pollution Genetic deficiency of A1AT enzyme	Allergy Emotional factors and excessive exertion in those predisposed to attacks
Underlying pathology	Hypertrophy of mucus-producing cells in bronchi; swelling and narrowing of respiratory passages	Inflammatory swelling and narrowing of bronchioles	Spastic constriction of respiratory airways; tissue swelling; elevated mucus secretion
Mucus production	Yes	Limited or absent	Yes
Cyanosis	Common	Rare	Varies with extent and duration of attack
Total lung capacity	Normal	Elevated owing to hyperinflation "Barrel chest"	May be elevated, even without symptoms of acute attack
Cor pulmonale	Frequent	Rare	May occur if asthmatic attack is sustained for more than 24 hours
Blood gas values	↓ pO_2; ↑ pCO_2 due to absence of compensatory hyperventilation	Usually within normal limits as a result of compensatory hyperventilation	Varies with extent and duration of attack; may remain within normal limits in mild to moderate attacks owing to compensatory hyperventilation

condition referred to as *bronchiectasis*. Lung *cancer* can also cause pulmonary obstruction.

Cystic Fibrosis Cystic fibrosis is a congenital disease that causes approximately 1 out of every 20 deaths in infancy and childhood. Characterized by production of abnormally thick mucus secretions, it results in obstruction of ducts in the pancreas, liver, and

lungs. Most often the restriction to ventilation posed by mucus accumulation results in debilitating respiratory complications.

Bronchiectasis Bronchiectasis is a disorder characterized by chronically enlarged, or dilated, bronchi. It most often develops secondary to an inflammatory weakening of the bronchial walls and is complicated by in-

TABLE 10.6 Obstructive Pulmonary Disorders

Obstructive Disorder	Causative Factors	Associated Pathophysiology	Characteristic Features
Chronic bronchitis ("blue bloaters")	Smoking Severe pollution	Hypertrophy of mucus glands and goblet cells Depressed ciliary activity Accumulation of mucus in the respiratory tract Swelling of the mucosa lining the respiratory tract Growth of bacteria within the normally sterile bronchi Ventilation-perfusion imbalance Hypoventilation	Chronic, productive cough Increased susceptibility to chest infection Frequent evidence of cor pulmonale Depressed pO_2 Elevated pCO_2
Emphysema ("pink puffers")	Smoking Bronchial irritants	Inflammatory swelling and narrowing of the bronchioles Enlargement of the alveoli and alveolar ducts Breakdown of the alveolar walls, with formation of air spaces, called bullae, within pulmonary tissue, and blebs on the surface of the lungs Trapping of air within the alveoli during expiration Minimal ventilation-perfusion imbalance Hyperventilation	Minimal sputum production Infrequent evidence of cor pulmonale Increased total lung capacity and residual volume Normal pO_2 until terminal stages Normal pCO_2 until terminal stages
Asthma	Allergens Bronchial infection Bronchial irritants Vigorous exercise Psychological stress	Spastic constriction of the bronchial airways Swelling of the mucosa lining the respiratory tract Increased production of mucus within the respiratory tract Work of ventilation increases, primarily during expiration Disorder reversible in nature	Dyspnea and wheezing Acute or prolonged attack can cause a decrease in pO_2 and an increase in pCO_2

Bronchiectasis	May arise secondary to:
	  lower respiratory
	    tract infection
	  neoplasm
	  tuberculosis
	  cystic fibrosis
		Chronic dilation of the bronchi
		Inflammation of the bronchial lining
		Production of copious quantities of purulent mucus scretions
			Expectoration of foul-smelling sputum
			Chronic cough
			Increased susceptibility to respiratory infection
			Pneumonia, cor pulmonale, and right heart failure are common complications during advanced stages of disease

creased susceptibility to respiratory infections. Specific causative factors vary, and include cystic fibrosis, whooping cough, influenza, tuberculosis, and cancer.

The most characteristic clinical manifestation of bronchiectasis is the production and expectoration of large amounts of foul-smelling mucus-pus secretions. Released by severely inflamed bronchial linings, these secretions ultimately obstruct the ventilation process. The degree to which alveolar gas diffusion is affected depends largely upon the extent of pulmonary tissue involvement.

Lung Cancer. Malignant growths in the lung most commonly develop on the surface of epithelial tissue lining the bronchi. Called *squamous cell carcinomas*, these neoplasms are frequently accompanied by coughing, secondary infection, and obstruction. Progressive invasion of healthy tissue causes escalation of both ventilation and diffusion impairment.

OBSTRUCTIVE PULMONARY DISORDERS: A SUMMARY Obstructive pulmonary disorders generally pose resistance to the passage of air through the respiratory tree. Characteristically, they increase the "work of ventilation" by forcing expiratory muscles to work harder. A comparative summary of some major obstructive disorders is presented in Table 10.6.

Because of the alveolar degeneration that typically accompanies obstructive disease, diffusion disorders invariably occur. The evolution and manifestations of diffusion disorders are elucidated subsequently in this chapter.

Ventilation Pathology: A Summary

A ventilation disorder is said to exist when the normal transport of gases between the alveoli and the atmosphere is disrupted. Most commonly, dysfunction accompanies disorders that (1) alter respiratory rate or rhythm, or (2) increase the "work of ventilation."

TABLE 10.7 **Ventilation Pathology**

Origin of Disease	Causative Disorders
Alterations in the normal rate or rhythm of ventilation	Cerebral edema Tumors of the CNS Poliomyelitis Myasthenia gravis Guillain-Barré syndrome Overdose of anesthesia or narcotics Hypersecretion of thyroxine, growth hormone, or epinephrine
Increase in the work of ventilation Restrictive pulmonary disorders	Kyphosis Scoliosis Abdominal distention Abdominal pain Flail chest Pneumothorax Pleural effusion COPD Bronchiectasis Pneumonia Tuberculosis Pneumoconioses
Obstructive pulmonary disorders	Chronic bronchitis Emphysema Asthma Bronchiectasis Cystic fibrosis Lung cancer

In most cases, disease falls into the latter category and is specifically induced by dysfunctions that are "restrictive" or "obstructive" in nature. A review of some major causes of ventilation disorders is presented in Table 10.7.

DIFFUSION PATHOLOGY

The respiratory system is designed to service cellular needs through cooperation between the ventilation and diffusion processes. Inspiration and expiration must be accompanied by adequate gas exchange between the alveoli and pulmonary capillaries, if homeostasis is to be maintained.

Disruption of diffusion can occur in a number of ways. Most typically, diffusion disorders are secondary to (1) disorders of alveolar ventilation, (2) disorders of alveolar perfusion, (3) ventilation-perfusion imbalances, or (4) diseases affecting the "respiratory membrane."

Disorders of Alveolar Ventilation

In order for air to enter or leave the alveoli, optimal ventilation must be sustained. Alveolar diffusion is thus facilitated by the existence of healthy pulmonary tissue that alternately expands and recoils in a normal rhythmic pattern. If respiratory disease of neural, restrictive, or obstructive origin occurs, the exchange of gases in the alveoli will ultimately be affected.

DISORDERS OF NEURAL ORIGIN

As described earlier, several disorders can affect the rate of respiration by modifying the neural mechanisms governing ventilation. These disorders are briefly described in the section on ventilation pathology and should be reviewed at this point. The rate of alveolar ventilation will be modified to the extent that respiratory rate is either depressed or elevated.

RESTRICTIVE DISORDERS

Disorders of a restrictive nature affect alveolar ventilation by decreasing the volume of air that can be inhaled or exhaled with each breath. Any of these disorders can thus affect the turnover of gases deep within the lungs. The wide range of dysfunctions that can cause pulmonary restriction are listed in Table 10.5.

OBSTRUCTIVE DISORDERS

Before air can enter the alveoli, it must first pass from the atmosphere down into the bronchioles of the respiratory tree. Exit is, likewise, predicated upon the existence of an open and functional airway.

As obstructive disorders evolve, they initially affect expiration more than inspiration. Inability to adequately expel air from the alveoli results in the trapping and accumulation of "old" gases deep within the lungs. The quantity of fresh new air that can enter the alveoli is thereby reduced. A summary of some primary disorders causing obstruction can be found in Table 10.6.

Disorders of Alveolar Perfusion

To facilitate optimal gas exchange, the alveoli of the lung must receive an adequate supply of blood. In analyzing the circulation of blood through pulmonary tissue, it is important to realize that there are two different vascular systems that service the lung: the *pulmonary* and the *bronchial* circulatory pathways.

Generally speaking, the pulmonary system is the one most directly involved with alveolar diffusion. It transports blood from the right ventricle through the pulmonary arteries and ultimately to the air sacs of the lungs, where gas exchange occurs. Blood rich in oxygen and low in carbon dioxide then returns to the left heart via the pulmonary veins, to be subsequently circulated throughout the body.

The bronchial system, on the other hand, is designed to carry nutrients and oxygen to the tissues of the respiratory tree. Since the vessels do not directly service the alveoli, they are essentially nonfunctional in respiratory gas exchanges. Bronchial arteries commonly arise from the intercostal artery, subclavian artery, and internal mammary arteries (on the right side) and from the upper thoracic aorta (on the left side). After servicing respiratory structures, blood can exit from the lungs via the bronchial veins (in the area of the hilum) or through the pulmonary veins (which empty into the left atrium) (see Figure 10.22). In the latter case, bronchial blood, which is high in carbon dioxide and low in oxygen content, contributes to a component of the circulation described as the *venous admixture*. By mixing with freshly diffused blood in the pulmonary veins, it slightly alters the composition of the blood that is returning to the left side of the heart.

Normally, only 2 per cent of total cardiac output travels through the bronchial circulatory system. When chronic pulmonary inflammation or neoplasms exist, however, a considerable increase in the number and size of bronchial arteries may be noted. Under these circumstances, the effects of venous admixture will be exacerbated and significant alterations in pO_2 and pCO_2 may occur.

The normal alveolar perfusion pattern can alternatively be modified by pulmonary vascular obstruction. To the extent that emboli or thrombi decrease circulation to certain alveoli, blood is shunted to other areas of pulmonary

tissue. In these cases, the extent of pO_2 and pCO_2 imbalance will be determined by the ability of functional alveoli to compensate for those that are underperfused.

Ventilation-Perfusion Imbalances

If homeostasis is to be maintained, alveolar ventilation ($\dot{V}$) must be matched by alveolar perfusion ($\dot{Q}$) (see Figure 10.23). Normally, reflex mechanisms function to decrease ventilation when perfusion is reduced, and vice versa. In certain cases, however, the balance between ventilation and perfusion ($\dot{V}/\dot{Q}$) can be disrupted. Characterized by either wasted perfusion or wasted ventilation, associated disorders may result in the onset of hypercapnia or hypoxia or both.

WASTED PERFUSION

In cases of wasted perfusion, pulmonary circulation is not optimally functional in respiratory gas exchange. Blood thus passes from pulmonary arteries into pulmonary veins without receiving adequate quantities of oxy-

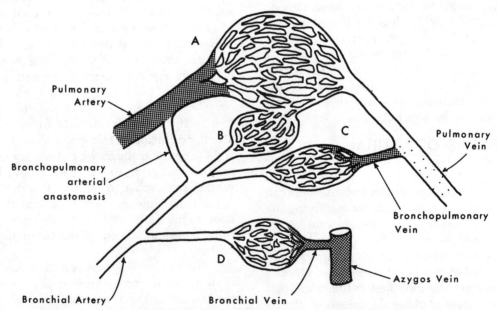

Figure 10.22 Relationship between the bronchial and pulmonary circulations. Note that the pulmonary artery supplies the pulmonary capillary network A. The bronchial artery supplies capillary networks B, C, and D. While networks B and C drain into pulmonary veins (contributing to venous admixture) network D feeds into true bronchial veins (azygos, hemiazygos, or intercostal veins). Shaded areas represent blood of low oxygen content. (From Murray, J. F.: The Normal Lung. Philadelphia, W. B. Saunders Company, 1976. Used by permission.)

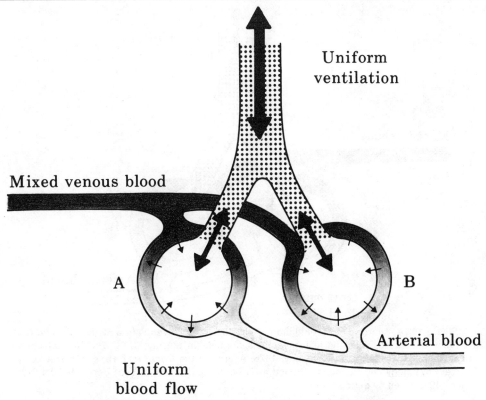

Uniform
ventilation

Mixed venous blood

A

B

Arterial blood

Uniform
blood flow

Figure 10.23 Ventilation-perfusion balance. Note that alveoli A and B are uniformly ventilated and perfused. (In Murray, J. F.: The Normal Lung. Philadelphia, W. B. Saunders Company, 1976. Adapted from Comroe, J. H., et al.: The Lung: Clinical Physiology and Pulmonary Function Tests, 2nd ed. Chicago, Year Book Medical Publishers, 1962. Used by permission.)

gen or losing sufficient amounts of carbon dioxide. Wasted perfusion can result from one of three major pathological patterns, as follows:

1. When total alveolar ventilation is depressed, but perfusion remains normal and uniformly distributed.

2. When ventilation is selectively depressed in only some alveoli, while perfusion remains normal and uniformly distributed.

3. When excessive quantities of blood are shunted past functional alveoli, thereby increasing the venous admixture.

A uniform depression in alveolar ventilation is most commonly associated with hypoventilation (see Figure 10.24). Caused by disorders such as myasthenia gravis, bulbar polio, central neural depression, and overdoses of anesthetics or sedatives, depressions in respiratory rate decrease air flow into the respiratory tract. Because insufficient intake does not provide enough volume for optimal

exhange, pO_2 will decrease while pCO_2 increases.

When there is a nonuniform decrease in ventilation, on the other hand, some alveoli receive adequate quantities of air while others are selectively deprived (see Figure 10.25). In these conditions, which are most frequently caused by diffuse obstructive disease and atelectasis, associated increases in pCO_2 and decreases in pO_2 may be partially compensated for by a reflex increase in respiratory rate.

While compensatory hyperventilation frequently alleviates hypercapnia, it is rarely functional in significantly elevating depressed pO_2 levels. Underlying reasons for this discrepancy include the following:

1. Carbon dioxide normally diffuses across the respiratory membrane in direct response to the concentration gradient existing between pulmonary blood and the alveolus. As compensatory hyperventilation occurs, alveolar pCO_2 decreases, and relatively greater

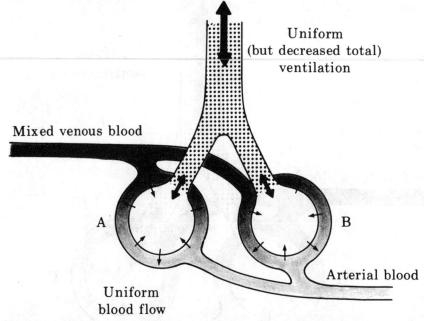

Figure 10.24   Uniform hypoventilation of alveoli. Note that ventilation of alveoli A and B is uniformly decreased, while perfusion remains normal. (In Murray, J. F.: The Normal Lung. Philadelphia, W. B. Saunders Company, 1976. Adapted from Comroe, J. H., et al.: The Lung: Clinical Physiology and Pulmonary Function Task, 2nd ed. Chicago, Year Book Medical Publishers, 1962. Used by permission.)

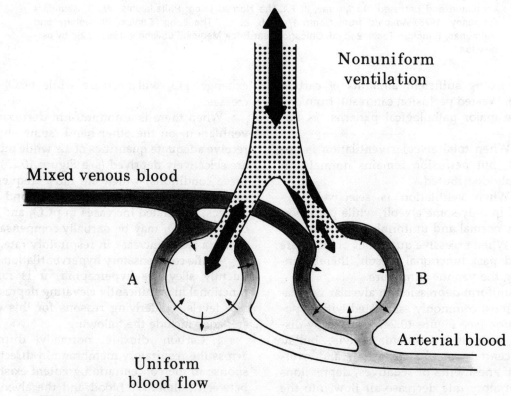

Figure 10.25   Nonuniform alveolar ventilation. Note that ventilation is selectively decreased in alveolus B. (In Murray, J. F.: The Normal Lung. Philadelphia, W. B. Saunders Company, 1976. Adapted from Comroe, J. H., et al.: The Lung: Clinical Physiology and Pulmonary Function Tests, 2nd ed. Chicago, Year Book Medical Publishers, 1962. Used by permission.)

amounts of carbon dioxide can pass from the pulmonary capillary into the alveolus to be expired.

2. Normally, oxygen is carried through the blood in chemical combination with hemoglobin. To the extent that hemoglobin is already saturated with oxygen, elevations in alveolar pO_2 will *not* significantly increase the oxygen concentration of pulmonary blood. Since hemoglobin is typically oxygen-saturated at normal alveolar pO_2 levels, compensatory hyperventilation cannot push sufficient quantities of extra oxygen into the pulmonary capillary.

In cases of nonuniform alveolar ventilation, one could thus expect to see a characteristic decrease in pO_2, with normal plasma CO_2 levels.

A form of wasted perfusion is also noted when venous admixture is increased second-ary to pulmonary disease (see Figure 10.26). In these cases, ventilation is adequate and uniform, but an excessive proportion of cardiac output totally bypasses the functional alveoli. A characteristic increase in pCO_2 and decrease in pO_2 will result.

WASTED VENTILATION

In some cases of respiratory disease, vascular obstruction caused by emboli or thrombi reduces pulmonary blood flow to certain alveoli (see Figure 10.27). Since ventilation is not typically depressed in these types of disorders, it can be said that a proportion of inspiratory and expiratory volume is effectively "wasted" and cannot serve to support the diffusion process. When underperfusion thus causes a decrease in alveolar functional capacity, the volume of gas that cannot participate in

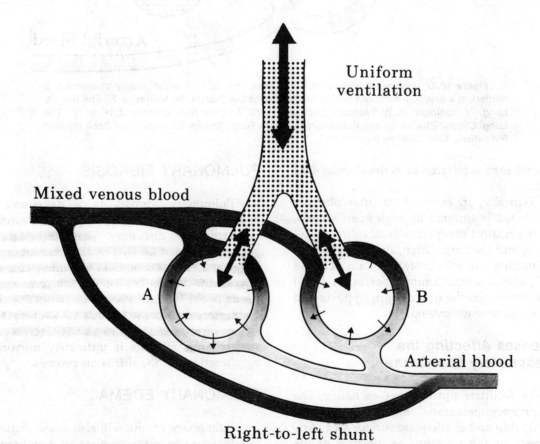

Figure 10.26   Right-to-left shunt. Note that a proportion of mixed venous blood bypasses alveoli A and B without contributing to respiratory gas exchange. (In Murray, J. F.: The Normal Lung. Philadelphia, W. B. Saunders Company, 1976. Adapted from Comroe, J. H., et al.: The Lung: Clinical Physiology and Pulmonary Function Tests, 2nd ed. Chicago, Year Book Medical Publishers, 1962. Used by permission.)

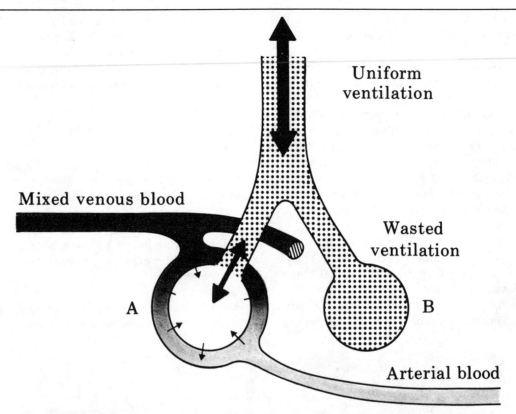

Figure 10.27 Wasted alveolar ventilation. Note that lack of blood supply to alveolus B renders this structure nonfunctional in respiratory gas exchange. (In Murray, J. F.: The Normal Lung. Philadelphia, W. B. Saunders Company, 1976. Adapted from Comroe, J. H., et al.: The Lung: Clinical Physiology and Pulmonary Function Tests, 2nd ed. Chicago, Year Book Medical Publishers, 1962. Used by permission.)

gas exchange is referred to as the *alveolar dead space.*

Typically, in cases of vascular obstruction, blood is shunted through open vessels, causing relative overperfusion of other alveoli throughout the lung. Often, this compensatory shunting will effectively maintain pO_2 and pCO_2 within normal limits. If perfusion deficit is extensive, on the other hand, hypoxia and hypercapnia may develop.

Diseases Affecting the "Respiratory Membrane"

To facilitate optimal gas exchange, the "respiratory membrane" must be both sufficiently thin and of adequate surface area. Any changes in the structure or function of the membrane can considerably alter the diffusion process. In the clinical setting, disruption is most often induced by either pulmonary fibrosis or pulmonary edema.

PULMONARY FIBROSIS

Pulmonary fibrosis is a degenerative process that frequently accompanies a variety of respiratory disorders. Diseases such as bronchiectasis, COPD, pneumonia, tuberculosis, and pneumoconioses are often characterized by the deposit of fibrous connective tissue in the lung. Subsequent changes in the respiratory membrane include a loss of elasticity, an increase in thickness, and a decrease in surface area. Fibrosis is ultimately mirrored by alterations in the diffusion process.

PULMONARY EDEMA

Pulmonary edema will also cause characteristic changes in the respiratory membrane. Increases in thickness and decreases in surface area occur as plasma shifts out of pulmonary capillaries. It is now generally believed that a considerable amount of fluid must leak into interstitial spaces before any liquid appears within the alveoli. Thus, rales and frothy sputum are often a relatively late manifestation of disease.

Pulmonary edema most frequently is the result of elevated capillary blood pressure or increased vascular permeability. Elevated pressure is commonly induced by left heart failure, as described in Chapter 9. Increases in permeability, on the other hand, can be induced by the inhalation of respiratory irritants (such as chlorine or sulfur dioxide) or by pleural inflammation (as evidenced in cases of pneumonia or pulmonary malignancy).

With the onset of edema, alveolar diffusion is considerably impeded. As fluid accumulates in the alveoli, respiratory membranes are structurally modified, and the patterns of gas exchange are affected. Disease is often reflected by a decrease in pO_2. Plasma CO_2 levels, on the other hand, are *not* significantly altered. This is primarily due to the fact that carbon dioxide normally diffuses across the alveolar membrane approximately 20 times more rapidly than oxygen. Hypoxemia is thus initiated much more readily than hypercapnia.

Diffusion Pathology: A Summary

Diffusion disorders are generally characterized by a disruption in the exchange of oxygen or carbon dioxide or both across the respiratory membrane. Since the diffusion of respiratory gases is dependent upon adequate alveolar ventilation and perfusion, dysfunction can arise secondary to a variety of disorders, as summarized in Table 10.8. Ultimately, homeostasis will be disrupted to the extent that disease causes the occurrence of hypoxia or hypercapnia or both.

RESPIRATORY INSUFFICIENCY OR FAILURE

Ventilation or diffusion disorders can cause varying degrees of physiological stress. If disease is characterized by a depression of pO_2 or elevation of pCO_2 during exercise, a state of *respiratory insufficiency* is said to exist. To the extent that dysfunction becomes severe and interferes with cellular oxygen supply or carbon dioxide elimination at rest, *respiratory failure* results. In truth, respiratory pathology is a continuum, with manifestations ranging from mild distress to critical dysfunction. Progressive changes can be monitored by tests and measures designed to assess respiratory status.

The Evolution of Respiratory Failure

In the initial stages of respiratory illness, alterations in blood gas levels are noted primarily during physical exertion. At times of

TABLE 10.8 **Diffusion Pathology**

Origin of Disease	Causative Disorders
Disruption of alveolar ventilation (see Table 10.7)	Disorders causing an alteration in the normal rate or rhythm of ventilation Restrictive pulmonary disorders Obstructive pulmonary disorders
Disruption of alveolar perfusion	Increased venous admixture Pulmonary embolus Pulmonary thrombus
Ventilation-perfusion imbalances	Hypoventilation Diffuse obstructive disease Pulmonary vascular obstruction
Diseases affecting the "respiratory membrane"	Pulmonary fibrosis Pulmonary edema

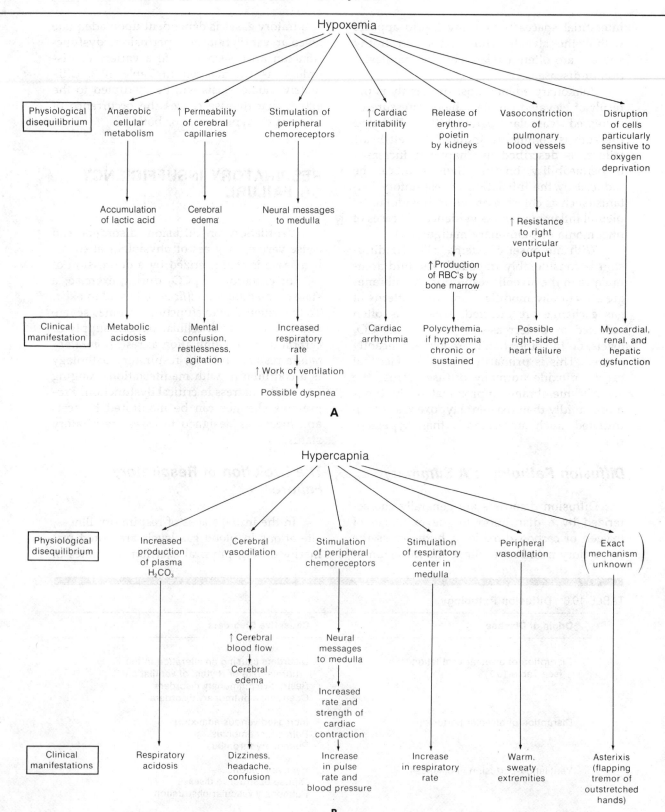

Figure 10.28   Evolution of physiological imbalance secondary to *(A)* hypoxemia and *(B)* hypercapnia.

normal activity, homeostasis can be maintained by cardiovascular or respiratory compensation mechanisms. Respiratory insufficiency is said to exist when adaptive increases in alveolar ventilation and perfusion serve to effectively counteract the effects of disease. Insufficiency is frequently associated with degenerative disorders such as emphysema, asthma, bronchitis, and pneumoconioses.

If dysfunction becomes more acute or further complications develop, compensation mechanisms will often fail to maintain homeostasis. As pO_2 falls to 50 mm. Hg or less, or pCO_2 increases to 50 mm. Hg or greater, respiratory failure is technically established. Failure can be induced by any aspect of ventilation or diffusion pathology discussed previously in this chapter.

Although depressed oxygen and elevated carbon dioxide levels are characteristic of respiratory failure, these changes do not necessarily occur simultaneously. Deviations from the norm depend largely upon the nature of underlying disorder. It is possible, for example, to have hypoxemia without hypercapnia. In these instances, decreases in pO_2 are due primarily to diseases affecting the respiratory membrane or to nonuniform alveolar ventilation (as described earlier). Specific disorders include pulmonary fibrosis, pulmonary edema, pneumonia, tuberculosis, and pneumoconioses.

Hypoxemia with hypercapnia, on the other hand, is frequently noted in cases of uniform hypoventilation, associated with disorders of neural origin, abnormalities of the chest cage, and COPD. In all situations, the severity of disease depends largely upon the extent to which respiratory gases deviate from the norm. A brief summary of some clinical manifestations of hypoxemia and hypercapnia can be found in Figure 10.28.

When respiratory disease terminates in elevated pulmonary blood pressure, resistance to the ejection of blood from the right ventricle can trigger right-sided failure. The resulting pathological condition, referred to as *cor pulmonale*, is characterized by evidence of venous congestion ranging from distended neck veins to peripheral edema. (see Chapter 9).

Cor pulmonale is induced most frequently by structural or functional changes in the small arteries and arterioles serving the lungs. Both obstructive and restrictive disease can cause degenerative pulmonary vascular changes that ultimately lead to elevated pulmonary blood pressure.

Further complicating the clinical picture is the tendency for pulmonary arterioles to constrict in response to hypoxemia or hypercapnia or both. As respiratory failure is established, reflex vasoconstriction in the lungs will typically cause an elevation of pulmonary blood pressure. The subsequent development of cor pulmonale will predictably aggravate the dysfunction associated with respiratory failure.

Measures of Respiratory Function

Two different types of tests are frequently utilized to evaluate and assess the respiratory status of a patient. Measures of *pulmonary volumes and capacities* and determinations of *arterial blood gas (ABG)* values both facilitate diagnosis in cases of respiratory disorders.

PULMONARY VOLUMES AND CAPACITIES

In evaluating pulmonary function, it is helpful to know how much air can be drawn into or eliminated from the lungs under specified conditions. The pulmonary volumes most frequently measured include:

1. *Tidal volume (TV)*, which is the volume of air inspired or expired with each normal breath. It is usually equivalent to 500 ml. in the average young male.

2. *Inspiratory reserve volume (IRV)*, which is the volume of air that can be forcibly inspired beyond the normal inspiration. It normally measures approximately 3000 ml. in the average young male.

3. *Expiratory reserve volume (ERV)*, which is the volume of air that can be forcibly expired beyond the normal expiration. It usually amounts to 1100 ml. in the young adult male.

4. *Residual volume (RV)*, which is the amount of air that remains in the lungs at all times and cannot be forcibly expired. It averages about 1200 ml. in the young adult male.

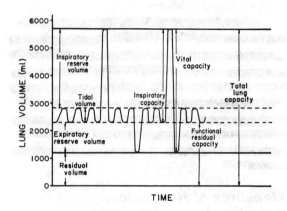

Figure 10.29 Pulmonary volumes and capacities. (From Guyton, A. C.: Textbook of Medical Physiology, 6th ed. Philadelphia, W. B. Saunders Company, 1981. Used by permission.)

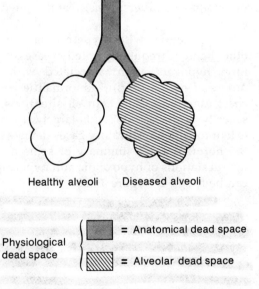

Figure 10.30 Dead space volume: a schematic presentation.

Evaluation of these four pulmonary volumes enables one to then calculate specific pulmonary capacities, as follows:

1. *Inspiratory capacity (IC)*, which equals tidal volume plus inspiratory reserve volume (about 3500 ml.). This is the amount of air that can be inspired with maximal effort.

2. *Functional residual capacity (FRC)*, which equals expiratory reserve volume plus residual volume (approximately 2300 ml.). This is the amount of air that usually remains in the lungs after a normal expiration.

3. *Vital capacity (VC)*, which equals inspiratory reserve volume plus tidal volume plus expiratory reserve volume (about 4600 ml.). This is the amount of air that can be expired with maximal effort after a forced inspiration.

4. *Total lung capacity (TLC)*, which equals tidal volume plus inspiratory reserve volume plus residual volume (approximately 5700 ml.). This is the total volume of air that will fill the lungs after a maximal inspiration.

The relationship between these pulmonary capacities and pulmonary volumes is illustrated in Figure 10.29.

The significance of these pulmonary tests lies in their ability to expose certain aspects of respiratory dysfunction. Diminished vital capacity, for example, can reflect paralysis of the respiratory muscles, pulmonary fibrosis, or pulmonary edema. Elevated total lung capacity or residual volume, on the other hand, is frequently indicative of hyperinflation induced by the "trapped air" of COPD.

In assessing the value of volume and capacity measures, it is important to remember that only air reaching the alveoli can act to facilitate gas exchange. It has, in fact, been established that a certain amount of inspired gas fills up the respiratory passageways without ever reaching the terminal air sacs. Described as *anatomical dead space*, this volume is normally equal to about 150 ml. in the average young male.

In cases of pulmonary disease, certain alveoli may become nonfunctional in the diffusion process. In these instances, the dead space concept is expanded to include air that reaches the alveoli but cannot actively serve in the exchange process (*alveolar dead space*). The sum total of anatomical and alveolar dead space is described as *physiological dead space*, and it is a more accurate measure of functional incapacity. The significance of dead space volume is visualized in Figure 10.30.

In reality, measures of respiratory volumes and capacities are diagnostically useful only to the extent that they reflect the volume of air per minute that actually reaches functional alveoli. This volume, defined as *alveolar ventilation*, is determined as follows:

Alveolar ventilation = Respiratory rate ×

(Tidal volume − Physiological dead space)

In the average adult male with a respiratory rate of about 12 per minute, a tidal volume of 500 ml., and a physiological dead space equal to anatomical dead space (150 ml.), alveolar ventilation will equal 12 × (500 ml. − 150 ml.) or 4200 ml. per minute. It is this volume of air that is specifically functional in oxygen and carbon dioxide exchanges between alveoli and pulmonary capillaries. In the event that alveolar ventilation is depressed, deviations in pO_2 and pCO_2 values will result.

ARTERIAL BLOOD GASES

Another means for the assessment of respiratory status is provided by laboratory measures of arterial pO_2, pCO_2, HCO^-_3, and pH. These values are often jointly referred to as *arterial blood gases (ABG's)*. Although a detailed explanation of the relationship between ABG's and acid-base imbalance can be found in Chapter 7, a brief clarification of the significance of pO_2, pCO_2, and pH values is presented in the following pages. Emphasis is placed upon utilization of arterial blood gases in the evaluation of respiratory disorders.

paO_2 The partial pressure of oxygen in arterial blood is specifically designated as paO_2. Reflecting the amount of oxygen *dissolved* in plasma, it is a good mirror of respiratory ventilation and diffusion. Under normal conditions, the paO_2 ranges from 80 to 104 mm. Hg, with an average value of 95 mm. Hg. Depressions in paO_2 are commonly associated with degeneration of the respiratory membrane or ventilation-perfusion imbalances.

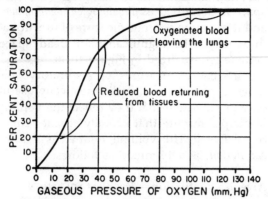

Figure 10.31 The oxygen-hemoglobin dissociation curve. (From Guyton, A. C: Textbook of Medical Physiology, 6th ed. Philadelphia, W. B. Saunders Company, 1981. Used by permission.)

In considering the significance of oxygen partial pressure, it is important to remember that only a small percentage of total oxygen is transported to cells dissolved in plasma water. The majority of transport, about 97 per cent, results from the *chemical combination* of oxygen with the hemoglobin in red blood cells:

$$Hb + O_2 \rightleftharpoons HbO_2$$

It is thus possible for cellular hypoxia to exist even in the face of adequate ventilation and diffusion. If hemoglobin concentration is depressed, or oxygen-hemoglobin association is impeded, cellular oxygen supply will predictably suffer.

The extent to which oxygen combines with hemoglobin varies with a number of factors. Oxygen-hemoglobin association, or per cent oxyhemoglobin saturation, is often related graphically to pO_2 values. The result is a plot of the *oxyhemoglobin dissociation curve*, illustrated in Figure 10.31.

It can be seen that the combination of oxygen with hemoglobin normally increases considerably as pO_2 moves from 0 to 50 mm. Hg. As pO_2 rises above 50 mm. Hg, however, increases have relatively less effect upon the degree of oxygen-hemoglobin association. When pO_2 approaches 80 mm. Hg, additional oxygen will dissolve primarily in the plasma and not combine with the hemoglobin of the red blood cell.

Several variables can affect or modify the normal oxyhemoglobin dissociation curve.

Primary among these are pCO_2, pH, and temperature. As pCO_2 increases, pH decreases, or temperature increases, hemoglobin will release oxygen with greater ease. Chemically, this can be indicated as follows:

$$Hb + O_2 \rightleftharpoons HbO_2$$
$$\uparrow pCO_2$$
$$\downarrow pH$$
$$\uparrow temperature$$

The shifting of this equation to the left favors dissociation of oxyhemoglobin into hemoglobin and free oxygen. This shift can be adaptive in nature when increasing cellular metabolic activity generates more carbon dioxide wastes and higher temperatures. Under these conditions, oxyhemoglobin releases greater quantities of oxygen to meet increased cellular needs.

Conversely, as pCO_2 decreases, pH increases, or temperature decreases, oxyhemoglobin will dissociate less readily. This can be summarized in chemical shorthand as follows:

$$\downarrow pCO_2$$
$$\uparrow pH$$
$$\downarrow temperature$$
$$Hb + O_2 \rightleftharpoons HbO_2$$

The shifting of this equation to the right promotes the binding of hemoglobin with oxygen and depresses the release of oxygen for tissue use. Cellular hypoxia can thus frequently accompany clinical conditions that promote excessive carbon dioxide loss or alkalosis or both.

In summary, it can be said that normal paO_2 values do not always reflect adequate cellular oxygenation. It is possible for oxygen to diffuse from alveoli into pulmonary capillaries, dissolve in plasma, and still not be transported effectively to service cellular needs. Whereas paO_2 readings are important in assessing cellular oxygen supply, the concentration and reactivity of hemoglobin must also be taken into consideration.

paCO₂/pH   The partial pressure of carbon dioxide in arterial blood is specifically designated as $paCO_2$. Reflecting the amount of carbon dioxide *dissolved* in plasma water, it is a good indicator of ventilation effectiveness. Since the majority of metabolically generated carbon dioxide is normally eliminated through the lungs, depressions in respiratory rate and obstructive disorders are frequently accompanied by carbon dioxide retention.

Under normal circumstances, $paCO_2$ averages 40 mm. Hg. Once again, it is important to realize that this value measures only dissolved carbon dioxide. Although only 7 per cent of total CO_2 is typically transported in this form, pCO_2 significantly affects acid-base balance in the following way:

$$\underset{\text{dissolved in plasma}}{CO_2} \quad + \quad H_2O \quad \rightleftharpoons \quad \underset{\text{carbonic acid}}{H_2CO_3}$$

It can be seen that elevations in dissolved CO_2 will trigger the formation of increasing quantities of carbonic acid. For this reason, respiratory disorders characterized by carbon dioxide retention typically initiate acidosis. Conversely, if hyperventilation causes plasma CO_2 levels to fall, relatively less carbonic acid is generated and alkalosis frequently results.

ARTERIAL BLOOD GASES: A SUMMARY

Arterial blood gas measurements facilitate the clinical assessment of respiratory and acid-base status. Used in conjunction with other evaluative tests, they can prove extremely valuable in the diagnostic process.

It can generally be said that paO_2 levels reflect the quantity of oxygen diffusing from alveoli into pulmonary capillaries. The degree of alveolar ventilation, on the other hand, is mirrored primarily by $paCO_2$ values. As respiratory disease develops, hypoxemia (depressed paO_2) and/or hypercapnia (elevated $paCO_2$) are characteristically noted.

RESPIRATORY PATHOLOGY: DISRUPTION OF CELLULAR NEEDS

In evaluating the effect of respiratory disease upon homeostasis, it is important to realize that respiratory dysfunction can disrupt the servicing of all four basic cellular life needs, as follows:

1. *The cellular need for oxygen:* Respira-

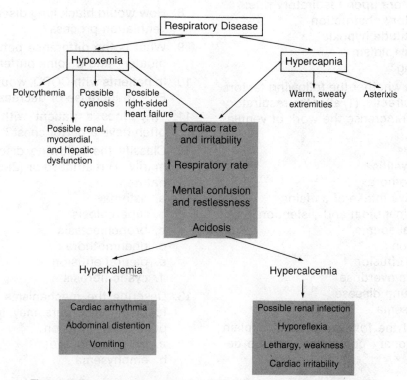

Figure 10.32 Systemic dysfunction triggered by respiratory pathology.

tory disease commonly results in a depression of pO_2 blood levels.

2. *The cellular need for nutrients:* The utilization of nutrients by cells is dependent upon the supply of adequate oxygen to support metabolism.

3. *The cellular need for elimination:* Respiratory dysfunction frequently interferes with the elimination of carbon dioxide from the alveoli.

4. *The cellular need for fluid-electrolyte and acid-base balance:* Since pCO_2 values affect plasma pH, acid-base imbalances can develop secondary to deviations in plasma carbon dioxide levels.

It can thus be said that respiratory activity services the cell in a wide variety of ways. Respiratory disorders can bring about many changes in the cellular environment. To the extent that disruptions in homeostasis affect the functional capacity of major organs, multisystemic dysfunction will result. The evolution of some major pathological patterns that could be triggered by respiratory disease is presented in Figure 10.32.

STUDY QUESTIONS

1. Why do the lungs inflate at birth?

2. A baby is born with infant respiratory distress syndrome. Explain to his parents, in simple terms, why he is in respiratory distress.

3. Differentiate between ventilation and diffusion.

4. Determine the effect of each of the following factors upon respiratory rate:
   a. respiratory obstruction
   b. high-altitude hypoxia
   c. hyperthyroidism
   d. vomiting

5. Determine whether the following factors will most directly: (1) alter the respiratory rate, or (2) increase the work of ventilation:
   a. scoliosis
   b. poliomyelitis
   c. pneumothorax
   d. excessive intake of caffeine
   e. abdominal bloat and distention
   f. cerebral edema
   g. pneumonia
   h. pleural effusion
   i. narcotic overdose
   j. black lung disease
   k. emphysema

6. In each of the following cases, explain why pulmonary compliance will be decreased:
   a. left heart failure
   b. knife wound in the chest
   c. rupture of the alveoli
   d. liver disease
   e. pleural inflammation

7. Why is it a good idea to require a tuberculin test of all individuals who will be handling food in a public or commercial enterprise?

8. How would black lung disease affect the ventilation process?

9. What is the difference between a "blue bloater" and a "pink puffer"?

10. In patients with COPD, would you expect ERV to increase or decrease, and why?

11. Why does a patient with emphysema often have a barrel chest?

12. Classify the following disorders as primarily (1) restrictive or (2) obstructive in nature:
    a. asthma
    b. tuberculosis
    c. bronchiectasis
    d. pneumothorax
    e. pleural effusion
    f. cystic fibrosis

13. Describe the mechanisms whereby the following disorders may interfere with pulmonary diffusion:
    a. left heart failure
    b. emphysema

c. asbestosis

d. cerebral edema

e. poliomyelitis

14. In cases of respiratory disorders, why is a decrease in pO_2 often noted before an elevation in pCO_2?

15. Describe the difference between respiratory insufficiency and respiratory failure.

16. From what you know about pulmonary pathology, predict the effect of:
    a. myasthenia gravis upon VC
    b. emphysema upon RV
    c. pulmonary edema upon pO_2
    d. chronic bronchitis upon pCO_2
    e. pneumothorax upon TLC

17. Which of the following factors will promote the *dissociation* of oxyhemoglobin into free oxygen and free hemoglobin:
    a. metabolic acidosis
    b. elevated body temperature
    c. hyperventilation, with excessive elimination of CO_2

Suggested Readings

Books

Addington, W. W.: Tuberculosis and other mycobacterial diseases. *In* Conn, H. F. (ed.): Current Therapy 1978. Philadelphia, W. B. Saunders Company, 1978.

Anderson, W. A. D., and Scotti, T. M.: Synopsis of Pathology, 10th ed. St. Louis, The C. V. Mosby Company, 1980, pp. 388–433.

Bates, D. V., et al.: Respiratory Function in Disease. Philadelphia, W. B. Saunders Company, 1971.

Baum, G. L. (ed.): Textbook of Pulmonary Diseases. Boston, Little, Brown & Company, 1974.

Becklake, M. R.: Physical and chemical irritants. *In* Beeson, P. B., McDermott, W., and Wyngaarden, J. B. (eds.): Cecil Textbook of Medicine, 15th ed. Philadelphia, W. B. Saunders Company, 1979, p. 983.

Berry, M. A.: Normal structure and function of the respiratory system. *In* Hudak, C. M., Lohr, T. S., and Gallo, B. M.: Critical Care Nursing, 2nd ed. Philadelphia, J. B. Lippincott Company, 1977, p. 211.

Brannin, P. K., and Kudla, M. S.: Management modalities: respiratory system. *In* Hudak, C.

M., Lohr, T. S., and Gallo, B. M.: Critical Care Nursing, 2nd ed. Philadelphia, J. B. Lippincott Company, 1977, p. 229.

Broughton, J. O.: Assessment skills for the nurse: respiratory system. *In* Hudak, C. M., Lohr, T. S., and Gallo, B. M.: Critical Care Nursing, 2nd ed. Philadelphia, J. B. Lippincott Company, 1977, p. 269.

Broughton, J. O.: Pathophysiology of the respiratory system. *In* Hudak, C. M., Lohr, T. S., and Gallo, B. M.: Critical Care Nursing, 2nd ed. Philadelphia, J. B. Lippincott Company, 1977, p. 221.

Burrows, B.: Diseases associated with airway obstruction. *In* Beeson, P. B., McDermott, W., and Wyngaarden, J. B. (eds.): Cecil Textbook of Medicine, 15th ed. Philadelphia, W. B. Saunders Company, 1979, p. 951.

Burrows, B., et al.: Respiratory Insufficiency. Chicago, Yearbook Medical Publishers, 1975.

Cherniack, R. M., Cherniack, L., and Naimark, A.: Respiration in Health and Disease, 2nd ed. Philadelphia, W. B. Saunders Company, 1972.

Cole, R. B.: Essentials of Respiratory Diseases. New York, MedCom, 1975.

Crofton, J., and Douglas, A.: Respiratory Diseases. Philadelphia, J. B. Lippincott Company, 1975.

Edwards, V., and Murphy, M. A.: Disruptions in the oxygen–carbon dioxide exchange mechanism. *In* Jones, D. A., Dunbar, C. F., and Jirovec, M. M.: Medical-Surgical Nursing, A Conceptual Approach. New York, McGraw-Hill Book Company, 1978, p. 1009.

Geschickter, C. F.: The Lung in Health and Disease. Philadelphia, J. B. Lippincott Company, 1973.

Goodwin, R. A.: Pulmonary tuberculosis. *In* Beeson, P. B., McDermott, W., and Wyngaarden, J. B. (eds.): Cecil Textbook of Medicine, 15th ed. Philadelphia, W. B. Saunders Company, 1979, p. 484.

Guyton, A. C.: Textbook of Medical Physiology, 5th ed. Philadelphia, W. B. Saunders Company, 1976, pp. 516–583.

Hole, J. W.: Human Anatomy and Physiology. Dubuque, Wm. C. Brown Company, 1978, pp. 496–528.

Kent, T. H., Hart, M. N., and Shires, T. K.: Introduction to Human Disease. New York, Appleton-Century-Crofts, 1979, pp. 125–139.

Killough, J. H.: Protective mechanisms of the lungs; pulmonary disease; pleural disease. *In* Sodeman, W. A., and Sodeman, T. M. (eds.):

Pathologic Physiology, Mechanisms of Disease, 6th ed. Philadelphia, W. B. Saunders Company, 1979, p. 451.

Luckmann, J., and Sorensen, K. C.: Medical-Surgical Nursing: A Psychophysiologic Approach, 2nd ed. Philadelphia, W. B. Saunders Company, 1980, pp. 1159–1222; 1263–1348.

Meyer, E. A.: Microorganisms and Human Disease. New York, Appleton-Century-Crofts, 1974, pp. 85–89; 124–129.

Michel, C. C.: The transport of oxygen and carbon dioxide by the blood. *In* Guyton, A. C. (ed.): MTP International Review of Science: Physiology, Vol. 2. Baltimore, University Park Press, 1974, p. 67.

Morgan, W. K. C., and Seaton, D.: Pulmonary ventilation and blood gas exchange. *In* Sodeman, W. A., and Sodeman, T. M. (eds.): Pathologic Physiology, Mechanisms of Disease, 6th ed. Philadelphia, W. B. Saunders Company, 1979, p. 427.

Murray, J. F.: Respiratory failure. *In* Beeson, P. B., McDermott, W., and Wyngaarden, J. B. (eds.): Cecil Textbook of Medicine, 15th ed. Philadelphia, W. B. Saunders Company, 1979, p. 1021.

Murray, J. F.: Respiratory structure and function. *In* Beeson, P. B., McDermott, W., and Wyngaarden, J. B. (eds.): Cecil Textbook of Medicine, 15th ed. Philadelphia, W. B. Saunders Company, 1979, p. 931.

Murray, J. F.: The Normal Lung. Philadelphia, W. B. Saunders Company, 1976.

Purtillo, D. T.: A Survey of Human Diseases. Menlo Park, Addison-Wesley Publishing Company, 1978, pp. 286–306.

Reynolds, H. Y.: Introduction to pneumonia. *In* Beeson, P. B., McDermott, W., and Wyngaarden, J. B. (eds.): Cecil Textbook of Medicine, 15th ed. Philadelphia, W. B. Saunders Company, 1979, p. 338.

Robbins, S. L., and Cotran, R. S.: Pathologic Basis of Disease, 2nd ed. Philadelphia, W. B. Saunders Company, 1979, pp. 814–879.

Ruppel, G.: Manual of Pulmonary Function Testing, St. Louis, The C. V. Mosby Company, 1975.

Selkurt, E. E.: Mechanics of pulmonary ventilation. *In* Selkurt, E. E. (ed.): Basic Physiology for the Health Sciences. Boston, Little, Brown & Company, 1975, p. 397.

Selkurt, E. E.: Nervous and chemical control of respiration. *In* Selkurt, E. E. (ed.): Basic Physiology for the Health Sciences. Boston, Little, Brown & Company, 1975, p. 439.

Selkurt, E. E.: Respiratory gas exchange and its transport. *In* Selkurt, E. E. (ed.): Basic Physiology for the Health Sciences. Boston, Little, Brown & Company, 1975, p. 419.

Shapiro, B. A.: Clinical Application of Blood Gases. Chicago, Yearbook Medical Publishers, 1973.

Thurlbeck, W. M.: Chronic Air Flow Obstruction in Lung Disease. Philadelphia, W. B. Saunders Company, 1976.

Tortora, G. J., and Anagnostakos, N. P.: Principles of Anatomy and Physiology, 2nd ed. San Francisco, Canfield Press, 1978, pp. 506–533.

Walter, J. B.: An Introduction to the Principles of Disease. Philadelphia, W. B. Saunders Company, 1977, pp. 469–493.

West, J. B.: Respiratory Physiology. Baltimore, Williams & Wilkins Company, 1974.

Articles

Adler, R. H.: Spontaneous pneumothorax. Hosp. Med., *1*:2, 1965.

Avery, M. E., et al.: The lung of the newborn infant. Sci. Am., *228*:74, 1973.

Betson, C.: Blood gases. Am. J. Nurs., *68*:1010, 1968.

Biddle, T. L.: Acute pulmonary edema. Hosp. Med., *13*:56, 1977.

Byrd, R. B.: Current concepts in diagnosing the cause of pleural effusion. Geriatrics, *32*:44, 1977.

Ciuca, R.: Cor pulmonale. Nursing 78, *8*:46, 1978.

DelBueno, D. J.: A quick review on using blood-gas determinations. RN, *41*:68, 1978.

Fitzmaurice, J. B., and Sashara, A. A.: Current concepts of pulmonary embolism: Implications for nursing practice. Heart Lung, *3*:209, 1974.

Foley, M. F.: Pulmonary function testing. Am. J. Nurs., *71*:1134, 1971.

Forster, R. E.: CO_2: chemical, biochemical, and physiological aspects. Physiologist, *13*:398, 1970.

Guz, A.: Regulation of respiration in man. Ann. Rev. Physiol., *37*:303, 1975.

Kroeker, E. J.: Atelectasis. Hosp. Med., *5*:67, 1969.

Lyons, H. A.: Obstructive emphysema. Hosp. Med., *7*:56, 1971.

Mead, J.: Respiration: pulmonary mechanics. Ann. Rev. Physiol., *35*:169, 1973.

Murray, J. F.: Mechanisms of acute respiratory failure. Am. Rev. Respir. Dis., *115*:1071, 1977.

Piiper, J., and Scheid, P.: Respiration: alveolar gas exchange. Ann. Rev. Physiol., *33*:131, 1971.

Snider, G. L.: Interpretation of the arterial oxygen and carbon dioxide partial pressures. Chest, *63*:801, 1973.

Staub, N. C.: Pulmonary edema. Physiol. Rev., *54*:678, 1974.

Staub, N. C.: The pathophysiology of pulmonary edema. Hum. Pathol., *1*:419, 1970.

Sweetwood, H.: Acute respiratory insufficiency: How to recognize this emergency . . . how to treat it. Nursing 77, 7:24, 1977.

Thomas, H. M., et al.: The oxyhemoglobin dissociation curve in health and disease. Am. J. Nurs., *57*:331, 1974.

Waldron, M. W.: Oxygen transport. Am. J. Nurs., *79*:272, 1979.

Chapter Outline

268

chapter 11

Renal Pathology

Chapter Objectives

At the completion of this chapter, the student will be able to:

1. Describe the basic structure and function of the kidneys and accessory organs in the renal system.
2. Trace renal blood flow.
3. Differentiate between filtration, reabsorption, and secretion, with respect to (a) basic functional mechanism, (b) modifying factors, and (c) ultimate result.
4. Describe the way in which aldosterone and ADH regulate urine formation.
5. Identify and describe four major diagnostic procedures utilized in the assessment of renal function.
6. Differentiate between acute renal failure and chronic renal failure, with respect to pathogenesis and clinical manifestations.
7. Distinguish between prerenal, intrarenal, and postrenal pathology as causes of acute renal failure.
8. Differentiate between (a) the syndrome of acute nephritis, (b) the syndrome accompanying tubular pathology, and (c) the prerenal syndrome as manifestations of acute renal failure.
9. Define uremia and trace the evolution of end-stage renal failure.
10. Differentiate between dialysis and transplant in the management of chronic renal failure.

INTRODUCTION

It is well established that the cells of the body require a fluid environment of ideal composition if life is to be supported. The urinary system plays a critical role in providing and maintaining this environment. Consisting of two kidneys, which function in the manufacture of urine, and accessory structures designed to transport and store urine on its voyage to the exterior, its major components are illustrated in Figure 11.1. As can be seen, the urine manufactured by the kidneys is conveyed to the bladder by two ureters. When sufficient volume has accumulated, the urine is then excreted through the urethra.

Most essential to the maintenance of homeostasis is the actual process of urine formation. In simple terms, urine is manufactured by microscopic subunits of the kidneys called nephrons. They process and modify the composition of urine so that it accommodates to ongoing changes in fluid-electrolyte and acid-base balance. If, for example, a patient with diabetes mellitus experiences acidosis, the nephrons respond by excreting more hydrogen ions. Conversely, in cases of hyponatremia, the kidneys attempt to conserve sodium by eliminating less of it in the urine. In most cases, deviations in the composition of extracellular fluid are compensated for by appropriate changes in urinary volume and content. Some of the basic mechanisms governing and regulating adaptive nephron activity are elucidated in Unit 2.

Since the kidneys are central to the maintenance of homeostasis, it therefore follows that disease of these structures can critically alter the cellular environment. At its extreme, renal disease almost always culminates in death.

In this chapter, a review of normal structure and function is followed by a close look at two different patterns of renal pathology.

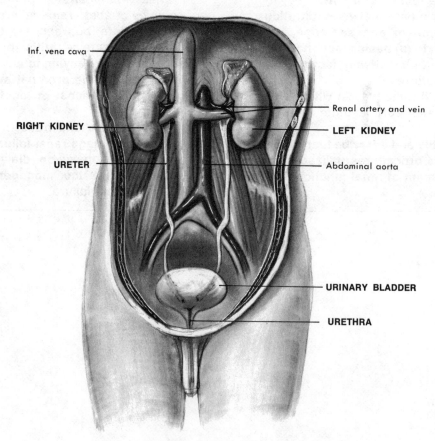

Inf. vena cava

Renal artery and vein

RIGHT KIDNEY

LEFT KIDNEY

URETER

Abdominal aorta

URINARY BLADDER

URETHRA

Figure 11.1   The *urinary system*

Acute renal failure is contrasted with *chronic renal failure* with respect to causative factors and characteristic clinical features.

RENAL PHYSIOLOGY

Although all components of the urinary system function to support homeostasis, the kidneys play by far the most significant role. For this reason, emphasis will be placed upon renal anatomy and physiology, with the structure and function of accessory organs (such as the ureters, bladder, and urethra) elucidated only briefly.

The Urinary System: An Overview

The kidneys, the major structures of the urinary system, are relatively protected from trauma by virtue of their location. Situated in the region of the lower back, they are positioned behind the peritoneum (retroperitoneal) and cushioned by fat. Sandwiched between the ribs and muscles posteriorly, and the intestines anteriorly, the right kidney is typically slightly lower than the left as a result of being pushed down by the mass and volume of the liver. The location of the kidneys is illustrated in Figure 11.2.

Once urine is manufactured by the nephrons, it emerges medially from the kidneys and passes into the ureters, a pair of narrow tubes approximately 10 to 12 inches in length. Propelled by a series of peristaltic muscular contractions, urine is conveyed to the bladder, where it is stored and ultimately eliminated.

The bladder is actually a muscular bag located in the lower abdominopelvic cavity. Anatomically it is divided into an upper *body* and lower *trigone,* as illustrated in Figure 11.3. When urine moves into the bladder, it initially accumulates owing to contraction of the *trigonal muscle* (also called the *internal sphincter*) located at the bladder base. As fluid pressure increases, the trigonal muscle automatically relaxes, while the *detrusor muscle* in the body of the bladder contracts. As a result, urine is pushed toward the urethra for expulsion from the body.

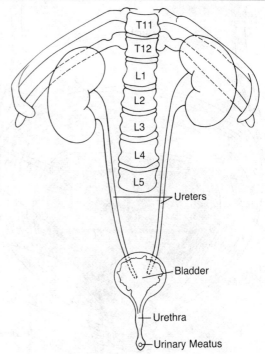

Figure 11.2 Location of the kidneys.

Before urinary elimination can occur, however, the *external sphincter muscle,* which is located in the upper or posterior urethra, must relax sufficiently to allow for fluid transport. This circular band of skeletal muscle is controlled voluntarily by neural messages from the higher brain centers. Unlike the detrusor or internal sphincter, its response is not regulated by automatic reflexes. Instead, when an individual wishes to urinate, muscular relaxation occurs and urine can then be eliminated through the urethra. It can thus be seen how interference with the functioning of the external sphincter could result in urinary incontinence, or the inability to voluntarily control urinary output.

In this chapter, abnormalities of *micturition,* or urinary expulsion, will be dealt with only to the extent that they affect or interfere with renal function.

The Kidneys: A Closer Look

To facilitate better understanding of the complex process of urine formation, an initial in-depth look at the structural organization of the kidney is advisable. The following elucidation of some key aspects of renal anatomy

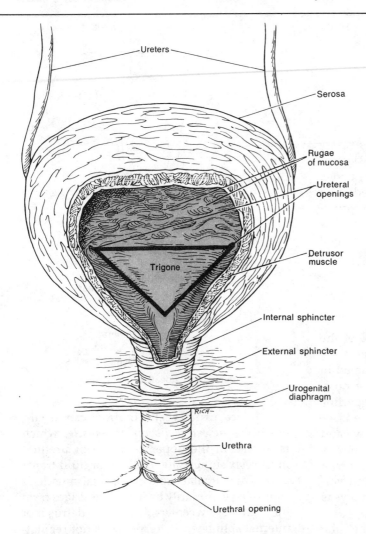

Ureters

Serosa

Rugae
of mucosa

Ureteral
openings

Trigone

Detrusor
muscle

Internal sphincter

External sphincter

Urogenital
diaphragm

RICH—

Urethra

Urethral opening

Figure 11.3 The urinary bladder and female urethra. (From Tortora, G. J., and Anagnostakos, M. P.: Principles of Anatomy and Physiology, 2nd ed. New York, Harper & Row, 1978. Used by permission.)

and blood supply should enhance comprehension and lay the groundwork for study of renal pathology.

RENAL ANATOMY

Each kidney is composed of approximately 1 million microstructures called nephrons, which are essentially responsible for urine formation. Nephrons, in turn, consist of five major parts, each having a functional role in the manufacture of urine: (1) the glomerular capsule, consisting of a tuft of capillaries called a glomerulus and Bowman's capsule (BC); (2) the proximal convoluted tubule (PCT); (3) the loop of Henle; (4) the distal convoluted tubule (DCT); and (5) the collecting duct or tubule (CD). The structure of the nephron is illustrated in Figure 11.4.

Functionally, Bowman's capsule serves as a receptacle for an ultrafiltrate of plasma derived from the glomerulus. All other nephron structures serve to modify the composition of this filtrate, so that by the time fluid enters the collecting ducts it has been effectively transformed into urine.

As a general rule, nephrons can be categorized as *cortical* or *juxtamedullary* according to their relative alignment within the kidney. A cross section of the kidney reveals an outer region of cortex and inner medulla, as illustrated in Figure 11.5. The medulla consists largely of triangular-shaped wedges, the points, or apices, of which are directed medially. These triangles, called *pyramids,* are separated from each other by areas of cortical material called *columns of Bertini*. They contain the collecting ducts of nephrons lined up in a

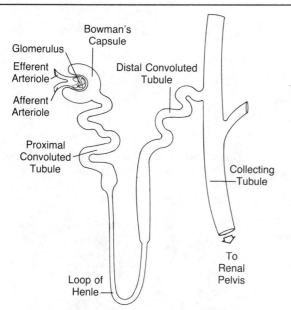

Figure 11.4 Structure of the nephron: a schematic drawing. (From Mulvihill, M. L.: Human Diseases: A Systemic Approach. Bowie, Md., Robert Brady Company, 1980. Used by permission.)

fairly uniform fashion so as to create a striated effect.

Whereas the majority of structural components in cortical nephrons are located primarily within the renal cortex (with the exception of the collecting ducts), juxtamedullary neph-

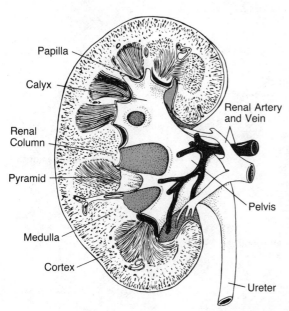

Figure 11.5 Coronal section through the right kidney. Redrawn for style from Textbook of A & P, Anthony & Thibodeau, 10th ed. Mosby, p. 540, Figure 20–2.

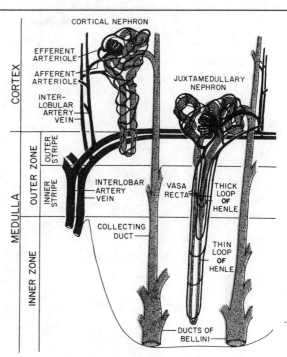

Figure 11.6 Diagram of a cortical nephron (left) and juxtamedullary nephron (right), showing relative location within the kidney. (From Guyton, A. C.: Textbook of Medical Physiology, 6th ed. Philadelphia, W. B. Saunders Company, 1981. Used by permission.)

rons contain loops of Henle, which typically extend deep into the renal medulla. Although limited in number, the juxtamedullary nephrons play a very significant role in the processing of urine, as will be explained later in this chapter. The relative location of these two types of nephrons is illustrated in Figure 11.6.

Once urine is formed in either the cortical or the juxtamedullary nephron, it is carried by collecting ducts, through openings in the tips of the pyramids, into cup-shaped receptacles called calyces. Calyces, in turn, merge into a large medial cavity known as the renal pelvis. It is from a slit in the renal pelvis, called the *hilus,* that blood vessels and nerves enter and leave the kidney and ureters exit to transport urine toward the bladder. The route taken by urinary filtrate in its movement through the kidneys is traced in Figure 11.7.

RENAL BLOOD FLOW

In order to function efficiently, the kidneys must receive an adequate blood supply

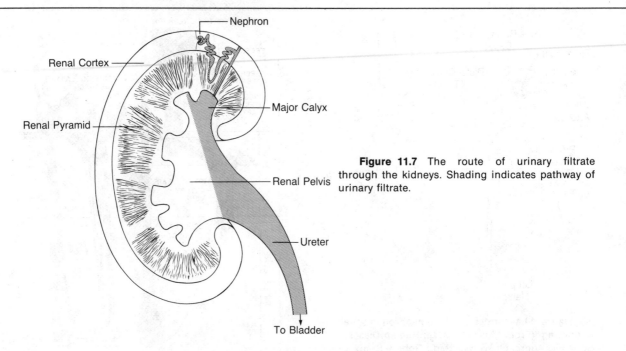

Figure 11.7 labels:
Nephron
Renal Cortex
Renal Pyramid
Major Calyx
Renal Pelvis
Ureter
To Bladder

Figure 11.7 The route of urinary filtrate through the kidneys. Shading indicates pathway of urinary filtrate.

from the systemic circulation. Ischemia, or inadequate circulation, can cause dysfunction on two levels:

1. Formation of urine is dependent upon filtration of a plasma ultrafiltrate out of the glomerular capillaries into Bowman's capsule. To the extent that glomerular blood flow is interrupted, urinary formation can be decreased.

2. Many cells in the walls of the PCT, loop of Henle, DCT, and CD must work actively to process glomerular filtrate and transform it into urine. To the extent that supplies of oxygen and nutrients are decreased, necrosis

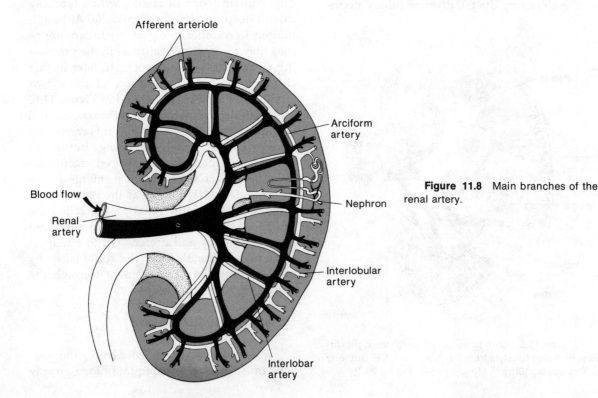

Figure 11.8 labels:
Afferent arteriole
Arciform artery
Blood flow
Nephron
Renal artery
Interlobular artery
Interlobar artery

Figure 11.8 Main branches of the renal artery.

of these functional cells can ensue. The result is urine of abnormal volume and composition.

In general, blood enters the kidneys through the renal arteries, which branch from the abdominal aorta. As illustrated in Figure 11.8, one renal artery enters each kidney at the hilus and branches into smaller vessels, which eventually give rise to the afferent arterioles. It is the afferent arterioles that directly feed the glomerular capillary tufts. Each glomerulus, in turn, services one Bowman's capsule in the kidney, providing the source for initial filtration of fluid into the nephron. Blood leaving the glomeruli subsequently enters the efferent arterioles, which branch into capillary structures of two major types: (1) the *peritubular capillaries,* which provide a network of small thin blood vessels to surround the PCT, loop of Henle, DCT, and collecting ducts; and (2) the *vasa recta,* which are specialized loops of peritubular capillary that dip deep into the medulla in a hairpin U configuration. These vessels are particularly important in modifying the composition of urine.

The relationship of the afferent and efferent arterioles to the peritubular capillaries is illustrated in Figure 11.9.

Blood, having moved through the peritubular capillaries or vasa recta, subsequently drains into larger venous vessels and finally into renal veins that exit through the hilus of the kidney.

Before turning from the subject of renal circulation, it is important to call attention to a structure that is closely associated with the afferent arteriole. Functioning in the regulation of blood pressure, this complex of cells lies in an area where the afferent arteriole and the distal convoluted tubule of the nephron come into direct contact. Consisting of (1) modified smooth muscle cells in the wall of the afferent arteriole, and (2) narrowed macula densa cells in the wall of the distal tubule, the structure is referred to as the *juxtaglomerular apparatus (JGA).*

Illustrated in Figure 11.10, the JGA functions to release renin when renal blood flow is depressed. Renin, in turn, ultimately triggers the formation of angiotensin II, which induces vasoconstriction and promotes the release of aldosterone. The renin-angiotensin mechanism, as discussed in Unit 2, plays a significant

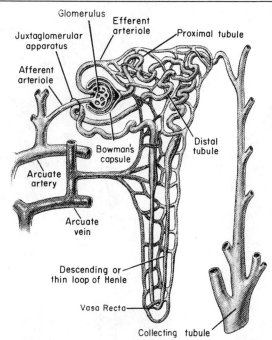

A, Anatomical representation of nephron and associated blood supply. (Modified from Smith: The Kidney: Structure and Function in Health and Disease. Oxford University Press. Used by permission.)

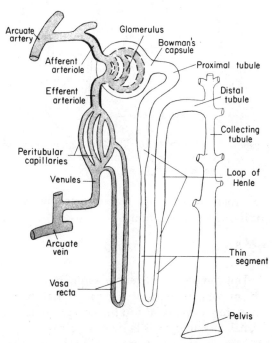

B, Schematic representation of nephron and associated blood supply. (From Guyton, A. C.: Textbook of Medical Physiology, 6th ed. Philadelphia, W. B. Saunders Co., 1981. Used by permission.)

Figure 11.9 The capillary network servicing the nephron.

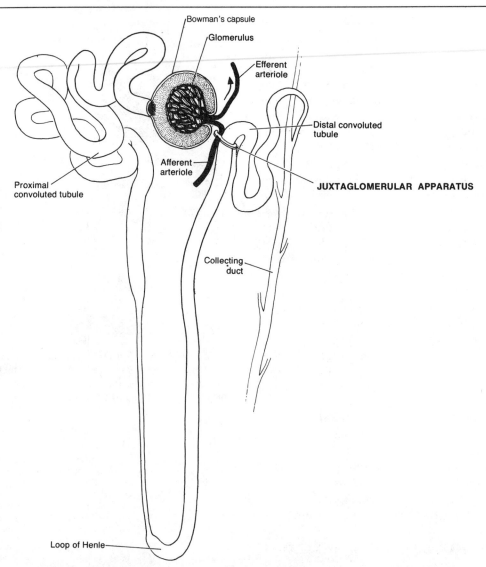

Figure 11.10 The juxtaglomerular apparatus. (From Tortora, G. J., and Anagnostakos, M. P.: Principles of Anatomy and Physiology, 2nd ed. New York, Harper & Row, 1978. Used by permission.)

dual role in altering blood pressure and modifying urinary content.

The Formation of Urine

The complexity of renal design and structure mirrors, in part, the intricate nature of kidney function. To aid in the comprehension of renal physiology, it is helpful to categorize the urinary formation process into two distinct phases: (1) *the filtration phase*, which involves the passage of a plasma ultrafiltrate out of the glomerulus into Bowman's capsule; and (2) *the modification phase*, which involves

alterations in the content of glomerular filtrate as it moves through the PCT, loop of Henle, DCT, and collecting ducts.

To ensure the optimal composition of urine, filtration and modification must work hand in hand. If all substances that initially filtered through the glomerulus into the nephron were ultimately eliminated as urine, extracellular fluid would rapidly be depleted of many essential constituents. Conversely, if the original glomerular filtrate were unable to receive additional substances derived directly from the peritubular capillaries, many potentially toxic components would remain within the body. It is therefore obvious that as glomerular filtrate passes through the nephron toward the renal pelvis, its composition must be selectively modified.

Since modification can occur in all portions of the nephron except for the glomerular capsule, this aspect of urine formation can basically be described as a tubular phenomenon. As one studies the complexities of modification, it becomes evident that changes in the composition of glomerular filtrate can occur by two distinctly different processes: (a) *reabsorption*, or the movement of certain materials out of the lumen of the nephron back into the peritubular capillaries, and (b) *secretion*, or the transport of select substances directly from the peritubular capillaries into the tubules of the nephron.

The basic mechanisms of urinary formation are illustrated in Figure 11.11. Each aspect is examined in more depth in the following pages.

FILTRATION

Filtration, or the movement of a plasma ultrafiltrate out of the glomerulus into Bowman's capsule, is the first step in the formation of urine. Although many factors can affect the rate, volume, and nature of glomerular filtration, the two most significant are (1) the filtration pressure, and (2) the status of the glomerular membrane.

FILTRATION PRESSURE Filtration pressure, which can be defined as the effective force driving fluid out of the glomerulus, is instrumental in affecting the rate and volume of glomerular filtration. Determined by interaction between many dynamic processes, its value is most significantly linked to:

1. *glomerular blood pressure,* which tends to push fluid out of the glomerulus into Bowman's capsule. It normally measures about 60 mm. Hg.

2. *glomerular colloid osmotic pressure,* which serves to draw fluid out of Bowman's capsule back into the glomerulus. It normally ranges around 32 mm. Hg.

3. *Bowman's capsule pressure,* which resists the movement of fluid out of the glomerulus into Bowman's capsule. It normally measures around 18 mm. Hg.

The interaction between these three forces is summarized diagrammatically in Figure 11.12. It can be seen that filtration pressure ultimately depends upon the degree to which blood pressure exceeds the combined effects of C.O.P. and Bowman's capsule pressure. In short, blood pressure in the glomerulus must

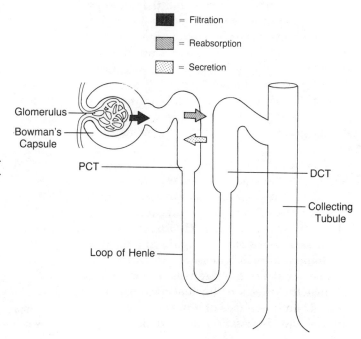

Figure 11.11 Renal filtration, reabsorption, and secretion: a schematic presentation.

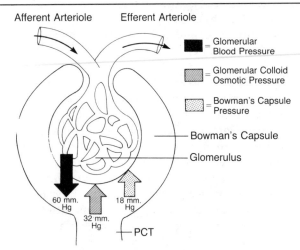

Figure 11.12 | = Glomerular Blood Pressure

| = Glomerular Colloid Osmotic Pressure

| = Bowman's Capsule Pressure

— Bowman's Capsule

— Glomerulus

60 mm. Hg   32 mm. Hg   18 mm. Hg

— PCT

Figure 11.12 Filtration pressure in the nephron: a schematic summary.

counteract both the osmotic forces in the glomerular capillary and the resistance posed by material already in Bowman's capsule. Mathematically, this relationship can be expressed as follows:

Filtration pressure = Glomerular blood pressure − (Glomerular C.O.P. + Bowman's capsule pressure)

or

$$60 \text{ mm. Hg} - (32 \text{ mm. Hg} + 18 \text{ mm. Hg})$$
$$60 \text{ mm. Hg} - (50 \text{ mm. Hg})$$

Filtration pressure = 10 mm. Hg

It is important to remember that although the filtration process is technically affected by all three pressures designated in the foregoing formula, the most significant clinical variations are noted in glomerular B.P. or C.O.P.

Glomerular Blood Pressure Blood pressure in the glomerulus varies as a function of several factors. Ultimately, however, it depends primarily upon the volume of blood entering the glomerulus.

As mentioned earlier, it is extremely important for the kidneys to be serviced with an adequate blood supply. Normally, about 21 per cent of total cardiac output flows through the kidneys per minute. If this amount is substantially reduced, a significant decrease in glomerular blood pressure can result.

Fortunately, the kidneys are protected against the effects of fluctuating renal blood flow. Even in the face of a 100 per cent rise in **arterial** blood pressure, glomerular filtration

pressure will typically increase by only 15 to 20 per cent. The reflex responses that guard against rapid changes in glomerular blood pressure are collectively referred to as *autoregulation* mechanisms.

Controlled primarily by afferent arterioles that feed the glomerulus, the autoregulation mechanism is illustrated in Figure 11.13. It can be seen that whereas dilation of the afferent arteriole promotes an increase in glomerular blood volume, vasoconstriction depresses the flow of blood through the glomerulus.

The way in which autoregulation works can best be illustrated by example. In cases in which hemorrhage causes a considerable reduction in blood volume, glomerular blood pressure and filtration pressure could dip to a

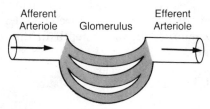

Afferent Arteriole   Glomerulus   Efferent Arteriole

Normal glomerular blood pressure

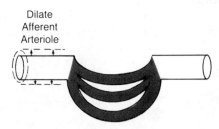

Dilate Afferent Arteriole

Glomerular blood pressure is increased

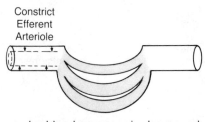

Constrict Efferent Arteriole

Glomerular blood pressure is decreased

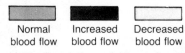

Normal blood flow   Increased blood flow   Decreased blood flow

Figure 11.13 Regulation of blood flow through the glomerulus.

critical low. As systemic blood pressure falls, however, the afferent arterioles of the nephron dilate. In this way, retention of blood in the glomerulus operates selectively against an excessive drop in renal pressure. Conversely, in cases of extracellular fluid excess, blood volume may increase to dangerously high levels. In these instances, constriction of afferent arterioles protects the glomeruli from excessive rises in blood pressure. At either extreme, autoregulation helps to prevent dramatic changes in glomerular pressure.

The exact mechanisms governing renal autoregulation have not yet been elucidated. Most current research, however, points to the JGA as playing a central role in the regulation of adaptive renal vasoconstriction and dilation.

Glomerular Colloid Osmotic Pressure   As discussed in Chapter 4, colloid osmotic pressure varies primarily with the plasma concentration of large protein molecules. It is these particles that remain within the vascular tree and exert the primary drawing force for fluids. Any systemic disorders causing a major disruption in plasma protein levels will, of course, precipitate changes in glomerular C.O.P. To the extent that proteins are lost, C.O.P. will drop; conversely, if plasma protein concentrations increase, C.O.P. will be elevated.

Although the *amount* of protein in the plasma is rarely found to increase clinically, it is significant that protein *concentration* is often elevated owing to loss of protein-free fluid. It has been noted, for example, that the longer fluid remains in the glomerulus, the more time there is for water and electrolytes to move into Bowman's capsule. A depressed rate of renal blood flow can therefore cause an elevation in glomerular C.O.P. as proteins retained in the glomerulus become increasingly concentrated.

Filtration Pressure: A Summary   Filtration pressure in the glomerulus is determined largely by the balance between glomerular B.P. and C.O.P. Any clinical conditions promoting a rise in B.P. or a fall in C.O.P. or both will increase filtration. Conversely, pathological conditions inducing a fall in B.P. or a rise in C.O.P. or both will be characterized by a decline in filtration pressure. The glomerular

TABLE 11.1   Changes in Glomerular Filtration Pressure

Underlying Mechanisms	Causative Disorders

Increase in glomerular blood pressure	Hypervolemia
	    Cushing's disease
	    SIADH
	    Renal failure
	    CHF
	Neurally induced dilation of the afferent arterioles

Decrease in glomerular blood pressure	Hypovolemia
	    Diabetes insipidus
	    Hemorrhage
	    Diarrhea and vomiting
	Hypotension

Decrease in glomerular colloid osmotic pressure	Albuminuria associated with renal disease Malnutrition and/or starvation Hepatic disease

pressure changes precipitated by certain clinical conditions are summarized in Table 11.1.

THE STATUS OF THE GLOMERULAR MEMBRANE   While filtration pressure can affect the rate and volume of urine formation, the status of the glomerular membrane more directly influences urinary composition. This membrane, through which all material must pass en route from the glomerulus into Bowman's capsule, consists of three major structural layers: (a) a capillary endothelial layer, (b) a mucopolysaccharide basement membrane, and (c) a layer of epithelial cells lining Bowman's capsule.

Illustrated in Figure 11.14, the membrane is approximately 100 to 1000 times more permeable than the normal capillary. This increased permeability, which facilitates the filtration process, is accounted for largely by specialized structural adaptations. Small holes in the capillary endothelium, called fenestrae, and "slit pores" between the epithelial cells lining Bowman's capsule aid in the formation of the initial urinary filtrate.

Even with increased permeability, however, the glomerular membrane will not allow large particles, such as blood cells or protein molecules, to pass into Bowman's capsule.

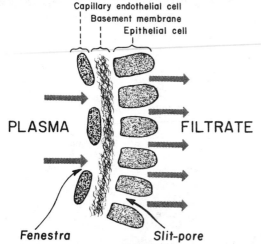

Capillary endothelial cell
Basement membrane
Epithelial cell

PLASMA   FILTRATE

Fenestra   Slit-pore

Figure 11.14   The functional structure of the glomerular membrane. The epithelial cells line Bowman's capsule. (From Guyton, A. C.: Textbook of Medical Physiology, 6th ed. Philadelphia, W. B. Saunders Company, 1981. Used by permission.)

Normally, therefore, the glomerular filtrate is similar in composition to interstitial fluid. It resembles plasma with respect to the concentration of electrolytes and smaller molecules. Larger particles, however, do not typically pass into Bowman's capsule.

If hemoglobin, blood cells, or albumin is found in significant amounts in the urine, a disorder of the glomerular membrane is most probably the cause. Disorders causing damage to the membrane will be discussed later in this chapter.

MODIFICATION

Although filtration is the significant first step in the formation of urine, the composition of the initial filtrate must be considerably modified, if homeostasis is to be maintained. The processes of reabsorption and secretion are thus largely responsible for producing urine of optimal volume and composition.

REABSORPTION   The reabsorptive process provides the necessary means for selectively retaining certain substances that initially filter into Bowman's capsule. Without reabsorption, the components of urinary filtrate that are needed by the body would be unable to move from tubular lumens back into the bloodstream. Many substances critical to physiological function would thus be eliminated in the urine.

Mechanisms of Reabsorption   Reabsorption of materials from the nephron can occur either passively (in response to the laws of diffusion) or through active transport (requiring the support of an energy-driven mechanism). In either case, the large majority of originally filtered water, and a significant amount of electrolytes and metabolites, are returned to the extracellular fluid each day via the reabsorptive process. The complexities of reabsorption can best be clarified by tracing examples of this phenomenon as evidenced in various portions of the nephron.

Once fluid has filtered into Bowman's capsule, it moves into the PCT, where approximately 65 per cent of all reabsorptive activity takes place. The cells composing the walls of these tubules are especially adapted to the active transport of sodium (Na^+). They actually remove a large percentage of sodium ions from the glomerular filtrate and pump it out of the tubular lumen. The majority of ions thus transported subsequently move into adjacent peritubular capillaries.

As sodium concentration builds up in the fluid surrounding the tubules, water moves out to dilute this sodium by the passive process of osmosis. Negatively charged chloride ions (Cl^-) also follow passively, to maintain electrical neutrality. The entire process is illustrated in Figure 11.15.

As a result of the combined reabsorption of sodium, chloride, and water, these substances are retained in extracellular fluid. Other physiologically significant constituents that are reabsorbed in the PCT include calcium, phosphate, vitamins, proteins, amino acids, and glucose. As glomerular filtrate leaves the PCT and flows on through the nephron, it can be seen that a considerable number of substances that are essential to the maintenance of cellular health have already been returned to the plasma.

In the area of the loop of Henle DCT and CD, the interstitial fluid surrounding the nephrons contains characteristically high concentrations of solute particles. This phenomenon is mediated by cells in the loop of Henle and vasa recta that work jointly, through active transport, to generate hypertonic interstitial fluid in the renal medulla. The process whereby this concentration occurs is illustrated in Figure 11.16.

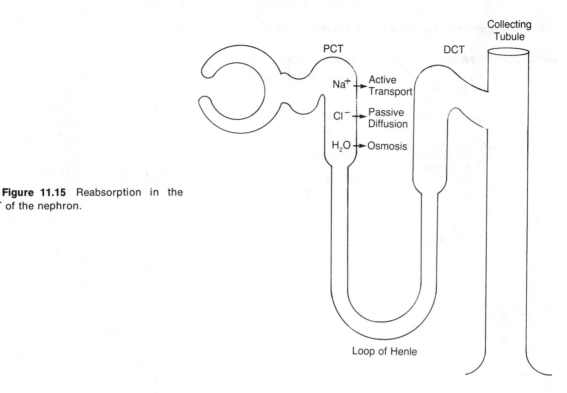

Figure 11.15 Reabsorption in the PCT of the nephron.

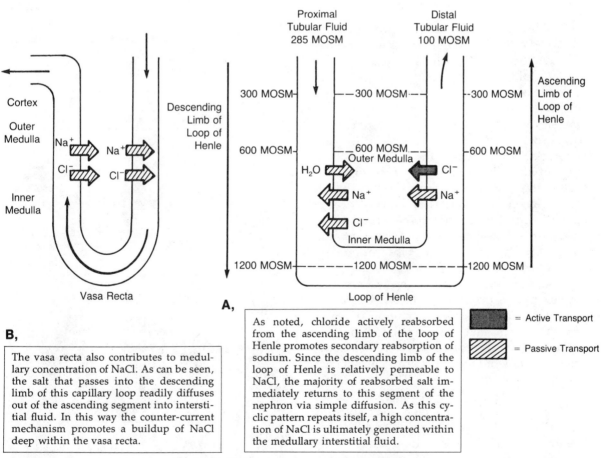

B,

The vasa recta also contributes to medullary concentration of NaCl. As can be seen, the salt that passes into the descending limb of this capillary loop readily diffuses out of the ascending segment into interstitial fluid. In this way the counter-current mechanism promotes a buildup of NaCl deep within the vasa recta.

A,

As noted, chloride actively reabsorbed from the ascending limb of the loop of Henle promotes secondary reabsorption of sodium. Since the descending limb of the loop of Henle is relatively permeable to NaCl, the majority of reabsorbed salt immediately returns to this segment of the nephron via simple diffusion. As this cyclic pattern repeats itself, a high concentration of NaCl is ultimately generated within the medullary interstitial fluid.

Figure 11.16 The counter-current mechanism.

281

TABLE 11.2   **Relative Concentrations of Select Substances in the Glomerular Filtrate (which approximates plasma) and in the Urine***

Constituent	Glomerular Filtrate (plasma) Concentration (in mEq./L.)	Concentration in Urine (in mEq./L.)
Na^+	142	128
K^+	5	60
Ca^{++}	4	4.8
Mg^{++}	3	15
Cl^-	103	134
HCO_3^-	28	14
$H_2PO_4^-$ HPO_4^{--}	2	50
SO_4^{--}	0.7	33
Glucose	100 mg per cent	0 mg per cent
Urea	26	1820
Uric acid	3	42
Creatinine	1.1	196
Inulin	—	—
Diodrast	—	—
PAH	—	—

*Adapted from Guyton, A. C.: Textbook of Medical Physiology. Philadelphia, W. B. Saunders Company, 1976.

Glomerular fluid, as it moves into the DCT and collecting tubules on its final journey through the medulla, is thus exposed to interstitial fluid of high solute concentration. Under these circumstances, water will move passively (by osmosis) out of the tubules into the surrounding hypertonic environment. In order for osmosis to occur, however, the hormone ADH must render the DCT and collecting tubules sufficiently permeable to water. Assuming normal endocrine support, by the time glomerular filtrate has moved through the nephron and is ready to be eliminated as urine, it will ideally have lost 99 per cent of its originally filtered water by reabsorption.

Results of Reabsorption It is important to note that, in some cases, the reabsorption of electrolytes from the nephron is balanced by osmosis of proportional amounts of water. To the extent that reabsorption of ions is balanced by reabsorption of water, the relative concentration of ions in urine and plasma will be approximately the same. This principle is verified by the comparative data presented in Table 11.2. It can be seen that sodium, chloride, and calcium are of similar concentration in both urine and plasma.

To further elucidate the phenomenon of equality in concentration, it is helpful to look at a hypothetical case, in which plasma contains only sodium and water in a ratio of 1:10. For every 100 molecules of water, there should be 10 particles of sodium. If these 100 molecules of water and 10 particles of sodium pass from the glomerulus into Bowman's capsule, selective reabsorption of sodium in the PCT could alter the original 1:10 ratio. To keep the sodium concentration from changing, 10 molecules of water would have to move passively from the lumen of the nephron into the surrounding interstitial fluid for every single particle of reabsorbed sodium. This is, in effect, what happens. In fact, throughout the entire length of the tubule, sodium retention is matched by osmosis of water in a 1:10 ratio. Thus, at the terminal end of the nephron, the fluid remaining to be excreted as urine should have a sodium concentration that is similar to our hypothetical plasma. Although the *volume* of glomerular filtrate may have decreased, the sodium *concentration* of the fluid has not been altered. This hypothetical case is illustrated in Figure 11.17.

Not all substances, however, are found in

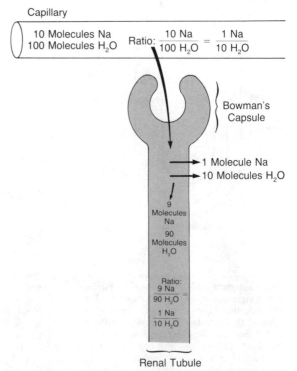

Figure 11.17 The production of isotonic urine: a hypothetical schematic presentation.

plasma and urine in equal concentrations. There are molecules, for example, that are reabsorbed to a much greater extent than is water. Their concentration can fall to essentially 0 mEq./L. in urine. Examples of substances that are reabsorbed almost completely out of the glomerular filtrate back into the extracellular fluid are glucose, amino acids, and proteins. It is significant to note that retention of these molecules is essential to the maintenance of normal cellular metabolism.

Conversely, certain constituents of glomerular filtrate are reabsorbed only marginally. Unable to move through tubular cells, they become increasingly concentrated in the urine as water moves out of the nephron by osmosis. It is the end products of protein metabolism, such as urea, uric acid, and creatinine, as well as potassium, sulfates, phosphates, and nitrates that tend to share this fate. In many cases, particularly with regard to potassium and nitrogen wastes, reabsorption or retention would induce a toxic plasma overload, with subsequent systemic disorders.

SECRETION It can be seen that the reabsorptive process provides a means of conserving many physiologically significant substances by selectively modifying the initial composition of glomerular filtrate. It is also important to be able to eliminate materials that did not originally enter the nephron via filtration. Such a mechanism is provided by the process of secretion.

Defined as the transport of substances from peritubular capillaries into nephron tubules, secretion is noted primarily in the DCT and collecting tubules. The secretory process is largely responsible for regulating the plasma concentration of potassium and hydrogen ions. Other chemicals or drugs commonly secreted by the nephron include penicillin, Diodrast, and phenolsulfonphthalein (PSP).

The Regulation of Urine Formation

If homeostasis is to be maintained, the processes of filtration, reabsorption, and secretion must be carefully regulated. Ultimately, the extracellular fluid concentration of many critical electrolytes, acids, and bases is determined by renal activity.

Ideally, the nephrons respond adaptively to diverse changes in the volume or composition of extracellular fluid. In cases of acidosis, for example, the nephrons act to *secrete* hydrogen ions as they accumulate excessively in the plasma fluid compartment. Conversely, if hypovolemia should develop, *reabsorption* of fluid can serve to offset a potentially serious imbalance.

Many mechanisms help to render the nephrons sensitive to changes in the cellular environment. Because the hormones *aldosterone* and *ADH* play a particularly significant role in supporting the adaptive function of the kidneys, the activity of these endocrine secretions will be reviewed briefly.

ALDOSTERONE

Aldosterone is a hormone secreted by specialized cells in the outer layer (cortex) of the adrenal glands. It is directly responsible for stimulating reabsorption of sodium ions and secretion of potassium and hydrogen ions in the distal convoluted tubules and collecting tubules of the nephron.

As a regulator of electrolyte concentration in the terminal segments of the nephron, aldosterone ultimately affects the elimination of sodium, potassium, and hydrogen. Elevated levels of aldosterone, for example, can promote excessive reabsorption of sodium, thereby considerably reducing the concentration of this ion in the urine. Depressed aldosterone output, on the other hand, results in excessive excretion of urinary sodium, with decreased amounts being conserved in the plasma.

In brief, aldosterone affects the cellular fluid environment by promoting (1) increases in the levels of sodium and water, and (2) decreases in the concentration of potassium or hydrogen or both. These changes are generated by, respectively: (1) direct stimulation of sodium reabsorption, followed by secondary osmosis of proportional amounts of water; and (2) selective secretion of potassium or hydrogen or both out of the extracellular fluid into the nephron.

Normally, aldosterone levels are respon-

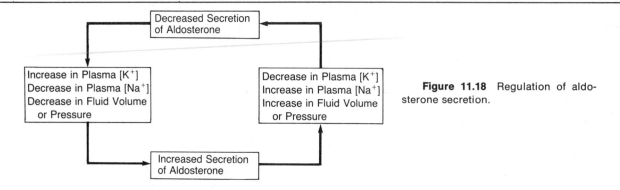

Figure 11.18   Regulation of aldosterone secretion.

sive to electrolyte changes and thus function in the ongoing maintenance of homeostasis. Several mechanisms operate to ensure that fluctuations in the release of this hormone remain adaptive. In general, aldosterone secretion will increase in response to (1) increasing concentrations of potassium or (less significantly) decreasing concentrations of sodium in the extracellular fluid. Changes in these electrolyte levels seem to directly stimulate the adrenal cortical cells to increase aldosterone output; (2) decreasing fluid volume or pressure or both. Depressions in fluid levels activate the renin-angiotensin mechanism, which, in turn, promotes aldosterone release.

Decreases in aldosterone output are initiated, in a similar manner, by either (1) decreasing concentrations of potassium or (less significantly) increasing concentrations of sodium in the extracellular fluid, or (2) increasing fluid volume or pressure or both. The feedback controls that regulate aldosterone secretion are depicted in Figure 11.18.

ANTIDIURETIC HORMONE (ADH)

Whereas aldosterone affects sodium reabsorption and potassium secretion, ADH functions to directly alter the permeability of the DCT and collecting tubule to water.

As a regulator of water permeability in the terminal segments of the nephron, ADH plays a primary role in determining the ultimate balance between fluid retention and elimination. To the extent that water levels are selectively altered, the concentration of solutes in the extracellular fluid will, of course, be secondarily affected.

Normally, the fluid surrounding the DCT

and collecting tubule is more concentrated in solutes than is the glomerular filtrate within the nephron. As a result, water will tend to move, by osmosis, out of the tubular lumen. The extent to which water can pass out of the nephron into surrounding interstitial fluid is determined primarily by ADH levels. Unless this hormone is secreted in sufficient quantity, the cells of the distal convoluted and collecting tubules remain effectively impermeable to water, and large quantities of fluid are lost in the urine. In short, the ability to concentrate urine, and subsequently conserve body water, depends, to a large extent, upon ADH release.

In general, antidiuretic hormone affects the cellular environment by increasing the volume of water in extracellular fluid while decreasing urinary output. Dilution of solutes in plasma and the interstitial compartment occurs secondarily.

Mechanisms to ensure adaptive release of ADH from the posterior pituitary gland are particularly responsive to (1) changes in extracellular fluid solute concentration, sodium in particular; and (2) alterations in the volume or pressure of fluid in the plasma compartment.

More specifically, as sodium plasma concentration increases, direct stimulation of receptors in the hypothalamus of the brain promotes increased release of ADH. Subsequent reabsorption of water from the nephron serves to offset the development of hypernatremia.

Alternatively, as fluid levels decrease in the cardiovascular system, strategically located stretch and pressure receptors initiate a feedback increase in ADH output. Subsequent retention of water helps to prevent the onset of hypovolemia.

Decreases in ADH release are caused, in

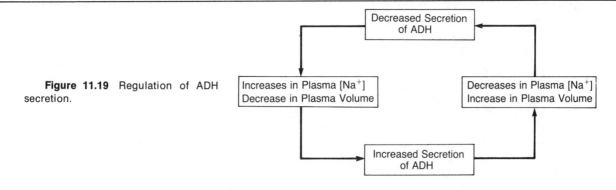

Figure 11.19 Regulation of ADH secretion.

the same fashion, by either depressed concentration of plasma sodium or increased extracellular fluid volume. The feedback regulation of ADH output is summarized in Figure 11.19.

THE REGULATION OF URINE FORMATION: A SUMMARY

It can be said that responsiveness of the nephron to a constantly fluctuating cellular environment is central to the maintenance of homeostasis. Adaptive changes in reabsorption and secretion are controlled largely by aldosterone and ADH. The comparative effects of these hormones upon functional activity within the nephron are presented in Figure 11.20.

Monitoring Renal Function

As one studies the urinary system, it becomes increasingly evident that renal disease can precipitate catastrophic changes in the cellular fluid environment. Because early diagnosis of disease and malfunction can be critically important, it is helpful to have an idea of some of the major diagnostic tools available to the clinician in assessing renal function. They include (1) renal clearance tests, (2) concentration and dilution tests, (3) measures of plasma creatinine and BUN levels, and (4) measures of protein in the urine.

RENAL CLEARANCE TESTS

In general, a clearance test is a measure of the rate of glomerular filtration. It thus provides an indication of the extent to which renal tissue is functioning effectively.

More specifically, clearance calculations are designed to determine the amount of plasma that had to be filtered through the glomerulus in order to deliver a measured quantity of a specific constituent into the urine. Clearance is evaluated by a specific formula, as follows:

$$\text{Plasma clearance (ml./minute)} = \frac{\text{Quantity of urine (ml./minute)} \times \text{Concentration in the urine}}{\text{Concentration in the plasma}}$$

In calculating plasma clearance, it is particularly important to use substances that are neither secreted nor reabsorbed to any great extent. In this way, one can be assured that elimination is primarily a function of glomerular filtration. Whatever is excreted in the urine must have been delivered to the nephron almost exclusively through the glomerular membrane. Both *inulin* and *mannitol* are substances that conform to this elimination pattern.

It has been determined that *approximately 125 ml. of filtrate must be delivered into Bowman's capsule per minute in order to effectively clear any given substance through the nephrons.* When a patient is being evaluated, controlled quantities of inulin or mannitol may be introduced intravenously, with concentration being measured in the plasma and the urine. Subsequent calculations using the plasma clearance formula provide a measure of functional glomerular filtration rate.

Although inulin and mannitol have been classic standards in clearance determinations, creatinine is being used with increasing fre-

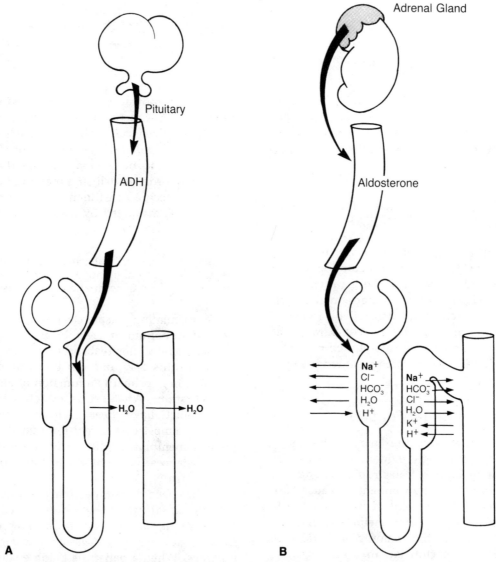

Figure 11.20 The effects of (A) ADH and (B) aldosterone upon reabsorption and secretion in the nephron.

quency in clinical testing. A natural product of muscle metabolism, creatinine is normally released into plasma by muscle at a controlled rate. Although a very small fraction of this substance is secreted by the nephron, its clearance serves as a very close approximation of glomerular filtration rate. Since creatinine does not have to be introduced intravenously, it provides an easier and faster means of measuring clearance than either inulin or mannitol.

CONCENTRATION AND DILUTION TESTS

Whereas clearance tests reflect glomerular filtration, concentration and dilution tests are designed to evaluate functional capacity of the renal tubules.

As mentioned earlier, the glomerular filtrate is considerably modified as it moves through the nephron from the PCT to the collecting tubules. Ideally, assuming normal output of the renal regulatory hormones (aldosterone and ADH), the ultimate volume and electrolyte concentration of urine should vary with cellular needs. Thus, under conditions of water deprivation the tubules should selectively reabsorb water, resulting in urine of lesser volume and greater solute concentration. Conversely, if excessive water is present in plasma, the tubules can compensate by putting out a large volume of watery urine.

The capacity of the nephron to adaptively concentrate or dilute urine is dependent upon functional activity of the tubular cells. To the extent that these cells are damaged or diseased, the solute concentration of urine can no longer fluctuate in response to changing levels of hydration in the body.

Often, tubular disease can be diagnosed in its early stages by subjecting a patient to artificially induced conditions of water deprivation or water excess. In the former case, the normal nephron should respond by selectively reabsorbing water and excreting urine of high solute concentration. In the latter case, renal compensation should result in the elimination of urine with higher water content and lower solute concentration. To the extent that tubu-

lar cells are nonfunctional, the artificial stress conditions will have relatively no effect upon the concentration of solutes in the urine. Solute concentration will remain constant regardless of changing physiological needs. The response of the nephron to concentration and dilution tests is summarized in Figure 11.21.

In determining the concentrating-diluting capacity of the nephron, *specific gravity* is a particularly helpful measure. Specific gravity is a measure of the relative buoyancy of a liquid, compared with water. Buoyancy, in turn, is dependent upon the concentration, size, and weight of solute particles in a given liquid. The normal specific gravity of urine, for example, ranges between 1.003 and 1.030, with a norm of 1.010 (compared with 1.000 of pure water). Elevated solute concentration will increase the specific gravity of urine, while dilute urine will have a lower specific gravity.

If tubular cells are functioning normally, water deprivation should result in a concentrated urine with a specific gravity of 1.025 or greater. Water excess, on the other hand, would precipitate output of dilute urine with a specific gravity of 1.003 or less. In cases of tubular disease, urinary specific gravity usually remains constant at approximately 1.010, regardless of changing levels in plasma hydration.

MEASURES OF PLASMA CREATININE AND BUN LEVELS

Both creatinine and blood urea nitrogen (BUN) are substances that are generated as end products of protein metabolism and are normally excreted in the urine. With the development of nephron disease, glomerular filtration rate for both creatinine and BUN decreases, and they begin to accumulate in the blood. An increase in the serum creatinine and BUN levels above the norms of 0.7 to 1.5 mg per cent and 10 to 20 mg. per cent, respectively, is called *azotemia*. This condition, which is an indication of renal failure, will be discussed in greater detail subsequently in this chapter.

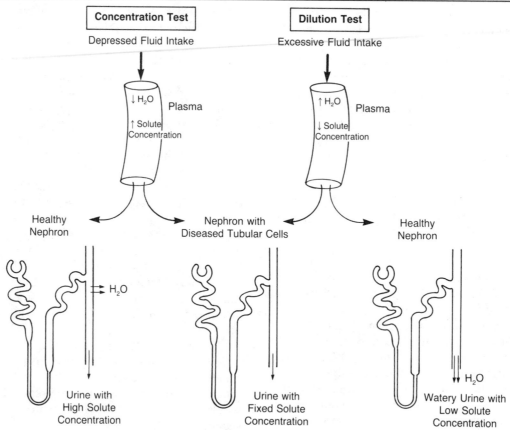

Figure 11.21 The response of the nephron to concentration and dilution tests.

MEASURES OF PROTEIN IN THE URINE

Under normal circumstances, plasma proteins are too large to filter through the glomerular membrane into Bowman's capsule. In certain diseases conditions, however, increasing permeability of the glomerular membrane results in abnormal fluxes of protein, such as albumin, into the urine. Under these circumstances, plasma protein levels will decline as urinary protein concentration increases. The functional changes evolving secondary to protein loss will be elucidated later in this chapter.

MONITORING RENAL FUNCTION: A SUMMARY

Many tests can be used to assess functional renal activity. In many cases, diagnostic evaluations are designed to evaluate one specific aspect of nephron physiology. Thus, whereas clearance tests are helpful in determining glomerular filtration rate, concentration and dilution tests are utilized to measure functional capacity of the renal tubular cells. A brief comparative summary of the diagnostic tests previously discussed is presented in Table 11.3. Used in conjunction with other indices of nephron activity and careful patient assessment, they can prove invaluable in the early diagnosis of renal disease.

TABLE 11.3 **Some Renal Diagnostic Tests**

Test	Designed to Evaluate
Clearance test	Rate of glomerular filtration
Concentration and dilution tests	Functional capacity of the renal tubular cells to adaptively retain and/or eliminate water
Plasma creatinine and BUN	Capacity to eliminate end products of protein metabolism
Protein in the urine	Permeability of glomerular membrane

RENAL PATHOLOGY

Because the renal system plays such a central role in the maintenance of homeostasis, disease of the kidneys characteristically results in disruption of the cellular environment.

Disease can be induced by a wide variety of processes, ranging from infection and inflammation to nonadaptive immune responses. Regardless of cause, however, renal disease usually results in the evolution of one of two major pathological syndromes:

1. *Acute renal failure (ARF)* — characterized by a sudden decline in renal function, with a decrease in urinary output to less than 400 ml. per day.

2. *Chronic renal failure (CRF)* — characterized by a slow and progressive deterioration of the nephrons, terminating in permanent destruction and atrophy of renal tissue.

In the following analysis of renal disease, each syndrome will be studied with respect to specific causative disorders and typical clinical course. Although the two syndromes are treated as separate entities, it is important to keep in mind that they are, in fact, closely intertwined. Several conditions, for example, can cause either acute or chronic renal failure, and are thus difficult to categorize. Perhaps more significantly, acute renal failure can precipitate a pattern of chronic disease, and vice versa, depending upon history and circumstances.

Acute Renal Failure (ARF)

Acute renal failure is a syndrome characterized by rapid onset of renal dysfunction. It, in turn, can be caused by a variety of disorders, which may be classified as *prerenal, intrarenal,* or *postrenal* in nature.

Prerenal disease is caused by any disorder external to the kidneys that decreases the flow of blood to the nephron. Ultimately, functional disorders develop secondary to renal ischemia or depression of glomerular filtration or both. Intrarenal disease is characterized by disease of the renal tissue itself. Although nephron damage is often caused by ischemia, it can also be initiated by immune diseases (such as acute glomerulonephritis) or infec-

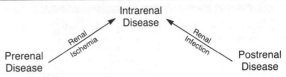

Figure 11.22 The relationship between mechanisms causing acute renal failure.

tious disorders (such as acute pyelonephritis). Postrenal disease, however, is characteristically caused by obstruction of the urinary tract. Usually precipitated by blockage of the ureters or urethra, it often results in urinary reflux back into the renal pelvis, with secondary intrarenal damage.

It is important to note that although ARF often originates with pre- or postrenal disease, almost all disorders eventually lead to subsequent intrarenal disease. Full-blown acute renal failure, in fact, reflects some degree of nephron damage. Thus, pre- and postrenal conditions feed the acute renal failure syndrome, as illustrated in Figure 11.22.

CAUSES OF ACUTE RENAL FAILURE

In discussing the causes of ARF, it is helpful to classify disorders as primarily prerenal, intrarenal, or postrenal in nature. It must be remembered, however, that, in reality, disease proceeds on a continuum, with much potential overlap among these conceptual categories.

Prerenal Pathology As mentioned earlier, prerenal disease is characterized by a decrease in blood flow to the kidneys. As might be expected, this type of disorder often arises secondary to cardiovascular malfunction. Disorders of any origin, however, that result in a decrease of cardiac output can precipitate prerenal disease. Specific causes are varied and extensive. They range from myocardial infarction to neurogenic shock and are summarized in Table 11.4.

As a result of diminished renal blood flow, the kidneys are affected in two primary ways. Initially, the glomerular filtration rate will be depressed, with a subsequent decrease in formation of urinary filtrate. Eventually, the basic survival needs of all nephron cells may

TABLE 11.4 **Causes of Prerenal Disease***

Renal arterial obstruction
    Embolus
    Thrombus
Hypovolemia
    Burns
    Hemorrhage
    Excessive diarrhea and vomiting
Hypotension
    Septic shock
    Neurogenic shock
Cardiac insufficiency

*Adapted from Jones, D. A., Dunbar, C. F., and Jirovec, M. M.: Medical-Surgical Nursing, A Conceptual Approach. New York, McGraw-Hill Book Company, 1978.

be compromised. Decreased supply of oxygen and nutrients, coupled with inefficient removal of metabolic wastes, will then precipitate secondary intrarenal damage.

INTRARENAL PATHOLOGY Intrarenal disease is characterized by primary destruction of renal tissue. Since the symptoms can vary to some extent with the causative disease, it is helpful to have some idea of the various pathways that can lead to intrarenal damage. Selected causative disorders that will be discussed in the following pages include: (1) acute poststreptococcal glomerulonephritis, (2) acute pyelonephritis, (3) renal poisoning, and (4) transfusion reactions.

Acute Poststreptococcal Glomerulonephritis Acute poststreptococcal glomerulonephritis is characterized by severe inflammation of the glomerular membrane secondary to an immune complex reaction.

The nonadaptive immune response that precipitates this disorder has been described in Chapter 8. Specifically, this form of glomerulonephritis is caused by the presence of group A beta-hemolytic streptococci in the bloodstream. These microorganisms are most commonly introduced with a streptococcal infection such as streptococcal sore throat, streptococcal tonsillitis, or scarlet fever. If the bacteria are not eradicated by appropriate medication, they serve as stimuli for the formation of immune complexes within one to three weeks after the onset of initial infection.

As immune complexes become trapped in certain sites throughout the body, they activate complement and initiate localized but severe inflammatory reactions. Since the glomeruli are prime target areas for deposit of these immune bodies, function of the nephron is characteristically affected.

Most typically, damage is centered in the glomerular membrane. Abnormal increases in the number of glomerular cells can often cause blockage and subsequently affect glomerular filtration. Heightened porosity of the membrane, on the other hand, results in considerable increases in glomerular permeability.

Fortunately, the disease normally runs its course in approximately ten days to two weeks. As the acute stage passes, nephrons usually regain functional capacity. Recovery is essentially complete in about 85 per cent of all cases.

Acute Pyelonephritis Pyelonephritis, unlike glomerulonephritis, is caused by direct attack of renal tissue by microorganisms. Most typically, the causative agent is a bacillus that originates in the colon and finds its way into the urethra, often as a result of improper hygiene. Because of the relatively close positioning of anal and urethral orifices in the female, pyelonephritis is a common disease in young girls. As bacteria travel up the urinary tract toward the kidneys, they frequently cause infection of the urinary tract (UTI) or the bladder (cystitis) or both.

Little girls, however, are not the only victims of pyelonephritis. Bacterial contamination of the urinary tract can occur under many circumstances, affecting males and females of any age. Certain conditions do facilitate the development of this disorder and thus increase the likelihood of ultimate renal involvement. *Urinary tract obstructions,* for example, can prevent the free flushing of any contaminated urine out of the lower urethra. *Instrumental examination* of the urinary tract can introduce harmful microorganisms into the normally sterile upper urethra, bladder, or ureters. Finally, abnormal *reflux* or urine from the lower urinary tract back into the kidneys (vesiculoureteral reflux) can accelerate renal contamination.

Regardless of cause or predisposing factors, pyelonephritis is characterized, in the acute stage, by damage progressing from the renal pelvis into the tubular cells. Destruction seems to occur particularly in the medulla, with relatively little glomerular involvement. Although inflammation accompanying the infectious process can lead to necrosis, acute pyelonephritis is usually resolved with minimal residual damage or scarring.

Renal Poisoning Not all intrarenal disorders are caused by infectious or immune processes. There are a number of chemical agents, for example, that can selectively and critically destroy renal tubular cells. Included among these are carbon tetrachloride, a standard component of commercial spot removers, and heavy metals such as mercury. A more complete list is presented in Table 11.5.

In almost all cases, functional changes result as damaged tubular cells slough off and block the nephron. In cases of renal poisoning, the potential for recovery varies. In some instances, repair can occur within three to four weeks. Such is the case with proximal tubular disease caused by mercury or carbon tetrachloride. Alternatively, however, damage can be irreversible, as when entire nephrons are destroyed by exposure to glycol.

Transfusion Reactions Transfusion reactions are caused by administration of red blood cells that are incompatible with an individual's own immune system. In these cases, the transfused red cells, acting as antigens, are subsequently clumped and destroyed by the recipient's antibodies. When red blood cells are broken down, free hemoglobin molecules are released into plasma. These molecules, small enough to pass through the glomerular membrane, filter into the nephron, where they become caught in the tubular lumens and block urine formation.

POSTRENAL PATHOLOGY Postrenal disease is caused by disorders that originate external to the kidneys, in areas designed to transport or store urine as it moves to be excreted.

Most commonly, postrenal disease is associated with obstructive disorders, which interfere with the elimination of urine while simultaneously facilitating the development of renal infection.

Causes of obstruction are varied and include scarring or fibrosis of the ureters or urethra secondary to previous damage or trauma, stones, neoplasms, and — in the older male — enlargement of the prostate gland.

CAUSES OF ACUTE RENAL FAILURE: A SUMMARY It can be seen that many different disorders may terminate in acute renal failure. Although the origin may be prerenal, intrarenal, or postrenal in nature, almost all conditions eventually lead to some degree of nephron damage. Very often, in fact, acute renal failure is characterized by a phenomenon described as acute tubular necrosis (ATN).

Whenever disease causes destruction of the proximal convoluted tubule, loop of Henle, distal convoluted tubule, or collecting tubule of the nephron, acute tubular necrosis is said to exist.

Clearly, almost all prerenal, intrarenal, and postrenal disease may eventually cause this type of dysfunction. The only major exception is acute poststreptococcal glomerulonephritis, in which the majority of damage is localized in the glomerulus.

The extent to which acute tubular necrosis develops is largely dependent upon the severity and duration of renal disease. Mild ischemia, for example, may cause slight decreases in glomerular filtration rate without actually resulting in tubular destruction. Even

---

TABLE 11.5 **Nephrotoxic Agents***

Solvents
    Carbon tetrachloride
    Methanol
    Ethylene glycol
Heavy metals
    Lead
    Arsenic
    Mercury
Antibiotics
    Kanamycin
    Gentamicin
    Polymyxin B
    Amphotericin B
    Colistin
    Neomycin
    Phenazopyridine
Pesticides
Mushrooms

*Adapted from Phipps, W. J., Long, B. C., and Woods, N. F. (eds.): Medical-Surgical Nursing, Concepts and Clinical Practice. St. Louis, The C. V. Mosby Company, 1979.

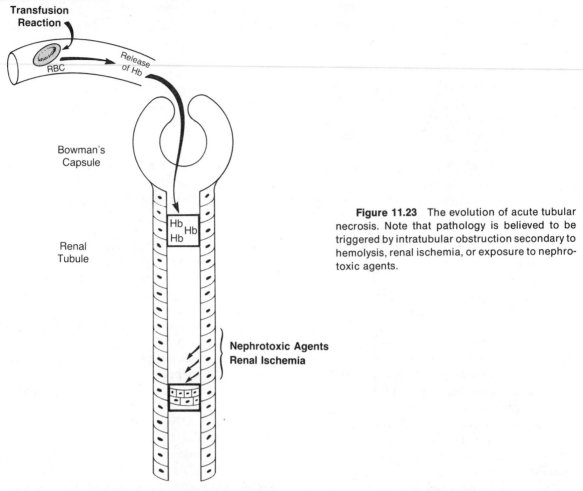

Figure 11.23   The evolution of acute tubular necrosis. Note that pathology is believed to be triggered by intratubular obstruction secondary to hemolysis, renal ischemia, or exposure to nephrotoxic agents.

renal poisoning or acute pyelonephritis does not always lead to extensive tubular damage. The mechanisms by which some major renal disorders can precipitate acute tubular necrosis are summarized diagrammatically in Figure 11.23.

CLINICAL COURSE OF ACUTE RENAL FAILURE

In cases of acute renal failure, it is not possible to identify a single pattern of signs and symptoms. Instead, clinical manifestations may vary considerably and depend upon the pathogenesis.

If damage is localized primarily in the glomerulus, for example, a clinical picture described as the *syndrome of acute nephritis* emerges. If, on the other hand, damage is present primarily in the tubules of the nephron, disease typically progresses through three characteristic stages: from *oliguria* to *diuresis* to *recovery*.

In some instances, acute renal failure can be secondary to disorders that destroy neither the glomerulus nor the tubular cells of the nephron. Most typically, this pattern is seen in cases of prerenal disease involving marginal ischemia. For discussion purposes, the characteristic clinical picture accompanying this aspect of renal disease will be referred to as the *prerenal syndrome.*

SYNDROME OF ACUTE NEPHRITIS. In cases of acute poststreptococcal glomerulonephrits, renal function is altered by extensive proliferation of epithelial cells in the glomeruli. The syndrome of acute nephritis evolves as increases in glomerular permeability cause hematuria and mild proteinuria. Simultaneous obstruction and swelling of glomerular capillaries are believed to be responsible for a decrease in glomerular filtration rate. Subsequent retention of fluids and electrolytes is usually manifested clinically by edema and mild hypertension.

SYNDROME ACCOMPANYING TUBU-LAR PATHOLOGY When renal disease leads to destruction of the tubular cells of the nephron (as typically occurs in cases of acute tubular necrosis), a characteristic response pattern is noted. It usually develops in three stages, progressing from oliguria to diuresis to recovery.

Oliguria Oliguria, defined as a urinary output of less than 400 ml. per day, is often an early indication of acute tubular necrosis. Usually lasting anywhere from one day to six weeks, the average duration is between seven and ten days. As the formation of urine declines, fluids, electrolytes, and the wastes of protein metabolism accumulate in extracellular fluid. Resulting disequilibrium is often characterized by (1) azotemia, (2) metabolic acidosis, (3) hyperkalemia, (4) hypernatremia (or hyponatremia if the patient is overhydrated), and (5) hypervolemia, with secondary manifestations of circulatory overload and pulmonary edema. Sustained oliguria can lead to critical systemic physiological changes. These imbalances, loosely referred to as the *uremic syndrome*, will be analyzed later in the chapter.

Because tubular cells are specifically functional in the conservation of both water and sodium, acute tubular necrosis is associated with characteristic changes in the nature of urinary filtrate. Although the *amount* of sodium entering Bowman's capsule is depressed during oliguria, its *concentration* in urine tends to be elevated because of deficient tubular reabsorption. Simultaneously, the concentration of most other urinary solutes will be *decreased* because of failure to adequately reabsorb filtered water (causing a decrease in specific gravity).

Diuresis As healing begins, improvement is reflected in the production of more than 400 ml. of urine per day. It is believed that the elevation in urinary output is promoted by high plasma levels of protein metabolic wastes generated by previous oliguria. Once filtration is re-established, large quantities of creatinine and urea tend to draw water and sodium along with them as they move through the nephron to be excreted. There is, in fact, a danger of excessive fluid and sodium loss during this stage, if output is not monitored carefully.

Although the glomerulus is operating sufficiently to faciliate urinary output, the tubular cells have not yet regained normal functional capacity. The ability to adaptively modify glomerular filtrate by appropriate retention of water and electrolytes is not yet evident. Concentration or dilution tests would thus reveal urine of depressed or fixed specific gravity.

Recovery Full recovery is characterized by healing of tubular epithelial cells. This process can take up to a year, but, most typically, functional activity is restored within several weeks. Unfortunately, not all individuals are restored to health. In approximately 50 per cent of these cases, failure to heal terminates in death.

PRERENAL SYNDROME As mentioned earlier, not all cases of renal disease are characterized by glomerular or tubular damage. Prerenal disease, characterized by marginal ischemia, presents its own clinical picture distinct from that of acute nephritis or acute tubular necrosis.

Often caused by hypovolemic or cardiogenic shock, the prerenal syndrome is characterized by a sluggish flow of fluid through the tubules of the nephron. A resulting increase in sodium reabsorption causes a depletion in urinary sodium (typically measures less than 5 mEq./L.). Simultaneously, however, the concentration of most other urinary solutes will be *increased* owing to excessive retention of water in plasma. An increase in the specific gravity of urine subsequently results.

To the extent that glomerular blood flow is sufficiently depressed, secondary release of ADH and aldosterone may occur. Resulting fluid retention may intensify manifestations of hypervolemia and edema. Plasma sodium concentration will be either normal or depressed, depending upon the relative reabsorption of sodium and water.

Because depressed renal blood flow causes a decrease in glomerular filtration rate, oliguria will typically develop. As a result, the prerenal syndrome is characterized by azotemia, with elevations in BUN and plasma creatinine levels. Since the tubular cells continue to be functional, however, the nephron retains its ability to adaptively concentrate and modify the glomerular filtrate in response to changing cellular needs.

TABLE 11.6   **Acute Renal Failure: Three Major Patterns**

Pathological Syndrome	Underlying Causative Mechanism	Characteristic Features
Syndrome of acute nephritis	Excessive proliferation of epithelial cells in the glomeruli; mild increase in glomerular permeability Most frequently associated with acute post-streptococcal glomerulonephritis	Mild proteinuria Hematuria Edema Mild hypertension
Syndrome associated with tubular disease	Destruction of the tubular cells in the nephron Induced in a variety of ways, including exposure to nephrotoxins, renal infection, prolonged renal ischemia, and transfusion reactions	Initial oliguria, associated with fluid and electrolyte imbalance and azotemia Diuresis following oliguria, characterized by excessive fluid loss Functional inability to adaptively modify urinary content
Prerenal syndrome	*Marginal* renal ischemia Most commonly caused by renal arterial obstruction, hypovolemia, hypotension, or cardiac insufficiency	Decrease in glomerular filtration rate, inducing subsequent azotemia and oliguria Possible fluid retention and edema Normal response to renal concentration and dilution tests

CLINICAL COURSE OF ACUTE RENAL FAILURE: A SUMMARY   In review, it can be seen that patients in acute renal failure can present widely varying clinical pictures. Symptoms depend, to a large extent, upon the nature of the causative disease.

The syndromes discussed in the previous pages reflect three major patterns of renal disorders. A comparative summary is presented in Table 11.6. It must be remembered, however, that many disorders may be characterized by a combination of these syndromes. In the end, the composite clinical picture is determined primarily by the specific nature of renal damage.

Chronic Renal Failure (CRF)

Chronic renal failure is characterized by progressive and irreversible destruction of renal tissue. Damage usually proceeds slowly, terminating in death when a sufficient number of nephrons have been rendered nonfunctional.

CAUSES OF CHRONIC RENAL FAILURE

A wide variety of renal disorders can cause chronic renal failure. To facilitate study, the diseases leading to CRF can generally be classified into two major groups: (1) those characterized by glomerular pathology, and (2) those characterized by tubular or interstitial pathology.

Although somewhat arbitrary, these categories do afford a useful conceptual framework. It is important to remember, however, that, disease rarely remains confined to one area of the nephron. Glomerular damage may eventually disrupt tubular-interstitial tissue, and vice versa. In the final stages of failure, all parts of the nephron are invariably affected by disease.

DISEASES CAUSING GLOMERULAR PATHOLOGY   A large number of glomerular diseases associated with chronic renal failure are initiated by nonadaptive immune responses. In these cases, disease derives primarily from one of two major mechanisms:

1. Nonglomerular antigens unite with antibodies and are carried to the glomeruli via the blood. Complement is activated, causing subsequent initiation of an inflammatory reaction. Glomerular destruction is believed to be caused primarily by enzymes released at the inflammatory site. Characteristic examples of this type of disease process include acute

poststreptococcal glomerulonephritis, and systemic lupus erythematosus (SLE).

2. Antibodies are formed to act directly against one's own glomerular protein. This autoimmune response causes destruction at the glomeruli and seems to be directed primarily against the basement membrane. A characteristic example is antiglomerular basement nephritis.

Manifestations of Chronic Glomerular Pathology Regardless of the initiating mechanism, glomerular destruction inevitably causes changes in the filtration process. The *nephrotic syndrome* typically develops as a result of underlying glomerular damage.

The nephrotic syndrome is caused primarily by a chronic inflammatory process that increases the porosity and permeability of the glomerular membrane. Subsequent loss of excessive amounts of protein (greater than 3.5 gm. per day) in the urine is a characteristic symptom.

As plasma protein levels decline, a chain reaction of physiological imbalance is initiated. Decreases in colloid osmotic pressure accompany the protein loss, causing a shift of fluid out of the plasma compartment into the interstitial fluid. Edema thus develops while plasma volume decreases.

The clinical picture is further complicated by secondary responses to plasma loss. Glomerular filtration rate, for example, is depressed as plasma volume falls. As a result, renin is released from the juxtaglomerular apparatus, leading to an increase in aldosterone output. Simultaneously, receptors responding to falling plasma volume trigger release of ADH. Both aldosterone and ADH significantly increase water retention, thereby aggravating the edematous condition.

In short, the nephrotic syndrome is characterized by protein in the urine (proteinuria), depressed plasma protein levels (hypoalbuminemia), and edema. The physiological basis for some of the symptoms is summarized diagrammatically in Figure 11.24.

Types of Chronic Glomerular Pathology In the study of chronic glomerular disease, it is common to distinguish between two general conditions. Typically, disorders are classified as primary or systemic. *Primary* disorders are those in which the initiating factors are direct-

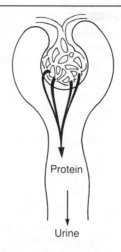

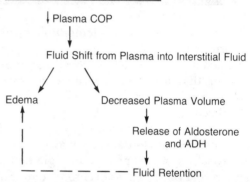

Figure 11.24 The nephrotic syndrome: underlying pathophysiology.

ed more or less exclusively against renal tissue. *Systemic* diseases are fairly general in nature and affect the nephrons only secondarily. Some classic examples of each type will be discussed in the following pages.

PRIMARY GLOMERULAR PATHOLOGY The most common example of primary glomerular pathology is represented by the broad entity referred to as *chronic glomerulonephritis (CGN)*. A major cause of chronic renal failure, this disease process is induced by a wide variety of specific disorders. The initiating factor, in most cases, is some form of immune disease. Progressive glomerular destruction terminates in atrophied nonfunctional kidneys, usually with end-stage involvement of all portions of the nephron.

In the early stages, different forms of glomerulonephritis vary with respect to causative factors and site of tissue damage. A few major differences are summarized in Table

TABLE 11.7 **Some Examples of Primary Glomerular Disease**

Disorder	Underlying Histological Changes	Causative Mechanism
Antiglomerular basement membrane nephritis	Injury of the glomerular basement membrane	Autoimmune response in which antibodies react against fixed antigens in the basement membrane
Membranous glomerulonephritis (MGN)	Thickening of the glomerular capillary wall	Immune response affecting the epithelial side of the basement membrane
Lipoid nephrosis, or minimal-change disease	Destruction of foot processes in glomerular epithelial cells	Unknown but postulated to be of an immune nature
Membranoproliferative glomerulonephritis (MPGN)	Alterations in the structure of the basement membrane; proliferation of associated mesangial cells	Believed to be caused by an immune complex mechanism

11.7. Any of these types of glomerulonephritis can terminate in CGN if damage is sufficiently sustained and severe. It is interesting to note, however, that in about 33 per cent of the cases, CGN occurs without any previous history of renal disease.

SYSTEMIC GLOMERULAR PATHOLOGY In many instances, disorders originating outside the renal system precipitate glomerular changes that can progress to chronic renal failure. Primary examples of this phenomenon include: (1) systemic lupus erythematosus (SLE), (2) serum sickness nephritis, and (3) diabetic glomerulosclerosis.

Systemic lupus erythematosus (SLE). SLE is an immunopathological condition characterized by the abnormal formation of antibodies against the DNA in one's own cells. Autoimmune in nature, it results in the formation of immune complexes that subsequently deposit throughout the body, causing considerable tissue destruction. The glomerulus, unfortunately, seems to be a major site of immune complex deposition. The pathological changes that result can produce classic cases of minimal change nephritis, diffuse proliferative glomerulonephritis, and diffuse membranous glomerulonephritis, as described earlier.

Serum sickness nephritis. Serum sickness nephritis, like SLE, is an immune disorder. In this case, immune complexes are formed in response to the introduction of a foreign protein and subsequently deposit in the glomerulus. The disease becomes chronic when the foreign protein (antigen) derives from a source that can be continuously reproduced within the body. Such is the case when the antigen is a living virus or bacterium. Cases of serum sickness nephritis have been identified in humans secondary to such diseases as bacterial endocarditis, syphilis, malaria, and leprosy.

Diabetic glomerulosclerosis. Unlike SLE or serum sickness nephritis, diabetes does not induce immunopathology. It does, however, cause characteristic glomerular damage, which typically includes thickening of the basement membrane and increases in glomerular permeability. It is believed that the vascular complications accompanying diabetes contribute to glomerular pathology. Regardless of the precise mechanism, however, it has been established that renal complications exist in 90 per cent of all patients who have had diabetes for more than ten years.

DISEASES CAUSING TUBULAR OR INTERSTITIAL PATHOLOGY Under normal circumstances, urinary filtrate is processed by the renal tubules. To the extent that these structures are damaged, the reabsorption and secretion of many critical constituents will be impeded. In many cases, an early indication of tubular damage is the excretion of large volumes of dilute urine. This occurs as the ability to selectively retain water or sodium or both is progressively lost.

Tubular-interstitial diseases are varied

and can be categorized according to initiating cause, as follows: (1) vascular, (2) infectious, (3) toxic, and (4) obstructive.

Vascular Causes Long-standing arterial hypertension causes characteristic changes in blood vessels. Disease often derives from hardening and narrowing of the vascular walls, with subsequent development of ischemia. When these changes, secondary to hypertension, affect the renal arteries and arterioles, the condition is specifically referred to as *nephrosclerosis*.

It will be remembered that the hypertension initiating this condition is most often of unknown orgin. Described as *primary*, or *essential, hypertension*, it is believed to be caused by a combination of genetic and environmental factors.

Regardless of origin, hypertension, once established, is inevitably aggravated by a secondary renal mechanism. Once blood pressure begins to rise and remains chronically elevated, subsequent narrowing of renal arteries and arterioles precipitates renal ischemia. Diminished blood flow, in turn, triggers the release of renin, which leads to: (1) systemic vasoconstriction, and (2) release of aldosterone, with secondary retention of both sodium and water. Renal nephrosclerosis induced by essential hypertension is thus further escalated by secondary hypertension of renal origin, as illustrated in Figure 11.25.

As a result of nephrosclerosis, progressive renal vascular occlusion may terminate in necrosis of functional kidney tissue. In many individuals, nephrosclerosis first appears in a *benign* form associated with chronic long-term arteriosclerosis. Rarely does benign nephrosclerosis precipitate a serious renal crisis. Occasionally, however, *malignant* nephrosclerosis develops owing to a sudden galloping and uncontrollable increase in blood pressure. In these instances, ischemia and necrosis can cause renal death.

Infectious Causes Chronic renal infections can also lead to chronic renal failure. *Chronic pyelonephritis* is a good example of this type of pathology. As described earlier, pyelonephritis is an infectious disorder characterized by inflammation and fibrosis of the renal pelvis and tubular-interstitial tissue of the medulla. The chronic phase is usually associated

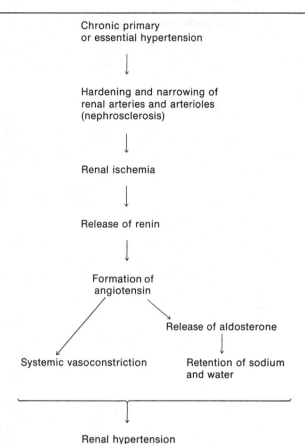

Figure 11.25 The evolution of renal hypertension

with ongoing obstructive or reflux disease. If infection recurs regularly, damage can be extensive and progressive. As increasing numbers of nephrons are affected by the disease process, chronic renal failure can set in, characterized by irreversible loss of kidney function.

Toxic Causes In dealing with the effect of toxins upon the kidneys, it is important to realize that varying responses can be induced by harmful chemicals. Some substances cause rapid destruction, leading to acute renal failure. Others are capable of inducing slow, cumulative tubular injury. If these changes are of sufficient magnitude, they will eventually culminate in chronic renal failure.

The most common example of long-term injury is found in cases of *chronic analgesic nephritis*. Associated with extensive exposure to high-level doses of analgesics (such as phenacetin, aspirin, and acetaminophen), it usually results in considerable tubular-interstitial damage. Fortunately, it is one of

TABLE 11.8 **Causes of Chronic Renal Failure**

Type of Disorder	Mechanism Inducing Disorder	Causative Diseases
GLOMERULAR PATHOLOGY		
Primary	Disease causes primary destruction of glomerular tissue; most often characterized by hypersensitivity reaction against glomerular protein	Chronic glomerulonephritis Antiglomerular basement nephritis Membranous glomerulonephritis Lipoid nephrosis Membranoproliferative glomerulonephritis
Systemic	Systemic disease acts to cause secondary glomerular damage	Acute poststreptococcal glomerulonephritis Systemic lupus erythematosus Serum sickness nephritis Diabetic glomerulosclerosis
TUBULAR-INTERSTITIAL PATHOLOGY		
Vascular	Narrowing and hardening of the arteries and arterioles supplying the kidneys	Chronic essential hypertension
Infectious	Inflammation and fibrosis of renal pelvis and medulla caused by pathogenic microbes	Chronic pyelonephritis
Toxic	Slow, cumulative tubular damage caused by chronic exposure to nephrotoxic agents	Long-term exposure to high levels of analgesics, lead, cadmium, uranium
Obstructive	Damage to the nephron caused by fluid back-pressure secondary to obstruction; often associated with infection	Renal calculi Renal tumors Urethral or ureteral strictures

the few types of chronic diseases in which improvement and recovery are possible with proper treatment and removal of the toxic agent. Other substances that can cause chronic renal failure, after prolonged exposure, include lead, cadmium, and uranium.

Obstructive Causes Obstruction in the urinary tract can lead to progressive damage to the nephron, as fluid back-pressure traumatizes tissue. When this obstruction is chronic, pathological changes can terminate in chronic renal failure. As would be expected, tissue damage will be accelerated to the extent that obstruction is coupled with infection.

Obstruction can be caused by any number of phenomena, including stones, clots, tumors, urethral or ureteral strictures, and enlargement of the prostate gland. Although symptoms vary with the degree, location, and nature of the obstruction, functional recovery is unlikely if the blockage persists for longer than four to six months.

CAUSES OF CHRONIC RENAL FAILURE: A SUMMARY It can be seen that a wide variety of diseases can initiate chronic

renal failure. Whether glomerular or tubular-interstitial in nature, they are all characterized by progressive changes that culminate in irreversible renal damage. A comparative review of the major disorders that often terminate in CRF is presented in Table 11.8.

CLINICAL COURSE OF CHRONIC RENAL FAILURE

Regardless of the initiating factors, chronic renal failure typically evolves progressively, through a number of characteristic stages, as follows:

1. *Decreased renal reserve* — At this stage, damage is marginal and the kidneys remain functional. Clinical symptoms may be detected only at times of stress.

2. *Renal insufficiency* — At this stage, 75 per cent of functional renal tissue has been destroyed. Glomerular filtration rate is decreased by approximately 25 per cent, accompanied by increases in BUN and serum creatinine. Tubular-interstitial damage often causes an increase in the elimination of urine

(polyuria) as ability to conserve water and sodium declines. Particularly characteristic is an increase in the nocturnal output of urine to 700 ml. or more (nocturia).

3. *End-stage renal failure, or uremia* — At this stage, 90 per cent of renal tissue has been destroyed. Glomerular filtration rate is decreased by approximately 90 per cent, and tubular cells are essentially nonfunctional. Because of the complexity of end-stage disease, this phase of chronic renal failure is well worth further exploration.

As glomerular filtration rate is significantly depressed, end-stage renal failure culminates in a complex clinical picture referred to as the *uremic syndrome*. Characteristically, changes in homeostasis are accompanied by progressive systemic dysfunction. It is believed that fluid-electrolyte and acid-base imbalances trigger secondary disease in many critical structures.

In studying uremia, it is helpful to differentiate between what we shall call *primary* and *secondary* symptoms. Primary symptoms are those changes in plasma chemistry that result directly from renal malfunction. Secondary symptoms, on the other hand, are manifested as systemic disorders that derive indirectly from alterations in the cellular fluid environment.

PRIMARY SYMPTOMS OF UREMIA

For the most part, primary symptoms of uremia are noted when the kidneys are unable to sustain their critical role in the maintenance of homeostasis. Resulting imbalances vary but usually include the following:

1. *Hyperkalemia*. Since approximately 80 per cent of potassium intake is normally excreted in the urine, it is easy to see why a depression of glomerular filtration would lead to excessive accumulation of plasma potassium. Hyperkalemia is further aggravated by the development of acidosis. It will be remembered that as the plasma concentration of hydrogen ions increases, H^+ shifts into the intracellular fluid in exchange for K^+. This exchange, illustrated in Figure 11.26, contributes to the existing potassium imbalance.

2. *Sodium and water imbalance*. Whereas excessive losses of water and sodium are often characteristic during later stages of renal insufficiency, end-stage disease is frequently as-

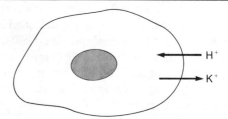

Figure 11.26 The generation of hyperkalemia secondary to acidosis.

sociated with sodium and water retention. As glomerular filtration critically declines, neither sodium nor water can pass sufficiently into Bowman's capsule. Their subsequent accumulation in extracellular fluid is often aggravated by the release of renin from the juxtaglomerular cells.

3. *Metabolic acidosis.* As normal functioning of the nephron is diminished, the ability to selectively monitor acid-base balance is progressively lost. Since cellular metabolism results in the generation of more acid than base, a relative excess of hydrogen ions occurs. Resulting metabolic acidosis is characterized by a depression of plasma bicarbonate, as this substance is used to buffer the accumulating hydrogen ions (see Chapter 7).

4. *Hyperuricemia*. With advancing renal disease, uric acid accumulates excessively in the plasma. Unable to be excreted, uric acid will often be deposited abnormally as salt crystals in joints and soft tissue. The resulting condition, which is associated with considerable pain, is referred to as gout.

5. *Azotemia.* Inability to efficiently excrete the wastes of nitrogen metabolism is accompanied by a characteristic increase in the plasma levels of urea, creatinine, phenols, and guanidines. It is believed that many of the secondary symptoms of uremia are in some way related to the toxic effects of these metabolic wastes.

SECONDARY SYMPTOMS OF UREMIA

Secondary symptoms generally develop in response to fluid-electrolyte and acid-base imbalances. Most often, their evolution parallels the progress of azotemia. Systemic changes are fairly widespread and include the following:

1. *Anemia.* Anemia is usually evident in the terminal stages of renal failure. It is caused largely by the inability of the diseased

nephron to produce sufficient erythropoietin. Since erythropoietin is an essential stimulus to the normal production of red blood cells, its lack results in a decline in the number of erythrocytes. The condition is exacerbated by the existing toxic fluid environment, which, for some reason, promotes early breakdown of red blood cells.

2. *Integumentary system*. Characteristically, the patient in advanced stages of renal failure shows alteration of skin color. Appearance ranges from waxy yellow (in whites) to yellow-brown (in browns) to ashen gray (in blacks). It is believed that the deposit of urinary pigments, such as urochrome, in the skin is largely responsible for this phenomenon.

When the BUN level is excessively high, fine white crystals of urea are noted on the skin surface in areas where perspiration is particularly heavy. This deposit is known as uremic frost. It is a manifestation of the body's attempt to rid itself of excess nitrogen wastes via the sweat glands when the nephrons are unable to adequately fulfill their excretory function.

3. *Cardiovascular system*. Most often, cardiovascular symptoms arise secondary to fluid retention. As renal failure evolves, associated elevations in extracellular fluid volume can increase the workload of the heart. Congestive heart failure will result if the myocardial muscle is sufficiently stressed.

4. *Respiratory system*. Characteristically, pulmonary edema will follow in the wake of congestive heart failure. As the pumping efficiency of cardiac muscle declines, end systolic volume will increase. In the left side of the heart, there is resistance to the normal flow of blood from pulmonary veins into the left atrium. Back-pressure causes excessive retention of fluid in the pulmonary vessels of the lungs, with subsequent flux out of capillaries into interstitial spaces. This mechanism, illustrated in Figure 11.27, is responsible for many secondary problems, including decreases in pulmonary compliance and depressed pulmonary diffusion.

Pulmonary edema is often superimposed upon altered ventilation patterns. Kussmaul respirations, for example, are frequently seen. The increases in rate and depth of respirations are evidence of attempts to compensate for the metabolic acidosis accompanying renal failure. It will be remembered that increased expiration of carbon dioxide can offset a drastic plasma pH change whenever nonvolatile acids accumulate internally.

5. *Digestive system*. It is believed that the

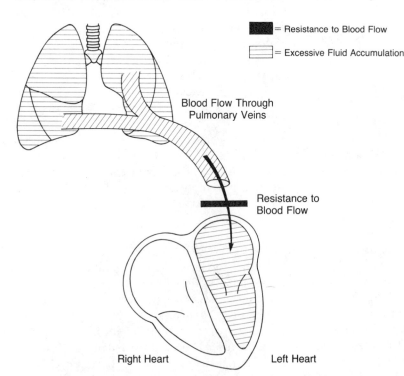

■ = Resistance to Blood Flow

▭ = Excessive Fluid Accumulation

Blood Flow Through Pulmonary Veins

Resistance to Blood Flow

Right Heart   Left Heart

Figure 11.27 The evolution of pulmonary edema.

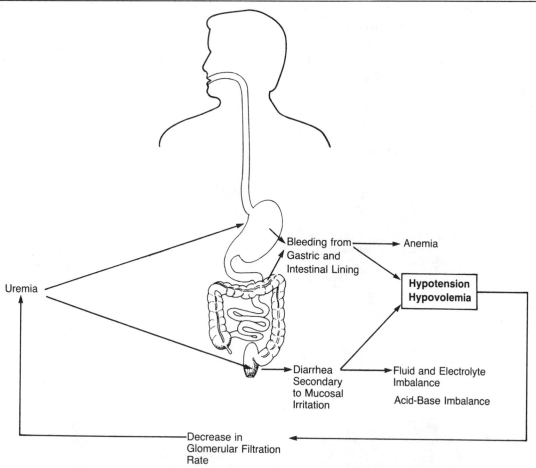

Figure 11.28 Involvement of the digestive system in the uremic syndrome.

gastrointestinal organs are directly affected by the azotemia of renal failure. Altered cellular fluid environment seems to induce mucosal ulcerations in the lining of the stomach and intestines. Subsequent bleeding can aggravate any existing anemia and if excessive, result in a depression of blood volume and blood pressure. If diarrhea, nausea, and vomiting should occur secondary to gastrointestinal irritation, the potential for dehydration is further increased. To the extent that fluid volume declines sufficiently, a cyclic and additional decrease in glomerular filtration rate may occur. The progressive involvement of the digestive system in the uremic syndrome is illustrated in Figure 11.28.

6. *Skeletal system.* The many skeletal disorders manifested during renal failure are collectively referred to as renal *osteodystrophy*. To fully understand the mechanisms underlying alterations in bone tissue, it is essential to review the calcium-parathormone feedback mechanisms (see Chapter 5).

Most frequently, skeletal disorders are of two major types:

a. *Osteomalacia.* Osteomalacia is a disorder due primarily to inadequate deposit of calcium in bone tissue. It is caused by deficiency of a form of vitamin D that is normally activated by the kidney. It will be remembered that vitamin D is essential to the absorption of calcium out of the gastrointestinal tract into the blood. As plasma calcium levels decline, ossification is affected.

b. *Osteitis fibrosa.* Osteitis fibrosa is a condition caused primarily by elevated levels of parathormone. Since parathormone promotes the breakdown and demineralization of bone, it results in considerably weakened skeletal tissue.

The mechanism whereby parathormone excess develops is relatively intricate and worthy of brief mention. In short, the endocrine change is triggered initially by a decrease in glomerular filtration rate accompanying renal failure. As urine formation is de-

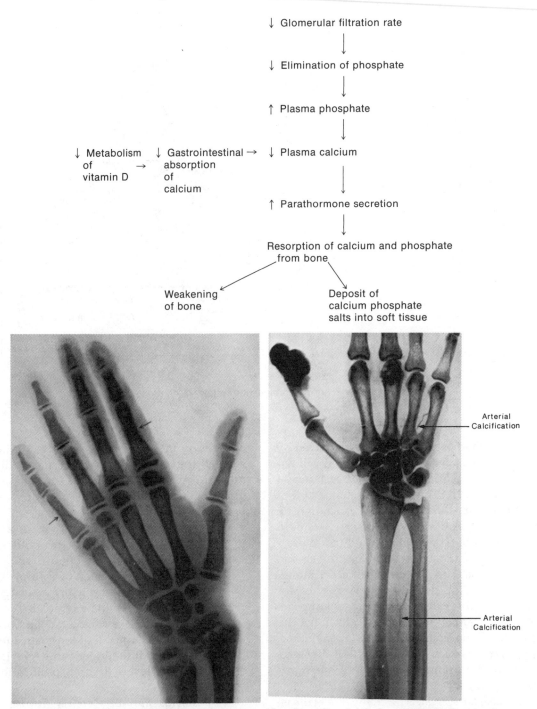

↓ Glomerular filtration rate

↓ Elimination of phosphate

↑ Plasma phosphate

↓ Metabolism of vitamin D → ↓ Gastrointestinal absorption of calcium → ↓ Plasma calcium

↑ Parathormone secretion

Resorption of calcium and phosphate from bone

Weakening of bone

Deposit of calcium phosphate salts into soft tissue

Arterial Calcification

Arterial Calcification

Figure 11.29 The evolution of osteodystrophy. (From Shanks, S. C., and Kerley, P., eds.: A Textbook of X-Ray Diagnosis, Vol. VI, Bones, Joints, and Soft Tissues, 4th ed. Philadelphia: W. B. Saunders Co., 1971. Used by permission.)

pressed, increasing levels of phosphate accumulate in the extracellular fluid. Chemical principles tell us that as phosphate levels increase, calcium concentration declines. Decreased plasma calcium, in turn, triggers the secretion of parathormone.

Parathormone serves, initially, to partially correct existing imbalances. By triggering the breakdown of bone, it causes the release of much-needed calcium into extracellular fluid. If this process lasts for a sufficient duration, however, hypercalcemia can be induced — with deposits of excess calcium salts in joints and soft tissue. The pathological chain of events underlying osteitis fibrosa is summarized in Figure 11.29.

CLINICAL COURSE OF CHRONIC RENAL FAILURE: A SUMMARY

As can be seen, the terminal stage of chronic renal failure is characterized by widespread systemic disease. Primary changes, resulting directly from renal malfunction, are accompanied by pathological alterations in many critical structures. The total picture of end-stage disease is summarized in Table 11.9.

MANAGEMENT OF CHRONIC RENAL FAILURE

Since chronic renal failure is, by definition, an irreversible condition, treatment op-

TABLE 11.9 **Some Primary Manifestations of Chronic Renal Failure**

Physiological Imbalance	Cause	Clinical Manifestations
Hyperkalemia	Decrease in glomerular filtration rate Metabolic acidosis	Cardiac arrhythmias Weakness Nausea Intestinal colic; diarrhea Muscular irritability Flaccid paralysis
Metabolic acidosis	Decrease in glomerular filtration rate	Compensatory Kussmaul respirations Hyperkalemia Hypercalcemia
Sodium and water retention	Decrease in glomerular filtration rate Release of renin	Hypervolemia Possible circulatory overload, with congestive heart failure
Hyperuricemia	Decrease in glomerular filtration rate	Gout
Osteodystrophy	Decrease in glomerular filtration rate Renal disease	Weakening of bone Deposit of calcium phosphate salts in soft tissue
Anemia	Decreased production of erythropoietin by diseased kidney Gastrointestinal bleeding	Pallor Hypoxemia Compensatory increase in cardiac and respiratory rate
Azotemia	Decrease in glomerular filtration rate	Anemia (secondary to hemolysis) Altered skin color Uremic frost Gastrointestinal bleeding and diarrhea (secondary to mucosal irritation) Anemia and hypovolemia (secondary to gastrointestinal bleeding and diarrhea)

tions are well defined. Either (1) the work of the kidneys must be artificially maintained by a process called *dialysis*, or (2) the damaged kidney must be replaced by a *transplant*. Each alternative has its pros and cons, and a comparative summary of the advantages and disadvantages can be found in Table 11.10. In the event that neither option is available or feasible, uremic syndrome will terminate in death.

DIALYSIS Dialysis is a procedure whereby particles dissolved in one fluid compartment are exchanged with particles dissolved in another fluid compartment across a selectively permeable membrane.

In essence, the purpose of dialysis is to functionally mimic renal activity by providing an artificial means of excreting wastes and maintaining fluid and electrolyte balance. During dialysis, fluid in the body is juxtaposed to an artificial fluid called a dialysate. The constituents of the dialysate are regulated to equal those in normal plasma. Water and dissolved particles move across the selectively permeable membrane from where they are in greater concentration to where they are in lesser concentration. As a result, if a substance is present in greater than ideal concentration in the body fluid, it will move into the dialysate, thence to be removed. Conversely, if a constituent is lacking in body fluid, it will move from the dialysate into body fluid. The basic process is illustrated in Figure 11.30.

In the treatment of chronic renal failure, the dialysis procedure can take two forms: (1) *hemodialysis,* in which the blood of a patient is passed through an artificial dialyzer contain-

TABLE 11.10 **Comparison of Dialysis and Well-Functioning Renal Transplant in the Management of End-Stage Renal Failure***

Effect on	With Dialysis	With Well-Functioning Transplant
Renal filtration	Only during dialysis	24 hours/day
Nutrition	Na, K, protein, and fluid restrictions	Possible Na restriction for up to one year after transplant
Erythropoietic system	Anemia, fatigue	Normal red blood cells and hematocrit
Skeletal system	Renal osteodystrophy Hyperparathyroidism	No further bone resorption Possible hyperparathyroidism Avascular necrosis
Nervous system	Peripheral, gastrointestinal, and genitourinary neuropathy	Neuropathy will not progress and may improve
Sexuality	Decreased libido Frequent impotence	Improved libido Impotence may persist
Liver	Increased risk of hepatitis from recurrent extracorporeal circulation and transfusion	10% incidence of hepatitis due to azathioprine therapy
Cardiovascular system	Risk of shunt infection, clotting, exsanguination, and frequent site changes Accelerated atherosclerosis Ventricular hypertrophy, heart failure Uremic pericarditis Cardiac tamponade	No need for vascular access Decrease in atherosclerotic process Ventricular size sometimes returns to normal
Muscular system	Decreased muscle mass due to dietary limits Decreased exercise tolerance	Myopathy which improves when steroid dosage decreases and patient's activity increases
Lungs	Risk of pulmonary edema, congestive heart failure	Pulmonary infections secondary to immunosuppressive therapy
Dependence	Dependent on machine to support life	Dependent on medications
Mortality	10% for first and second years, 36% for third year and increasing	20% for first year, then decreases

*From Hudak, C. M., Lohr, T. S., and Gallo, B. M.: Critical Care Nursing, 2nd ed. Philadelphia, J. B. Lippincott Company, 1977. Used by permission.

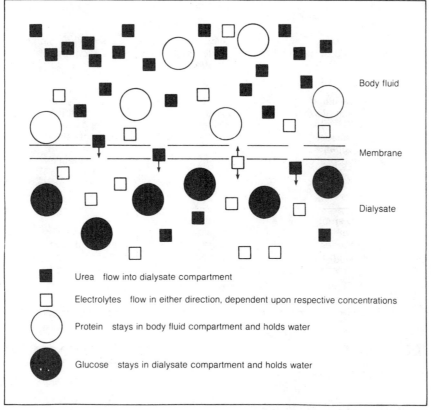

Figure 11.30 Dialysis process. (From Jones et al: Medical-Surgical Nursing. A Conceptual Approach. New York, McGraw-Hill Book Company, 1978. Used by permission.)

ing a selectively permeable membrane and the dialysate fluid; and (2) *peritoneal dialysis,* in which the dialysate fluid flows directly through the peritoneal cavity, with the wall of the intestines serving as the selectively permeable membrane.

TRANSPLANT In many cases of terminal renal failure, it may be decided that transplant is a preferable option to long-term dialysis. This involves introduction of a donor kidney into the body of the patient; the procedure is subject to failure if rejection occurs.

As mentioned in Chapter 8, rejection of a transplanted organ is normally precipitated by T cell immunity mechanisms attacking the transplanted structure as a foreign protein. Ideally, of course, compatible tissue matching will minimize the chances of failure. Living relatives usually provide the best sources for transplant. Very often, however, this is not a viable option, and an appropriate nonrelated cadaver donor must be found.

Postoperatively, immunosuppressive drugs help to reduce the potential for rejection. Unfortunately, these drugs simultaneously increase susceptibility to infection. A high percentage of early deaths are thus frequently associated with the infectious process.

RENAL FAILURE: DISRUPTION OF CELLULAR NEEDS

Because of the central role played by the kidneys in maintaining fluid-electrolyte and acid-base balance, it is easy to see why renal disease would precipitate serious disruptions in homeostasis.

Certainly, the uremic syndrome, as manifested in terminal stages of acute and chronic renal failure, reflects the systemic dependence upon normal renal function.

As renal activity decreases, all basic cellular needs are compromised. A summary of some of the mechanisms whereby disruption occurs can be found in Figure 11.31.

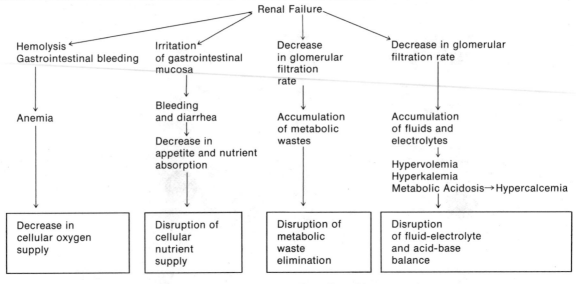

Figure 11.31   Renal failure: disruption of homeostasis

STUDY QUESTIONS

1. Define or describe the following terms:
   a. ureter
   b. trigonal muscle
   c. detrusor muscle
   d. micturition
   e. glomerular capsule
   f. juxtamedullary nephron
   g. hilus
   h. vasa recta
   i. JGA
   j. reabsorption

2. Why does heart failure frequently cause secondary renal disease?

3. Determine the effect each of the following factors might have upon filtration pressure in the nephron:
   a. cardiac failure
   b. hypovolemia
   c. hypertension

4. Predict the effect of each of the following factors upon (1) urinary volume, (2) urinary sodium concentration, and (3) urinary potassium concentration:
   a. Cushing's disease
   b. diabetes insipidus
   c. SIADH
   d. Addison's disease

5. Mr. Thompson is admitted to the hospital with renal dysfunction. The following laboratory tests are ordered. What is their significance?
   a. concentration and dilution tests
   b. renal clearance test
   c. plasma creatinine and BUN levels
   d. specific gravity of urine
   e. protein in the urine

6. Categorize the following disorders as causative of prerenal, intrarenal, or postrenal disease:
   a. acute poststreptococcal glomerulonephritis
   b. enlargement of the prostate
   c. cardiac failure
   d. ureteral stones
   e. transfusion reaction
   f. mercury poisoning
   g. anaphylactic shock

7. Mr. McDermott is admitted to the hospital in acute renal failure. Answer the following:
   a. List at least five disease conditions that might cause acute renal failure.
   b. Assuming the existence of acute tubular pathology, briefly describe the progressive evolution of disease.
   c. Assuming the existence of acute glomerular pathology, briefly describe the progressive evolution of disease.

8. Mrs. Watson is diagnosed as having chronic renal failure. Answer the following:
   a. List at least five causes of chronic renal failure.

b. Identify five predictable manifestations of CRF, and describe their evolution.

9. Differentiate between the nephrotic syndrome and the uremic syndrome in renal pathology.

10. Mr. Farrell recently purchased a dry cleaning establishment. After working in the store for a few weeks, he suddenly developed oliguria. At the time of admission, his urinary output was approximately 180 ml. per 24 hours, with a BUN of 100 mg. per cent and serum creatinine of 8.5 mg per cent. Urinalysis revealed an increase in the concentration of sodium and a specific gravity of 1.005.

a. Do you predict that he is suffering from acute or chronic renal failure, and why?

b. Is the condition most likely of prerenal, intrarenal, or postrenal origin?

c. Why are BUN and creatinine elevated?

d. Why is urinary sodium elevated?

e. Why is the specific gravity of urine depressed?

f. Would you assume the existence of renal atrophy?

11. Mrs. Baker was in a fire and suffered extensive burns over 13 per cent of her body. Oliguria developed within 24 hours of admission, with urinalysis showing a specific gravity of 1.035 and depressed sodium concentration.

a. Is the condition most likely of prerenal, intrarenal, or postrenal origin, and why?

b. Why is urinary sodium depressed?

c. Why is specific gravity of urine increased?

Suggested Readings

Books

Alfrey, A. C.: Chronic renal failure: manifestations and pathogenesis. *In* Schrier, R. W. (ed.): Renal Failure and Electrolyte Disorders. Boston, Little, Brown & Company, 1976, p. 331.

Alfrey, A. C., and Butkus, D. E.: Renal failure: pathophysiology and management. *In* Hudak, C. M., Lohr, T. S., and Gallo, B. M.: Critical Care Nursing, 2nd ed. Philadelphia, J. B. Lippincott Company, 1977, p. 319.

Brenner, B. M.: Structure and function of the kidneys. *In* Beeson, P. B., McDermott, W., and Wyngaarden, J. B. (eds.): Cecil Textbook of Medicine, 15th ed. Philadelphia, W. B. Saunders Company, 1979, p. 1316.

Brenner, B. M., Deen, W. M., and Robertson, C. R.: Glomerular filtration. *In* Brenner, B. M., and Rector, F. C., Jr. (eds.): The Kidney. Philadelphia, W. B. Saunders Company, 1976, p. 251.

Bricker, N. S.: Acute renal failure. *In* Beeson, P. B., McDermott, W., and Wyngaarden, J. B. (eds.): Cecil Textbook of Medicine, 15th ed. Philadelphia, W. B. Saunders Company, 1979, p. 1367.

Bricker, N. S.: The pathophysiology of chronic renal disease. *In* Beeson, P. B., McDermott, W., and Wyngaarden, J. B. (eds.): Cecil Textbook of Medicine, 15th ed. Philadelphia, W. B. Saunders Company, 1979, p. 1346.

Burg, M. B.: The renal handling of sodium chloride. *In* Brenner, B. M., and Rector, F. C., Jr. (eds.): The Kidney. Philadelphia. W. B. Saunders Company, 1976, p. 272.

Burgess, A.: The Nurse's Guide to Fluid and Electrolyte Balance, 2nd ed. New York, McGraw-Hill Book Company, 1979, pp. 159–165.

Chapman, W. H., Bulger, R. E., et al.: The Urinary System. Philadelphia, W. B. Saunders Company, 1973.

Deetjen, P., Boylan, J. W., and Kramer, K.: Physiology of the Kidney and of Water Balance. New York, Springer-Verlag, Inc., 1975.

Dirks, J. H., Seely, J. F., and Levy, M.: Control of extracellular fluid volumes and the pathophysiology of edema formation. *In* Brenner, B. M., and Rector, F. C., Jr. (eds.): The Kidney. Philadelphia, W. B. Saunders Company, 1976, p. 495.

Glassock, R. J.: Mechanisms of renal injury. *In* Beeson, P. B., McDermott, W., and Wyngaarden, J. B. (eds.): Cecil Textbook of Medicine, 15th ed. Philadelphia, W. B. Saunders Company, 1979, p. 1323.

Golden, A., and Maher, J.: The Kidney. Baltimore, The Williams & Wilkins Company, 1977.

Grant, M. M.: The kidney and fluid and electrolyte imbalances. *In* Jones, D. A., Dunbar, C. F., and Jirovec, M. M.: Medical-Surgical Nursing, A Conceptual Approach. New York, McGraw-Hill Book Company, 1978, p. 493.

Guyton, A. C.: Textbook of Medical Physiology, 5th ed. Philadelphia, W. B. Saunders Company, 1976, pp. 438–513.

Handler, J. S., and Orloff, J.: The mechanism of action of antidiuretic hormone. *In* Orloff, F., and Berliner, R. W. (eds.): Handbook of Physiology, Sec. 8. Baltimore, The Williams & Wilkins Company, 1973, p. 791.

Hole, J. W.: Human Anatomy and Physiology. Dubuque, Wm. C. Brown Company, 1978, pp. 654–672.

Kent, T. H., Hart, M. N., and Shires, T. K.: Introduction to Human Disease. New York, Appleton-Century-Crofts, 1979, pp. 190–207.

Kerr, D. N. S.: Chronic renal failure. In Beeson, P. B., McDermott, W., and Wyngaarden, J. B. (eds.): Cecil Textbook of Medicine, 15th ed. Philadelphia, W. B. Saunders Company, 1979, p. 1351.

Kerr, D. N. S.: Investigation of renal function. In Beeson, P. B., McDermott, W., and Wyngaarden, J. B. (eds.): Cecil Textbook of Medicine, 15th ed. Philadelphia, W. B. Saunders Company, 1979, p. 1336.

Kunin, C. M.: Urinary tract infections and pyelonephritis. In Beeson, P. B., McDermott, W., and Wyngaarden, J. B. (eds.): Cecil Textbook of Medicine, 15th ed. Philadelphia, W. B. Saunders Company, 1979, p. 1409.

Ladides, J.: Fundamentals of Urology. Philadelphia, W. B. Saunders Company, 1976.

Levinsky, N. G., and Alexander, E. A.: Acute renal failure. In Brenner, B. M., and Rector, F. C., Jr. (eds.): The Kidney. Philadelphia, W. B. Saunders Company, 1976, p. 806.

Luckmann, J., and Sorensen, K. C.: Medical-Surgical Nursing, A Pathophysiologic Approach, 2nd ed. Philadelphia, W. B. Saunders Company, 1980, pp. 911–1012.

Maude, D.: Kidney Physiology and Kidney Disease: An Introduction to Nephrology. Philadelphia, J. B. Lippincott Company, 1977.

Miller, P. L.: Assessment of urinary function. In Phipps, W. J., Long, B. C., and Woods, N. F. (eds.): Medical-Surgical Nursing, Concepts and Clinical Practice. St. Louis, The C. V. Mosby Company, 1979, p. 1227.

Miller, P. L.: Problems of the urinary system. In Phipps, W. J., Long, B. C., and Woods, N. F. (eds.): Medical-Surgical Nursing, Concepts and Clinical Practice. St. Louis, The C. V. Mosby Company, 1979, p. 1301.

Pitts, R. F.: Physiology of the Kidney and Body Fluids, 3rd ed. Chicago, Year Book Medical Publishers, 1974.

Purtillo, D. T.: A Survey of Human Diseases. Menlo Park, Addison-Wesley Publishing Company, 1978, pp. 338–352.

Reed, G. M., and Sheppard, V. F.: Regulation of Fluid and Electrolyte Balance: A Programmed Instruction in Clinical Physiology, 2nd ed. Philadelphia, W. B. Saunders Company, 1977, pp. 254–273.

Robbins, S. L., and Cotran, R. S.: Pathologic Basis of Disease, 2nd ed. Philadelphia, W. B. Saunders Company, 1979, pp. 1115–1183.

Robinson, R. R.: The major renal syndromes. In Beeson, P. B., McDermott, W., and Wyngaarden, J. B. (eds.): Cecil Textbook of Medicine, 15th ed. Philadelphia, W. B. Saunders Company, 1979, p. 1331.

Shires, D. L.: Renal diseases: water and electrolyte balance. In Sodeman, W. A., and Sodeman, T. M. (eds.): Pathologic Physiology, Mechanisms of Disease, 6th ed. Philadelphia, W. B. Saunders Company, 1979, p. 392.

Stroot, V. R., Lee, C. A., and Schaper, C. A.: Fluids and Electrolytes: A Practical Approach. Philadelphia, F. A. Davis Company, 1977, pp. 132–140.

Suki, W. M., and Eknoyan, G.: Tubulo-interstitial diseases. In Brenner, B. M., and Rector, F. C., Jr. (eds.): The Kidney. Philadelphia, W. B. Saunders Company, 1976, p. 1113.

Tanner, G. A.: Kidney function. In Selkurt, E. E. (ed.): Basic Physiology for the Health Sciences. Boston, Little, Brown & Company, 1975, p. 455.

Tortora, G. H., and Anagnostakos, N. P.: Principles of Anatomy and Physiology, 2nd ed. San Francisco, Canfield Press, 1978, pp. 598–620.

Wrong, O. M.: Glomerulonephritis. In Beeson, P. B., McDermott, W., and Wyngaarden, J. B. (eds.): Cecil Textbook of Medicine, 15th ed. Philadelphia, W. B. Saunders Company, 1979, p. 1390.

Wrong, O. M.: Nephrotic syndrome. In Beeson, P. B., McDermott, W., and Wyngaarden, J. B. (eds.): Cecil Textbook of Medicine, 15th ed. Philadelphia, W. B. Saunders Company, 1979, p. 1387.

Articles

Adler, S.: Managing chronic renal failure. Consultant, 16:41, 1976.

Cronin, R., et al.: Acute renal failure: Diagnosis, pathogenesis and management. Hosp. Med., 12:26, 1976.

Crowe, L., et al.: Evaluating renal function: Current status of clinical tests. Postgrad. Med., 62:58, 1977.

Donadio, J.: Glomerulonephritis: Approach to diagnosis and treatment. Hosp. Med., 14:36, 1978.

Eknoyan, G.: Axioms on acute oliguria. Hosp. Med., 13:32, 1977.

Flanagan, M.: Acute urinary retention. Hosp. Med., 12:60, 1976.

Freedman, P., and Smith, E.: Acute renal failure. Heart Lung, 4:873, 1975.

Gault, P.: How to break the kidney stone cycle. Nursing '78, *8*:24, 1978.

Hepinstall, R.: Interstitial nephritis: A brief review. Am. J. Pathol., *83*:213, 1976.

Hollenberg, N., and Adams, D.: The renal blood supply in oliguria states: When is the kidney ischemic? Am. Heart J., *91*:255, 1976.

Klein, K., and Karokawa, K.: Metabolic and endocrine alterations in end-stage renal failure. Postgrad. Med., *64*:99, 1978.

Klopper, J., et al.: Measurement of glomerular filtration rate. N. Engl. J. Med., *296*:284, 1977.

Kokko, J.: The role of renal concentrating mechanisms in the regulation of serum sodium concentration. Am. J. Med., *62*:165, 1977.

Kussman, M., et al.: The clinical course of diabetic nephropathy. JAMA, *236*:1861, 1976.

Landes, R.: Urinary tract infection — More than a one-time thing. Consultant, *15*:32, 1975.

Landsman, M.: The patient with chronic renal failure: A marginal man. Ann. Intern. Med., *82*:268, 1975.

Lange, K., and Treser, G.: Acute poststreptococcal glomerulonephritis. Clin. Nephrol., *1*:55, 1973.

Leman, J.: Acute renal failure. Am. Fam. Physician, *18*:146, 1978.

Lenaghan, D., et al.: The natural history of reflux and long-term effects of reflux on the kidney. J. Urol., *15*:728, 1976.

Merrill, J. P.: Glomerulonephritis. N. Engl. J. Med., *290*:257, 1974.

Mitchell, J.: Axioms on uremia. Hosp. Med., *14*:6, 1978.

Nortman, D., and Coburn, J.: Renal osteodystrophy in end-stage renal failure. Postgrad. Med., *64*:123, 1978.

Simon, N., et al.: Chronic renal failure: Pathophysiology and medical management. Cardiovasc. Nurse, *12*:7, 1976.

Smith, E., and Freedman, P.: Dialysis: Current status and future. Heart Lung, *4*:879, 1975.

Szwed, J.: Pathophysiology of acute renal failure: Rationale for signs and symptoms. Crit. Care Q., *1*:1, 1978.

Chapter Outline

chapter 12

Gastrointestinal Pathology

Chapter Objectives

At the completion of this chapter, the student will be able to:

1. Describe the basic structure and function of the gastrointestinal tract.
2. Define the relationship between the main and accessory organs of the digestive system.
3. Describe the evolution and characteristic features of esophageal disease.
4. Differentiate between gastric obstruction, neoplasms, and inflammatory disorders, with respect to development and manifestations.
5. Distinguish between gastritis and peptic ulcers, with respect to causative factors and characteristic pathological course.
6. Differentiate between digestive-absorptive and obstructive-paralytic disorders of the small intestine, with respect to causative factors and clinical manifestations.
7. Identify two major differences between nontropical sprue and regional enteritis.
8. List and describe three clinical laboratory tests commonly used to confirm the presence of malabsorption.
9. Differentiate between inflammatory disorders, neoplasms, and motility disorders of the large intestine, with respect to development and clinical manifestations.
10. Distinguish between diverticulitis and ulcerative colitis, with respect to characteristic pathological course and clinical manifestations.
11. Identify some complications associated with diarrhea and constipation.
12. Differentiate between (a) acute and chronic pancreatitis, and (b) hepatitis and cirrhosis, with respect to causative factors and clinical manifestations.
13. Trace the evolution of jaundice secondary to (a) excessive production of bilirubin, and (b) insufficient excretion of bilirubin.
14. Define the term *portal hypertension* and describe its clinical significance.
15. Describe five ways in which gastrointestinal disease may disrupt the servicing of cellular needs.

INTRODUCTION

Although the intake of an adequately balanced diet is a significant first step in the maintenance of physiological health, the majority of ingested foods must be broken down into small particles before they can be utilized to service cellular needs.

The digestive system functions specifically in the processing of nutrients and the elimination of nondigestible fecal wastes. Consisting of a series of hollow organs through which ingested food is sequentially transported (the gastrointestinal tract), and a number of accessory structures that facilitate functional activity, the system is described briefly in Chapter 2.

Ultimately, the generation of cellular energy is dependent upon the absorption of digested nutrients out of the gastrointestinal tract into the bloodstream. Only in this way can the metabolic furnaces be continuously fired by a steady supply of fuel. The close relationship between digestion and metabolism is illustrated in Figure 12.1.

In the following pages, emphasis is placed upon the way in which the digestive system functions to support cellular survival. Toward this end, a more detailed overview of normal structure and function is followed by an elucidation of gastrointestinal pathology. A clarification of the intricacies and implications

of metabolic dysfunction will be reserved for Chapter 15.

NORMAL ANATOMY AND PHYSIOLOGY: AN OVERVIEW

Generally speaking, the digestive system consists of two types of structures:

1. *Main organs*, which constitute the gastrointestinal (or GI) tract. Consisting of the mouth, pharynx, esophagus, stomach, small intestine, and large intestine, this series of organs presents one continuous tube within which food is processed and transported.

2. *Accessory organs*, which are located external to the gastrointestinal tract. Although these structures do not directly accommodate ingested food, they do manufacture and release a number of enzymes and secretions essential to the digestive process. The salivary glands, liver, gallbladder, and pancreas are categorized as accessory organs.

The way in which these two types of structures function together to promote the breakdown of ingested nutrients is summarized in Figure 12.2. It can be seen that whereas accessory organs enhance the primary functional activity of the digestive system, the majority of critical changes occur within the gastrointestinal tract. For this reason, subsequent analysis emphasizes the main organs,

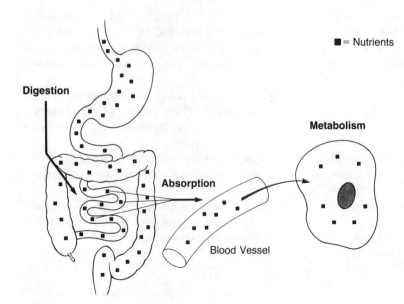

■ = Nutrients

Digestion

Metabolism

Absorption

Blood Vessel

Figure 12.1 The supply of cellular fuel: a schematic illustration.

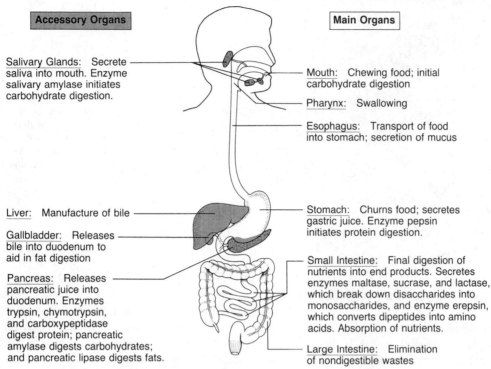

Figure 12.2 The function of the digestive system: main and accessory organs.

with specific elucidation of their (1) structure, (2) function, and (3) relationship to accessory organs.

Structure of the Gastrointestinal Tract

Although the organs of the gastrointestinal tract differ in appearance and function, they are all composed of the same basic types of tissue. While modifications exist to support differential function, the basic design consists of four structural layers that constitute the walls of all organs. From inside to outside they are:

1. *the tunica mucosa*, which is the innermost layer of tissue in the gastrointestinal tract. Coming into direct contact with nutrients passing through the lumen of the digestive organs, the mucosa consists primarily of epithelial cells designed to protect, secrete, or absorb. A small amount of smooth muscle tissue and an abundant supply of blood and lymph vessels are also found in this layer.

2. *the tunica submucosa*, which is composed primarily of loose connective tissue and supplied by a large number of blood vessels.

Interlaced within this layer are autonomic nerve fibers forming *Meissner's plexus* and functioning to regulate contractility of the gastrointestinal tract.

3. *the tunica muscularis*, which is composed of an inner circular and an outer longitudinal sheet of muscle. Consisting primarily of smooth muscle, this layer also contains skeletal muscle in areas where voluntary control of swallowing or elimination is necessary. Muscular contraction is regulated and coordinated by autonomic neural fibers forming the *plexus of Auerbach* within the tunica muscularis.

4. *the tunica serosa*, which is the outermost layer of tissue in the gastrointestinal tract. Composed primarily of connective and epithelial cells, this layer is specifically described as *visceral peritoneum* when covering organs located within the abdominopelvic cavity.

The relationship between the four basic structural layers of the gastrointestinal tract is illustrated in Figure 12.3.

In considering the orientation and alignment of tissues within the gastrointestinal tract, it is helpful to describe some of the

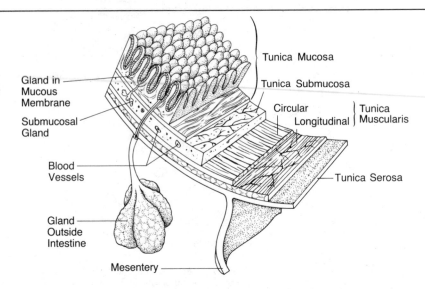

Tunica Mucosa

Gland in Mucous Membrane

Tunica Submucosa

Submucosal Gland

Circular

Longitudinal | Tunica Muscularis

Blood Vessels

Tunica Serosa

Gland Outside Intestine

Mesentery

Figure 12.3 The four basic structural layers of the gastro-intestinal tract are illustrated by a section of small intestine: tunica mucosa, tunica submucosa, tunica muscularis, and tunica serosa.

modifications that facilitate optimal systemic function.

In the mouth, pharynx, and esophagus, for example, epithelial tissue is layered, or stratified, to afford maximal protection against abrasive particles of food. As mentioned earlier, these areas also contain skeletal muscle in the tunica muscularis, so that voluntary control over the swallowing mechanism can be maintained. Further specialization can be

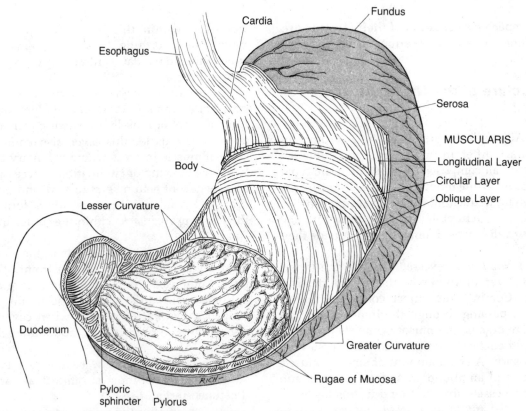

Cardia

Fundus

Esophagus

Serosa

MUSCULARIS

Body

Longitudinal Layer

Circular Layer

Oblique Layer

Lesser Curvature

Duodenum

Greater Curvature

Rugae of Mucosa

Pyloric sphincter   Pylorus

Figure 12.4 Basic anatomical subdivisions of the stomach. (From Tortora, G. J., and Anagnostakos, N. P.: Principles of Anatomy and Physiology, 2nd ed. New York, Harper & Row, 1978. Used by permission.)

seen at the gastroesophageal junction. A thickening of the tunica muscularis in this area results in the formation of the *gastroesophageal sphincter,* which serves to monitor the transport of nutrients into the gastric lumen and prevent reflux.

The stomach, whose basic anatomical subdivisions are illustrated in Figure 12.4, is an area where ingested nutrients are broken down both physically and chemically. The churning of food within this organ is facilitated by the addition of a third layer of inner oblique muscle to the tunica muscularis, while a modification of circular muscle at the small intestinal junction (the *pyloric sphincter)* controls the exit of nutrients into the lower gastrointestinal tract.

Particularly significant to gastric functional activity is the modification of the tunica mucosa in the stomach. Typically found in folds, or *rugae,* when the organ is relatively empty, the epithelial cells of the mucosal layer are organized into specialized gastric glands within the fundus of the stomach. As illustrated in Figure 12.5, secretion is dependent upon *parietal cells,* which produce hydrochloric acid and intrinsic factor, *zymogenic or chief cells,* which produce enzymes, and *mucus or neck cells,* which secrete mucus.

Once nutrients have been partially digested within the gastric lumen, they pass into the small intestine for further processing. As illustrated in Figure 12.6, the small intestine is divisible into three major segments:

1. *the duodenum,* an initial C-shaped por-

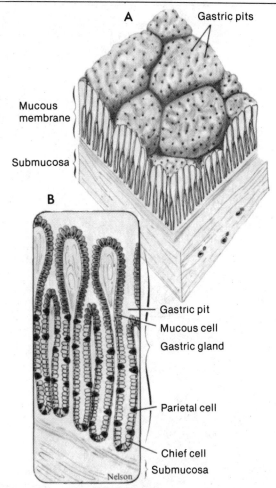

Figure 12.5 The gastric mucosa. Note that the mucous membrane illustrated in *A* contains a variety of specialized cells, as identified in *B*. (From Hole, J. W.: Human Anatomy and Physiology. Dubuque, Wm. C. Brown Company, 1978. Used by permission.)

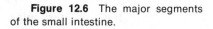

Figure 12.6 The major segments of the small intestine.

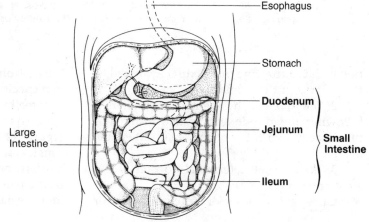

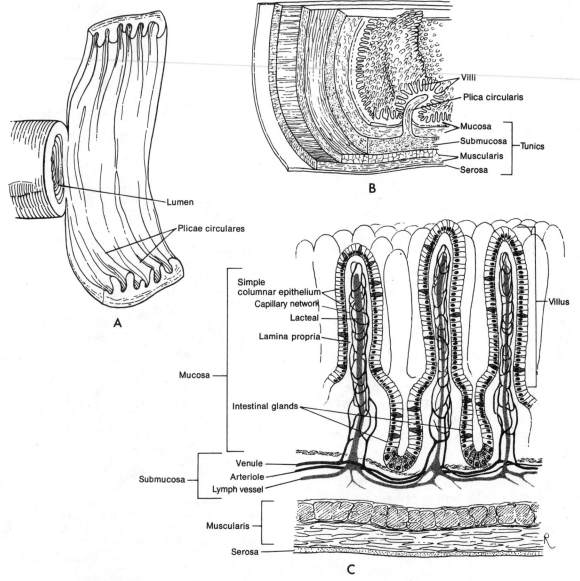

Figure 12.7 The lining of the small intestine. *A*, Section of small intestine cut open to expose plicae circulares. *B*, Villi in relation to the tunics of the small intestine. *C*, Enlarged aspect of several villi. (From Tortora, G. J., and Anagnostakos, N. P.: Principles of Anatomy and Physiology, 2nd ed. New York, Harper & Row, 1978. Used by permission.)

tion of small intestine that is directly linked to the pylorus of the stomach.

2. *the jejunum*, the segment immediately following the duodenum, constituting approximately two fifths of the small intestinal length.

3. *the ileum*, the terminal portion of the small intestine.

Once again, the major structural layers of the gastrointestinal tract are modified to facilitate specific functional activity. In the case of the small intestine, adaptations are particularly noted in the tunica mucosa. As illustrated in Figure 12.7, the absorptive surface area is considerably increased by the organization of mucosal and submucosal tissue into specialized circular folds called *plicae circularis*. Further specialization is evidenced in the form of

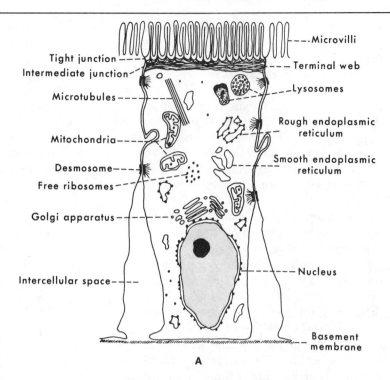

Microvilli

Tight junction

Terminal web

Intermediate junction

Microtubules

Lysosomes

Rough endoplasmic reticulum

Mitochondria

Smooth endoplasmic reticulum

Desmosome

Free ribosomes

Golgi apparatus

Nucleus

Intercellular space

Basement membrane

A

Figure 12.8 *A* and *B,* Columnar epithelial cells in villi of small intestine. Note microvilli forming brush border within lumen of intestine. (*A* from Sodeman, W. A., and Sodeman, T. M.: Sodeman's Pathologic Physiology: Mechanisms of Disease, 6th ed. Philadelphia, W. B. Saunders Company, 1979. Used by permission. *B* from Leeson, T. S., and Leeson, C. R.: Histology, 3rd ed. Philadelphia, W. B. Saunders Company, 1977. Used by permission.)

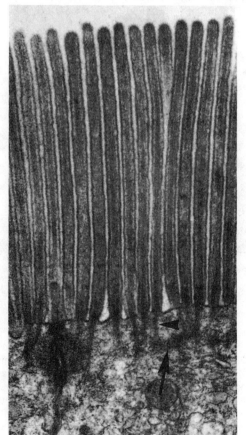

B

small finger-like projections called *villi,* which extend into the intestinal lumen to give the lining a velvety appearance and texture. Structured from mucosal epithelial cells, these villi contain an internal network of blood and lymph vessels. As illustrated in Figure 12.8, the surface area of the lining is maximized by the presence of a microscopic brush border on many individual cells of the villi. These cellular "fringes," called microvilli, come into contact with luminal content and enhance absorptive capacity.

Although a number of structural modifications facilitate the absorption of nutrients, digestion is a necessary prelude to the transport of particles out of the gastrointestinal tract into the bloodsteam. The chemical breakdown of food within the small intestine is facilitated, in part, by chemicals released from the intestinal glands, or *crypts of Lieberkühn,* within the mucosal layer. As illustrated in Figure 12.9, enzymes are released directly from the tunica mucosa, while protective mucus is secreted by *Brunner's glands* in the tunica submucosa. Modifications of the tunica muscularis into the *ileocecal valve* at the junction of the small and large intestines further promote digestion by controlling the exit of food from the ileum into the cecum.

Whereas the small intestine functions primarily in the breakdown and absorption of ingested nutrients, the large intestine is mainly involved in processing nondigestible wastes and eliminating them through the lower bowel in the form of feces. Comprising four major segments (the cecum, colon, rectum, and anal canal), the basic structure of the large intestine is illustrated in Figure 12.10. It can·be seen that the colon is further divisible into ascending, transverse, and descending portions, reflecting the direction of intraluminal transport.

Once again, by examining tissue structure it is possible to see evidence of modifications designed to facilitate functional activity. In the large intestine, for example, the tunica mucosa is composed primarily of columnar epithelial cells adapted to secrete lubricating

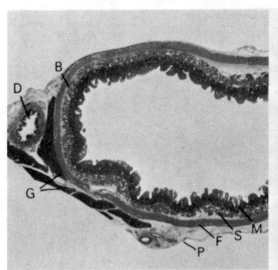
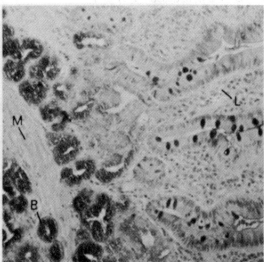

Figure 12.9.   Left, this transverse section of the duodenum also shows part of the pancreas (G) and the common bile duct (D). In the duodenum, the serosa (P), muscularis (F), submucosa (S), and mucosa (M) are seen. In the submucosa are glands of Brunner (B), and the mucosa shows villi protruding from the surface and intestinal glands (darkly staining). Right, only mucosa and part of submucosa are seen. Note the broad villi, with a core of cellular lamina propria (L) and covered by simple columnar epithelium with scattered goblet cells (pink-staining). Opening into intestinal glands are the submucosal glands of Brunner (B), lying in submucosa with their ducts passing through the muscularis mucosae (M). These glands secrete a mucus with a high bicarbonate content. (From Leeson and Leeson: *A Brief Atlas of Histology.* Philadelphia: W. B. Saunders Co., 1979. Used by permission.)

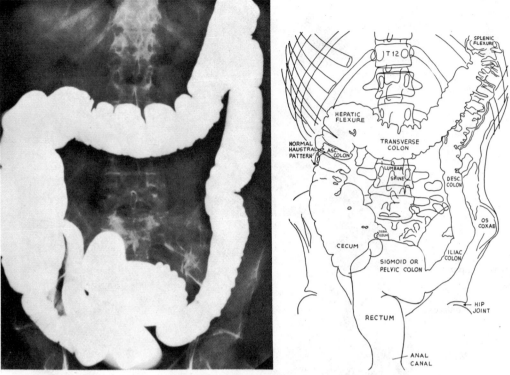

Figure 12.10 Major segments of the large intestine. (From Meschan, I.: *Synopsis of Analysis of Roentgen Signs in General Radiology*, p. 591, A): W. B. Saunders Company, 1976. Used by permission.)

mucus. Stratified, or layered, epithelium is found only in the anal region, where it functions protectively against the frequent abrasion encountered in this area.

Further modification is noted in the tunica muscularis of the large intestine. Unlike its continuous and noninterrupted counterparts in other organs of the gastrointestinal tract, the longitudinal muscular coat is segmented into three discrete muscular bands, as illustrated in Figure 12.11. These bands, called *taeniae coli*, are shorter than the intestines, resulting in a puckering of the colon into characteristic pouch-like sacs called *haustra*. Although the presence of haustra facilitates slow churning of intestinal contents, fecal elimination is regulated by the activity of two sphincter muscles in the anal canal. Consisting of thickened bands of circular muscle fibers, the smooth muscle *internal sphincter* is controlled by autonomic neural reflexes, while the *external sphincter* is composed of voluntarily regulated skeletal muscle. The relative loca-

tion of these sphincter muscles is illustrated in Figure 12.12.

Function of the Gastrointestinal Tract

As is the case throughout the body, the structure of the digestive system is intimately related to functional activity. Digestion, absorption, and fecal elimination are, in fact, interdependent activities that rely upon a well-integrated relationship between all digestive organs. To better clarify its activity, the gastrointestinal tract will be arbitrarily subdivided into four major functional segments, as follows: (1) the mouth, pharynx, and esophagus; (2) the stomach; (3) the small intestine; and (4) the large intestine.

THE MOUTH, PHARYNX, AND ESOPHAGUS

It is within the mouth that the digestive process is initiated. While food is physically

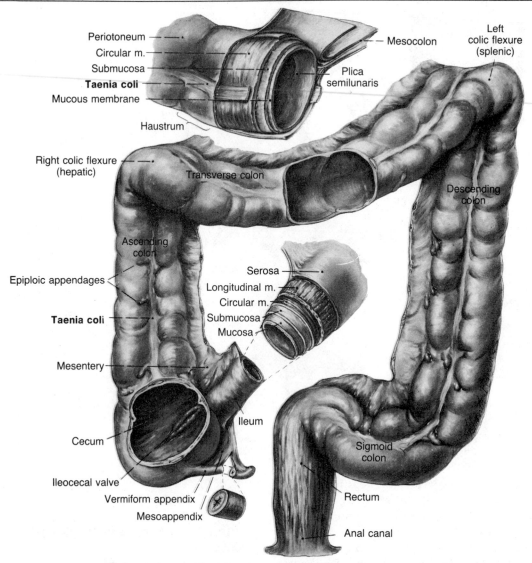

Figure 12.11   A section through the large intestine showing taenia coli. (From Jacob, S. W., Francone, C. A., and Lossow, W. J.: Structure and Function in Man, 4th ed. Philadelphia, W. B. Saunders Company, 1978. Used by permission.)

broken down by activity of the teeth and tongue, moisture is provided by accessory salivary glands, as illustrated in Figure 12.13. The secretions produced by these glands lubricate ingested nutrients and promote the chemical breakdown of carbohydrates. The release of saliva (triggered by the sight, smell, thought, or taste of food) is regulated by neural reflexes that respond automatically to these stimuli. Saliva is particularly useful in facilitating the smooth passage of nutrients from the mouth into the pharynx and esophagus.

Swallowing, or *deglutition*, is a complex process regulated by a series of neural reflexes. Transport of nutrients from the mouth into the esophagus is aided by two mechanisms; as illustrated in Figure 12.14: (1) utilization of the uvula and soft palate to guard against the movement of food from the mouth into the nasopharynx, and (2) utilization of the epiglottis to guard against the entry of nutrients into the respiratory tract.

Having entered the esophagus, the bolus of food is propelled downward by a wave of peristaltic muscular contraction. Additionally

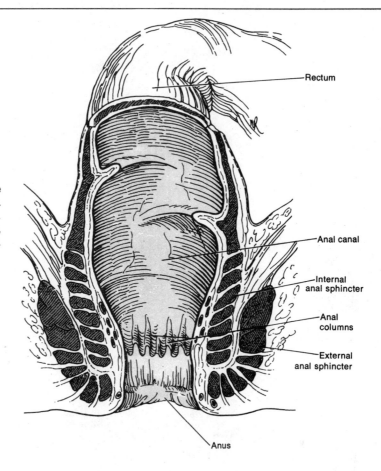

Figure 12.12 Relative location of the internal and external anal sphincters. (From Tortora, G. J., and Anagnostakos, N. P.: Principles of Anatomy and Physiology, 2nd ed. New York, Harper & Row, 1978. Used by permission.)

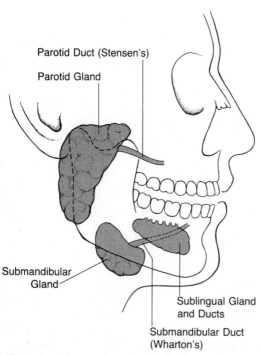

Figure 12.13 The salivary glands and their ducts.

aided by the force of gravity, luminal contents pass through the gastroesophageal sphincter and into the fundus of the stomach within 5 to 15 seconds.

THE STOMACH

A good deal of digestive activity occurs within the stomach. Nutrients are mixed with gastric juice and churned into a semiliquid state referred to as *chyme*. Within two to six hours gastric contents pass through the pyloric sphincter and into the duodenum of the small intestine.

As a result of gastric digestion, proteins are broken down into smaller proteoses and peptones. The enzyme *pepsin*, which catalyzes protein hydrolysis, is initially released by zymogenic, or chief, cells in the form of an inactive precursor called pepsinogen. It is the acidity of gastric juice that promotes the conversion of pepsinogen into functional pepsin.

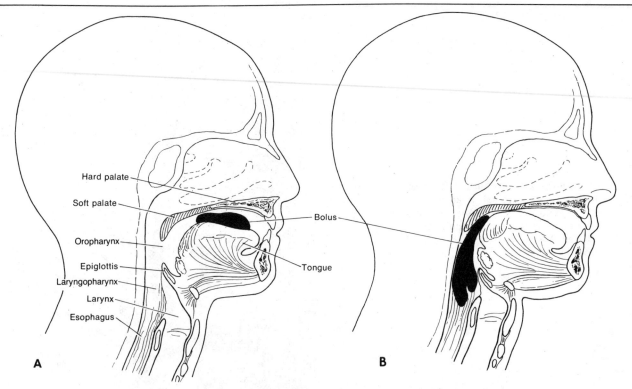

Figure 12.14 Deglutition. *A*, Position of structures prior to swallowing. *B*, During swallowing, the tongue rises against the palate, the nose is closed off, the larynx rises, the epiglottis seals off the larynx, and the bolus is passed into the esophagus. (From Tortora, G. J., and Anagnostakos, N. P.: Principles of Anatomy and Physiology, 2nd ed. New York, Harper & Row, 1978. Used by permission.)

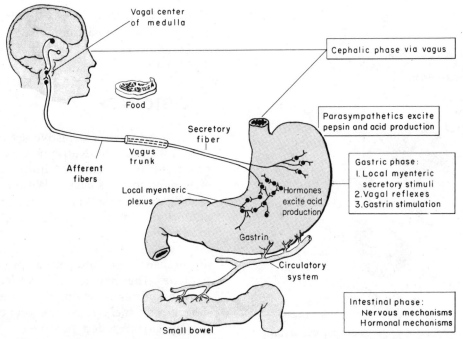

Figure 12.15 The regulation of gastric secretion. (From Guyton, A. C.: Physiology of the Human Body, 5th ed. Philadelphia, W. B. Saunders Company, 1979. Used by permission.)

As illustrated in Figure 12.15, control of gastric secretion primarily occurs in one of three ways:

1. *The cephalic phase* — triggered by the sight, smell, thought, or taste of food, a neural reflex is initiated that promotes the release of hydrochloric acid, pepsingogen, and mucus. This response, which accounts for approximately 10 per cent of gastric secretion, is mediated by branches of the vagus nerve.

2. *The gastric phase* — triggered by the entry of food into the pylorus of the stomach, a neural reflex initiates release of the hormone *gastrin*. The gastrin secreted by gastric mucosal glands passes into the bloodstream and is subsequently transported throughout the body. Eventually returning to the stomach, it promotes the release of approximately 2000 ml. of gastric juice daily and thereby accounts for approximately 66 per cent of total gastric secretion. Increases in the secretion of gastric juice is often caused by the excessive release of gastrin. This phenomenon is commonly noted when the pyloric mucosa is exposed to excessive quantities of bile salts, protein foods, or alcohol.

Supporting the gastrin mechanism are reflexes triggered by stretch of the visceral walls subsequent to the entry of food. Neural messages conveyed to the medulla initiate additional stimulation of gastric secretion.

3. *The intestinal phase* — triggered by the entry of chyme into the small intestine, an intestinal hormone capable of stimulating gastric secretion is believed to be released into the bloodstream. This mechanism, however, is of minimal significance and accounts for only a small fraction of gastric mucosal output.

In reality, the major effect of the small intestine upon gastric activity is one of suppression. Intestinal distention triggers the *enterogastric reflex*, which, in turn, depresses the release of gastric juice. This mechanism is potentiated by the secretion of certain intestinal hormones, such as secretin and cholecystokinin (pancreozymin). Released in response to the presence of acidic chyme in the intestinal lumen, they are carried by the circulatory system to the stomach, where they inhibit gastric mucosal secretion.

Considering the corrosive nature of gastric secretions, one would expect the wall of the stomach to be partially or totally digested by the combined action of the hydrochloric acid and proteolytic enzyme found in gastric juice. Clearly, survival would not be possible under such circumstances. The protective mechanism responsible for inhibiting the back-diffusion of hydrogen ions from the gastric lumen into visceral tissue is described as the *gastric mucosal barrier*. As illustrated in Figure 12.16, it consists of a dual line of defense:

1. The mucus secreted by neck cells in the tunica mucosa serves to coat the gastric lining and protect the stomach wall from acidic erosion.

2. The relatively tight junctional relationship existing between adjacent gastric mucosal cells further serves to inhibit back-diffusion of hydrogen ions.

THE SMALL INTESTINE

Functional activity within the small intestine includes digestion and absorption. Ulti-

Figure 12.16 The gastric mucosal barrier. Note that the gastric mucosa is protected from acid erosion by a mucus covering and the existence of tight intercellular junctions.

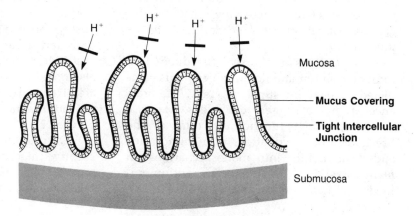

Gastric Lumen

Mucosa

Mucus Covering

Tight Intercellular Junction

Submucosa

TABLE 12.1   **Digestion Within the Small Intestine**

Nutrient Particle	Acted Upon By	Converted Into
CARBOHYDRATES		
Dextrin	Pancreatic amylase (secreted by pancreas)	Disaccharide maltase
Maltose	Maltase (secreted by intestinal glands)	Monosaccharide glucose
Sucrose	Sucrase (secreted by intestinal glands)	Monosaccharides glucose and fructose
Lactose	Lactase (secreted by intestinal glands)	Monosaccharides glucose and galactose
PROTEINS		
Protein	Carboxypeptidase (secreted by pancreas)	Amino acids
Protein	Trypsin and chymotrypsin (secreted by pancreas)	Proteoses and peptones
Proteoses and peptones	Trypsin and chymotrypsin (secreted by pancreas)	Dipeptides and amino acids
Dipeptides	Erepsin (secreted by intestinal glands)	Amino acids
FATS		
Neutral fats	Bile	Emulsified fat particles
Emulsified fats	Pancreatic lipase (secreted by pancreas)	Fatty acids and glycerol

mately, nutrient particles are broken down into small end products that can pass into the bloodstream and be utilized by cells to support metabolism.

DIGESTION IN THE SMALL INTES-TINE   As nutrients pass from the pylorus of the stomach into the small intestine, they trigger the release of secretions from certain accessory organs. Pancreatic enzymes, for example, are transported to the duodenum through the duct of Wirsung. They serve to break proteins and large polypeptides into smaller polypeptides, digest starches into disaccharides, and reduce fats to glycerol and fatty acids. Bile, on the other hand, is released from the gallbladder into the duodenum through the common bile duct. Manufactured in the liver, it functions to physically reduce large fat globules to smaller particles that can be more readily digested and absorbed. The relationship of these accessory organs to the gastrointestinal tract will be clarified later in this chapter.

As nutrients move from the duodenum into the jejunum and ileum, digestion is completed by small intestinal enzymes. The presence of chyme triggers the release of these enzymes, which function to catalyze the breakdown of polypeptides into amino acids and disaccharides into monosaccharides. In many cases, final digestion occurs within epithelial cells of the mucosa as nutrients are being absorbed from the lumen into the villi. A summary of the major digestive activity occurring within the small intestine is presented in Table 12.1.

ABSORPTION IN THE SMALL INTES-TINE   Once nutrients are digested, they must pass from the intestinal lumen into the bloodstream before they can become available for cellular utilization. This transport of nutrients into the circulatory system, referred to as *absorption*, involves both active and passive mechanisms.

Whereas the absorption of sodium is an active process, necessitating the generation of cellular energy, water and chloride generally follow sodium passively. It is postulated that the active transport of monosaccharides and amino acids from the intestinal lumen into the bloodstream is linked in some way to the sodium carrier mechanism. Evidence suggests that the carrier molecules involved in sodium absorption also serve in the transport of monosaccharides and amino acids. To the extent that sodium absorption is blocked, a decline is also noted in both monosaccharide and amino acid transport. An illustration of the postulated sodium transport carrier can be found in Figure 12.17.

Despite the hypothetical nature of absorptive mechanisms, the fate of absorbed particles has been well established. Monosaccharides and amino acids are generally

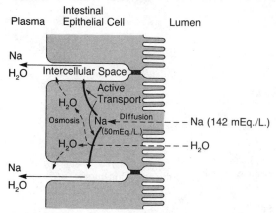

Figure 12.17 An illustration of the mechanism postulated to be responsible for the active transport of sodium from the lumen of the small intestine into the bloodstream.

transported directly into the blood vessels of the villi, to be carried to the liver via the portal vein. Fats, on the other hand, are absorbed in the form of *micelles* (small water-soluble particles surrounded by bile salts) into the epithelial cells of the villi. Intracellular reorganization

results in the formation of protein-coated lipid droplets called *chylomicrons*. The majority of these particles pass into the lacteals of the villi and are transported, through the lymph system, into the thoracic duct. Ultimately, they enter the bloodstream at the junction of the left internal jugular and left subclavian veins. The fate of absorbed nutrient particles is summarized in Figure 12.18.

In evaluating the absorptive process, it is important to realize that many substances are selectively absorbed in particular segments of the small intestine. Localized mucosal damage can thus inhibit absorption of specific nutrients and cause a limited type of malabsorption. A brief overview of the major absorptive areas within the small intestine is presented in Figure 12.19.

It should be noted that bile salts are absorbed primarily from the terminal ileum and returned, via the bloodstream, to the liver. This phenomenon, described as the *enterohepatic circulation of bile*, provides a means for conserving biliary constituents. In this

Figure 12.18 The circulation of absorbed nutrients. Note that chylomicrons are absorbed differentially into lymphatic vessels and transported to the thoracic duct before being emptied into the bloodstream at the junction of the left internal jugular and left subclavian veins.

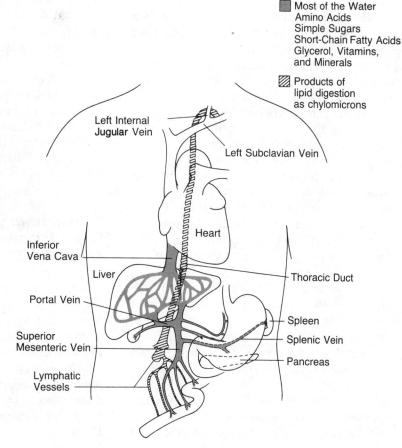

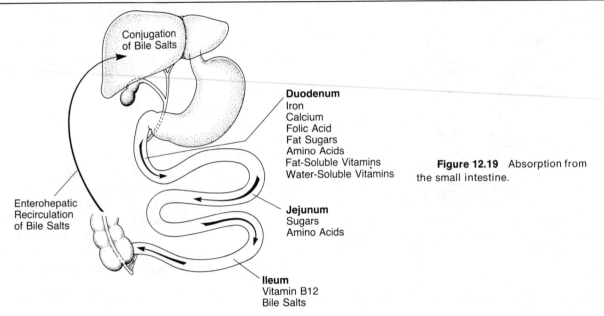

Figure 12.19   Absorption from the small intestine.

way, fecal elimination is avoided, and bile salts can be reused by the liver in the manufacture of new bile.

THE LARGE INTESTINE

The majority of substances passing from the ileum into the cecum are earmarked for elimination. Within the large intestine, nondigestible wastes are processed into feces, certain vitamins are synthesized, and water and electrolytes are absorbed.

Absorption occurs primarily in the proximal half of the colon. As is the case in the small intestine, active transport of sodium is accompanied by passive absorption of water and chloride. In the colon, however, chloride can additionally be absorbed through active transport, in exchange for the active secretion of bicarbonate to maintain electrical neutrality. The presence of HCO_3^- in the intestinal lumen accounts, in part, for the relative alkalinity of large intestinal contents.

To a large extent, functional activity inside the colon is facilitated by bacteria that normally live within the confines of the large intestine. Referred to as normal flora, these rod-shaped microorganisms are responsible for the manufacture of vitamins K, B_{12}, thiamine and riboflavin. They also aid in the production of normal feces by processing nondigestible nutrient wastes. Undigested proteins, for example, are typically converted into

indole, skatole, and hydrogen sulfide. Carbohydrates remaining in the colon, on the other hand, undergo fermentation. The hydrogen, carbon dioxide, and methane gases generated by this process are a primary source of colonic flatus. They account for the distention and discomfort that frequently accompany the ingestion of certain carbohydrate foods, such as beans and peas.

Bacteria additionally function in the breakdown of bilirubin (derived from bile) into *stercobilinogen* and *urobilinogen*. These simple pigments are responsible for the characteristic brown color of feces and are conspicuously absent when bile cannot enter the duodenum. Biliary obstruction is, in fact, characterized by the formation of abnormal, pasty, clay-colored stools.

Relationship of the Gastrointestinal Tract to Accessory Organs

A number of accessory organs facilitate digestive activity within the gastrointestinal tract by releasing secretions directly into one of the main organs of the digestive system. Primary examples are the pancreas and liver, which promote nutrient breakdown by emptying enzymes and bile, respectively, into the duodenum of the small intestine. The relative location of these organs is illustrated in Figure 12.20.

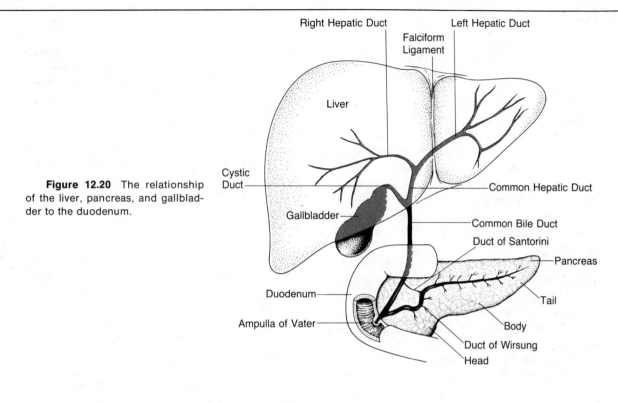

Figure 12.20 The relationship of the liver, pancreas, and gallbladder to the duodenum.

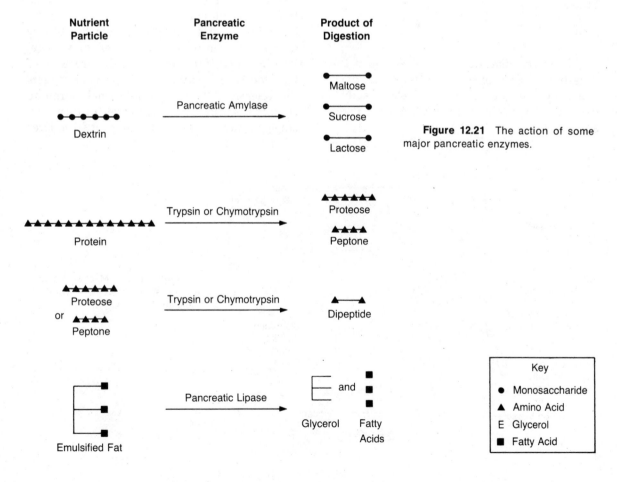

Figure 12.21 The action of some major pancreatic enzymes.

THE PANCREAS

The pancreas is both an endocrine and an exocrine gland. In the former capacity, it secretes insulin and glucagon directly into the bloodstream. These hormones function in the regulation of carbohydrate metabolism, as discussed in Chapters 2 and 15.

As an organ that functions in the digestive process, the pancreas releases a varied number of enzymes into the duodenum via the duct of Wirsung. As shown in Figure 12.21, the hydrolysis of carbohydrate, fat, and protein molecules is catalyzed by pancreatic enzymes.

The secretion and release of pancreatic juice is regulated primarily by hormones produced by the small intestinal mucosa. It is believed that the presence of partially digested proteins within the duodenum triggers the release of cholecystokinin (pancreozymin) and secretin into the bloodstream. These substances, in turn, circulate through the pancreas to initiate the secretion of enzymes and bicarbonate into the duct of Wirsung.

THE LIVER

The liver, like the pancreas, supports the digestive mission of the gastrointestinal tract. It also mediates a broad range of related activities essential to cellular survival. Among these are:

1. *The manufacture of several major plasma proteins.* The liver produces albumin (which functions in the maintenance of colloid osmotic pressure) and clotting proteins, such as fibrinogen and prothrombin. To the extent that plasma protein levels are significantly depressed secondary to hepatic dysfunction, fluid shifts or excessive bleeding can result.

2. *Nutrient metabolism.* The essential role played by the liver in the metabolism of all nutrients is elucidated in Chapter 2.

3. *Vitamin storage.* Hepatic cells are specifically functional in the storage of vitamins A, D, and B_{12}.

4. *Storage of iron.* Within the liver, iron is characteristically combined with apoferritin to produce a ferritin storage molecule that is subsequently deposited in hepatic tissue.

5. *Detoxification.* As blood travels through the liver, hepatic cells extract and inactivate a wide variety of toxic substances, such as alcohol and drugs.

In addition to these vital activities, the liver functions specifically within the digestive system as the producer of bile. Essential to the breakdown of fat, bile is secreted by hepatic cells and transported, via the biliary duct system, into the gallbladder for storage. As illustrated in Figure 12.22, the presence of fatty foods in the duodenum normally triggers the release of the small intestinal hormone cholecystokinin. This substance, in turn, circulates to the gallbladder, where it stimulates

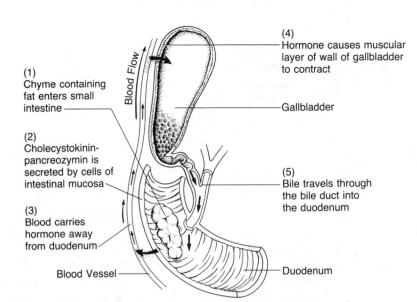

(1) Chyme containing fat enters small intestine

(2) Cholecystokinin-pancreozymin is secreted by cells of intestinal mucosa

(3) Blood carries hormone away from duodenum

Blood Flow

Blood Vessel

(4) Hormone causes muscular layer of wall of gallbladder to contract

Gallbladder

(5) Bile travels through the bile duct into the duodenum

Duodenum

Figure 12.22   Mechanism governing the release of bile from the gallbladder.

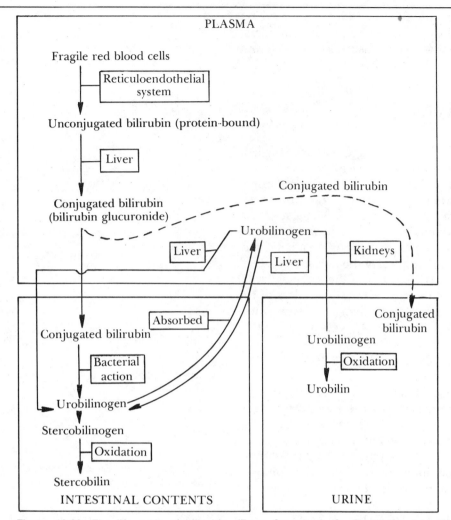

PLASMA

Fragile red blood cells

Reticuloendothelial system

Unconjugated bilirubin (protein-bound)

Liver

Conjugated bilirubin (bilirubin glucuronide)

Conjugated bilirubin

Liver

Urobilinogen

Liver

Kidneys

INTESTINAL CONTENTS

Conjugated bilirubin

Absorbed

Bacterial action

Urobilinogen

Stercobilinogen

Oxidation

Stercobilin

URINE

Conjugated bilirubin

Urobilinogen

Oxidation

Urobilin

Figure 12.23 The life cycle of bilirubin. (From Guyton, A. C.: Textbook of Medical Physiology, 6th ed. Philadelphia, W. B. Saunders Company, 1981. Used by permission.)

the ejection of bile into the cystic duct. Bile then travels through the common bile duct and into the duodenum through the sphincter of Oddi.

Once released into the gastrointestinal tract, bile promotes the emulsification and absorption of fats within the small intestine. Bile is composed primarily of cholesterol, bilirubin pigment, and bile salts. The last constituent is most directly responsible for emulsifying fats into small particles as an essential prelude to digestion and absorption.

In considering bile formation, it is important to take a closer look at the way in which bilirubin pigment becomes a functional part of bile. Derived from hemoglobin that is released when old red blood cells are broken

down in reticuloendothelial tissue throughout the body, bilirubin is formed from the heme portion of erythrocyte pigment. In order to be incorporated into bile, it must first be transported to the liver, where hepatic cells conjugate the bilirubin by attaching it to a protein. In the form of *conjugated bilirubin*, it is ultimately ejected into the duodenum as part of bile and transformed into stercobilinogen or urobilinogen by bacteria residing within the large intestine. The life cycle of bilirubin is summarized diagrammatically in Figure 12.23.

Under certain circumstances, the body is unable to eliminate sufficient quantities of bilirubin, and it accumulates in the bloodstream, resulting in a condition known as *jaundice*. Characterized by a yellowish discoloration of the skin, jaundice can develop secondary to a wide range of clinical disorders. A detailed discussion of jaundice can be found further on in this chapter.

PATHOLOGY

In the case of the digestive system, it is difficult to categorize disease from a functional perspective. Since disorders of diverse origin can ultimately interfere with digestion or absorption or both, it is most beneficial to classify dysfunctions organically. In the following pages, pathological conditions are related specifically to major areas of the digestive system, as follows: (1) disorders of the esophagus, (2) disorders of the stomach, (3) disorders of the small intestine, (4) disorders of the large intestine, and (5) disorders of accessory organs.

Disorders of the Esophagus

The esophagus is a muscular tube that functions primarily in the transport of food from the oropharynx to the stomach. Disorders in this structure are most commonly related to one of two phenomena: (1) failure to propel food normally through the eosphagus, or (2) inflammation of the mucosal lining.

FAILURE TO PROPEL FOOD

Under normal circumstances, ingested nutrients are rapidly and smoothly transported from the mouth through the esophagus into the stomach. To ensure optimal direction and timing, specialized circular bands of muscle are located at the superior and inferior ends of the esophagus. As illustrated in Figure 12.24, a ring of skeletal muscle (the cricopharyngeus muscle) controls the entry of substances from the oropharynx, while the gastroesophageal muscle regulates the passage of nutrients between the esophagus and the stomach.

When the swallowing mechanism propels a bolus of food into the esophagus, the cricopharyngeus muscle relaxes. Nerve fibers in Auerbach's plexus coordinate peristalsis, and nutrients are rapidly transported toward the

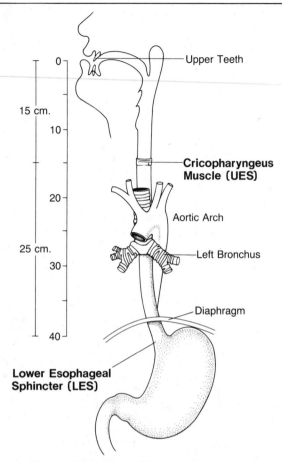

Figure 12.24 Bands of muscle that regulate the transport of nutrients through the esophagus.

stomach. Temporary relaxation of the gastroesophageal muscle normally allows ingested food to pass from the esophagus into the gastric lumen.

Under certain circumstances, the swallowing mechanism may be disrupted, resulting in a condition called *dysphagia*. Indicative of pharyngeal or esophageal dysfunction, dysphagia is often associated with systemic neural or neuromuscular disease. Common causative disorders include myasthenia gravis, bulbar polio, muscular dystrophy, and botulism.

Dysphagia can also be initiated by a disorder arising within the esophagus itself. Obstructive tumors or depressed contractility, for example, could considerably disrupt the normal swallowing mechanism. The latter phenomenon is particularly evident in cases of *achalasia*. This disorder is characterized by lack of peristalsis in the lower two thirds of the esophagus and failure of the gastroesophageal sphincter to relax during swallowing. Commonly associated with degeneration of the neural fibers in Auerbach's plexus, achalasia is accompanied by gastric regurgitation. Malnutrition can result if nutrient transport into the lower gastrointestinal tract is significantly reduced.

INFLAMMATION OF THE MUCOSAL LINING

The epithelial cells lining the esophagus are protected from excessive irritation in two primary ways: (1) Mucus secreted by the tunica mucosa serves to coat and protect the esophageal lining, and (2) contraction of the gastroesophageal sphincter prevents backflow of acidic chyme into the esophagus.

Under certain circumstances, however, the esophagus may be exposed to gastric reflux. This phenomenon is commonly associated with *hiatus hernia* and results in an esophageal inflammation known as *esophagitis*.

Hiatus hernia is a condition characterized by protrusion of a portion of the stomach into the thoracic cavity through a weakening in the wall of the diaphragm. As illustrated in Figure 12.25, these hernias can be of two distinct types.

In the more common direct, or sliding, hiatus hernia, the gastroesophageal junction protrudes into the thorax. There is associated incompetence of the gastroesophageal sphincter, with subsequent gastric reflux and esophagitis.

Alternatively, the hiatus hernia can be of the rolling, or paraesophageal, variety. In

these instances, the gastroesophageal junction remains below the diaphragm, while a portion of the fundus of the stomach protrudes into the thoracic cavity. Reflux esophagitis is not evident, but compression of the herniated tissue may lead to ischemia.

Disorders of the Stomach

When ingested nutrients pass into the stomach, protein digestion is initiated and luminal contents are reduced to a semiliquid state referred to as chyme. Because the stomach prepares food for entry into the small intestine, gastric dysfunction can disrupt both the digestive and the absorptive processes. Disorders can generally be classified as obstructive, neoplastic, or inflammatory.

OBSTRUCTIVE DISORDERS

Most frequently, gastric obstruction is associated with narrowing and hypertrophy of the pyloric sphincter. This condition, technically referred to as *pyloric stenosis*, interferes with the passage of chyme from the stomach into the duodenum and accordingly reduces cellular nutrient availability.

Most typically evidenced as a congenital disorder of unknown origin, pyloric stenosis affects male infants approximately four times as frequently as females. Within one to two weeks after birth, vomiting and regurgitation begin, causing failure to thrive. Unless the defect is corrected surgically, severe malnutrition will develop.

Although most frequently noted in infants, pyloric stenosis can also occur in adults. Characteristically, the condition arises sec-

Figure 12.25 Two major types of hiatus hernia: *A*, Sliding or direct hiatus hernia. *B*, rolling or paraesophageal hiatus hernia.

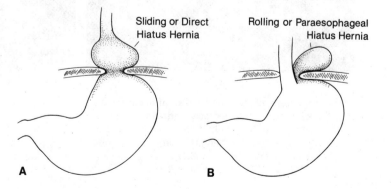

ondary to inflammation associated with ulcers, gastric cancer, or pancreatic cancer.

GASTRIC NEOPLASMS

Abnormal gastric tissue growths can vary considerably, both structurally and symptomatically. Whereas benign neoplasms are essentially "silent," or asymptomatic, malignancies ultimately cause severe malfunction.

Benign growths, for the most part, are categorized as *adenomas* or *leiomyomas*. Adenomas are primarily small polyps that protrude into the gastric lumen; leiomyomas are usually small submucosal growths or nodules that are rarely symptomatic.

Gastric malignancies, on the other hand, are most frequently classified as *carcinomas*.

Once a leading cause of death in the United States, these neoplasms now rank sixth in cancer mortality. For unknown reasons, their incidence has declined considerably in recent years.

Carcinomas can arise anywhere in the stomach but are most often found in the pyloric region. Although they may take a variety of forms, gastric malignancies are frequently of the *fungating* or *ulcerative* type. In the former case, growth is characterized by a fairly good-sized intraluminal mass. In the latter, the carcinoma consists of an erosion of the mucosal lining (see Figure 12.26). Regardless of diversity in structural characteristics, metastasis is uniformly common. Both intra-abdominal seeding and spread to the lungs and the liver are frequently noted. Diffuse clinical manifestations include loss of weight,

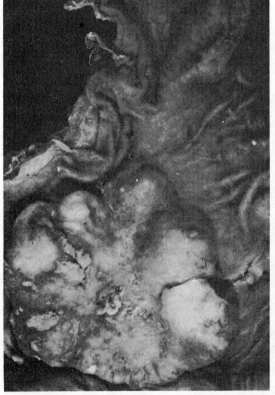 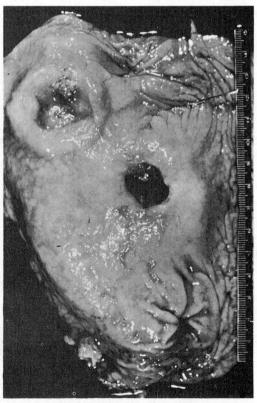

| A | B |

Figure 12.26 Carcinomas of the stomach. *A*, A fungating cancer of the stomach showing beginning central necrosis and excavation. *B*, Ulcerative pattern of gastric carcinoma. A late stage with diffuse infiltration of the wall and two distinct crater formations, one to the left with typical beaded overhanging margins, and one to the right with deep excavation. (From Robbins, S. L., and Cotran, R. S.: Pathologic Basis of Disease, 2nd ed. Philadelphia, W. B. Saunders Company, 1979. Used by permission.)

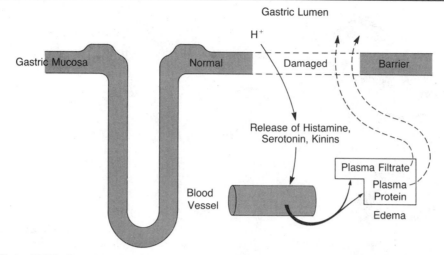

Figure 12.27 Results of back diffusion of acid through the damaged gastric mucosal barrier.

abdominal pain, anorexia, vomiting, and alterations in bowel habits.

INFLAMMATORY DISORDERS

Inflammation of the stomach most commonly involves the mucosal lining and is characterized by varying degrees of irritation or erosion or both. Whereas generalized, superficial inflammation is described as *gastritis*, deeper necrosis associated with acidic digestion of visceral tissue is specifically referred to as a *peptic ulcer*. Some major differences between these two types of inflammatory conditions will be pointed out in the following pages.

GASTRITIS The diffuse inflammatory irritation of gastric mucosa, generally referred to as gastritis, may be either acute or chronic.

In acute gastritis, degenerative changes are usually superficial and result from exposure to irritants such as alcohol, aspirin, steroids, and bile acids. The effect of these chemicals upon the "gastric mucosal barrier" is believed to play a particularly critical role in causing the dysfunction.

As illustrated in Figure 12.27, degeneration of the tunica mucosa paves the way for back-diffusion of hydrogen ions into the gastric tissue. Resulting interstitial acidity trig-

gers the release of vasoactive chemicals such as histamine, serotonin, and kinins. In the presence of these substances, a characteristic inflammatory response occurs, with associated infiltration of lymphocytes, plasma cells, and eosinophils. Clinical manifestations become increasingly evident as localized edema and necrosis cause cellular disruption.

Unlike acute gastritis, chronic gastritis usually develops for unknown reasons. Degenerative changes typically culminate in atrophy of many functional cells within the tunica mucosa. Ultimately, this disorder can result in a decrease or absence of hydrochloric acid production (*hypochlorhydria* or *achlorhydria*) or depression of intrinsic factor secretion or both.

To the extent that acidity within the gastric lumen is diminished or absent, digestive function will be disrupted. Since the activity of pepsin is dependent upon the presence of an acid environment, gastric digestion is virtually eliminated with achlorhydria.

The additional deficit of intrinsic factor during advanced stages of chronic gastritis will cause the evolution of pernicious anemia. As indicated in Figure 12.28, degeneration of parietal mucosal cells results in decreased absorption of vitamin B_{12}. In these cases, the maturation of erythrocytes is impeded, and cellular oxygen supply is subsequently compromised.

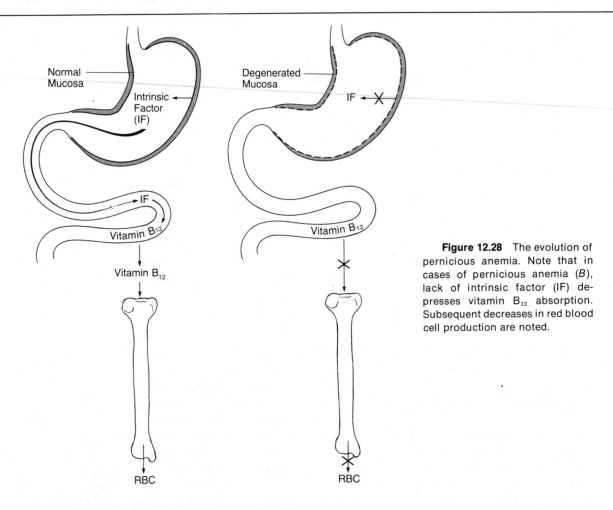

Figure 12.28 The evolution of pernicious anemia. Note that in cases of pernicious anemia (*B*), lack of intrinsic factor (IF) depresses vitamin B_{12} absorption. Subsequent decreases in red blood cell production are noted.

PEPTIC ULCERS When acidic gastric secretions cause the degeneration and necrosis of gastrointestinal mucosa, a peptic ulcer is said to exist. Although initiated by secretions generated within the stomach, ulcers can occur throughout the digestive tract. As illustrated in Figure 12.29, they are most commonly found in the lower esophagus, pylorus of the stomach, or duodenum of the small intestine.

Normally, those areas that are frequently exposed to gastric acidity are protected from erosion by the presence of the "gastric mucosal barrier." Heavy mucus secretions and tight intercellular junctions reduce the destructive effects of hydrogen ions. In spite of these protective mechanisms, however, ulcers can develop when (1) gastric acid secretion is excessively elevated, or (2) the gastric mucosal barrier is significantly disrupted.

In cases of *gastric ulcers*, gastric secretions

are characteristically depressed. Disease is thus associated with disruption of the mucosal barrier, and frequently caused by excessive exposure to alcohol, aspirin, or (in cases of duodenal reflux) bile acids. To the extent that

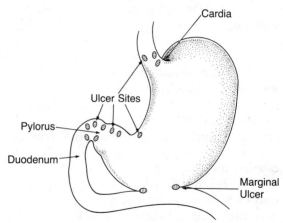

Figure 12.29 The location of peptic ulcers.

gastric ulcers trigger pyloric hypertrophy, symptoms of obstructive pyloric stenosis may also be noted.

Duodenal ulcers, on the other hand, are most commonly associated with hypersecretion of acidic gastric juice. A characteristic increase in parietal cell mass is possibly due to hyperstimulation by the vagus nerve, although this hypothesis has not been confirmed. In rare cases, elevations in hydrochloric acid secretion are associated with the *Zollinger-Ellison (Z-E) syndrome*. The disorder in these instances results from an abnormal secretion of gastrin by adenomas of non-beta islet cells in the pancreas.

Whenever gastric or duodenal ulcers are caused by prolonged psychological or physiological stress, the resulting condition is referred to as *stress ulcer*. Most commonly occurring in the stomach, stress ulcers are usually secondary to one of two distinct phenomena: (1) serious brain injury, or (2) other sources of physiological stress, such as cardiovascular shock, hypoxia, burns, or excessive intake of certain drugs.

Stress ulcers associated with brain injury are called *Cushing's ulcers*. In these cases, a neural disorder is believed to trigger excess vagal stimulation of gastric secretion, and lesions develop secondary to hyperacidity. If, on the other hand, ulcers are caused by other physiological stressors, disruption of the gastric mucosal barrier is believed to be the primary causative mechanism.

A comparative summary of the major types of ulcers can be found in Figure 12.30.

CLINICAL MANIFESTATIONS OF GASTRIC INFLAMMATION Whenever inflammation of the gastric mucosa exists, one can expect associated symptoms of epigastric pain and anorexia, possibly accompanied by nausea and vomiting. Nutritional status will be compromised to the extent that discomfort decreases the desire or ability to ingest food.

Additional manifestations of dysfunction will vary according to the specific nature of the illness. Pernicious anemia, for example, is frequently associated with chronic gastritis. As a result of deficient erythrocyte maturation, symptoms of cellular hypoxia will predictably occur.

In cases of peptic ulcers, on the other hand, bleeding often complicates the clinical picture. Commonly originating in the duodenum, hemorrhage can cause a variety of symptoms, depending upon the severity and extent of blood loss. In milder cases, fecal elimination of blood will result in anemia, as erythrocytes and hemoglobin are passed out of the body. If hemorrhage is more severe, vomiting of blood may occur, causing a considerable depletion of plasma volume. At the extreme, hematogenic shock may result, as described in Chapter 9.

A less frequent, but nonetheless critical, complication of ulcers is *perforation*. In these cases, total erosion of the visceral wall results

	Duodenal Ulcer	Gastric Ulcer	Stress Ulcer
Location	90% in bulb of duodenum	90% in antrum and lesser curvature	Multiple erosions most commonly in stomach
Pathogenesis	1. Hyperacidity is the significant factor	1. Normal or low hydrochloric acid production	1. If caused by head injuries, note increase in hydrochloric acid secretion
	2. Often associated with alcoholic cirrhosis, chronic pancreatitis, emotional stress, smoking	2. Disruption of gastric mucosal barrier is the significant factor	2. All other causes seem to be associated with disruption of gastric mucosal barrier
Common Complications	1. Hemorrhage in posterior wall of duodenal bulb 2. Obstruction	Difficult to treat	1. Hemorrhage 2. Perforation

Figure 12.30 Some major distinctions among duodenal, gastric, and stress ulcers.

in emptying of gastrointestinal contents into the abdominopelvic cavity. Immediate and acute pain is noted as gastric acid causes inflammation of the peritoneal membranes. Abdominal rigidity reflects cessation of functional activity, and death is inevitable unless immediate surgical repair is done.

Disorders of the Small Intestine

It is within the small intestine that the majority of nutrients undergo terminal digestive breakdown and are subsequently absorbed into the bloodstream. Dysfunction of this segment of the gastrointestinal tract can thus seriously disrupt homeostasis by depriving the cells of much-needed nutrient supply.

Generally speaking, the pathogenesis of small intestinal disorders can be categorized as (1) digestive-absorptive, or (2) obstructive-paralytic.

In the following pages, examples of each type of dysfunction will be accompanied by a description of clinical manifestations.

DIGESTIVE-ABSORPTIVE DISORDERS

Within the small intestine, digestion and absorption must work hand in hand to facilitate the servicing of cellular needs. Clearly, ingested nutrients must be broken down chemically before they can pass across the small intestinal wall into the bloodstream.

Although considerable overlap may exist between digestive and absorptive disorders, a distinction should be made between the two. For this reason, digestive and absorptive dysfunctions will be discussed separately.

DISORDERS OF DIGESTION Most often, digestive dysfunction within the small intestine is linked to either pancreatic or biliary deficiency. Although diseases of the major accessory organs are discussed in detail subsequently in this chapter, some related digestive disturbances will be briefly clarified at this point.

In cases of pancreatic inflammation, cancer, or resection, deficiency of enzyme secretion can considerably suppress nutrient digestion. Digestion is further inhibited as a result of Z-E syndrome, when hyperacidity within the intestinal lumen causes (1) inactivation of pancreatic enzymes, and (2) precipitation of bile salts.

Functional activity within the small intestine is also affected by diseases of the liver or biliary tract. In these cases, interference with the introduction of bile into the duodenum causes a disruption of fat emulsification and digestion.

Also influencing small intestinal digestion is the way in which chyme is fed from the stomach into the duodenum. When nutrients bypass the duodenum, for example, they do not always mix effectively with pancreatic juice or bile. Under these circumstances, rate of transit through the intestinal lumen is increased and nutrient breakdown may be considerably impeded. A typical example of this phenomenon can be noted in patients with a *Billroth II gastrectomy*. As illustrated in Figure 12.31, this surgical procedure involves removal of a portion of the stomach, with attachment of remaining gastric tissue directly to the jejunum.

DISORDERS OF ABSORPTION Although digestive dysfunctions may ultimately

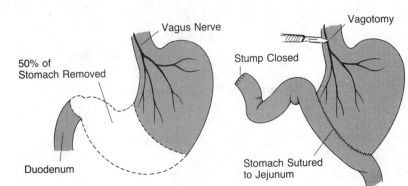

50% of Stomach Removed

Vagus Nerve

Duodenum

Vagotomy

Stump Closed

Stomach Sutured to Jejunum

Figure 12.31 Billroth II gastrectomy.

interfere with small intestinal absorption, the following discussion will emphasize those disorders that specifically impede the transport of digested nutrients from the gastrointestinal lumen into the bloodstream. Primary examples of this type include nontropical sprue (celiac disease) and regional enteritis (Crohn's disease).

Nontropical Sprue Nontropical sprue is a disorder caused by sensitivity to the protein gluten, which is a common constituent of grains such as wheat, rye, barley, and oats. Although the way in which this condition develops has not yet been clarified, the effects are relatively predictable. Characteristic atrophy of the villi causes a marked decrease in small intestinal absorption of most nutrients. Fortunately, treatment is relatively simple and involves removal of the causative agent from the diet. Since gluten may be found in such a wide variety of foods (such as ice cream, salad dressings, canned foods, candy, and beer), the nutritional intake of the patient must be very carefully monitored.

In cases of celiac disease, associated cellular degeneration often causes lactase deficiency. An enzyme found within certain cells that line the small intestine, lactase catalyzes the chemical breakdown of the milk sugar lactose. In its absence, an intolerance to milk develops. As undigested lactose moves into the large intestine, it exerts an osmotic attraction for water, causing fluid to move from the bloodstream into the gastrointestinal lumen. Subsequent bloat, cramping, and colonic irritation are followed by severe diarrhea.

While lactase deficiency often evolves secondary to nontropical sprue, it can also develop as the result of a genetic defect. In these instances, dysfunction is most frequently noted in blacks, Orientals, and Cypriot Greeks.

Regional Enteritis Regional enteritis, or Crohn's disease, is a chronic inflammatory disorder. Most commonly affecting the terminal ileum, it can also occur in other portions of the gastrointestinal tract, including the large intestine, stomach, and esophagus. Although the underlying causative mechanism is unknown, a hypersensitivity response is believed to be involved.

In cases of regional enteritis, lesions are first noted in lymph nodes adjacent to the

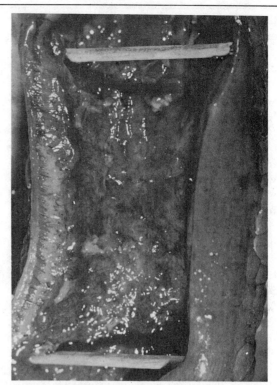

Figure 12.32 Crohn's disease of the ileum. A close-up of a segment of thickened bowel wall. Note the wooden pegs required to keep the lumen exposed. (From Robbins, S. L., and Cotran, R. S.: Pathologic Basis of Disease, 2nd ed. Philadelphia, W. B. Saunders Company, 1979. Used by permission.)

affected area. Subsequent lymphatic obstruction is postulated to cause thickening of the submucosa, while progressive degeneration results in hardening of the small intestinal wall and obstruction of the gastrointestinal lumen (see Figure 12.32). Ultimately, inflammation and necrosis of the mucosa may be most directly responsible for the malabsorption that characteristically ensues.

CLINICAL MANIFESTATIONS OF DIGESTIVE-ABSORPTIVE DISORDERS Any pathological condition causing disruption of the digestive or absorptive processes will ultimately decrease cellular nutrient supply. When cells are deprived of their metabolic fuel, energy output declines. Subsequent weakness and weight loss are thus primary indications of dysfunction.

More specific manifestations of digestive or absorptive disorders vary with the nature of the illness. Lack of protein absorption, for example, causes a decrease in colloid osmotic pressure, with subsequent shifts of fluid out of the plasma compartment (see Chapter 4). Deficient iron absorption can result in anemia, whereas excessive calcium loss causes characteristic symptoms of skeletal muscle irritability and tetany. To the extent that large volumes of nonabsorbed fluids and electrolytes are introduced into the large intestine, diarrhea will result. A summary of some of the primary manifestations of malabsorption is presented in Table 12.2.

Although a variety of clinical symptoms often provide early evidence of absorptive dysfunction, the existence of malabsorption is frequently confirmed by diagnostic testing. Some commonly used procedures are:

1. *Laboratory test for the presence of fat in the feces.* Steatorrhea, or the elimination of excessive quantities of fat in the feces, is a characteristic indication of malabsorption. If more than 6 grams of fat are excreted daily through the lower gastrointestinal tract, dysfunction of the absorptive process must be suspected. Feces frequently appear bulky, frothy, pale, and greasy. The laboratory test used to confirm the presence of fecal fat is commonly performed on 72-hour stool samples, to minimize the possibility of random error.

2. D-*Xylose absorption test.* D-Xylose is a 5-carbon sugar unique in its ability to be absorbed without any preliminary digestion. As illustrated in Figure 12.33, it typically passes into the bloodstream from the lumen of the proximal small intestine and is then transported through the liver to the kidneys for excretion. Assuming normal absorption and renal function, approximately 20 per cent of ingested D-xylose should be eliminated by the kidneys within five hours after intake. The usual procedure is to administer the sugar after 12 hours of fasting and to subsequently test urine for the presence of D-xylose.

3. *Barium x-ray study.* Although not a definitive or specific test, the introduction of a radiopaque barium solution into the digestive tract helps the clinician to visualize the internal contours of certain gastrointestinal organs. In classic cases of malabsorption, the characteristic feathery appearance of barium within

TABLE 12.2 **Some Primary Manifestations of Malabsorption**

Clinical Manifestation	Pathophysiology
Muscle wasting; small stature	Protein malabsorption
Weight loss	Malabsorption of fats, carbohydrates, and protein; calorie deficit
Bone pain; skeletal deformity	Malabsorption of vitamin D and calcium; protein malabsorption
Tetany; positive Chvostek and Trousseau signs	Hypocalcemia, secondary to calcium malabsorption
Tendency to bleed and bruise	Malabsorption of vitamin K, with subsequent disruption of the clotting mechanism
Edema	Malabsorption of amino acids, with secondary decrease in plasma colloid osmotic pressure
Anemia	Malabsorption of iron, folic acid, and vitamin B_{12}
Steatorrhea	Fat malabsorption
Neuritis; dermatitis	Malabsorption of B complex vitamins and folic acid
Abdominal distention	Typically associated with secondary lactase deficiency. The fermentation of undigested lactose produces excessive quantities of gastrointestinal flatulence
Diarrhea	Mucosal irritation; poor absorption of fluids, bile acids, and fatty acids creates laxative effect
Muscle cramps; weakness	Sodium depletion secondary to diarrhea
Muscle flaccidity; cardiac arrhythmias	Potassium depletion secondary to diarrhea

the small intestine is absent, and clumping of the test solution is seen. In Crohn's disease, a narrowing of the small intestinal lumen is evident. This phenomenon is referred to as the *string sign* (see Figure 12.34).

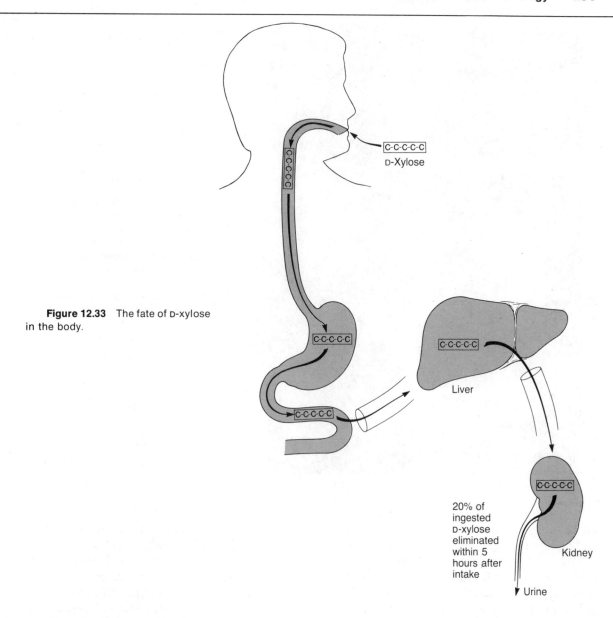

Figure 12.33 The fate of D-xylose in the body.

OBSTRUCTIVE-PARALYTIC DISORDERS

In certain cases, gastrointestinal disorders can be characterized by interference with the propulsion of nutrients through the small intestinal lumen. Most commonly, such disorders are caused by one of two phenomena: (1) obstruction of the small intestinal lumen, or (2) disruption of small intestinal peristalsis. In the following pages, an elucidation of obstructive and paralytic dysfunction is followed by an analysis of their clinical manifestations.

OBSTRUCTIVE DISORDERS Obstruction of the small intestine can occur in a number of ways. Inflammatory hyperplasia, as noted in Crohn's disease, for example, will ultimately reduce the luminal opening through which nutrients can pass. Neoplasms as well can cause obstruction if they grow large enough to pose a barrier to transport. Certain mechanical or structural alterations may also be significant sources of small intestinal occlusion.

Hernias are primary examples of obstruction caused by mechanical factors. They are defined as the protrusion of viscera through

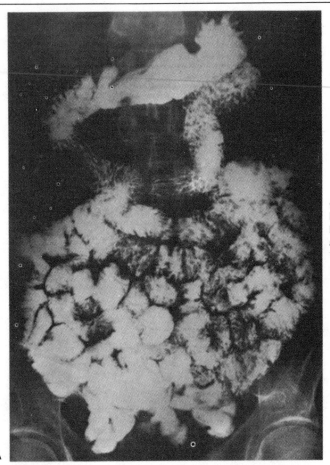

A

Figure 12.34 Barium x-ray studies of the gastrointestinal tract. *A,* Normal intestinal tract. Note characteristic feathery appearance of barium within the lumen. (From Williams, P. L., and Warwick, R.: Gray's Anatomy, 36th ed. New York, Churchill Livingstone, 1980. Used by permission.)

(Illustration continued on opposite page.)

an opening in the muscular wall of the body, and some typical defects are illustrated in Figure 12.35. It can be seen that in cases involving the small intestine, gastrointestinal tissue typically projects out of the abdomino-pelvic cavity in one of three major areas: (1) the abdominal muscle in the vicinity of the groin, (2) the inguinal canal, or (3) the femoral ring (which normally accommodates the external iliac arteries and veins).

Regardless of the particular location, obstruction can result to the extent that pressure surrounding the intestinal loop interferes with nutrient transport. When restriction is severe enough to cut off blood supply to the involved viscera, a *strangulated hernia* is said to exist. This phenomenon is characterized by total obstruction and constitutes a medical emergency. If it is not repaired surgically, ischemia will lead to death and necrosis of gastrointestinal tissue (see Figure 12.36).

Other forms of mechanical obstruction are frequently noted in middle-aged patients after abdominal surgery. In these cases, the postoperative growth of fibrous bands of connective tissue (described as *postoperative adhesions*) can bind adjacent gastrointestinal tissue and ultimately cause obstruction. Adhesions may also lead to *volvulus*, a characteristic twisting of the small intestine that is illustrated in Figure 12.37.

Another potential source of small intestinal occlusion is *intussusception*, or the telescoping of one portion of the intestine into another. Illustrated in Figure 12.38, it is most commonly noted in infants and young children and is frequently evident at the ileocecal junction.

PARALYTIC DISORDERS Assuming lack of obstruction, propulsion of nutrients through the small intestine can be disrupted

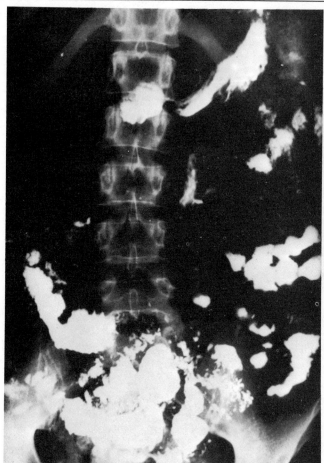

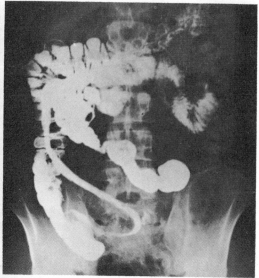

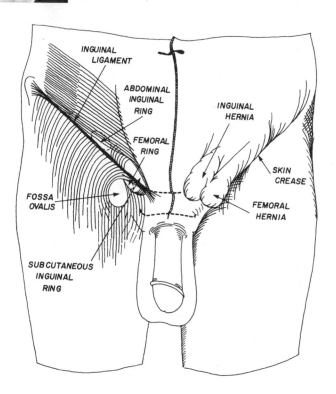

Figure 12.34 *Continued* *B*, X-ray of the small intestine in a classic case of malabsorption. Note clumping of barium solution within the lumen. (From Sodeman, W. A., and Sodeman, T. M.: Sodeman's Pathologic Physiology: Mechanisms of Disease, 6th ed. Philadelphia, W. B. Saunders Company, 1979. Used by permission.) *C*, X-ray of small intestine in case of Crohn's disease. Note narrowing of small intestinal lumen in terminal ileum. (From Beeson, P. B., et al.: Cecil Textbook of Medicine, 15th ed. Philadelphia, W. B. Saunders Company, 1979. Used by permission.)

Figure 12.35 Areas involved in femoral and inguinal hernias. (From Artz, C. P., Cohn, I., and Davis, J. H.: A Brief Textbook of Surgery. Philadelphia, W. B. Saunders Company, 1976. Used by permission.)

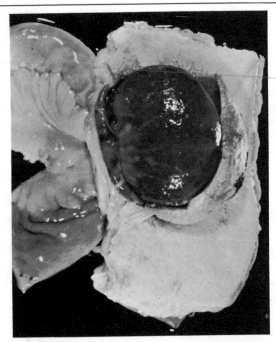

Figure 12.36 Strangulated inguinal hernia. A knuckle of small intestine trapped in an inguinal hernial sac is demonstrated en bloc with the encircling skin of the inguinal region in situ. The sac has been opened to demonstrate the hemorrhagic condition of the contents. (From Robbins, S. L., and Cotran, R. S.: Pathologic Basis of Disease, 2nd ed. Philadelphia, W. B. Saunders Company, 1979. Used by permission.)

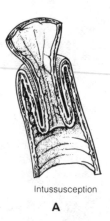

Intussusception

A

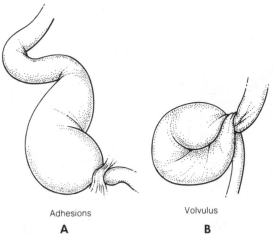

Adhesions

A

Volvulus

B

Figure 12.37 Adhesions and volvulus may both trigger intestinal obstruction. A, Adhesions. Note binding of gastrointestinal tract by bands of connective tissue. B, Volvulus. Note twisting and enlargement of intestinal loop. (From Jones, D. A., Dunbar, C. F., and Jirovec, M. M. (eds.): Medical-Surgical Nursing: A Conceptual Approach. New York, McGraw-Hill Book Company, 1978. Used by permission.)

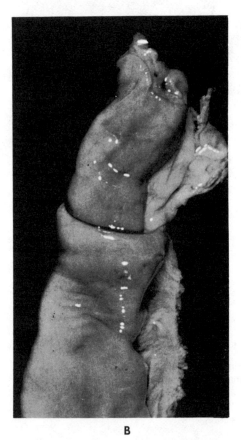

B

Figure 12.38 Intussusception. A, Note the way in which one portion of the bowel telescopes into another. B, Intussusception of the small intestine viewed externally. (A from Jones, D. A., Dunbar, C. F., and Jirovec, M. M. (eds.): Medical-Surgical Nursing: A Conceptual Approach. New York, McGraw-Hill Book Company, 1978. Used by permission. B from Robbins, S. L., and Cotran, R. S.: Pathologic Basis of Disease, 2nd ed. Philadelphia, W. B. Saunders Company, 1979. Used by permission.)

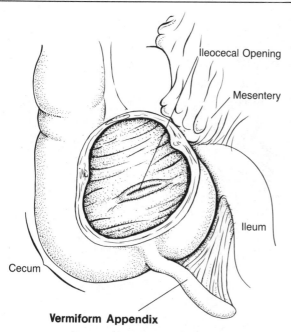

Ileocecal Opening

Mesentery

Ileum

Cecum

Vermiform Appendix

Figure 12.39 The appendix.

by any disorder that reduces or inhibits peristalsis. Failure of intestinal contractility is generally described as *paralytic ileus*. It frequently occurs secondary to mechanical obstruction or as a temporary complication of abdominal surgery. Peritonitis or ischemia can also trigger this dysfunction.

Peritonitis is an inflammation of the membranes lining the abdominopelvic cavity. Often caused by the leakage of gastrointestinal contents into the abdomen, it is frequently associated with a perforated ulcer or ruptured appendix. As illustrated in Figure 12.39, the appendix is a hollow worm-like structure that extends from the cecum of the large intestine. If it becomes infected or inflamed, necrosis can set in, causing rupture and release of inflammatory toxins into the abdominopelvic cavity. Under these circumstances, the small intestine may be secondarily affected, as paralytic ileus sets in.

As mentioned earlier, ischemia can also disrupt gastrointestinal contractility. Normally, the majority of blood servicing the small intestine is carried through the *superior mesenteric artery* and leaves the organ via the *superior mesenteric vein*, as illustrated in Figure 12.40.

Blood supply to the intestine may be inter-

rupted for a number of reasons. Approximately 60 per cent of the time, pathogenesis is the result of atherosclerotic narrowing of the vascular lumen. Less frequently, thrombi or emboli are the cause.

Regardless of the mechanism, dysfunction is characterized by initial mucosal ischemia and necrosis. Smooth muscle paralysis and intestinal dilation typically follow, ultimately causing the development of paralytic ileus.

CLINICAL MANIFESTATIONS OF OBSTRUCTIVE-PARALYTIC DISORDERS

Whenever the flow of nutrients through the small intestinal lumen is suppressed, symptoms of pain, distention, and constipation are characteristically noted.

In cases of obstruction, luminal contents predictably accumulate behind the occlusion, as illustrated in Figure 12.41. While blockage proximal to the stomach commonly results in the vomiting of gastric content, lower obstruction can cause ejection of vomitus that is more fecal in nature. In either case, intestinal contractility will usually increase initially in attempts to propel nutrients through the obstructed area. Ultimately, however, peristalsis is depressed, and paralytic ileus ensues.

Whenever the transport of nutrients through the intestinal lumen is seriously disrupted, fluid imbalances commonly result. Hypotension is, in fact, a potential complication of obstructive-paralytic disorders for three major reasons:

1. Normal secretion of fluids and electrolytes into the intestinal lumen is maintained, while a decrease in absorption is noted. Under these circumstances, fluid derived from the vascular compartment accumulates excessively within the gastrointestinal tract.

2. Inflammatory changes in the wall of the small intestine cause increases in permeability, with subsequent leakage of fluid and bacteria into the abdominopelvic cavity.

3. Vomiting, secondary to obstruction, can further reduce fluid content in the body.

When fluid shifts cause a large volume of plasma to be displaced into the intestinal lumen or the peritoneal spaces or both, blood pressure will be decreased. In these cases, associated symptoms of hypotension and shock

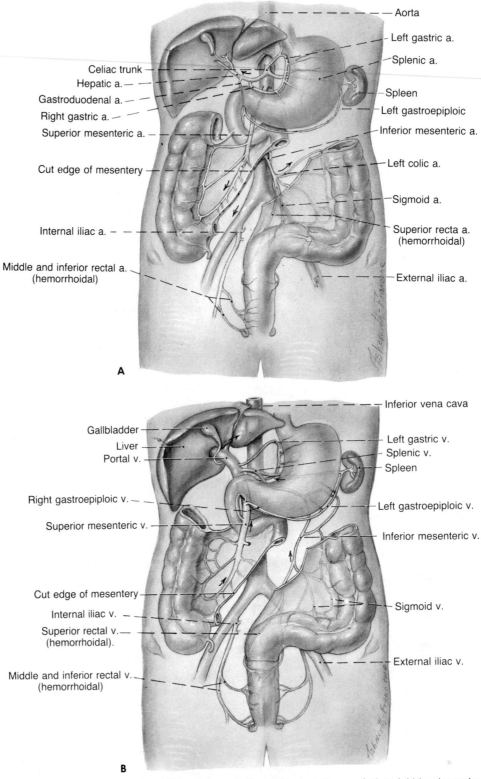

Figure 12.40   Circulation of blood through the abdominal viscera. *A*, Arterial blood supply to the abdominal viscera. *B*, Veins servicing the abdominal viscera. (From Jacob, S. W., Francone, C. A., and Lossow, W. J.: Structure and Function in Man, 4th ed. Philadelphia, W. B. Saunders Company, 1978. Used by permission.)

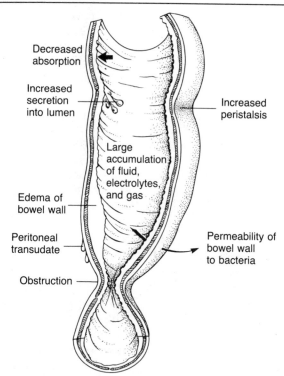

Figure 12.41 The pathophysiology of intestinal obstruction. (From Nadrowski, L. F.: Pathophysiology and current treatment of intestinal obstruction. Rev. Surg., *31*(6): 381–404, 1974. Used by permission.)

may be noted. Absorption of intestinal bacteria and toxins will further complicate the clinical picture by adding elements of sepsis to the condition.

Disorders of the Large Intestine

Whereas the small intestine is mainly involved with digestion and absorption, the large intestine functions primarily in the processing, storage, and elimination of fecal material.

A pathological condition within this segment of the gastrointestinal tract is usually associated with one of three major phenomena: (1) inflammatory disorders, (2) neoplasms, or (3) motility disorders.

Although they are arbitrarily classified for study purposes, it must be remembered that there can be considerable overlap among these categories in the clinical setting. In the following pages, the evolution and clinical manifestations of each disease entity are discussed separately.

INFLAMMATORY DISORDERS

The two most common inflammatory disorders of the large intestine are diverticulitis and ulcerative colitis. Whereas diverticulitis is noted most frequently in the sigmoid colon, ulcerative colitis is a more diffuse condition that can affect extensive segments of the intestinal mucosa.

DIVERTICULITIS Diverticulitis is a disorder that characteristically begins with the formation of small sac-like mucosal outcroppings through the intestinal wall, as illustrated in Figures 12.42 and 12.43. These pouches, called diverticuli, are often asymptomatic and remain undiagnosed in a large majority of patients. When diverticuli are present, the resulting condition is referred to as *diverticulosis*. The likelihood of developing this disorder is believed to be minimal in individuals who ingest sufficient quantities of bulk or roughage — hence, the value of a high-bran diet.

Under certain circumstances, diverticuli can become inflamed, leading to a condition known as *diverticulitis*. Pain and bleeding frequently result, associated with possible perfo-

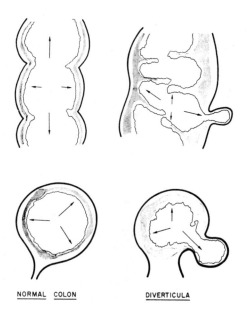

Figure 12.42 The pathogenesis of diverticular disease. (From Ranson, J. H. C., et al.: Am. J. Surg., *123*: 185, 1972. Used by permission.)

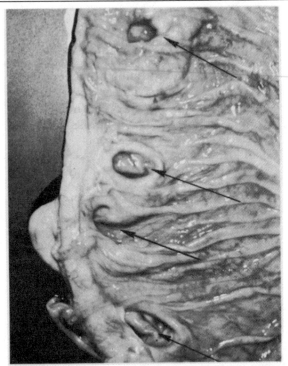

Figure 12.43 Diverticulosis of colon. Openings into diverticuli are seen in the mucosa (arrows). (From Purtilo, D. T.: Survey of Human Disease. Reading, Mass., Addison-Wesley Publishing Company, 1978. Used by permission.)

ration and peritonitis. In chronic cases, long-term inflammation may culminate in fibrosis, adhesions, and eventual intestinal obstruction. Characteristic symptoms include distention, constipation, and the formation of narrow stools.

ULCERATIVE COLITIS Ulcerative colitis is an inflammatory condition characterized by edema and congestion of the mucosal tissue lining the large intestine. Degenerative changes promote ready bleeding, and involvement of the submucosa is frequently noted as the disease progresses. Although genetic factors and autoimmunity have been suggested as possible causative factors, the initiating mechanisms have not been established with any degree of certainty.

Symptoms commonly accompanying the acute form of ulcerative colitis include fever, bloody stools, pain, nausea, and severe diarrhea. When the disease pattern is more chronic in nature, manifestations are similar but often milder. If inflammation is prolonged, loss of blood and mucus can lead to anemia and hypoproteinemia.

Similar to ulcerative colitis in many re-

TABLE 12.3 **Differential Diagnosis of Crohn's Disease and Ulcerative Colitis***

	Crohn's Disease of Colon	Chronic Ulcerative Colitis
CLINICAL		
Diarrhea	Most common symptom, but usually of moderate severity	Most common symptom but more severe and often of extreme degree
Rectal bleeding	Uncommon and never severe	Almost always during active phase
Abdominal pain	Common	Unusual
Fever	Common and often persistent	Only during acute attack
Abdominal mass	Frequent in right lower quadrant	Absent
Perianal disease	Frequent, often an early feature and persistent	Unusual
Sigmoidoscopy	May be negative, or scattered ulcers	Always reveals diffuse ulcerative disease
Rectal biopsy	May reveal granulomas	Active inflammation, often "crypt abscesses"
Toxic megacolon	Rarely occurs	5–10% of severe cases
Carcinoma	Rarely occurs	Risk increases proportionate to duration of diseases; 4–6% in prolonged cases
RADIOLOGICAL		
Site	Rectum rarely involved, distribution often segmental and discontinuous, right colon a common site	Rectum always involved, extends proximally in continuous pattern into left colon and beyond
Symmetry	Eccentric distribution with unequal involvement of colon circumference	Entire circumference involved
Terminal ileum	Often involved	Usually normal, occasional "backwash ileitis"

*From Conn, H. F., and Conn, R. B.: Current Diagnosis. Philadelphia, W. B. Saunders Company; 1977. Used by permission.

spects is Crohn's disease, as it occurs in the large intestine. Although most commonly a disorder of the small intestine, regional enteritis occasionally affects the large bowel. In these cases, the differential diagnosis is often quite difficult. A comparative summary of some characteristic distinctions between ulcerative colitis and Crohn's disease is presented in Table 12.3.

NEOPLASMS

Neoplasms, or abnormal tissue growths in the large intestine, may be either benign or malignant.

As illustrated in Figure 12.44, the benign tumors may take a variety of forms. Most common are the *pedunculated adenomas* (also called adenomatous polyps or polypoid adenomas). These growths, which project from the mucosa into the lumen, are circular and project from a thin stalk. Although much controversy exists as to whether they are precursors of cancer, the general consensus seems to be that they are essentially harmless.

Villous adenomas, on the other hand, are benign tumors that more often evolve into malignant growths. Occurring less frequently than the polypoid neoplasms, they are generally nodular, with characteristic finger-like projections noted on histological examination.

While benign adenomas of all types are usually asymptomatic, malignant tumors have a variety of manifestations.

Cancer of the colon is the second leading cause of all cancer deaths in the United States. Although most large intestinal malignancies are *adenocarcinomas* (derived from glandular epithelium), the specific form often varies as a function of location. Polypoid or flat, bulky growths are more common in the cecum or ascending colon, whereas *annular* (or ringlike) lesions are frequently noted in the rectum or sigmoid colon.

In cases of colonic cancer, location also considerably influences symptoms. As noted in Figure 12.45, intestinal contents are usually soft and liquid in the ascending, or right, colon. As a result, luminal material can flow around potential obstructions with relative ease, and clinical manifestations of occlusion are not usually evident until the malignancy is far advanced.

In the descending, or left, colon, however, intestinal contents are typically semisolid.

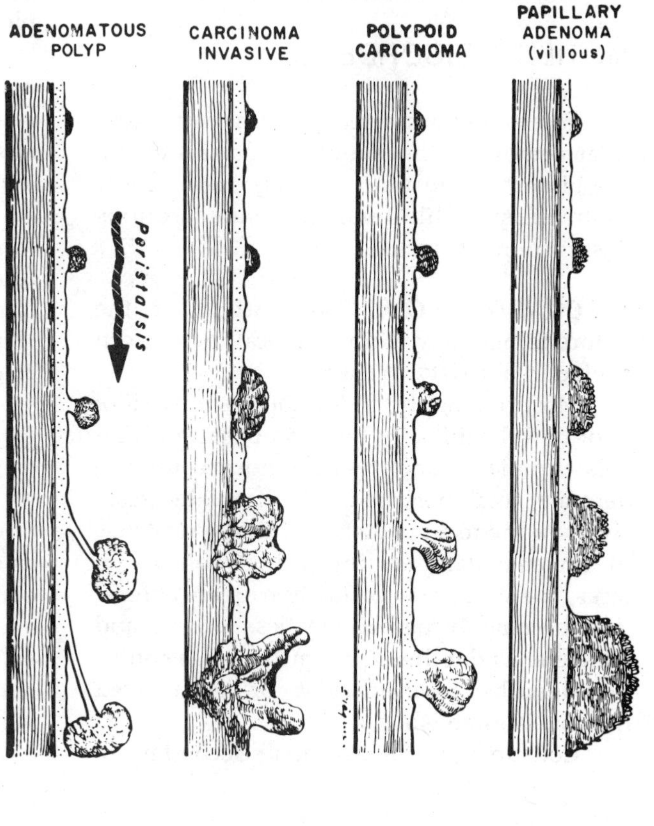

Figure 12.44 Benign tumors of the colon. (From Welch, C. E., and Hedberg, S.: Polypoid Lesions of the Gastrointestinal Tract, 2nd ed. Philadelphia, W. B. Saunders Company, 1974. Used by permission.)

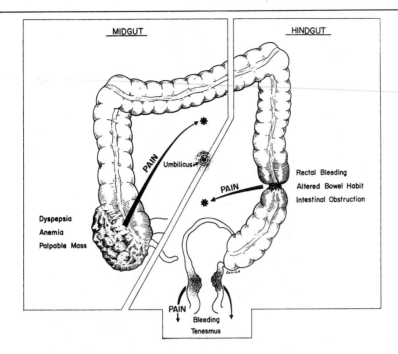

MIDGUT | HINDGUT

PAIN
Umbilicus

Rectal Bleeding
Altered Bowel Habit
Intestinal Obstruction

PAIN

Dyspepsia
Anemia
Palpable Mass

PAIN
Bleeding
Tenesmus

Figure 12.45 Symptoms of carcinoma in the right and left colon. (From Sabiston, D. C.: Davis-Christopher Textbook of Surgery, 11th ed. Philadelphia, W. B. Saunders Company, 1977. Used by permission.)

In these cases, characteristic annular lesions tend to obstruct fecal transport. Pain, distention, and diarrhea may be noted owing to reflex response to the malignant growth. Evidence of obstruction is additionally reflected in characteristically narrow, ribbon-like stools.

MOTILITY DISORDERS

To ensure normal fecal elimination, muscular activity in the tunica muscularis of the large intestine must be optimally regulated. If contractility is inhibited or accelerated, serious dysfunction can result.

CONSTIPATION Constipation, or the failure to normally eliminate fecal matter, can evolve in a variety of ways.

Most commonly, it develops as a result of poor bowel habits. To the extent that individuals chronically suppress the normal urge to defecate, fecal material can accumulate excessively in the rectum. As rectal tissue stretches to accommodate an increasing volume of feces, the reflex that normally triggers defecation becomes progressively less strong and effective. Under these circumstances, a condition described as *atonic colon*, or desensitized rectum, is established.

Constipation can also occur secondary to neural disorders. When the segment of the spinal cord (S2–S4) that normally integrates the defecation reflex is damaged, fecal elimination will be suppressed. Other neural conditions associated with constipation include megacolon (a congenital lack of the myenteric plexus in the sigmoid colon), absence of colonic neural ganglia, and a disorder described as spastic, or irritable, colon. In cases of spastic colon, constriction of the large intestinal smooth muscle often alternates with spasms that cause intermittent bouts of diarrhea.

As constipation evolves, for whatever reason, characteristic changes are noted in the feces. They become increasingly hard and dry, often causing voluntary retention, with associated aggravation or initiation of atonic colon.

The fecal changes that commonly accompany constipation can best be explained by taking a closer look at large intestinal function. As mentioned earlier, a substantial volume of fluid is usually absorbed from the large intestine back into the bloodstream preceding fecal elimination. Of the approximately 500 to 600 ml. of fluid that pass through the ileocecal valve daily, about 400 to 500 ml. are normally reabsorbed. This leaves approximately 100 ml. remaining as a characteristic constituent of fecal material. It is significant to note that most absorption occurs in the right colon, while the rectum is relatively impermeable to both water and electrolytes.

Whenever fecal elimination is disrupted, more time is available for fluid absorption. For this reason, hard, dry stools are characteristically associated with constipation. Because of these fecal changes, a number of secondary rectal-anal disorders can develop.

Hemorrhoids, for example, are varicose veins of the anal canal. Developing as a rule in individuals over 25 years of age, they frequently accompany disorders that disrupt venous return from the hemorrhoidal veins. Causative factors include constipation as well as enlargement of the prostate gland and congestion associated with pregnancy or rectal tumors.

Constipation can also cause the development of *anal fissures*, or cracks in the lining of the anus. Brought about by the forcing of hard, dry feces through the anal lumen, fissures cause discomfort and burning after defecation. To the extent that fear of pain initiates fecal retention, constipation can be aggravated by this condition.

DIARRHEA Unlike constipation, diarrhea is characterized by the rapid and frequent movement of fecal material through the lower gastrointestinal tract. Although it is commonly associated with inflammatory bowel disorders (as discussed earlier), diarrhea can also be caused by infection or excessive parasympathetic stimulation of the large intestine.

A viral or bacterial infection of the gastrointestinal tract is referred to as *enteritis*. Usually affecting the distal ileum and large intestine most extensively, infection causes mucosal irritation, with subsequent increases in mucus secretion and intestinal motility. These mechanisms combine to flush the infectious agent out of the intestinal tract and provide a means of rapidly eliminating the pathogenic microbe from the system.

Further promoting diarrhea in cases of infectious disorders is the phenomenon of volume overload. When pathogens affect the small intestine, resulting increased motility and decreased absorption time cause large volumes of liquefied nutrients to pass into the large intestine at a rapid rate. Since the colon

is able to absorb only approximately 125 ml. of fluid per hour, increased influx can frequently result in watery diarrhea. This situation is classically noted in cases of *cholera*, in which toxins cause the transport of massive quantities of sodium and water into the lumen of the bowel.

In the absence of infection, diarrhea can be induced by excessive parasympathetic neural stimulation. This branch of the autonomic nervous system characteristically causes increases in gastrointestinal secretion and motility.

In certain individuals, tension or stress is believed to trigger parasympathetic stimulation of the digestive tract. The result is a condition referred to as *irritable colon*. Symptoms include abdominal pain associated with alternating bouts of constipation and diarrhea. Increased mucus production is frequently noted, along with excessive expulsion of flatus.

The elimination of colonic gases is promoted by rapid transit of fecal material through the large intestine. Normally, a large proportion of the flatus produced by colonic bacteria is reabsorbed into the bloodstream preceding defecation. When gastrointestinal motility increases, the time available for gaseous absorption is reduced. Under these circumstances, flatus is expelled in excessive amounts through the anus.

Generally, the most serious physiological consequences of diarrhea result from associated loss of fluid and electrolytes. Symptoms of hypovolemia characteristically occur, accompanied by manifestations of sodium, potassium, and bicarbonate depletion. Since bicarbonate is a base, metabolic acidosis frequently results. A brief elucidation of some of the fluid and electrolyte imbalances that commonly accompany diarrhea can be found in Table 12.4.

Disorders of the Accessory Organs

Whereas a large majority of gastrointestinal disorders originate in the main organs of the digestive tract, dysfunction of certain accessory structures can also disrupt the digestive-absorptive processes. In the following pages, disorders of the pancreas and the

TABLE 12.4 **Fluid and Electrolyte Imbalances that Commonly Accompany Diarrhea**

Diarrhea May Cause	Which Results In
Hypovolemia	Dry mucous membranes Loss of skin turgor Weight loss Late signs of decreased blood pressure/circulatory collapse
Sodium depletion	Headache/confusion Weakness/giddiness Muscular twitching/convulsions
Potassium depletion	Muscular weakness/fatigue Cardiac arrhythmias Hyperreflexia Anorexia, nausea, and vomiting Apathy/drowsiness/irritability
Bicarbonate depletion	Metabolic acidosis, with associated headache, nausea, vomiting, sensorium changes, and hyperventilation Secondary hypercalcemia may result in cardiac arrhythmias and muscular flaccidity

TABLE 12.5 **Pancreatic Enzymes***

Enzyme	Function
Amylase	Catalyzes the hydrolysis of starch and glycogen to maltose or maltotriose. Contains calcium. Excreted in the urine.
Lipase	Hydrolyzes fats into mono-, di-, and triglycerides and free fatty acids.
Proteases Trypsinogen Chymotrypsinogen Procarboxypeptidase Proaminopeptidase	Splits proteins to peptides and a few amino acids. The proteases are secreted in an inactive form; otherwise they would act on pancreatic tissue and cause destruction. Once in the intestine, intestinal enterokinase acts on trypsinogen, converting it to trypsin. Trypsin then acts on the other proteases to convert them to active enzymes.

*From Luckmann, J., and Sorensen, K. C.: Medical-Surgical Nursing: A Psychophysiologic Approach. Philadelphia: W. B. Saunders Company, 1980. Used by permission.

liver and biliary tract are discussed. Special emphasis is placed upon causative mechanisms and resulting physiological imbalances.

DISORDERS OF THE PANCREAS

The pancreas is a relatively small accessory organ that plays a significant role in the digestive process. Functioning as an exocrine gland, it releases potent enzymes into the gastrointestinal tract that promote the breakdown of all nutrients into their respective end products (see Table 12.5).

Normally, these enzymes are not activated until they reach the duodenum, at which point they catalyze the chemical breakdown of carbohydrates, proteins, and fats. In cases of pancreatic inflammation, however, proteolytic and lipolytic enzymes become functional within the pancreas itself. Autodigestion results, characterized by considerable cellular destruction and necrosis.

Inflammation of the pancreas is frequently initiated by alcoholism or biliary duct obstruction and may be manifested in either the acute or the chronic form. Regardless of the specific nature of the illness, degeneration usually results in edema, necrosis, and hemorrhage of pancreatic tissue.

ACUTE PANCREATITIS Acute pancreatitis is commonly triggered by biliary duct obstruction. As noted in Figure 12.46, back-up of enzymes and bile into the pancreas can easily occur when these substances are unable to enter the duodenum through the papilla of Vater. It is believed that autodigestion is in some way promoted by the reflux of bile into the pancreatic duct.

In the evolution of acute pancreatitis, necrosis and edema are followed by hemorrhage. Subsequent abscess formation is also common. In about 25 per cent of the cases, jaundice occurs as a consequence of biliary duct compression by the swollen head of the pancreas. *Pancreatic ascites* is an additional complication usually associated with alcoholism. Most frequently caused by rupture of pancreatic tissue, it is characterized by the release of secretions into the abdominopelvic cavity.

Adult respiratory distress syndrome has also been cited as a less common complication

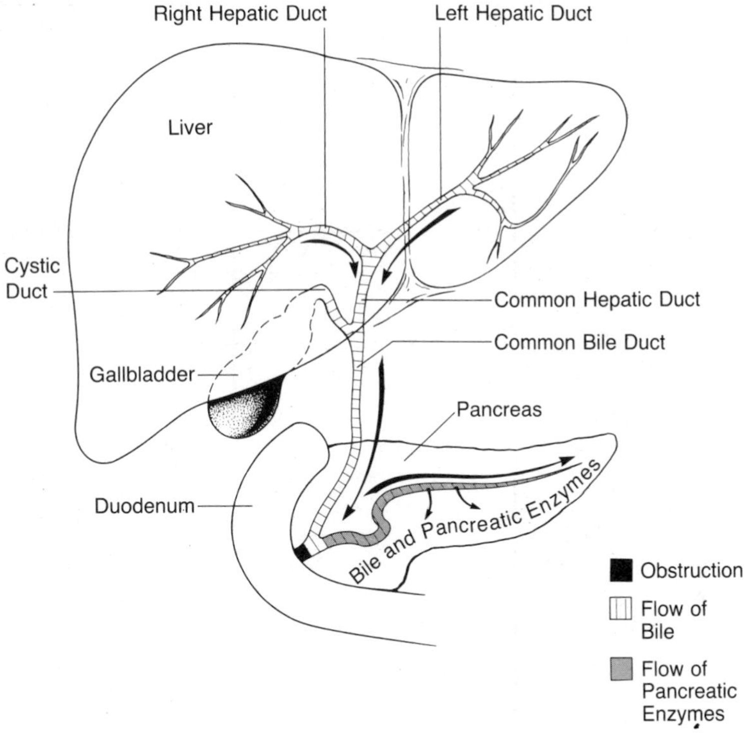

Figure 12.46 Backup of enzymes and bile into the pancreas secondary to biliary duct obstruction.

of acute pancreatitis. In these cases, the escape of pancreatic lipase and proteases into the bloodstream is believed to be responsible for the digestion and breakdown of pulmonary capillary membranes. Resulting pulmonary edema ultimately disrupts the exchange of gases within the lungs, causing respiratory dysfunction.

In addition to these specific manifestations of acute pancreatitis, more general symptoms include severe pain, nausea, and vomiting. As enzymes are released from the diseased pancreas into the bloodstream, laboratory tests will reveal elevations in serum amylase and lipase.

Hypocalcemia may also be associated with acute pancreatitis. It is postulated that this phenomenon is due to a shift of calcium out of plasma into degenerating pancreatic tissue during early stages of inflammation. If calcium is significantly depleted, symptoms of skeletal muscle irritability, tetany, and cardiac arrhythmias will develop.

CHRONIC PANCREATITIS Following acute pancreatic inflammation, degenerative disease may persist. In these cases, cellular necrosis is followed by fibrous repair, and the disease condition is described as chronic pancreatitis.

Most commonly associated with alcoholism or malnutrition or both, chronic pancreatitis is frequently characterized by the deposit of calcium salts or protein plugs or both into pancreatic ductal tissue. Obstruction of the common bile duct may occur secondarily, causing the onset of juandice. Massive abdominal distention will also be evident if secretions leak from the inflamed organ into the abdominopelvic cavity.

Ultimately, fibrotic degeneration may cause physiological disruption as the secretion of pancreatic enzymes and hormones is suppressed. Clinical manifestations reflect underlying organic dysfunction and include: (1) steatorrhea, caused by failure to adequately digest and absorb fats; (2) increased tendency to bruise and bleed, caused by failure to adequately absorb fat-soluble vitamin K, (3) increase of protein nitrogen in the stools, caused by failure to adequately digest and absorb proteins; and (4) glucose intolerance–diabetes mellitus, caused by failure to adequately secrete insulin.

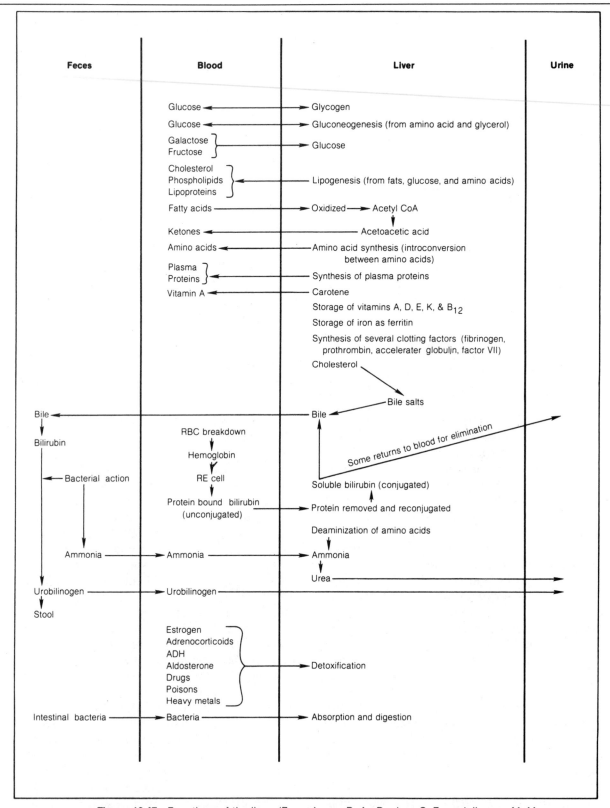

Figure 12.47 Functions of the liver. (From Jones, D. A., Dunbar, C. F., and Jirovec, M. M. (eds.): Medical-Surgical Nursing: A Conceptual Approach. New York, McGraw-Hill Book Company, 1978. Adapted from Jirovec, M.: Metabolism. Boston, Boston University Print Shop, 1974. Used by permission.)

DISORDERS OF THE LIVER AND BILIARY TRACT

The liver is an organ that services cellular needs in many different ways. Most directly influencing digestion through the production of bile, it also plays a critical role in the metabolism of nutrients and the detoxification of foreign substances in the blood. Some major functional activities of the liver are summarized in Figure 12.47.

In categorizing disorders of the liver and biliary system, two major pathological mechanisms can be cited: (1) disruption of bile production and excretion, and (2) disruption of hepatic cellular function.

DISRUPTION OF BILE PRODUCTION AND EXCRETION

Bile produced by the liver is normally stored in the gallbladder and secreted, via biliary ducts, into the duodenum. Disease of the liver, gallbladder or biliary tract can thus significantly affect the digestion and absorption of fat in the gastrointestinal tract.

To understand the mechanisms underlying biliary pathology, it is important to review the life cycle of bilirubin, as outlined previously in this chapter. If bilirubin is excessively produced, or insufficiently excreted, jaundice will develop.

Excessive Production of Bilirubin When red blood cells are destroyed, or hemolyzed, too rapidly, an overload of unconjugated bilirubin is released into the circulatory system. To the extent that the liver is unable to incorporate sufficient quantities of this bilirubin into bile, bilirubin will accumulate in the bloodstream to cause a pale yellow skin discoloration. Since, under these circumstances, the release of bile is not obstructed, brown fecal pigment will continue to be formed by intestinal bacteria.

Evidence of increased hemolysis is often noted in newborns who have elevated numbers of immature red blood cells. Accelerated rupture of these erythrocytes is frequently complicated by the existence of immature liver cells that are unable to efficiently extract and conjugate bilirubin. This situation can be seriously damaging only when plasma bilirubin levels exceed 20 mg. per cent. In these cases,

deposit of bilirubin within certain areas of the brain can cause neural degeneration.

In the adult, excessive hemolysis often arises secondary to sickle cell anemia, pernicious anemia, and transfusion or drug reactions. Although jaundice will occur, critical physiological disequilibrium usually stems from associated hypoxemia.

Insufficient Excretion of Bilirubin Under certain circumstances, dysfunction is characterized by the inability of bile to enter the duodenum. In these cases, *conjugated bilirubin* is reabsorbed from the liver back into the bloodstream and causes a yellow-orange to yellow-green skin discoloration. Since the quantity of bile pigment within the gastrointestinal tract is characteristically decreased, associated manifestations will include: (1) disruption of the digestion or absorption of fat and fat-soluble vitamins (such as vitamins A, D, E, and K); and (2) decreased production of stercobilinogen and urobilinogen, resulting in pale or clay-colored feces.

Jaundice arising secondary to obstruction (*obstructive jaundice*) is caused primarily by one of two phenomena: (1) Compression of biliary ducts within the liver. In these cases, dysfunction is most often associated with the interstitial swelling that typically accompanies hepatic cellular disease, such as hepatitis and cirrhosis. (2) Occlusion of biliary ducts external to the liver. In these instances, dysfunction commonly arises secondary to pancreatic cancer or biliary stone formation. The mechanisms underlying these phenomena are illustrated in Figure 12.48.

Stones in the biliary ducts (or *cholelithiasis*) are generally precipitates of one or more bile components. Commonly containing bilirubin, cholesterol, or calcium, they almost always form in the gallbladder. Frequently, however, they pass into the biliary ducts and cause obstruction of the cystic or common bile duct. Although the exact cause of stone formation is unknown, cholelithiasis is often associated with conditions such as diabetes, pancreatitis, cirrhosis of the liver, and cancer of the gallbladder.

DISRUPTION OF HEPATIC CELLULAR FUNCTION

Although disease of the liver can cause widespread imbalance in the body,

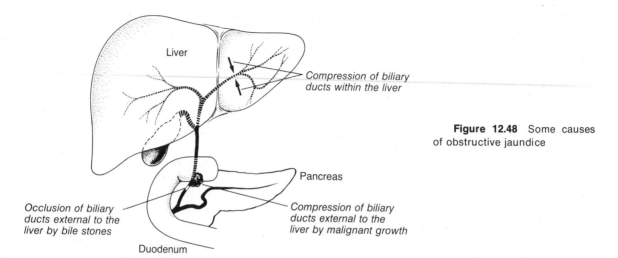

Figure 12.48 Some causes of obstructive jaundice

the organ is amazingly resilient under adverse conditions. Hepatic tissue is possessed of remarkable regenerative capacity and is thus able to withstand severe physiological stress. Even when disease is well established, causing degeneration of 80 to 90 per cent of hepatic cells, the liver is still capable of sustaining an effective level of functional activity. In cases of organic failure, however, homeostasis is critically disrupted, and death results.

Most often, dysfunction of the liver is caused by either hepatitis or cirrhosis. Some major differences between these two disorders are clarified in the following pages.

Hepatitis Hepatitis is an inflammatory disorder that results from the exposure of hepatic cells to toxic agents such as alcohol, carbon tetrachloride, and acetaminophen (in excessive doses). Viral pathogens may also cause hepatitis, specifically triggering the onset of either *hepatitis A* or *hepatitis B*. Some general distinctions between these two disease types are summarized in Table 12.6.

It can be seen that in cases of hepatitis A, viruses originating in contaminated water or shellfish frequently enter the body through the fecal-oral route. In cases of hepatitis B, the major sources of infection are contaminated blood transfusions or contaminated needles and syringes utilized in the administration of drugs.

Regardless of the origin of the condition, hepatitis generally affects the liver by causing inflammation, necrosis, and release of the enzymes SGOT and SGPT from damaged hepatic cells. The presence of these enzymes in plasma

TABLE 12.6 **Differential Features of Viral Hepatitis**

	Hepatitis A	**Hepatitis B**
Also known as	Infectious or short-incubation hepatitis	Serum or post-transfusion hepatitis
Incubation time	15–45 days	28–160 days
Transmission	Usually by fecal-oral route. Contaminated water or milk is a common source of infection; poor sanitation and overcrowding predispose. May be transmitted parenterally.	Usually by parenteral route. Contaminated blood and vaccines are common sources of infection. Also may be transmitted by fecal-oral route.
Pathology	Hepatic cellular degeneration and necrosis, followed by cellular regeneration. Inflammatory cell infiltration, with accumulation of plasma cells, lymphocytes, neutrophils, and eosinophils.	
Clinical manifestations	Usually mild flu-like symptoms without jaundice (anicteric) or with (icteric). Symptoms include lethargy, irritability, anorexia, nausea, vomiting, fever, diarrhea or constipation, and abdominal pain. If jaundice does occur, it typically abates within two weeks in children and four to six weeks in adults.	
Differential diagnosis	Negative response to hepatitis-B (Australian) antigen	Positive response to hepatitis-B (Australian) antigen

can, in fact, be utilized to confirm a diagnosis of hepatitis, particularly when associated with characteristic symptoms, such as malaise, weakness, anorexia, headache, and low-grade fever.

Jaundice typically occurs after the seventh day and lasts for approximately four to six weeks. Barring complications, recovery usually begins around one to two weeks after the

---

TABLE 12.7 **Major Signs and Symptoms of Hepatitis and Their Underlying Causes**

Signs and Symptoms	Underlying Causes
Jaundice, clay-colored feces, dark urine (containing bilirubin and urobilinogen)	Conjugated bilirubin is not excreted properly into intestine, leading to elevated serum levels, staining of skin (jaundice), a low level of bile pigment in stools (clay-colored feces), and increased amounts of conjugated bilirubin excreted into the kidneys. Urinary urobilinogen is elevated because small amounts of urobilinogen being produced in the intestine are eliminated by the kidneys instead of the liver.
Pruritus	Accumulation of bile salt in the skin.
Tiredness, weakness	Energy metabolism in liver is at a low level.
Fever	Pyrogens are released in inflammatory process.
Pain in right upper abdomen	Glisson's capsule is stretched owing to swelling of inflamed liver.
Loss of appetite, nausea, vomiting	Visceral reflexes may reduce peristalsis. Changes in stomach or bowel may be responsible.
Bleeding (in extreme cases)	Prothrombin synthesis by injured liver cells is decreased. Fat-soluble vitamin K absorption is reduced owing to reduced bile in intestine.
Anemia	Red blood cell life is shorter because of changes in liver enzymes; in extreme cases, bleeding and hemorrhage can occur.

---

onset of jaundice and is complete in two to six weeks. A summary of the pathophysiology underlying some primary clinical manifestations of hepatitis is presented in Table 12.7.

Cirrhosis Cirrhosis is a chronic disease of the liver characterized by fibrous degeneration of hepatic tissue. Unlike hepatitis, it is almost always preceded by long-term exposure to stress, and it culminates in irreversible cellular damage.

THE EVOLUTION OF CIRRHOSIS Approximately 50 per cent of the time, cirrhosis arises secondary to chronic alcoholic hepatitis and is specifically referred to as *Laennec's cirrhosis*. In these cases, damage is attributed primarily to the toxic effects of ethanol upon hepatic cells. Less commonly, cirrhosis can evolve subsequent to viral hepatitis, toxic hepatitis, or biliary stasis.

Regardless of the cause, cirrhosis is characterized by a number of progressive changes: (1) necrosis affecting approximately two thirds of the liver; (2) permanent replacement of some necrotic cells with fibrous connective scar tissue; and (3) generation of large nodules of hepatic cells to replace some damaged tissue.

As a result of these structural alterations, the internal architecture of the liver is considerably changed. Frequently, available blood supply does not adequately service new cells, and additional damage is caused by ischemia. To the extent that veins within the liver are compressed by nodular growths, venous return is also decreased. Under these circumstances, congestion may also cause an elevation in portal capillary blood pressure, with the subsequent development of edema in the wall of the intestine.

THE CLINICAL MANIFESTATIONS OF CIRRHOSIS Usually, cirrhosis evolves slowly and may remain asymptomatic for a long period. Early indications of dysfunction include weakness, anorexia, dull pain, nausea, and vomiting. Ultimately, hepatic degeneration will culminate in serious physiological disruption throughout the body. The causative mechanisms primarily responsible for advanced manifestations of disease include: (1) hepatic cellular failure, and (2) portal hypertension.

HEPATIC CELLULAR FAILURE Since the cells of the liver are so actively involved in a wide variety of functional processes, hepatic necrosis can trigger severe physiological disequilibrium.

Blood disorders, for example, are common manifestations of cirrhosis. As hepatic cells fail, less prothrombin and fibrinogen are produced. With associated decreases in the secretion of bile, the absorption of fat-soluble vitamin K is also decreased. Blood will thus clot less readily, and symptoms of nosebleeds, bleeding from the gums, and excessive menstrual bleeding may be noted.

Decreased production of albumin will additionally cause a drop of colloid osmotic pressure, with the subsequent evolution of edema. Elevations in the levels of aldosterone and ADH further aggravate fluid imbalances. Normally, these hormones are inactivated by the liver and prepared for elimination from the body. In cases of hepatic disease, however, they accumulate excessively in plasma, resulting in hypervolemia.

Jaundice is also present in a large proportion of patients with cirrhosis and evolves through mechanisms described earlier in this chapter. In advanced stages of the disease, however, *hepatic coma* emerges as one of the most critical disturbances resulting from hepatic cellular dysfunction.

Hepatic coma, also referred to as *hepatic encephalopathy*, results primarily from reduction in detoxification secondary to necrosis of the liver cells. In cases of hepatic cellular failure, a number of toxic chemicals that would typically be extracted and inactivated by the liver remain instead in plasma. Ammonia, for example, is produced by bacterial action within the large intestine. Under normal circumstances, it would pass into the bloodstream and be converted into urea by hepatic cells. As a result of cirrhosis, however, ammonia accumulates in plasma, causing disruption in cerebral metabolism. Resulting changes in personality and behavior are usually accompanied by muscular twitching. Subsequent confusion will be followed by coma and death if the syndrome cannot be reversed. A summary of some of the major effects of hepatic cellular failure can be found in Table 12.8.

PORTAL HYPERTENSION   Portal hypertension, which is defined as an increase in the pressure of blood within the portal vein, is generally associated with resistance to blood flow through the liver.

TABLE 12.8   Some Major Manifestations of Hepatic Cellular Failure

Clinical Manifestation	Causative Mechanisms

Bleeding
  Nosebleeds
  Bleeding from the gums
  Excessive menstrual bleeding
	Decreased production of prothrombin and fibrinogen
	Decreased production of bile, with associated depression in the absorption of fat-soluble vitamin K

Edema	Decreased production of plasma proteins, with a subsequent decrease in colloid osmotic pressure
Jaundice	Compression of biliary ducts within the liver secondary to interstitial swelling Reabsorption of conjugated bilirubin from the liver back into the bloodstream

Hepatic coma
  Personality and behavior changes
  Confusion, coma, and death
	Failure of hepatic detoxification mechanisms
	Accumulation of ammonia in plasma

To fully understand the phenomenon of portal hypertension, it is necessary to review hepatic circulation. As illustrated in Figure 12.49, blood is normally transported to the liver by two distinct routes:

1. One third of hepatic blood supply is transported from the abdominal aorta through the hepatic artery to the liver.

2. Two thirds of hepatic blood supply is carried from the stomach, spleen, and intestine through the portal vein to the liver.

Ultimately all blood traveling through the liver drains into the hepatic veins and is subsequently emptied into the inferior vena cava.

In most cases, portal hypertension develops secondary to hepatic inflammation and fibrosis. Under these circumstances, interstitial swelling poses resistance to hepatic circulation, and blood is shunted into collateral vessels. As illustrated in Figure 12.50, the submucosal esophageal veins are frequently utilized to bypass the liver and transport blood from the portal vein into the vena cava. As pressure increases within the esophageal vessels, they dilate and are specifically referred to as *esophageal varices*. At the extreme, rupture and profuse hemorrhage can result.

The transport of blood around the liver

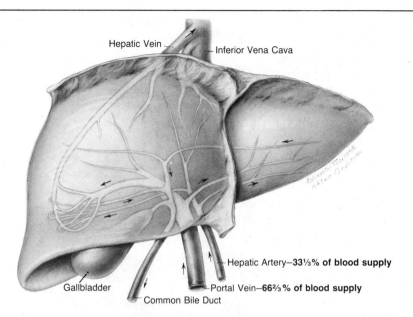

Figure 12.49 Flow of blood through the liver. (From Jacob, S. W., Francone, C. A., and Lossow, W. J.: Structure and Function in Man, 4th ed. Philadelphia, W. B. Saunders Company, 1978. Used by permission.)

Hepatic Vein — Inferior Vena Cava

Hepatic Artery—33⅓% of blood supply

Portal Vein—66⅔% of blood supply

Gallbladder

Common Bile Duct

can cause plasma composition to be considerably altered. Normally, hepatic cells extract large quantities of ammonia and glucose from the blood. When the liver is bypassed, these substances remain elevated in the systemic circulation, causing hyperglycemia and possible hepatic coma.

As portal hypertension evolves, a characteristic decrease in venous return causes an increase in capillary blood pressure within the liver. Subsequent increases in lymph formation are accompanied by the leakage of a plasma-like filtrate directly through the liver capsule and into the peritoneal cavity. The resulting condition, characterized by bloat and distention, is called *ascites* (see Figure 12.51).

To the extent that the spleen is enlarged as a result of portal venous congestion, an increase in the reticuloendothelial destruction of red blood cells, white blood cells, and platelets occurs. Varying degrees of anemia, infection, and hemorrhage may thus be associated with *hypersplenism*. A summary of some of the major clinical manifestations of portal hypertension is presented in Table 12.9.

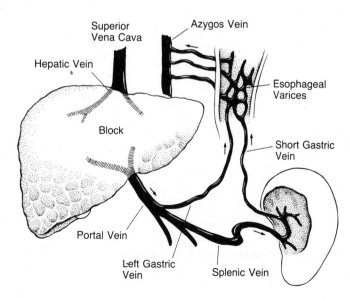

Figure 12.50 Hemodynamic changes in liver cirrhosis leading to the development of esophageal varices.

Superior Vena Cava

Azygos Vein

Hepatic Vein

Esophageal Varices

Block

Short Gastric Vein

Portal Vein

Left Gastric Vein

Splenic Vein

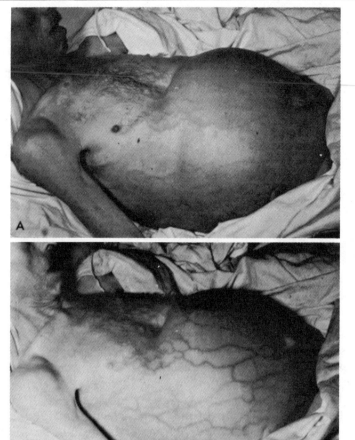

Figure 12.51   Ascites. *A*, Patient with advanced cirrhosis of liver shows marked ascites. *B*, Infrared photography is used to demonstrate multiple collateral vessels that are present. (From Schiff, L. (ed.): Diseases of the Liver, 4th ed. Philadelphia, J. B. Lippincott Company, 1975. Used by permission.)

TABLE 12.9   **Some Major Manifestations of Portal Hypertension**

Clinical Manifestation	Causative Mechanism
Ascites	Increased resistance to blood flow through the liver Increased formation of lymph within the liver Decrease in colloid osmotic pressure secondary to depressed plasma protein formation Elevated levels of ADH and aldosterone associated with hepatocellular disease
Esophageal varices	Increased resistance to blood flow through the liver Development of collateral vascular channels to bypass the congested liver
Splenomegaly	Resistance to the exit of blood from the splenic vein Congestion of the spleen secondary to fluid back-pressure

GASTROINTESTINAL PATHOLOGY: DISRUPTION OF CELLULAR NEEDS

Because the digestive system plays such a significant role in the breakdown and absorption of ingested nutrients, disease may considerably disrupt cellular metabolism. Additionally, gastrointestinal dysfunction can interfere with the servicing of cellular needs in a wide variety of peripheral ways. Gastric vomiting, for example, frequently causes metabolic alkalosis, and the malabsorption of iron may be associated with hypoxemia. A summary of some of the major ways in which pathological conditions can disrupt homeostasis is presented in Table 12.10.

TABLE 12.10 **Disruption of Homeostasis Associated With Gastrointestinal Disease**

Cellular Need Being Disrupted	Underlying Pathophysiological Mechanism	Causative Clinical Disorders
Oxygen	Bleeding $\longrightarrow$ loss of RBC's	Peptic ulcers Ulcerative colitis
	$\downarrow$ Production of intrinsic factor $\longrightarrow$ $\downarrow$ absorption of vitamin B_{12} $\longrightarrow$ $\downarrow$ in RBC production	Gastritis
	$\downarrow$ Production of fibrinogen and prothrombin $\longrightarrow$ $\downarrow$ absorption of fat-soluble vitamin K $\longrightarrow$ $\uparrow$ bleeding $\longrightarrow$ loss of RBC's	Hepatocellular disease associated with cirrhosis
	Splenomegaly $\longrightarrow$ $\uparrow$ breakdown of RBC's	Portal hypertension
Nutrients	Interference with the transport of nutrients from the pharynx to the stomach	Dysphagia Achalasia Pyloric stenosis
	Anorexia, nausea and/or vomiting	Obstruction Acute pancreatitis Peptic ulcer Hepatitis Cirrhosis Gastrointestinal cancer
	Hepatocellular disease or biliary obstruction $\longrightarrow$ $\downarrow$ in the production or secretion of bile $\longrightarrow$ interference with fat digestion	Hepatitis Cirrhosis Biliary stones
	Malabsorption	Celiac disease Crohn's disease
Elimination	Failure to eliminate nondigestible gastrointestinal wastes	Diverticulitis Colonic cancer Atonic colon Megacolon
	Failure of the liver to adequately detoxify plasma $\longrightarrow$ $\uparrow$ ammonia in bloodstream	Cirrhosis $\longrightarrow$ hepatic coma
Fluid-electrolyte and acid-base balance	Excess vomiting $\longrightarrow$ hypovolemia and metabolic alkalosis	Obstruction Acute pancreatitis Peptic ulcer Hepatitis Cirrhosis Gastrointestinal cancer
	Excess diarrhea $\longrightarrow$ hypovolemia, Na^+, K^+, and HCO_3^- depletion and metabolic acidosis	Ulcerative colitis Enteritis
	Obstructive-paralytic disorders of the small intestine $\longrightarrow$ fluid shifts out of plasma into the gastrointestinal lumen and peritoneal spaces $\longrightarrow$ hypovolemia	Neoplasms Strangulated hernia Adhesions Volvulus Intussusception Paralytic ileus

STUDY QUESTIONS

1. Define or describe the following terms:
   a. tunica mucosa
   b. taeniae coli
   c. uvula
   d. enterogastric reflex
   e. villi
   f. plexus of Auerbach
   g. gastric mucosal barrier
   h. ileum
   i. external anal sphincter
   j. urobilinogen and stercobilinogen
   k. gastroesophageal sphincter
   l. chyme
   m. enterohepatic circulation of bile
   n. parietal cells
   o. the gastric phase of gastric secretion

2. Explain why hepatic disease might be associated with the following clinical manifestations:
   a. edema
   b. increased bleeding time
   c. increased sensitivity to alcohol
   d. indigestion associated with the intake of fatty foods

3. Mr. Walters is admitted to the hospital with a diagnosis of *dysphagia.* Explain the nature of this disorder and identify some possible causative conditions.

4. Further tests on Mr. Walters (see above) reveal the existence of achalasia. Explain the relationship between achalasia and dysphagia.

5. Mr. Rizer is suffering from a direct, or sliding, hiatus hernia, while Mr. Croft has a hiatus hernia of the rolling, or paraesophageal, variety. Why is it that Mr. Rizer often suffers from considerable heartburn after a meal whereas Mr. Croft can enjoy food without associated discomfort?

6. Bobby Taylor is born with pyloric stenosis. The pediatrician recommends immediate corrective surgery, but the parents are reluctant to sign the consent form. Explain to them why it is not a good idea to delay surgery.

7. Explain why anemia may result from (a) chronic gastritis, and (b) peptic ulcers.

8. What mechanism is responsible for the bloat, cramping, and diarrhea characteristically associated with milk intolerance?

9. Explain why the following clinical symptoms might be associated with malabsorption:
   a. edema
   b. anemia
   c. tetany
   d. diarrhea
   e. steatorrhea

10. A patient is being given a D-xylose absorption test to confirm the existence of malabsorption. She asks why you are testing her urine when all of her symptoms are intestinal. Explain the nature of this test.

11. Determine whether the following disorders would cause: (1) digestive-absorptive, or (2) obstructive-paralytic disease of the small intestine:
    a. lactose deficiency
    b. regional enteritis (Crohn's disease)
    c. volvulus
    d. inguinal hernia
    e. nontropical sprue (celiac disease)
    f. peritonitis
    g. Billroth II gastrectomy
    h. postoperative adhesions
    i. Zollinger-Ellison (Z-E) syndrome
    j. intestinal ischemia
    k. obstruction of the biliary tract

12. Explain why obstructive-paralytic disorders of the small intestine frequently cause the development of hypotension.

13. Are the following symptoms primarily indicative of (1) diverticulitis, or (2) ulcerative colitis:
    a. bloody stools
    b. constipation
    c. diarrhea
    d. narrow stools

14. Would you always expect carcinoma of the colon to cause manifestations of gastrointestinal obstruction? Explain.

15. Identify each of the following factors as (1) causing constipation, (2) resulting from constipation, (3) causing diarrhea, or (4) resulting from diarrhea.

a. anal fissures
b. metabolic acidosis
c. atonic colon
d. hypovolemia
e. enteritis
f. excessive expulsion of flatus
g. megacolon
h. cholera
i. hemorrhoids

16. Mr. Dawley is an alcoholic. Describe the evolution and clinical manifestations of two gastrointestinal disorders that are frequently associated with alcoholism.

17. Mr. Parker is admitted to the hospital with severe pain in the URQ (upper right quadrant). He is running a low-grade fever and is worried about the abnormal pasty color of his feces and the yellowish discoloration he has noted in the whites of his eyes. What diagnosis do you expect, and why?

Suggested Readings

Books

Alyn, I. B.: Disturbances in hepatic function. *In* Jones, D. A., Dunbar, C. F., and Jirovec, M. M.: Medical-Surgical Nursing, A Conceptual Approach. New York, McGraw-Hill Book Company, 1978, p. 640.

Anderson, W. A. D., and Scotti, T. M.: Synopsis of Pathology, 10th ed. St. Louis, The C. V. Mosby Company, 1980, pp. 436–473; 525–573.

Bolt, R. J.: Pathophysiology of gallbladder disease. *In* Sodeman, W. A., and Sodeman, T. M. (eds.): Pathologic Physiology, Mechanisms of Disease, 6th ed. Philadelphia, W. B. Saunders Company, 1979, p. 915.

Brooks, F. P.: Diseases of the pancreas. *In* Beeson, P. B., McDermott, W., and Wyngaarden, J. B. (eds.): Cecil Textbook of Medicine, 15th ed. Philadelphia, W. B. Saunders Company, 1979, p. 1550.

Burgess, A.: The Nurse's Guide to Fluid and Electrolyte Balance, 2nd ed. New York, McGraw-Hill Book Company, 1979, pp. 167–178.

Christensen, J.: Motility. *In* Frohlich, E. D. (ed.): Pathophysiology, Altered Regulatory Mechanisms in Disease, 2nd ed. Philadelphia, J. B. Lippincott Company, 1976, p. 461.

Davenport, H. W.: Mechanisms of gastric and pancreatic secretion. *In* Frohlich, E. D. (ed.): Pathophysiology, Altered Regulatory Mechanisms in Disease, 2nd ed. Philadelphia, J. B. Lippincott Company, 1976, p. 481.

Durham, N.: Problems of the lower gastrointestinal tract. *In* Phipps, W. J., Long, B. C., and Woods, N. F. (eds.): Medical-Surgical Nursing, Concepts and Clinical Practice. St. Louis, The C. V. Mosby Company, 1979, p. 1280.

Durham, N.: Problems of the upper gastrointestinal tract. *In* Phipps, W. J., Long, B. C., and Woods, N. F. (eds.): Medical-Surgical Nursing, Concepts and Clinical Practice. St. Louis, The C. V. Mosby Company, 1979, p. 1187.

Faloon, W. W.: Hepatic mechanisms. *In* Frohlich, E. D. (ed.): Pathophysiology, Altered Regulatory Mechanisms in Disease, 2nd ed. Philadelphia, J. B. Lippincott Company, 1976, p. 531.

Gall, E. A., and Mostofi, F. K. (eds.): The Liver. Baltimore, The Williams & Wilkins Company, 1973.

Greenberger, N. J., and Winship, D. H.: Gastrointestinal Disorders: A Pathophysiologic Approach. Chicago, Year Book Medical Publishers, 1976.

Grossman, M. E.: Peptic ulcer: pathogenesis and pathophysiology. *In* Beeson, P. B., McDermott, W., and Wyngaarden, J. B. (eds.): Cecil Textbook of Medicine, 15th ed. Philadelphia, W. B. Saunders Company, 1979, p. 1502.

Guyton, A. C.: Textbook of Medical Physiology, 5th ed. Philadelphia, W. B. Saunders Company, 1976, pp. 850–901; 936–943.

Hartman, C. E.: Disturbances in elimination. *In* Jones, D. A., Dunbar, C. F., and Jirovec, M. M.: Medical-Surgical Nursing, A Conceptual Approach. New York, McGraw-Hill Book Company, 1978, p. 611.

Hole, J. W.: Human Anatomy and Physiology. Dubuque, Wm. C. Brown Company, 1978, pp. 407–442.

Iber, F. L.: Normal and pathologic physiology of the liver. *In* Sodeman, W. A., and Sodeman, T. M. (eds.): Pathologic Physiology, Mechanisms of Disease, 6th ed. Philadelphia, W. B. Saunders Company, 1979, p. 885.

Janowitz, H. D.: Chronic inflammatory diseases of the intestine. *In* Beeson, P. B., McDermott, W., and Wyngaarden, J. B. (eds.): Cecil Textbook of Medicine, 15th ed. Philadelphia, W. B. Saunders Company, 1979, p. 1560.

Jeffries, G. H.: Diseases of the liver. *In* Beeson, P. B., McDermott, W., and Wyngaarden, J. B. (eds.): Cecil Textbook of Medicine, 15th ed. Philadelphia, W. B. Saunders Company, 1979, p. 1637.

Johnson, L. R. (ed.): Gastrointestinal Physiology. St. Louis, The C. V. Mosby Company, 1977.

Kent, T. H., Hart, M. N., and Shires, T. K.: Introduction to Human Disease. New York, Appleton-Century-Crofts, 1979, pp. 151–188.

Kirsner, J. B., and Winans, C. S.: The stomach. In Sodeman, W. A., and Sodeman, T. M. (eds.): Pathologic Physiology, Mechanisms of Disease, 6th ed. Philadelphia, W. B. Saunders Company, 1979, p. 799.

Knoebel, L. K.: The gastrointestinal system I. The mouth, esophagus, and stomach. In Selkurt, E. E. (ed.): Basic Physiology for the Health Sciences. Boston, Little, Brown & Company, 1975, p. 219.

Knoebel, L. K.: The gastrointestinal system II. The exocrine pancreas, biliary system, and small and large intestines. In Selkurt, E. E. (ed.): Basic Physiology for the Health Sciences. Boston, Little, Brown & Company, 1975, p. 245.

Luckmann, J., and Sorensen, K. C.: Medical-Surgical Nursing, A Pathophysiologic Approach, 2nd ed. Philadelphia, W. B. Saunders Company, 1980, pp. 1385–1532.

McSherry, C. K.: Cholecystitis and cholelithiasis. In Conn, H. F. (ed.): Current Therapy, 1978. Philadelphia, W. B. Saunders Company, 1978.

Purtillo, D. T.: A Survey of Human Diseases. Menlo Park, Addison-Wesley Publishing Company, 1978, pp. 309–335.

Robbins, S. L., and Cotran, R. S.: Pathologic Basis of Disease, 2nd ed. Philadelphia, W. B. Saunders Company, 1979, pp. 918–1113.

Safer, N. G.: Disturbances in digestion. In Jones, D. A., Dunbar, C. F., and Jirovec, M. M.: Medical-Surgical Nursing, A Conceptual Approach. New York, McGraw-Hill Book Company, 1978, p. 583.

Schiff, L. (ed.): Diseases of the Liver, 4th ed. Philadelphia, J. B. Lippincott Company, 1975.

Sherlock, S.: Diseases of the Liver and Biliary System, 5th ed. Philadelphia, F. A. Davis Company, 1975.

Skinner, D. B.: The esophagus. In Sodeman, W. A., and Sodeman, T. M. (eds.): Pathologic Physiology, Mechanisms of Disease, 6th ed. Philadelphia, W. B. Saunders Company, 1979, p. 785.

Skinner, D. B., et al. (eds.): Gastroesophageal Reflux and Hiatal Hernia. Boston, Little, Brown & Company, 1972.

Sleisenger, M. H., and Fordtran, J. S. (eds.): Gastrointestinal Diseases, 2nd ed. Philadelphia, W. B. Saunders Company, 1977.

Sleisenger, M. H.: Malabsorption. In Beeson, P. B., McDermott, W., and Wyngaarden, J. B. (eds.): Cecil Textbook of Medicine, 15th ed. Philadelphia, W. B. Saunders Company, 1979, p. 1523.

Snodgrass, P. J.: Pathophysiology of the pancreas. In Sodeman, W. A., and Sodeman, T. M. (eds.): Pathologic Physiology, Mechanisms of Disease, 6th ed. Philadelphia, W. B. Saunders Company, 1979, p. 928.

Sodeman, W. A., and Watson, D. W.: The large intestine. In Sodeman, W. A., and Sodeman, T. M. (eds.): Pathologic Physiology, Mechanisms of Disease, 6th ed. Philadelphia, W. B. Saunders Company, 1979, p. 860.

Soergel, K. H., and Hofman, A. F.: Absorption. In Frohlich, E. D. (ed.): Pathophysiology, Altered Regulatory Mechanisms in Disease, 2nd ed. Philadelphia, J. B. Lippincott Company, 1976, p. 499.

Tortora, G. H., and Anagnostakos, N. P.: Principles of Anatomy and Physiology, 2nd ed. San Francisco, Canfield Press, 1978, pp. 538–570.

Watson, D. W., and Sodeman, W. A.: The small intestine. In Sodeman, W. A., and Sodeman, T. M. (eds.): Pathologic Physiology, Mechanisms of Disease, 6th ed. Philadelphia, W. B. Saunders Company, p. 825.

Way, L. W.: Diseases of the gallbladder and bile ducts. In Beeson, P. B., McDermott, W., and Wyngaarden, J. B. (eds.): Cecil Textbook of Medicine, 15th ed. Philadelphia, W. B. Saunders Company, 1979, p. 1618.

Way, L. W.: Portal hypertension. In Dunphy, J. E., and Way, L. W. (eds.): Current Surgical Diagnosis and Treatment. Los Altos, Lange Medical Publications, 1977.

Articles

Altshuler, A., and Hilden, D.: The patient with portal hypertension. Nurs. Clin. North Am., 12:317, 1977.

Barkin, J. S.: Ascites as a complication of chronic pancreatic disease. Postgrad. Med., 64:195, 1978.

Bates, M.: Hiatus hernia. Nurs. Mirror, 141:50, 1975.

Beachley, M. C., and Turner, M. A.: Diverticular disease of the gastrointestinal tract. Curr. Concepts Gastroenterol., 2:30, 1978.

Brady, P. G.: Small intestinal syndromes: Guide to diagnosis. Hosp. Med., 15:41, 1979.

Brooke, B. N. (ed.): Crohn's disease. Clin. Gastroenterol., 1:261, 1972.

Buhac, I., and Balint, J.: Diarrhea and constipation. Am. Fam. Physician, 12:149, 1975.

Cameron, J. L., Zuidema, G. D., and Margolis, S.: A pathogenesis for alcoholic pancreatitis. Surgery, *77*:754, 1975.

Duodenal ulcer: Important considerations in the pathogenesis. Hosp. Med., *15*:20, 1979.

Fromm, D.: Stress ulcer. Hosp. Med., *14*:58, 1978.

Gelb, A. M.: Reflux esophagitis: Myths and realities. Consultant, *16*:44, 1976.

Hanson, R. F., and Pries, J. M.: Synthesis and enterohepatic circulation of bile salts. Gastroenterology, *73*:611, 1977.

Hunter, G., and Gaisford, W.: Guide to the diagnosis and management of obstructive jaundice. Hosp. Med., *13*:82, 1977.

Iber, F. L.: Axioms on biliary tract disease. Hosp. Med., *15*:51, 1979.

Ivey, K. J.: Gastric mucosal barrier. Gastroenterology, *61*:247, 1971.

Javitt, N. B.: Hyperbilirubinemic and cholestatic syndromes. Postgrad. Med., *65*:120, 1979.

Johnston, I. D. A.: Duodenal ulcers. Nurs. Mirror, *136*:24, 1973.

Keusch, G.: Bacterial diarrheas. Am. J. Nurs., *73*:1028, 1973.

Kretchmer, N.: Lactose and lactase. Sci. Am., *227*:1, 1972.

Lessene, H., and Fallon, H.: Alcoholic liver disease. Postgrad. Med., *53*:101, 1973.

Mendeloff, A. I.: What has been happening to duodenal ulcer? Gastroenterology, *67*:1020, 1974.

Moody, F. G., and Cheung, L. Y.: Stress ulcers: Their pathogenesis, diagnosis, and treatment. Surg. Clin. North Am., *56*:1469, 1976.

Peterson, A. M.: Acute viral hepatitis. Nurse Practitioner, *4*:9, 1979.

Pierce, L.: Anatomy and physiology of the liver in relation to clinical assessment. Nurs. Clin. North Am., *12*:259, 1977.

Regan, P. T.: Acute pancreatitis: diagnosis and treatment. Hosp. Med., *15*:30, 1979.

Roth, J. L.: Introduction: Colon diverticular disease. Postgrad. Med., *60*:75, 1976.

Sethbhakdi, S.: Pathogenesis of colonic diverticulosis. Postgrad. Med., *60*:76, 1976.

Sherlock, S.: Chronic hepatitis. Postgrad. Med., *65*:81, 1979.

Stahlgren, L. H., and Morris, N. W.: Intestinal obstruction. Am. J. Nurs., *77*:999, 1977.

Trapnell, J. E.: Acute pancreatitis. Nurs. Mirror, *139*:52, 1974.

Wormsley, K. G.: The pathophysiology of duodenal ulceration. Gut, *15*:59, 1974.

Chapter Outline

chapter 13

Neural Pathology

Chapter Objectives

At the completion of this chapter, the student will be able to:

1. Describe the basic structure and function of a neuron.
2. Describe the organization of the peripheral nervous system.
3. Trace the transmission of: (1) a sensory impulse, and (2) a motor impulse as they travel between the central nervous system and the periphery.
4. Differentiate between the spinal cord and the brain with respect to basic structure and function.
5. Identify two major causes of cerebral pathology.
6. Trace normal cerebral blood flow and define cerebral ischemia.
7. Differentiate between cerebral ischemia caused by: (1) thrombi, (2) emboli, (3) hemorrhage, and (4) pathology external to the central nervous system, with respect to development and clinical manifestations.
8. Explain the difference between a TIA and a CVA.
9. Identify and describe four major causes of increasing intracranial pressure.
10. Describe the clinical manifestations associated with increasing intracranial pressure.
11. Identify and describe five major causes of spinal cord pathology.
12. Distinguish between UMN and LMN lesions, with respect to cause and predictable clinical manifestations.
13. Differentiate between an UMN and a LMN bladder or bowel.
14. Given the location of a spinal cord lesion, be able to predict some associated clinical symptoms.

INTRODUCTION

The nervous system consists of many specialized cells, called neurons, organized into a brain, spinal cord, and peripheral nerves. The central nervous system (CNS) comprises the brain and spinal cord, whereas the peripheral nervous system (PNS) consists primarily of neurons carrying messages toward and away from the CNS.

In the maintenance of homeostasis, all components of the nervous system function together to direct and integrate many essential and adaptive responses. It is neural activity that frequently mediates appropriate reactions to both external and internal change. A burn on the hand, for example, will precipitate limb withdrawal, whereas hypercapnia characteristically triggers compensatory increases in respiratory rate. Since neural mechanisms are responsible for many aspects of physiological control, neural abnormalities can initiate a wide range of multisystemic dysfunction.

In the following pages, a basic review of normal structure and function is followed by an elucidation of neural pathology. Since the vast majority of critically debilitating disorders originate in the central nervous system, emphasis is placed upon diseases of the brain and spinal cord. Peripheral dysfunction is discussed only to the extent that it relates to cranial or spinal disorders.

BASIC ANATOMY AND PHYSIOLOGY: A REVIEW

The understanding of neural pathology is particularly enhanced by a good foundation in the basics of normal anatomy and physiology. Traditionally a difficult system to master conceptually, the nervous system poses an intricate challenge to even the most avid learner. To enhance clarity, in the following pages the structure and function of individual neurons are related to the organization and behavior of peripheral nerves, the spinal cord, and the brain.

The Neuron

The neuron, as the functional unit of the nervous system, is designed to transmit neural impulses. As illustrated in Figure 13.1, a typical neuron consists of a cell body from which emanate a number of extensions or "processess."

Whereas the body of the cell mediates essential metabolic reactions, it is the cytoplasmic extensions that function most specifically in impulse transmission. Processes called dendrites typically carry messages toward the cell body, whereas a single axon or "nerve fiber" is characteristically responsible for the transmission of impulses away from the cell toward other neurons.

Under certain circumstances, some axons, and a limited number of dendrites, are covered and protected by a fatty myelin sheath, as illustrated in Figure 13.2. In large numbers, myelinated fibers appear white to the naked eye and make up the "white matter" of the CNS. Conglomerates of nonmyelinated dendrites or cell bodies, on the other hand, typically constitute the "gray matter" of the brain and spinal cord.

The presence of myelin can, at times, be a good indicator of neural regenerative capacity. Although, as a general rule, neurons do not regenerate very successfully after injury, myelinated axons in the peripheral nervous system are occasionally capable of self-repair. Assuming survival of the cell body, regrowth is specifically mediated by the *neurolemma* membrane, a thin layer of modified Schwann cells that normally produces the fatty myelin sheath. Because the neurolemma membrane is not present in the neurons of the brain or spinal cord, any damage to the central nervous system is usually permanent.

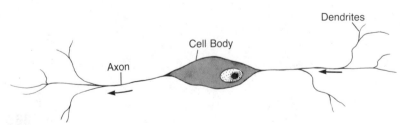

Figure 13.1 The structure of a neuron.

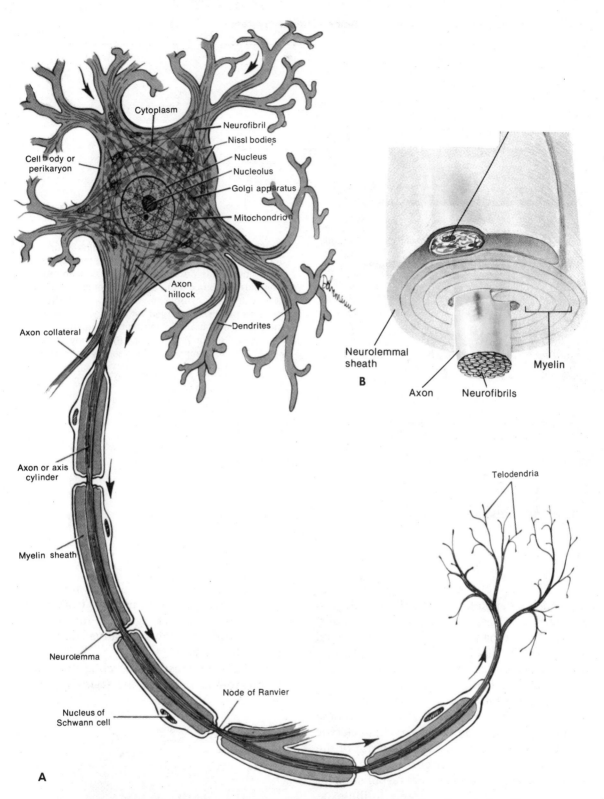

Figure 13.2 Myelinated axon. *A*, Note that the myelin sheath is not continuous along the length of the axon but is separated into discrete segments by the nodes of Ranvier. (From Tortora, G. J., and Anagnostakos, N. P.: Principles of Anatomy and Physiology, 2nd ed. New York, Harper & Row, 1978. Used by permission.) *B*, Note that myelin consists of layers of membrane wound continuously around the axon fiber. (From Hole, J. W.: Human Anatomy and Physiology. Dubuque, Wm. C. Brown Company, 1978. Used by permission.)

367

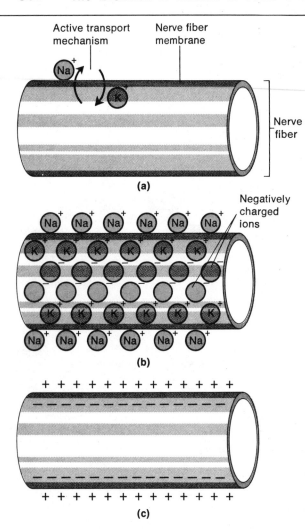

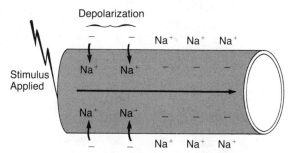

Figure 13.3 Membranes of a resting neuron. (a) Sodium ions are actively transported to the outside of a nerve fiber, while potassium ions are concentrated on the inside. (b) Since there are many negatively charged ions within the cytoplasm, the surface of the fiber becomes positively charged with respect to the inside, and such a membrane (c) is said to be polarized. (From Hole, J. W.: Human Anatomy and Physiology. Dubuque, Wm. C. Brown Company, 1978. Used by permission.)

Since the physiological significance of neurons is dependent upon their ability to conduct impulses, it is important to understand the mechanisms that facilitate neural transmission. Elucidation of the conduction process is perhaps best illustrated by tracing an impulse as it moves from one neuron to another along the conduction pathway.

As shown in Figure 13.3, the membrane of a resting neuron normally carries an electric charge on its surface, with the exterior of the cell being positively charged relative to the interior. The ionic distribution responsible for this *polarized* state is due largely to the existence of an active pump within the cell membrane that functions to selectively eject sodium ions into the interstitial fluid while retaining potassium ions intracellularly. Since the intracellular accumulation of nondiffusible

negative ions (such as chloride, proteinate, and phosphate) is not sufficiently balanced by positive potassium charges, the inside of the neuron tends to carry a negative charge relative to the outside.

Whenever a resting neuron is stimulated, its membrane becomes increasingly perme-

Figure 13.4 Depolarization of a nerve fiber.

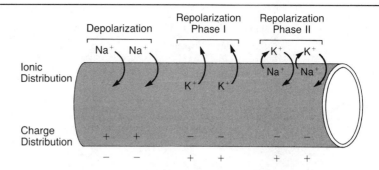

Figure 13.5 Repolarization of a nerve fiber. Note that potassium initially leaks into the interstitial fluid (Phase I), followed by the re-establishment of resting conditions (Phase II).

able to sodium (Na$^+$), and Na$^+$ fluxes into the intracellular compartment. As these positive ions move into the cell, the outer surface of the membrane becomes negatively charged, and the neuron is said to be *depolarized*. Technically, a nerve *impulse* is generated when altered ionic permeability causes a wave of electronegativity to sweep across the surface of a neuron, as illustrated in Figure 13.4.

Once depolarized, a neuron cannot respond to any subsequent stimuli until the resting state has been re-established. *Repolarization* of a nerve cell occurs as a result of two major changes:

1. Intracellular potassium (K$^+$) initially leaks into the interstitial fluid, causing the outer surface of the neural membrane to become increasingly positive.

2. The membrane pump pulls Na$^+$ out of the intracellular fluid in exchange for K$^+$, and resting conditions are thereby re-established. The repolarization process is summarized diagrammatically in Figure 13.5.

In order to insure continuity of neural transmission, mechanisms must exist to facilitate the conduction of an impulse from one neuron to another. To understand how messages can pass between adjacent neurons, it is helpful to look closely at the anatomical and physiological linkages existing between nerve cells.

Neurons characteristically articulate with one another in junctional areas called *synapses*. As can be seen in Figure 13.6, the small synaptic gap that separates two nerve cells from each other is specifically referred to as the *synaptic cleft*. Neurons are frequently categorized according to their functional relationship to this synaptic cleft. If they carry impulses howard the gap, they are considered to be *presynaptic*; if they carry messages away

from the gap, they are said to be *postsynaptic*.

Generally, as an impulse travels through the axon of a presynaptic neuron, it terminates at small structures called *synaptic knobs*. These knobs, in turn, release chemicals (called *neurotransmitters*) that react with postsynaptic dendrites, and alter their selective ionic permeability (Fig. 13.7).

If a neurotransmitter causes an increase in sodium permeability, it will facilitate postsynaptic impulse transmission and is therefore

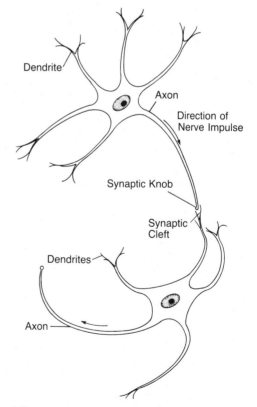

Figure 13.6 A synapse. When an impulse travels from one neuron to another, it must cross a synaptic cleft.

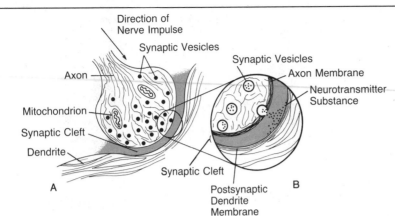

Figure 13.7 Synaptic transmission. Note that when a nerve impulse arrives at the synaptic knob of an axon (*A*), it stimulates the release of a neurotransmitter substance into the synaptic cleft (*B*).

described as *excitatory*. Chemicals functioning in this fashion include norepinephrine, serotonin, dopamine, and acetylcholine (ACH), with the last being encountered most frequently. In cases of ACH-induced impulse conduction, return to the resting state is regulated by the release of an ACH enzyme (acetylcholinesterase). Secreted by the postsynpatic neuron, this enzyme destroys acetylcholine

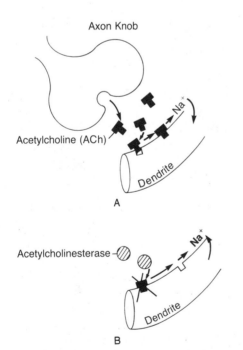

Figure 13.8 The function of acetylcholinesterase in neural repolarization. When ACH reacts with receptor sites on the dendrite membrane (*A*) permeability to Na⁺ is increased and depolarization occurs. Repolarization is mediated secondary to inactivation of ACH by acetylcholinesterase, (*B*), as indicated by X.

and promotes repolarization, as illustrated in Figure 13.8.

Not all neurotransmitters, however, are supportive of conduction. Those chemicals that depress synaptic transmission are referred to as *inhibitory* and include gamma-aminobutyric acid (GABA), glycine, and dopamine (in select areas of the brain). They are believed to function by promoting the leakage of K^+ out of the neuron, thereby facilitating the accumulation of positively charged potassium ions on the surface of the resting membrane. Neurons exposed to this electrolyte shift manifest an increased external positive charge and are described as *hyperpolarized*. In this state, they are relatively more resistant to depolarization, and thus are less responsive to stimulation.

In considering the characteristics of individual neurons, it is important to remember that these cells serve as the building blocks for a larger integrated nervous system. Normally supported, surrounded, and interconnected by specialized connective tissue called *neuroglia*, neurons generally relate to each other in such a way as to create functional neural pathways throughout the body. Because they bind neurons together in an ordered fashion, glial cells are paticularly essential to the creation of systemic structural unity. The neuroglia, additionally, is of specific clinical significance, since it is the primary site of tumor formation in the nervous system.

The Peripheral Nervous System

External to the brain and spinal cord, conglomerates of axons, dendrites, or den-

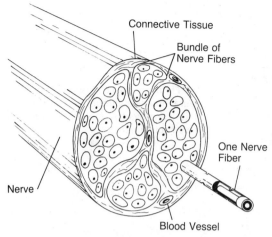

Figure 13.9 The basic structural organization of a nerve. A nerve is a bundle of nerve fibers held together by connective tissue.

drites and axons are bound together by membrane sheaths into structures called *nerves*. The nerve is the basic functional unit of the peripheral nervous system and acts as an information pipeline — carrying information to and from the central nervous system. The basic structural organization of a nerve is illustrated in Figure 13.9.

Peripheral nerves can generally be classified, with respect to activity, in the following manner:

1. *Somatic afferent nerves* — which carry information from the skin, skeletal muscle, and joints toward the central nervous system.

2. *Somatic efferent nerves* — which carry information from the central nervous system to skeletal muscle.

3. *Visceral afferent nerves* — which carry information from smooth muscle, glands, and cardiac muscle tissue toward the central nervous system.

4. *Visceral efferent nerves* (alternatively called *autonomic nerves*) — which carry information from the central nervous system to smooth muscle, glands, and cardiac muscle.

Since nerves are, ultimately, composites of a large number of different axons and dendrites, varying types of information can often be carried within one structure. Both afferent and efferent messages, for example, are frequently transmitted simultaneously — rendering functional categorization somewhat difficult. In general, nerves that carry impulses both toward and away from the central nervous system are described as "mixed" nerves. Their structure is illustrated diagrammatically in Figure 13.10.

In order to function effectively as part of an integrated system, all peripheral nerves must be connected, either directly or indirectly, to the central nervous system. Those major nerves that enter or leave the spinal cord or brain are described as *spinal nerves* or *cranial nerves*, respectively. The many auxiliary nerves that transmit messages between peripheral organs and spinal or cranial nerves complete the information network and facilitate functional integration. In the following pages, some of the major distinctions between spinal and cranial nerves will be more specifically elucidated.

SPINAL NERVES

Thirty-one pairs of spinal nerves normally emerge from the vertebral column through narrow spaces between the vertebrae called

Figure 13.10 A "mixed" nerve. Note that impulses are traveling simultaneously toward and away from the spinal cord within the mixed nerves.

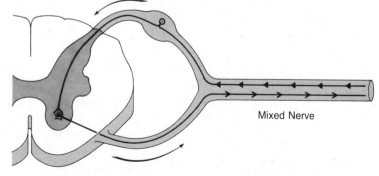

Spinal Cord

Mixed Nerve

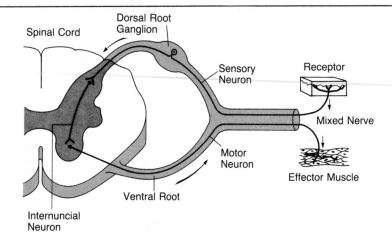

Figure 13.11 Transmission of neural impulses through the dorsal (posterior) and ventral (anterior) roots of a mixed spinal nerve.

intervertebral foramina. Since all spinal nerves contain both afferent and efferent fibers, they are described as mixed nerves and carry both motor and sensory messages.

At a point very close to the spinal cord itself, however, afferent and efferent fibers separate into a posterior and anterior root, respectively. As illustrated in Figure 13.11, sensory (afferent) impulses enter the cord via the posterior, or dorsal, root, whereas motor (efferent) messages emerge through the anterior, or ventral, root.

The composite spinal nerve that results from the merging of motor and sensory fibers is named according to its level of origin. The spinal nerves predictably mirror the pattern of vertebral organization; thus, there are eight pairs of cervical nerves, twelve pairs of thoracic nerves, five pairs of lumbar nerves, five

pairs of sacral nerves, and one pair of coccygeal nerves.

To facilitate the integration of information among discrete spinal nerves, many complex interconnections are necessary. By understanding some of the anatomical linkages that exist between peripheral nerves, comprehension of functional activity can be considerably enhanced.

Shortly after emerging from the cord, for example, spinal nerves divide into anterior and posterior branches called *rami.* The *dorsal ramus* primarily services the dorsal surface of the trunk, whereas the *ventral ramus* supplies both motor and sensory fibers to all extremities as well as to the lateral and ventral trunk (Fig. 13.12).

The ventral rami, moreover, feed into intricate braided networks of nerve fibers

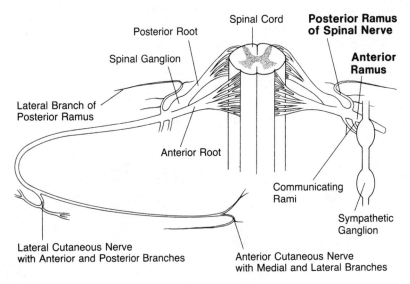

Figure 13.12 The distribution of a spinal nerve. Note that the mixed spinal nerve divides into an anterior and a posterior ramus.

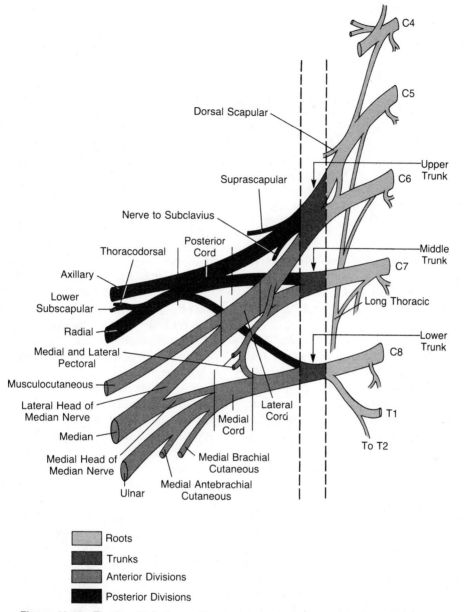

Figure 13.13   The brachial plexus. The roots of spinal nerves C5–C8 and T1 are merely continuations of the ventral rami. These roots unite to form the upper, middle, and lower trunks, which subsequently divide into an anterior and a posterior division.

called *plexi*. The four major plexi (cervical, brachial, lumbar, and sacral) are each associated with specific spinal nerves and serve as focal centers for the reception of sensory information and dispersal of motor impulses (Fig. 13.13).

To clarify the way in which information travels sequentially through spinal nerves toward and away from the cord, it is helpful to

trace the transmission of a typical motor and sensory message from point of origin to ultimate destination.

SPINAL NERVES: SENSORY TRANS-MISSION   If you were to receive a burn on the upper chest, sensory fibers in the skin would first transmit impulses to the cervical plexus. From the plexus, neural messages

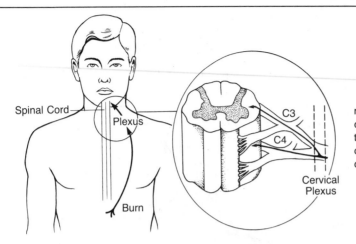

Figure 13.14 Schematic presentation of neural transmission secondary to a burn on the chest. Note that impulses are conducted from the cervical plexus through the posterior roots of spinal nerves C3 and C4 into the spinal cord.

would subsequently travel into the ventral ramus of the C3 or C4 spinal nerve and thence into the spinal cord through the posterior root of the nerve. The specified pathway is illustrated in Figure 13.14.

In considering sensory conduction, it is important to note that each spinal nerve (except C1) services a specific segment of the skin, called a *dermatome*. It is thus possible to devise a map correlating superficial sensation in a particular area of the body with activity of a designated spinal nerve, as illustrated in Figure 13.15. Because of this relative anatomical specificity, superficial loss of sensation can frequently be associated with dysfunction of a particular spinal nerve. Since there is a certain amount of functional overlap between dermatomes, however, exact localization of a neural deficit is not always possible.

SPINAL NERVES: MOTOR TRANS-MISSION   Whereas sensory fibers carry information toward the central nervous system, motor impulses generally stimulate responses by triggering either muscular or glandular activity.

In considering motor transmission, it is important to distinguish between two distinctly different neural pathways:

1. The neural pathway responsible for the innervation of structures that are under voluntary control (such as skeletal muscles). In these cases, impulses are transmitted by somatic efferent nerves.

2. The neural pathway responsible for the innervation of involuntary structures (such as smooth muscle, cardiac muscle, and glands).

In these cases, impulses are transmitted by visceral efferent, or autonomic, nerves.

Somatic Efferent Nerves   Somatic efferent nerves generally transmit impulses through the traditional ramus/plexus pathway previously described. To initiate contraction of the biceps femoris muscle of the posterior thigh, for example, a message must originate in the anterior roots of spinal nerves L4–S3. Impulses are subsequently transmitted to the ventral rami, and thence to the sacral plexus. The sciatic nerve emerging from the plexus ultimately stimulates the skeletal muscle, thereby triggering the desired response. This pathway is summarized diagrammatically in Figure 13.16.

Visceral   Efferent   Nerves   Autonomic nerve fibers differ from somatic efferent nerves in several respects. Characteristically, they emerge from the central nervous system in select cranial nerves, as well as through the anterior roots of spinal nerves T1–T12, L1–L2, and S2–S4. Those fibers exiting through the thoracic and lumbar nerves are specifically referred to as thoracolumbar and make up the *sympathetic* branch of the autonomic nervous system. Neurons emerging at the base of the cranium or from the sacral cord, on the other hand, are designated as craniosacral and are part of the *parasympathetic* division of the autonomic nervous system.

Although mixed with somatic fibers at their point of origin, all autonomic fibers eventually branch away to carry impulses toward synapse centers called *ganglia*. Autonomic neurons are generally categorized according to whether they carry impulses

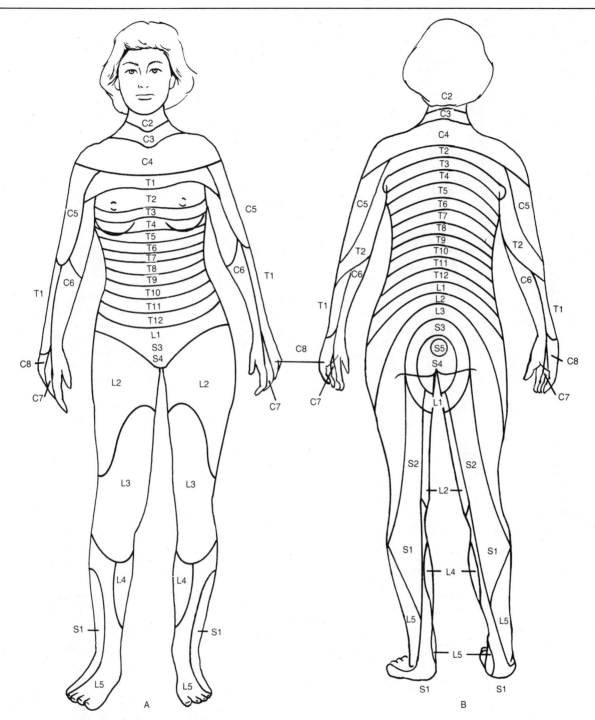

Figure 13.15 Distribution of spinal nerves within dermatomes. Anterior view (*A*) and posterior view (*B*).

toward or away from these ganglia. The *preganglionic fibers* transmit information to a ganglion, whereas the *postganglionic fibers* conduct impulses from the ganglion to the ultimate target structure.

The relationship between autonomic neurons and their synapse centers is depicted in Figure 13.17. It can be seen that sympathetic ganglia are found fairly close to the central nervous system. They are organized into ver-

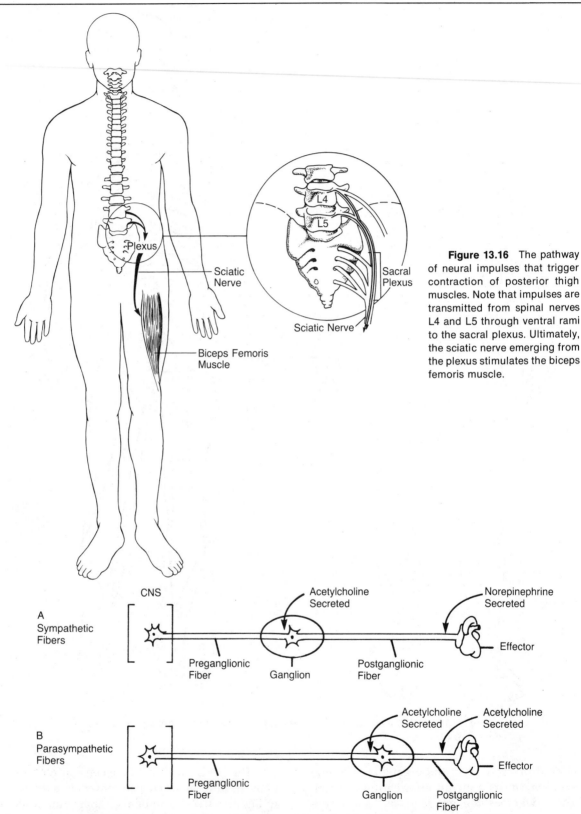

Figure 13.16   The pathway of neural impulses that trigger contraction of posterior thigh muscles. Note that impulses are transmitted from spinal nerves L4 and L5 through ventral rami to the sacral plexus. Ultimately, the sciatic nerve emerging from the plexus stimulates the biceps femoris muscle.

Figure 13.17   The relationship between autonomic neurons and their synapse centers. Note the relatively short sympathetic preganglionic fiber (A) and short parasympathetic postganglionic fiber (B). (Modified from Hole, J. W.: Human Anatomy and Physiology. Dubuque, Wm. C. Brown Company, 1978.)

tical chains either lateral or anterior to the spinal cord. Parasympathetic ganglia, on the other hand, are located relatively close to their target organs and are thus serviced by long preganglionic and short postganglionic fibers.

In considering functional aspects of the autonomic nervous system, it is important to realize that involuntary structures in the body are simultaneously innervated by both sympathetic and parasympathetic neurons. Whereas postganglionic sympathetic fibers release norepinephrine to mediate organic response, postganglionic parasympathetic neurons secrete ACH as a neurotransmitter. Since these neurotransmitters characteristical-

TABLE 13.1 **The Functions of the Autonomic Nervous System***

Organ	Sympathetic Stimulation	Parasympathetic Stimulation
EYE		
Iris	Stimulates radial fibers (dilates pupil)	Stimulates circular fibers (constricts pupil)
Ciliary muscle	Inhibits (flattens lens)	Stimulates (bulges lens)
GLANDS		
Salivary	Vasoconstriction may diminish secretion	Stimulate copious secretion high in enzyme content
Lacrimal	None	Stimulate secretion
Sweat	Copious sweating	None
Adrenal medulla	Secretion of epinephrine	None
HEART		
Sinoatrial (SA) node	Increased rate	Decreased rate
Muscle	Increased force of contraction	None
LUNGS		
Bronchi	Dilation	Constriction
STOMACH		
Wall	Decreased motility and tone	Increased motility and tone
Glands	Stimulate secretion of alkaline juice with low enzyme activity	Stimulate secretion of acid juice with high enzyme activity
INTESTINE		
Smooth muscular wall	Decreased motility and tone	Increased motility and tone
Anal sphincter	Contraction	Inhibition
PANCREAS	Vasoconstriction may diminish secretion	Stimulates secretion of pancreatic enzymes
URINARY BLADDER		
Smooth muscular wall	Relaxes	Contracts
Sphincter	Contracts	Relaxes
PENIS	Ejaculation	Erection (vasodilation)
ARRECTOR PILI MUSCLES OF HAIR FOLLICLES	Contraction	None
ARTERIOLES		
Skin	Constrict	None
Skeletal muscle	Dilate	None
Splanchnic vessels	Constrict	None

*Adapted from Jacob, S. W., Francone, C. A., and Lossow, W. J.: Laboratory Manual for Structure and Function in Man, 4th ed. Philadelphia, W. B. Saunders Company, 1978, p. 278.

ly evoke opposing response patterns in any given organ, activity is ultimately determined by the joint effect of contrasting neural messages.

The influence of autonomic stimulation upon physiological regulation can, perhaps, best be clarified by example. Sympathetic stimulation of the heart, for instance, will trigger an increase in cardiac rate, whereas parasympathetic innervation will induce a decrease in cardiac activity. Gastrointestinal secretions and motility, on the other hand, are stimulated by parasympathetic fibers and depressed by sympathetic neurons. In general, it can be said that sympathetic innervation supports the mobilization of emergency "fight or flight" response patterns, whereas parasympathetic stimulation characteristically causes a more stable and moderate type of physiological activity. A tabular summary of the effect of autonomic stimulation upon major organs in the body is presented in Table 13.1.

CRANIAL NERVES

Whereas spinal nerves carry messages directly to and from the spinal cord, the 12 pairs of cranial nerves articulate with the central nervous system at the base of the brain. The cranial nerves are identified both by roman numeral (which reflects their relative position,

anterior to posterior) and by name and are depicted in Figure 13.18.

Unlike spinal nerves, some cranial nerves contain only sensory fibers (such as the olfactory, optic, and vestibulocochlear nerves), whereas others are "mixed." A summary of the major functions of each nerve is presented in Table 13.2.

It can be seen that many aspects of sensation and skeletomuscular activity in the upper thorax, head, and neck are mediated by cranial nerves. It is also important to note that parasympathetic autonomic fibers are carried in some cranial nerves. A primary example of this phenomenon can be found in the *vagus nerve* (cranial nerve X), which branches to serve the pharynx, larynx, and heart, as well as the esophagus, stomach, and small intestine.

The Central Nervous System

Although both cranial and spinal nerves provide an essential link between peripheral structures and the central nervous system, it is the brain and spinal cord that function in the integration, coordination, and interpretation of most neural messages.

In the following pages, a closer look is taken at the structure and function of the central nervous system. The spinal cord and

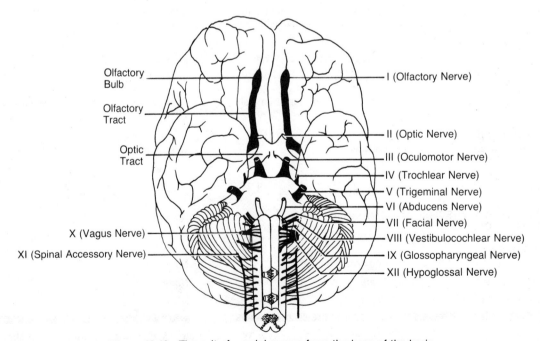

Figure 13.18   The exit of cranial nerves from the base of the brain.

TABLE 13.2 **Functions of Cranial Nerves***

Number and Name	Type of Nerve	Site of Origin	Site of Termination	Function
I. Olfactory	Sensory (afferent)	Sensory receptors in the nasal mucosa	Olfactory in the brain	Smell
II. Optic	Sensory (afferent)	Sensory cells in the retina	Occipital lobe of the cerebrum	Vision and associated reflexes
III. Oculomotor	Motor (efferent)	Gray matter in the mid-brain	Levator palpebrae, superior, medial, and inferior rectus, and inferior oblique muscles	Movement of the eyeball, pupillary constriction and accommodation
IV. Trochlear	Motor (efferent)	Gray matter in the mid-brain	Superior oblique muscles	Movement of the eyeball
V. Trigeminal	Sensory (afferent)	Ophthalmic branch: Eye, lacrimal gland, nose, forehead	Sensory: Midpons, below the fourth ventricle	General sensations from the anterior surface of the face, mouth, nose, and tongue
	Sensory (afferent)	Maxillary branch: Teeth and gums of the upper jaw, upper lip, cheek	Motor: Muscles of mastication	Mastication, swallowing; movement of the soft palate, auditory tube, ear ossicles, and tympanic membrane
	Mixed	Mandibular branch: Sensory from teeth and gums of lower jaw, chin, lower lip, tongue. Motor from the midpons		
VI. Abducent	Motor (efferent)	Lower pons beneath fourth ventricle	Lateral rectus muscle	Movement of the eyeball
VII. Facial	Motor (efferent)	Lower pons	Muscles of face and forehead; parasympathetic fibers to lacrimal, submandibular, and sublingual glands	Facial expression; lacrimation, salivation, and vasodilatation
	Sensory (afferent)	Anterior two thirds of tongue, external ear, and facial glands	Geniculate ganglion in temporal bone	Taste; sensation from external ear and glands
VIII. Vestibulocochlear	Sensory (afferent)	Cochlear branch: Sensory receptors in cochlea	Temporal lobe of the cerebrum	Hearing
		Vestibular branch: Sensory receptors in the semicircular canals and vestibule	Cerebellum	Equilibrium
IX. Glossopharyngeal	Motor (efferent)	Medulla	Muscles of the pharynx, parotid gland via parasympathetic fiber	Swallowing movements, vasodilatation, and salivation
	Sensory (afferent)	Tonsils, mucous membrane of the pharynx, external ear and posterior one third of the tongue, pressoreceptors and chemoreceptors in the carotid body	Medulla	Taste, general sensation to the posterior tongue, tonsils, and upper pharynx; cardiovascular and respiratory effects from receptors in the carotid sinus and carotid body
X. Vagus	Sensory (afferent)	Mucous membrane lining respiratory and digestive tracts	Medulla	Taste and general sensation from larynx, neck, thorax, and abdomen
	Motor (efferent)	Medulla	Muscles of pharynx and larynx	Swallowing, movement of pharynx and larynx
			Parasympathetic fibers to thoracic and abdominal viscera	Inhibitory fibers to the heart; secretion of gastric glands and pancreas; vasodilator fibers to abdominal viscera
XI. Accessory	Motor	Cranial portion: Medulla	Pharyngeal and laryngeal muscles	Movement of the soft palate, pharynx, and larynx
		Spinal portion: Upper cervical region of the spinal cord	Sternocleidomastoid and trapezius muscles	Shoulder and head movement
XII. Hypoglossal	Motor	Medulla	Muscles of the tongue	Speaking and swallowing, tongue movement

*From Jones, D. A., Dunbar, C. F., and Jirovec, M. M. (eds.): Medical-Surgical Nursing: A Conceptual Approach. New York, McGraw-Hill Book Company, 1978, p. 1071.

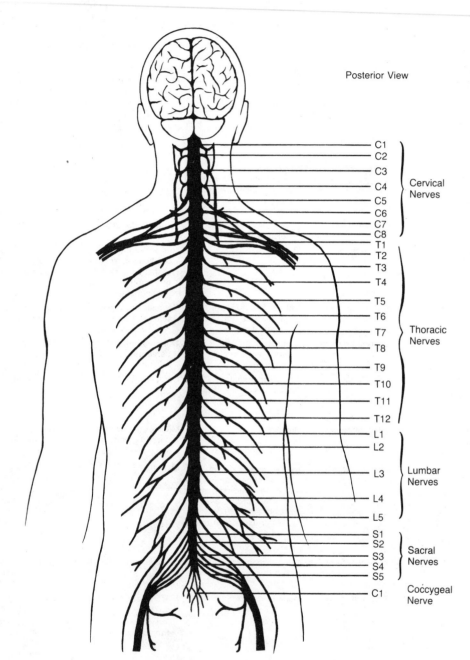

Posterior View

Cervical Nerves
C1
C2
C3
C4
C5
C6
C7
C8

Thoracic Nerves
T1
T2
T3
T4
T5
T6
T7
T8
T9
T10
T11
T12

Lumbar Nerves
L1
L2
L3
L4
L5

Sacral Nerves
S1
S2
S3
S4
S5

Coccygeal Nerve
C1

Figure 13.19 The spinal nerves.

brain are each reviewed briefly, with special emphasis upon those aspects that will most directly facilitate ultimate comprehension of neural pathology.

THE SPINAL CORD

The spinal cord is a cylindrical column of neural tissue that extends from the base of the brain down to the level of the second lumbar vertebra. It emerges from the cranium through a hole in the occipital bone called the *foramen magnum* and consists of a series of 31 vertically arranged segments, each giving rise to a pair of spinal nerves. The relative orientation of the spinal cord is illustrated in Figure 13.19.

The cord is encased by bony vertebrae and is further protected by surrounding membranes and fluid. The membranes around the cord, called *meninges,* provide a continuous covering for the brain as well and can be categorized into three distinct layers:

1. *The pia mater* — a thin membrane located directly on the surface of the cord.

2. *The dura mater* — a relatively thicker membrane serving as the outermost covering of the cord.

3. *The arachnoid mater* — a delicate, spi-dery membrane located between the pia and the dura mater.

A comparative view of the meninges is presented in Figure 13.20.

Although the three meninges are positioned relatively close to one another, narrow spaces do exist between the individual membranes. These spaces can be identified, by relative location, as follows:

1. *The epidural space* — found between the dura mater and the inner surface of the bony vertebrae. This space is characteristically filled with fat, connective tissue, and blood vessels.

2. *The subdural space* — found between the dura and the arachnoid mater. This space typically contains a watery serous fluid.

3. *The subarachnoid space* — found between the arachnoid and the pia mater. This space contains cerebrospinal fluid, the formation of which will be discussed subsequently in this chapter.

An illustrative summary of the relationships between these intermeningeal spaces is presented in Figure 13.21.

Although the cord is protected by this intricate composite of bone, fluid, and membranes, its internal structural organization is

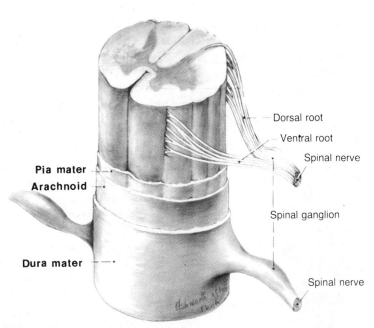

Pia mater
Arachnoid

Dura mater

Dorsal root
Ventral root
Spinal nerve

Spinal ganglion

Spinal nerve

Figure 13.20 The meninges surrounding the spinal cord. (From Jacob, S. W., Francone, C. A., and Lossow, W. J.: Structure and Function in Man, 4th ed., Philadelphia, W. B. Saunders Company, 1978. Used by permission.)

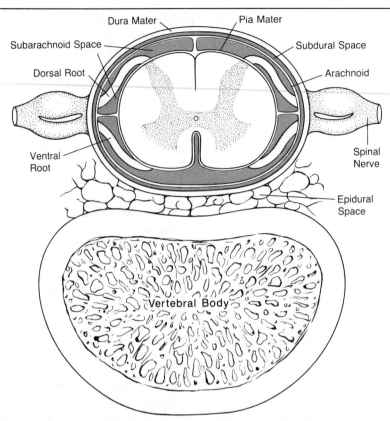

Figure 13.21 The intermeningeal spaces. Note the relative positions of the subdural, subarachnoid, and epidural spaces. (Modified from Jacob, S. W., Francone, C. A., and Lossow, W. J.: Structure and Function in Man, 4th ed. Philadelphia, W. B. Saunders Company, 1978.)

deceptively simple. As illustrated in Figure 13.22, the spinal cord contains an inner segment of butterfly-shaped gray matter surrounded by white matter composed of myelin-

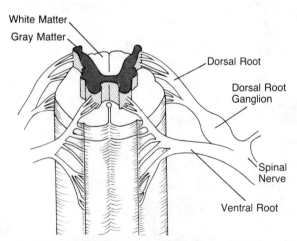

Figure 13.22 The gray and white matter of the spinal cord.

ated axons. Functionally, the white matter serves primarily to convey information up and down the cord between the peripheral nervous system and the brain, whereas the gray matter acts as a coordinating center for reflex and other activities. In the following pages, a closer look is taken at the anatomy and physiology of the spinal cord.

CONDUCTION PATHWAYS The white matter of the cord is composed primarily of bunches of myelinated axons that function to conduct impulses to and from the brain. The cord thus mediates essential linkages between higher cerebral centers and the periphery.

Structurally, the conduction pathways within the cord can be divided into three general areas — the anterior white column, the posterior white column, and the lateral white column — as illustrated in Figure 13.23. Within each column, moreover, are distinct bundles of fibers. Those fibers carrying infor-

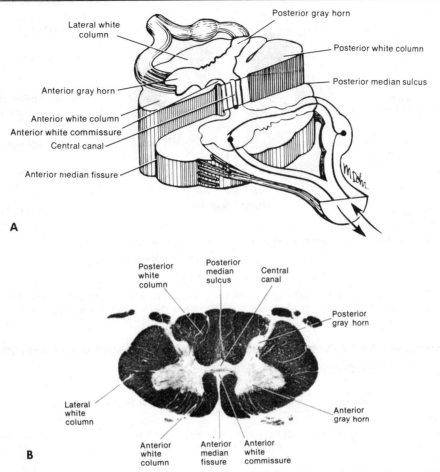

Figure 13.23 *A*, Selected conduction pathways within the spinal cord. (From Tortora, G. J., and Anagnostakos, N. P.: Principles of Anatomy and Physiology, 2nd ed. New York, Harper & Row, 1978. Used by permission.) *B*, Photograph of the spinal cord at the seventh cervical segment, as a magnification of 7×. (Courtesy of Murray L. Barr, The Human Nervous System. New York, Harper & Row, 1974.)

mation toward the brain are called *ascending tracts*, whereas those transmitting messages down the cord are referred to as *descending tracts* (Fig. 13.24). The names and functions of some major tracts are summarized in Table 13.3.

It should be noted that, in most cases, sensory information traveling up the right side of the cord crosses over to the left side in the area of the lower brain, and is thus eventually conveyed to opposing upper cerebral centers. In this way, pain in the right hand is ultimately interpreted by the left brain, and vice versa. Conversely, many motor impulses originating in the left brain cross to the right side of the cord in the area of the medulla —

subsequently to initiate response on the left side of the body.

Because of this crossover of impulses, technically called *decussation*, lesions in one side of the brain typically cause clinical symptoms on the opposite side of the body. Severe ischemia in the right cerebrum, for example, will characteristically result in a left-sided motor or sensory deficit.

In considering the transmission of impulses through the cord, it`is important to remember that many different neurons characteristically work together to create a given conduction pathway. Thus, sensory information arriving at the lumbar level of the cord is often conveyed to the brain by a

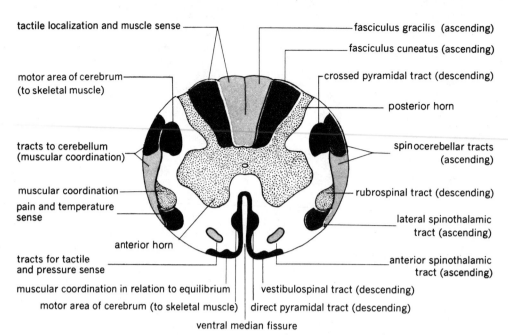

tactile localization and muscle sense

fasciculus gracilis (ascending)

fasciculus cuneatus (ascending)

crossed pyramidal tract (descending)

motor area of cerebrum (to skeletal muscle)

posterior horn

tracts to cerebellum (muscular coordination)

spinocerebellar tracts (ascending)

muscular coordination

rubrospinal tract (descending)

pain and temperature sense

lateral spinothalamic tract (ascending)

anterior horn

anterior spinothalamic tract (ascending)

tracts for tactile and pressure sense

muscular coordination in relation to equilibrium

vestibulospinal tract (descending)

motor area of cerebrum (to skeletal muscle)

direct pyramidal tract (descending)

ventral median fissure

Figure 13.24   Some selected tracts of the spinal cord. (From De'Coursey, R. M.: The Human Organism, 4th ed. New York, McGraw-Hill Book Company, 1974. Used by permission.)

TABLE 13.3   **Major Tracts (Pathways) of the Spinal Cord***

Tract	Spinal Cord Location	Site of Origin	Site of Termination	Function
ASCENDING TRACTS				
Fasciculus gracilis (T7 and below) Fasciculus cuneatus (T6 and above)	Posterior white columns	Spinal ganglions on the same side of the cord	Medulla	Touch, two-point discrimination, position sense, motion, weight perception
Spinocerebellar posterior	Lateral white columns	Neuromuscular receptors on the same side of the cord	Cerebellum	Unconscious proprioception (muscle sense)
Spinocerebellar anterior	Lateral white columns	Neuromuscular receptors on the same *and* opposite sides of the cord	Cerebellum	Coordination of posture and limb movement
Spinothalamic lateral	Lateral white columns	Cell bodies in the posterior horn on the opposite side of the cord	Thalamus	Pain and temperature sensation on the opposite sides of the body
Spinothalamic anterior	Anterior white columns	Cell bodies in the posterior horn on the opposite side of the cord	Thalamus	Touch and pressure on the opposite sides of the body
DESCENDING TRACTS Pyramidal				
Lateral corticospinal	Lateral white columns	Voluntary motor areas of the cerebral cortex (fibers cross in the medulla)	Anterior gray or anterolateral columns in the spinal cord	Voluntary movement, especially of the arms and legs
Anterior corticospinal	Anterior or ventral columns	Voluntary motor areas of the cerebral cortex (uncrossed fibers)	Anterior gray or anterolateral columns in the spinal cord	Voluntary movement of the trunk muscles
Extrapyramidal Rubrospinal	Lateral white columns	Red nucleus of the midbrain (fibers cross immediately)	Anterior gray or anterolateral columns in the spinal cord	Muscle tone and coordination; posture
Vestibulospinal	Anterior or ventral columns	Vestibular nuclei in the medulla	Anterior gray or anterolateral columns in the spinal cord	Equilibrium and posture

*From Jones, D. A., Dunbar, C. F., and Jirovec, M. M. (eds.): Medical-Surgical Nursing: A Conceptual Approach. New York, McGraw-Hill Book Company, 1978, p. 1077.

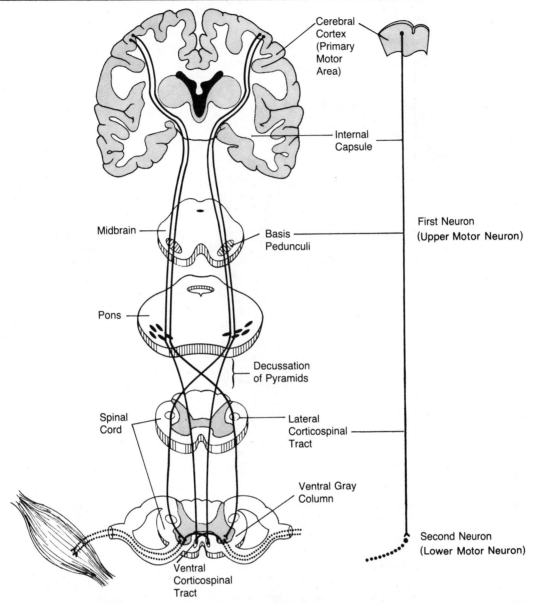

Cerebral Cortex (Primary Motor Area)

Internal Capsule

First Neuron (Upper Motor Neuron)

Midbrain

Basis Pedunculi

Pons

Decussation of Pyramids

Spinal Cord

Lateral Corticospinal Tract

Ventral Gray Column

Second Neuron (Lower Motor Neuron)

Ventral Corticospinal Tract

Figure 13.25 Upper and lower motor neurons. Note that upper motor neurons are contained totally within the central nervous system, while lower motor neurons emerge from the spinal cord to stimulate skeletal muscle.

vertically arranged series of synapsing cells. Whereas the relative position of sensory neurons within the cord is not of major significance, the distinction between *upper motor neurons (UMN's)* and *lower motor neurons (LMN's)* in the descending tracts does have clinical relevance.

As illustrated in Figure 13.25, upper motor neurons originate in the cortex or brain stem and are contained totally within the central nervous system. Lower motor neurons,

on the other hand, originate in the central nervous system but have fibers that extend peripherally to terminate on skeletal muscle. Although dysfunction of either upper or lower motor neurons can generally affect voluntary muscular contraction, it is the location of motor neurons within the cord that will ultimately determine the nature of evolving disorder. Some major disorders associated with UMN and LMN lesions are summarized in Figure 13.26.

Classification	Site of Lesion	Associated Disorders
Upper Motor Neuron Pathology	Motor Cortex	Birth Injuries (Cerebral Palsies) Inflammation Trauma Neoplasms
	Internal Capsule of Brain	Vascular Lesions (CVA, Thrombosis, Embolism, Hemorrhage) Inflammations Trauma Neoplasms
	Brain Stem	Multiple Sclerosis Parkinson's Disease Vascular Lesions Inflammations Trauma Neoplasms
	Spinal Cord	Demyelinating Diseases Inflammations Trauma Neoplasms
Lower Motor Neuron Pathology	Anterior Horn Cell of Spinal Cord	Poliomyelitis Polyneuritis Amylotrophic Lateral Sclerosis
	Neural Component of Myoneural Junction	Myasthenia Gravis

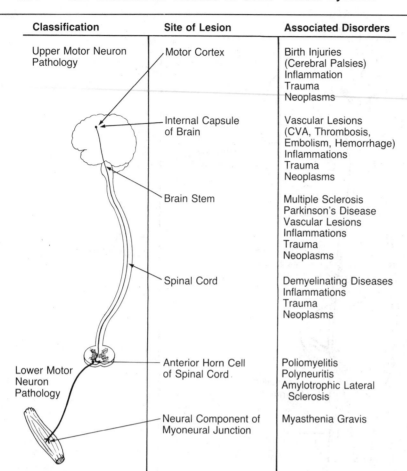

Figure 13.26 Some major disorders associated with upper motor neuron and lower motor neuron lesions.

REFLEX CENTER Whereas the white matter of the spinal cord functions to transmit messages toward and away from the brain, the internal gray matter serves as a center for reflex activity.

A reflex can generally be defined as an automatic response to a given stimulus. Adaptive in nature, it functions to protect the body from sudden changes in the internal or external environment. Execution of a reflex act involves the utilization of a programmed neural pathway called the *reflex arc*. As illustrated in Figure 13.27, the major anatomical components of this arc include:

1. *A receptor* — a nerve ending or structure sensitive to a specific environmental change.

2. *A sensory neuron* — a neuron that carries information from the receptor to the CNS.

3. *A reflex center* — an area in the gray matter of the cord where sensory and motor neurons synapse.

4. *A motor neuron* — a neuron that carries information from the spinal cord to the effector organ.

5. *An effector* — a muscle or gland triggered by the motor neuron to initiate the reflex response.

An understanding of the reflex act can perhaps best be facilitated by tracing the evolution of a simple stretch reflex. For example, the patellar, or knee jerk, reflex is initiated by a tap on the patellar ligament and results in the extension of the lower leg. As illustrated in Figure 13.28, the stretch sensation caused by a knee tap is transmitted to the spinal cord by sensory fibers in a spinal nerve. Information is conveyed through the posterior root of the spinal nerve into the gray matter of the cord, where synapse with an efferent neuron occurs. Motor impulses are subsequently initiated and travel through the anterior root out into a mixed spinal nerve, where they ultimately trigger contraction of the quadriceps femoris muscle.

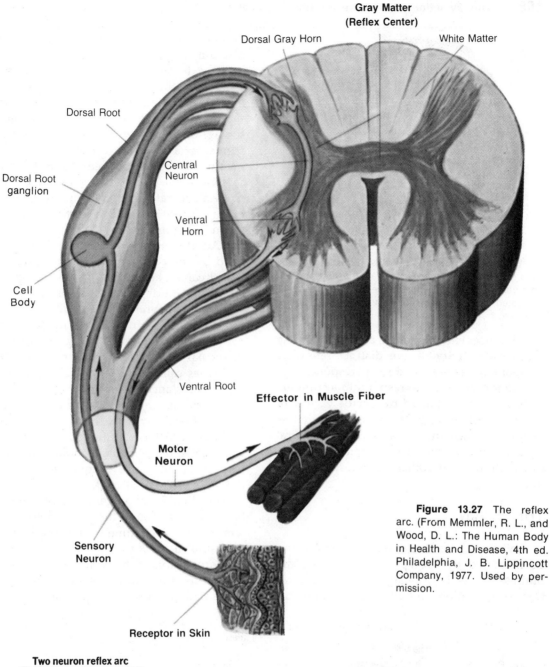

**Gray Matter
(Reflex Center)**

Dorsal Gray Horn

White Matter

Dorsal Root

Dorsal Root
ganglion

Central
Neuron

Ventral
Horn

Cell
Body

Ventral Root

Effector in Muscle Fiber

**Motor
Neuron**

Sensory
Neuron

Receptor in Skin

Figure 13.27 The reflex arc. (From Memmler, R. L., and Wood, D. L.: The Human Body in Health and Disease, 4th ed. Philadelphia, J. B. Lippincott Company, 1977. Used by permission.

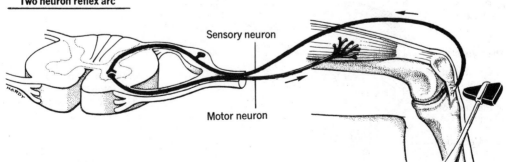

Two neuron reflex arc

Sensory neuron

Motor neuron

Figure 13.28 Knee jerk or stretch reflex. A tap on the patellar ligament causes reflex extension of the lower leg. Note that only two neurons are involved in the reflex pathway. (From Chaffee, E. E., and Lytle, I. M.: Basic Physiology and Anatomy, 4th ed. Philadelphia, J. B. Lippincott Company, 1980. Used by permission.)

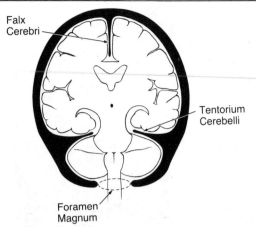

Figure 13.29 Significant folds in the dura mater. Note that the falx cerebri separates the right and left cerebral hemispheres, whereas the tentorium cerebelli is located between the cerebrum and the cerebellum.

Because reflex responses depend upon the functional activity of five distinct reflex arc components, exaggerated reflex response (*hyperreflexia*) or failure to respond to a stimulus (*areflexia*) can be caused by a wide variety of disorders. Although reflex evaluations are frequently utilized in the assessment of neural status, results are most valid when analyzed in conjunction with other diagnostic procedures.

THE BRAIN

Whereas a number of reflex responses can be mediated by the spinal cord alone, the brain serves as the primary center for integration, coordination, initiation, and interpretation of most neural messages. Housed in the cranium, this intricate structure is protected by an extension of the three meninges that also cover the spinal cord. The outermost fibrous dura mater is of particular anatomical significance, since folds of this membrane serve as landmark separations between certain segments of the brain. The *falx cerebri*, for example, is located between the right and left cerebral hemispheres, whereas the *tentorium cerebelli* separates the cerebrum from the cerebellum. These dura mater partitions are illustrated in Figure 13.29.

Additional protection for the brain is supplied by the clear watery cerebrospinal fluid that circulates around the central nervous system. This fluid provides a soft cushion for vulnerable neural tissue and is initially formed deep within the brain in spaces called ventricles. As illustrated in Figure 13.30, cerebrospinal fluid is secreted by specialized capillaries called *choroid plexuses*. Under normal circumstances, it will flow from the lateral ventricles into the third ventricle and thence into the fourth ventricle through the aqueduct of Sylvius. After passing out of the fourth ventricle into the subarachnoid space, cerebrospinal fluid circulates continuously around the brain and spinal cord.

Ideally, 150 ml. of cerebrospinal fluid will be circulating around the central nervous system at any given time. Since approximately 840 ml. of fluid is secreted daily, a considerable proportion of this volume must be reabsorbed to offset any potential build-up of interstitial pressure. Fluid normally returns to

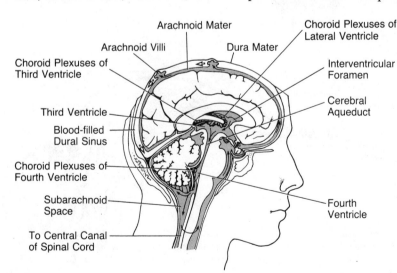

Figure 13.30 The formation and circulation of cerebrospinal fluid. Note the location of choroid plexuses, from which cerebrospinal fluid is derived.

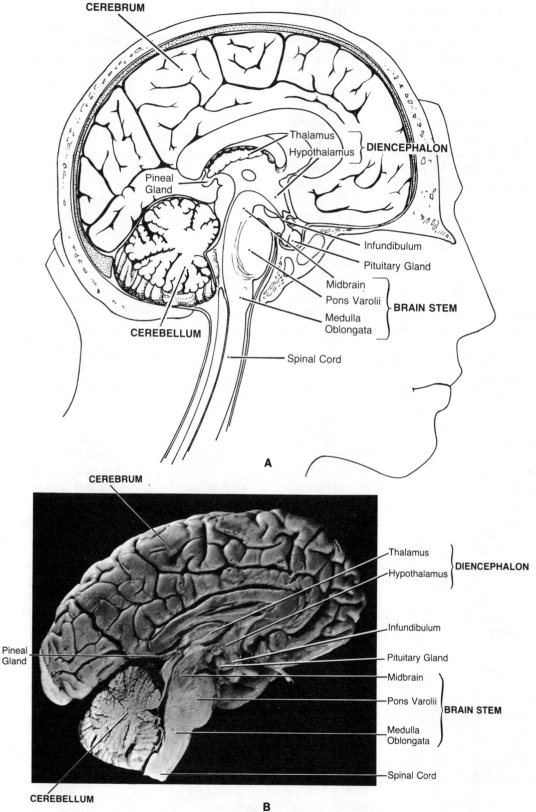

Figure 13.31 Structure of the brain. Illustration (A) and photograph (B) of the human brain, indicating location of the cerebrum, cerebellum, diencephalon, and brain stem. (B from Gardner, E., Gray, D. J., and O'Rahilly, R.: Anatomy: A Regional Study of Human Structure, 4th ed. Philadelphia, W. B. Saunders Company, 1975. Used by permission.)

the circulatory system through specialized arachnoid villi in the area of the central venous sinuses.

Because of its complex nature, the structure and function of the brain are best elucidated by considering the organ segmentally. For study purposes it is helpful to subdivide the brain into several major parts, including the *brain stem,* the *diencephalon,* the *cerebellum,* and the *cerebrum,* as illustrated in Figure 13.31.

The brain stem, consisting of the *medulla, pons,* and *midbrain (mesencephalon),* is located at the base of the brain. It transmits impulses between the cord and higher cerebral centers and also functions in the mediation of certain critical autonomic reflexes. The medulla, in particular, contains control centers that regulate cardiac rate, vascular tone, and respiratory rate.

Located above the brain stem, the diencephalon consists of the *thalamus* and the *hypothalamus.* The thalamus serves as a center for the reception, and subsequent relay, of sensory information, and the hypothalamus functions more diffusely as a vital link between the nervous and endocrine systems. It is specifically through the hypothalamus that many autonomic neural responses are mediated and that basic characteristics such as temperature, rage, sexual drive, hunger, thirst, and sleep/wakefulness are regulated.

Unlike the brain stem and diencephalon, which are only marginally involved with voluntary activity, the cerebellum functions primarily in the coordination and integration of skeletal muscle contraction. Consisting of two hemispheres bound together by bundles of neural fibers, the cerebellum is a butterfly-shaped structure located beneath the cerebrum and posterior to the brain stem. Because of the significance of the cerebellum in mediating smooth, unified muscular activity, dysfunction in this area frequently results in spastic, tremorous, and/or dissociated voluntary muscular responses.

The cerebrum is the largest functional area of the brain. It consists of an outer layer of gray matter called *cortex* and an inner accumulation of white matter. Cortical surface area, moreover, is considerably increased by the convoluted arrangement of surface neurons. Deep downfolds of cortex are referred to as *fissures,* and the longitudinal fissure serves to separate the cerebrum into two major hemispheres, each of which is subdivided into four lobes. As illustrated in Figure 13.32, the frontal, parietal, temporal, and occipital lobes are named, respectively, for the cranial bones under which they lie.

It is among the cells of the cerebrum that the majority of complex neural activity is mediated. Although many aspects of cerebral function can be clearly elucidated, (Fig. 13.33 and Table 13.4), questions about the human brain will continue to puzzle scientists for years to come. Until further advances are made in the area of neurophysiology, the scientific basis for traits such as memory, emotion, intelligence, logic, and conscience must remain primarily conjectural.

Although the majority of structures in the brain can be fit rather neatly into one of the four identified anatomical subdivisions, certain areas do exist that defy categorization. The *reticular formation* and *basal ganglia,* for

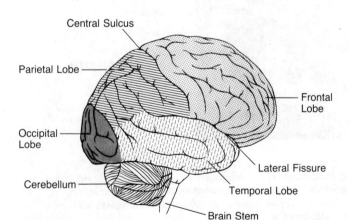

Figure 13.32 The four lobes of the right cerebral hemisphere.

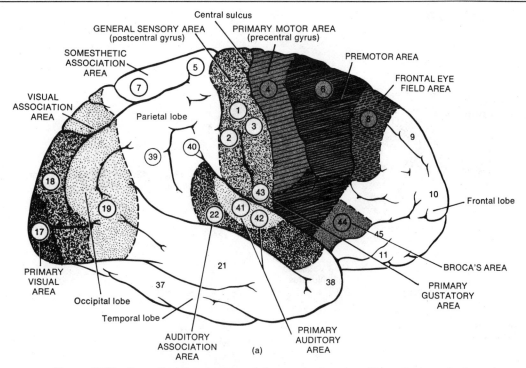

Figure 13.33 Some functional areas of the cerebral cortex. (From Tortora, G. J., and Anagnostakos, M. P.: Principles of Anatomy and Physiology, 2nd ed. New York, Harper & Row, 1978. Used by permission.)

TABLE 13.4 **Functional Areas of the Cerebrum**

General Nature of Area	Location	Function
Sensory	Areas 1, 2, and 3 — parietal lobe	General sensory area — receives impulses from skin, muscles, and visceral receptors; localizes origin of sensation
	Areas 5 and 7 — parietal lobe	Somesthetic association area — integrates and interprets sensations; storage of sensory memories
	Areas 17 — occipital lobe	Primary visual area — receives sensory impulses from the eyes; interpretation of shape and color
	Areas 18 and 19 — occipital lobe	Visual association area — relates past to present visual experience
	Areas 41 and 42 — temporal lobe	Primary auditory area — interpretation of pitch and rhythm
	Area 22 — temporal lobe	Auditory association area — distinction between speech, music, and noise; interpretation of speech
	Area 43 — parietal cortex	Primary gustatory area—interpretation of taste sensations
Motor	Area 4 — frontal lobe	Primary motor area — initiates skeletal muscle contraction
	Area 6 — frontal lobe	Premotor area — controls skilled movements such as writing
	Area 44 — frontal lobe	Broca's area — translation of thoughts into speech
Association	Lateral surfaces of the frontal, parietal, temporal, and occipital lobes	Concerned with memory, judgment, intelligence, personality, emotions, and logic

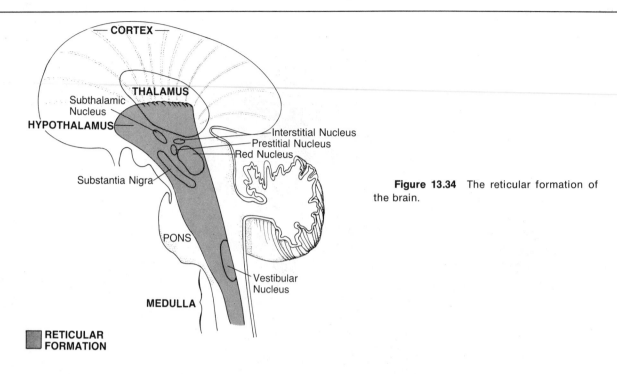

Figure 13.34 The reticular formation of the brain.

example, consist of neurons that are scattered diffusely throughout several different segments of brain tissue.

As illustrated in Figure 13.34, the reticular formation is superimposed upon areas of the medulla, pons, mesencephalon, and diencephalon. The reticular formation contains both sensory and motor fibers and generally serves to promote the transmission of motor impulses, thereby causing an increase in skeletal muscular tone. A small portion of the reticular formation located in the lower medulla, however, is inhibitory in nature. This area will predictably initiate a loss of muscular tone. If the inhibitory impulses are interrupted by pathological changes, as frequently happens

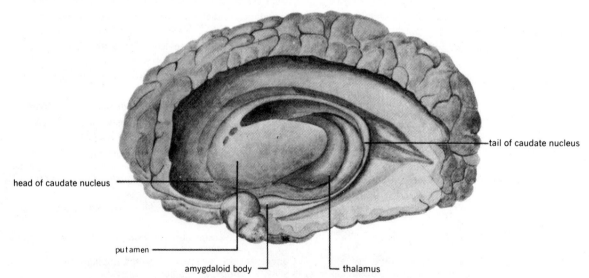

Figure 13.35 The basal ganglia of the brain. (From McClintic, R. J.: Basic Anatomy and Physiology of the Human Body. New York, John Wiley & Sons, 1975. Used by permission.)

secondary to cerebral ischemia, increased spasticity of skeletal muscle is noted.

In mediating its characteristic response patterns, the reticular formation often functions in conjunction with the basal ganglia (Fig. 13.35). These ganglia consist of isolated accumulations of gray matter deep within the brain and cause a decrease in muscular tone when innervated by the inhibitory center of the reticular formation. The ganglia can, alternatively, be directed by the cerebral cortex to facilitate subconscious skeletal muscular contraction. In these instances, muscular tone is increased.

Basic Neural Anatomy and Physiology: A Summary

In summary, it can be said that the nervous system ideally functions as a well-integrated information network. Designed to facilitate adaptive response to internal and external environmental changes, the system consists of many functional units called neurons organized into peripheral nerves, a spinal cord, and a brain.

To support cellular survival, all aspects of the nervous system must work together to mediate integrated and coordinated neural transmission. In essence, this means that certain basic conduction units are critical to the maintenance of homeostasis. Included among these are:

1. The synaptic connections between and among individual neurons in the body.

2. The peripheral nervous system networks, which convey information toward and away from the central nervous system.

3. The conduction tracts in the white matter of the spinal cord, which transmit impulses toward and away from the brain.

4. The synaptic centers in the gray matter of the spinal cord, which help to mediate reflex responses.

5. The intricate neural connections within the brain, which serve to facilitate the integration, coordination, initiation, and interpretation of other impulses.

Because of the inherently interdependent nature of the nervous system, disruption at any of these levels can precipitate neural pathology.

NEURAL PATHOLOGY

Because the nervous system regulates and influences so many major functional activities in the body, neural pathology can directly or indirectly initiate diffuse multisystemic dysfunction. Since neural disorders are potentially so varied and complex, it is helpful to set well-defined limits for the study of disease. In the following pages, emphasis will be placed upon two very discrete and significant areas: (1) pathology of the brain and (2) pathology of the spinal cord.

Pathology of the Brain

As briefly indicated earlier, the brain is an extremely intricate and complicated organ that serves as a primary regulator of varied functional activities. Most frequently, disorders of the brain develop secondary to ischemia, increases in intracranial pressure, or both. In subsequent pages, the mechanisms underlying each of these pathological processes will be further elucidated, with particular emphasis on causative factors and clinical manifestations.

ISCHEMIA

Because the brain is extremely sensitive to lack of oxygen and glucose, the maintenance of cerebral circulation is of primary importance. Under normal circumstances, the brain receives approximately one sixth of total cardiac output and uses about 20 per cent of available plasma oxygen. Because of the excessive metabolic demands of neurons in the brain, circulatory deprivation sustained for only three to ten minutes can lead to permanent cellular damage.

To support cerebral blood flow (CBF), autoregulatory mechanisms exist that facilitate the ongoing circulation of blood through the brain. As ischemia develops, decreases in available oxygen, and increases in carbon dioxide and metabolic wastes, will have direct vasodilator effects upon cerebral vessels. In this way, the brain is partially protected against sudden oxygen deprivation. If circulatory depression is severe, however, autoregulation becomes increasingly less effective, and ischemia will ultimately result in spite of compensatory adjustments.

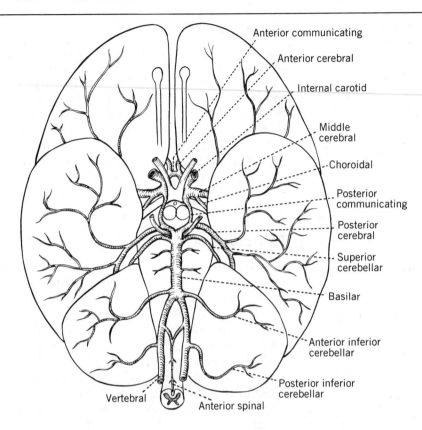

Anterior communicating

Anterior cerebral

Internal carotid

Middle cerebral

Choroidal

Posterior communicating

Posterior cerebral

Superior cerebellar

Basilar

Anterior inferior cerebellar

Posterior inferior cerebellar

Vertebral

Anterior spinal

Figure 13.36 Arterial blood supply to the brain. (From Patton, H. D., et al.: Introduction to Basic Neurology. Philadelphia, W. B. Saunders Company, 1976. Used by permission.)

In the following pages, a brief introduction to normal cerebral circulation precedes a more detailed elucidation of the causative mechanisms and clinical symptoms associated with cerebral ischemia.

CEREBRAL CIRCULATION Blood is normally transported to the brain through a circulatory pathway illustrated in Figure 13.36. It can be seen that oxygenated blood is carried to the brain by the anterior internal carotid arteries and the posterior vertebral arteries. These vessels eventually communicate at the base of the brain to form the *circle of Willis*, from which emanate derivative penetrating arteries that transport blood deep into cerebral tissue.

Any decrease of blood flow through this vascular system can lead to cerebral ischemia. The extent of resulting neural damage is generally influenced by the degree of collateral circulation, the site of the causative vascular lesion, and the quantity of neural tissue subsequently deprived of oxygen. Some major

cerebral areas supplied by specific arterial vessels are illustrated in Figure 13.37.

CAUSES OF CEREBRAL ISCHEMIA Although cerebral ischemia can be caused by a variety of disorders, deficient cerebral blood flow is most commonly induced by one of three major mechanisms:

1. Occlusion of cerebral vessels.
2. Hemorrhage in cerebral vessels.
3. Circulatory deficit induced by disorders external to the central nervous system.

In cases in which pathological changes are caused by occlusion or hemorrhage of cerebral vessels, disorders are generally described as *cerebrovascular* in nature. In these instances, the specific manifestations of ischemia are largely dependent upon the site of associated neural damage. On the other hand, if ischemia is induced by dysfunction external to the nervous system (in the heart or lungs, for example), oxygen deprivation will affect the cerebrum in a more diffuse and generalized

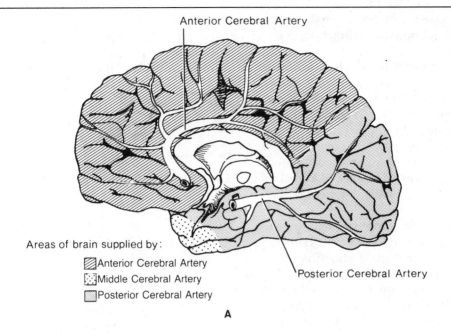

Anterior Cerebral Artery

Areas of brain supplied by:

▨ Anterior Cerebral Artery
⠂⠂ Middle Cerebral Artery
▦ Posterior Cerebral Artery

Posterior Cerebral Artery

A

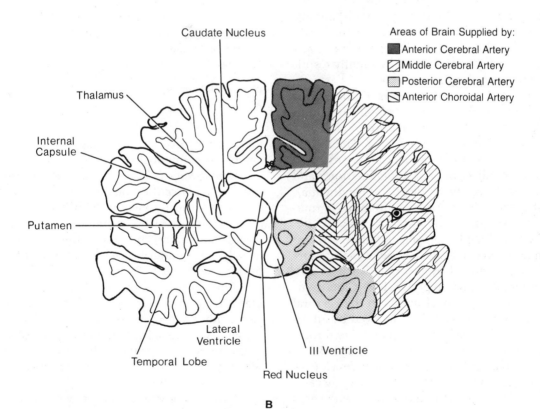

Caudate Nucleus

Areas of Brain Supplied by:

▦ Anterior Cerebral Artery
▨ Middle Cerebral Artery
▦ Posterior Cerebral Artery
◩ Anterior Choroidal Artery

Thalamus

Internal
Capsule

Putamen

Lateral
Ventricle

III Ventricle

Temporal Lobe

Red Nucleus

B

Figure 13.37 *A*, The medial surface of the cerebral hemisphere, showing the course of the anterior and posterior cerebral arteries and the area of the brain supplied by each. *B*, The cerebral hemispheres and the vascular supply, in coronal section. (From Beeson, P. B., et al.: Cecil Textbook of Medicine, 15th ed. Philadelphia, W. B. Saunders Company, 1979. Used by permission.)

way. In these cases, metabolic, renal, gastro-intestinal, and pulmonary dysfunction is also frequently noted.

Occlusion of Cerebral Vessels   Occlusion of cerebral vessels is most commonly caused by the deposit of a *thrombus* or an *embolus* within the cerebral arteries. Cerebral ischemia is induced by thrombi approximately 40 per cent of the time, with emboli being the second most frequent cause of cerebrovascular obstruction. In either case, blockage of a cerebral vessel can result in considerable neural damage.

Although specific symptoms will depend largely upon the site and extent of occlusion, the general clinical picture is also affected by the nature of the obstruction. Thrombi, for example, tend to develop most frequently in patients over 50. Onset of symptoms typically occurs during sleep or soon after waking, with increases in intensity often occurring for a period of 48 hours thereafter. Emboli, on the other hand, generally affect younger patients, although most individuals are over 40. Occlusion is usually more abrupt, can occur at any time of the day or night, and frequently results in more extensive tissue death.

In considering the factors inducing the formation of thrombi or emboli, it is important to note that disease external to the nervous system is often involved. The formation of thrombi, for example, can be promoted by hemorrhage, arterial inflammation, and increased viscosity of blood (polycythemia). Most frequently, however, thrombus formation is associated with atherosclerosis. As described in Chapter 9, degenerative vascular changes evolve over the course of many years and are accelerated by disorders such as diabetes mellitus and hypertension. Clots typically form at junctional points in the cerebral circulation that have been narrowed by atherosclerotic deposits. Some major sites of thrombus formation are illustrated in Figure 13.38.

Whereas thrombi most often develop in conjunction with chronic vascular disease, emboli can originate in individuals who show little evidence of atherosclerosis. In these cases, clot formation is usually associated with cardiac arrhythmia, myocardial infarction, endocarditis, or valvular dysfunction. Occlusion typically occurs when clots moving through

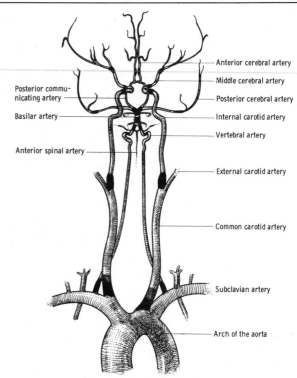

Figure 13.38   Some common sites of atherosclerosis and obstruction in cerebral vessels (indicated by darkened areas on arterial diagram). (From Beeson, P. B., et al.: Cecil Textbook of Medicine, 15th ed. Philadelphia, W. B. Saunders Company, 1979. Used by permission.)

the cerebral circulation are deposited in small vessels, thereby obstructing blood flow.

Hemorrhage in Cerebral Vessels   Approximately 10 per cent of the time, cerebral ischemia is induced by bleeding within the tissue of the brain, described as *intracerebral hemorrhage*. Pathological changes, in these cases, are usually of sudden onset, with symptoms peaking within 1 to 24 hours.

Although hemorrhage can be due to bleeding from a vein or capillary, it is most commonly caused by rupture of an arterial vessel. Any sustained elevation in arterial blood pressure or weakness in the arterial wall will thus increase the risk of developing a cerebrovascular hemorrhage.

Often involved in the development of intracerebral bleeding are small sac-like weak spots in the arterial walls, called *aneurysms*. Believed to be present at birth, they are commonly noted in specific areas of the cerebral circulation, as illustrated in Figure 13.39.

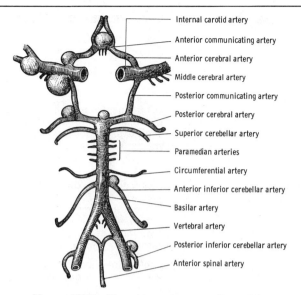

Internal carotid artery
Anterior communicating artery
Anterior cerebral artery
Middle cerebral artery
Posterior communicating artery
Posterior cerebral artery
Superior cerebellar artery
Paramedian arteries
Circumferential artery
Anterior inferior cerebellar artery
Basilar artery
Vertebral artery
Posterior inferior cerebellar artery
Anterior spinal artery

Figure 13.39 The more common sites of berry aneurysm. The size of the aneurysm at the various sites is directly proportional to the frequency at that site. (From Beeson, P. B., et al.: Cecil Textbook of Medicine, 15th ed. Philadelphia, W. B. Saunders Company, 1979. Used by permission.)

Although hemorrhage, for whatever reason, will characteristically disrupt blood flow to cerebral tissue, it can also result in the localized development of inflammatory edema. For this reason, bleeding is often accompanied by increases in intracranial pressure, a phenomenon discussed subsequently in this chapter.

Pathology External to the Central Nervous System Although occlusion and hemorrhage are the most common causes of cerebral ischemia, it has been noted that cerebrovascular pathology is frequently associated with diseases originating outside the central nervous system. Atherosclerosis, for example, will typically accelerate thrombus formation, whereas hypertension often triggers intracerebral hemorrhage. Since cerebral circulation is ultimately predicated upon the funtional activity of many different systems, oxygen deprivation can be initiated by pathology of diverse origin. Some primary examples would include:

1. Cardiac pathology characterized by insufficient cardiac output.

2. Vascular pathology characterized by hypotension.

3. Systemic pathology characterized by hypovolemia.

Although the volume of cerebral blood flow is of critical importance, the composition of plasma supplying the brain is of equal significance. If oxygen or glucose content is depressed neural damage may result, even when optimal quantities of blood are circulating through the brain. Any disorder that seriously compromises pO_2 levels or glucose concentration can thus seriously affect cerebral activity. Some major examples of this type of dysfunction are:

1. Respiratory pathology, characterized by depressed alveolar gas exchange.

2. Skeletomuscular pathology, which indirectly affects respiratory function.

3. Anemias, characterized by inadequate transport of oxygen through the blood.

4. Endocrine disorders, characterized by hypoglycemia.

In conclusion, it can be said that a variety of systemic disorders may indirectly affect the quantity or quality of cerebral circulation. A brief tabular summary of some major disorders and the way in which they alter blood flow through the brain is presented in Table 13.5.

MANIFESTATIONS OF CEREBRAL ISCHEMIA When blood supply to the brain is significantly depressed, anoxia will trigger neural dysfunction and cellular necrosis, with the ultimate formation of an area of *cerebral infarction*. In these cases, characteristic clinical symptoms will depend largely upon the site and extent of tissue damage.

Most commonly, severe ischemia is induced by cerebrovascular disease. In these instances, the resulting pathological condition is referred to as a *cerebrovascular accident (CVA)*, otherwise known as a *stroke*. Since CVA's affect approximately 500,000 Americans a year, causing 200,000 deaths, they constitute one of the major clinical disorders in this country — touching the lives of a large number of people.

In cases in which the development of cerebral ischemia is a progressive, degenerative phenomenon associated with atherosclerosis, early warning signs are frequently detectable. These episodes of temporary,

TABLE 13.5 **Causes of Cerebral Ischemia**

Pathophysiological Mechanism	Causative Clinical Pathology	Characteristic Manifestations
OCCLUSION OF CEREBRAL VESSELS		
Thrombus	Atherosclerosis Hemorrhage Arterial inflammation Polycythemia	Most frequent in patients over 50 Onset of symptoms typically during sleep, or soon after waking Symptoms usually increase in intensity for 48 hours after onset
Embolus	Cardiac arrhythmia Myocardial infarction Endocarditis Valvular dysfunction	Patients generally over 40, but younger than 50 Onset of symptoms typically abrupt, and often more severe than those associated with thrombi
INTRACEREBRAL HEMORRHAGE	Hypertension Aneurysms	Pathology of sudden onset, with symptoms peaking within 24 hours Frequently associated with cerebral edema and increases in intracranial pressure
PATHOLOGY EXTERNAL TO THE CNS		
Cardiac pathology	Cardiac failure Valvular dysfunction Pericarditis Cardiac arrhythmias	Varies with nature of causative pathology
Vascular pathology	Vasogenic shock Atherosclerosis	
Pathology causing hypovolemia	Burns Hemorrhage Diarrhea and vomiting Diabetes insipidus	
Pathology characterized by depressed pO_2	Anemias Myasthenia gravis Narcotic overdose Scoliosis/kyphosis Atelectasis Chronic obstructive pulmonary disease (COPD) Bronchiectasis Pulmonary edema	
Pathology causing hypoglycemia	Adenoma of the islets of Langerhans Insulin shock Addison's disease Alcoholism	

reversible cerebral ischemia, called *transient ischemic attacks (TIA's)*, usually last from 5 to 30 minutes and are characterized by a variety of potential symptoms. Manifestations include muscular weakness, numbness, impaired speech or comprehension, impaired hearing, altered visual acuity, vertigo, and sudden depression of postural tone causing a "drop attack" without loss of consciousness.

In contrast, a "completed stroke" results from prolonged ischemia with irreversible neural damage. Symptoms in these cases reflect the site of the causative lesion.

If ischemia is limited to the cerebral hemispheres, common indications include weakness or paralysis of skeletal muscles on the side opposite to (or contralateral to) the infarction. To the extent that upper motor neurons (UMN's) are functionally disrupted, initially flaccid muscle can, after a period of time,

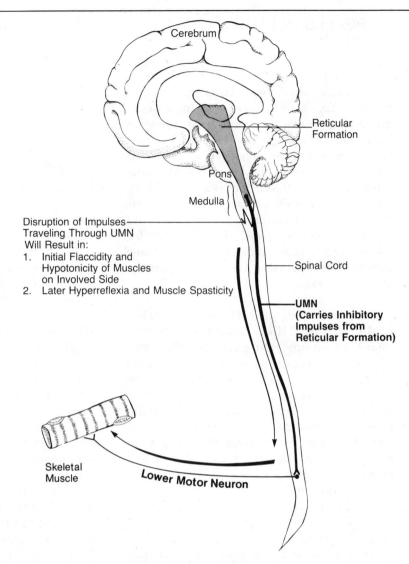

Cerebrum

Reticular
Formation

Pons

Medulla

Disruption of Impulses
Traveling Through UMN
Will Result in:
1. Initial Flaccidity and
   Hypotonicity of Muscles
   on Involved Side
2. Later Hyperreflexia and Muscle Spasticity

Spinal Cord

UMN
(Carries Inhibitory
Impulses from
Reticular Formation)

Skeletal
Muscle

Lower Motor Neuron

Figure 13.40 Disruption of impulses traveling through upper motor neurons.

show evidence of increases in muscle tone with corresponding hyperreflexia. This phenomenon is due primarily to the disruption of inhibitory impulses that originate in the lower reticular formation and are normally transmitted by upper motor neurons. A diagrammatic summary of resulting abnormalities is presented in Figure 13.40. Depending upon the area of cerebral ischemia, skeletal muscle changes will often be accompanied by altered patterns of vision and loss of the ability to speak or understand or both. Necrosis of the brain stem, on the other hand, is typically characterized by dizziness, double vision, sensory impairment, weakness, and altered states of consciousness. A brief summary of some of the major clinical manifestations of a CVA is found in Table 13.6.

TABLE 13.6   **Some Major Clinical Manifestations of a CVA**

Location of Causative Lesion	Clinical Manifestations
Cerebrum	Weakness and paralysis of skeletal muscles on the side opposite to the lesion (followed by hyperreflexia and muscle spasticity in cases of UMN pathology) Loss of ability to speak and/or understand Altered patterns of vision
Brain stem	Dizziness Double vision Sensory impairment Weakness Altered state of consciousness

INCREASES IN INTRACRANIAL PRESSURE

Although cerebral ischemia can initiate considerable neural dysfunction, pathological changes may also be triggered by increases in intracranial pressure. Intracranial pressure, which normally ranges between 4 and 15 mm. Hg, is defined as the pressure exerted within the cranial cavity by the blood, cerebrospinal fluid, and brain tissue that normally fill the bony cranium. As intracranial pressure is increased, tissue compression can lead to the death, or necrosis, of neural cells. In the following pages, some major causes and manifestations of increasing intracranial pressure are elucidated.

CAUSES OF INCREASING INTRA-CRANIAL PRESSURE Since the cranium is essentially an unyielding vault, it offers very little room for expansion of the soft tissue housed within it. As a result, any factor that causes an increase in volume of the brain, blood, or cerebrospinal fluid will predictably cause a certain degree of neural compression. Increases in intracranial pressure are most frequently associated with one of four major phenomena:

1. Head injuries.
2. Cerebrovascular disease.
3. Brain tumors.
4. Infectious disorders.

Regardless of the original source of trauma, edema has been found to play a significant role in the development of intracranial swelling. As cellular stress develops, a characteristic inflammatory response is normally triggered. Subsequent increases in blood flow and vascular permeability will predictably cause increasing intracranial pressure.

Head Injuries In cases of head injury (also referred to as craniocerebral trauma), bleeding may be an additional source of intracranial pressure elevation. Underlying pathophysiology depends, to a large extent, upon the specific type of damage incurred.

In "closed head injuries," in which the cranium is not physically disrupted, initial damage frequently takes one of two forms:

1. *A concussion* — in which temporary disruption of cerebral neural synapses is

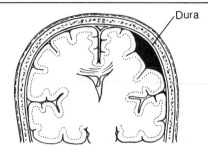

Figure 13.41   A subdural hematoma. (From Luckmann, J., and Sorensen, K. C.: Medical Surgical Nursing: A Psychophysiological Approach, 2nd ed. Philadelphia, W. B. Saunders Company, 1980. Used by permission.)

noted, without any true structural tissue damage. Unless the concussion is accompanied by an inflammatory reaction, it will not typically cause increased intracranial pressure.

2. *A contusion* — in which brain tissue is actually bruised. Small intracerebral hemorrhages and localized sites of edema are often noted, along with possible increases in intracranial pressure.

Although the damage caused by closed head injuries is frequently reversible, the clinician must watch carefully for any indications of delayed intracranial bleeding. Most commonly, this type of hemorrhage results in the formation of an aggregate of blood and fluid described as either a *subdural* or an *epidural hematoma*, according to location.

As illustrated in Figure 13.41, the subdural hematoma is a collection of blood between the dura and arachnoid membranes covering the brain. It frequently occurs secondary to cerebral contusion and is due to the rupture of veins in the subdural space. As fluid and disintegrating blood cells accumulate under the dura, the high concentration of osmotically active particles serves to draw water from the subarachnoid space. This phenomenon accelerates neural compression and may ultimately promote herniation of brain tissue through the foramen magnum.

An epidural hematoma most commonly results from a tear in the wall of the middle meningeal artery. It is characterized by the accumulation of blood in the space between the dura and the cranium and usually results in herniation through the tentorium, as illustrated in Figure 13.42. Death will ensue unless the hematoma is surgically removed.

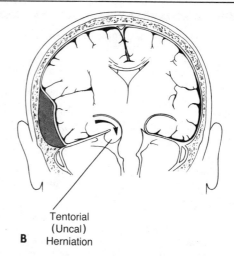

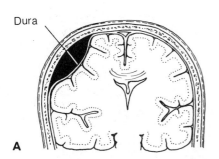

Dura

A

Tentorial
(Uncal)
Herniation

B

Figure 13.42 An epidural hematoma (*A*) may commonly result in tentorial herniation (*B*). Note the displacement of the uncus (or medial gyrus of the temporal lobe) through the tentorial notch. (*A* from Luckmann, J., and Sorensen, K. C.: Medical Surgical Nursing: A Psychophysiological Approach, 2nd ed. Philadelphia, W. B. Saunders Company, 1980. Used by permission.)

Although hematomas are frequently associated with a closed head wound, they are also noted in some cases in which the skull has been fractured. With a depressed skull fracture in particular, fragments of bone may exert pressure upon or penetrate the brain itself. In these cases, intracerebral hematoma can be a frequent complication, as illustrated in Figure 13.43.

Cerebrovascular Disease As previously discussed, cerebrovascular pathology is typically characterized by occlusion or intracerebral hemorrhage, or both. In either case, the resulting cellular stress will often trigger an inflammatory response. As edema develops, considerable neural damage can occur at the site of the swelling. In cases of cerebrovascular disease, therefore, ischemia may predictably

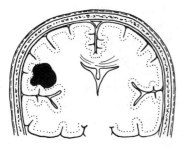

Figure 13.43 Intracerebral hematoma. (From Luckmann, J., and Sorensen, K. C.: Medical Surgical Nursing: A Psychophysiological Approach, 2nd ed. Philadelphia, W. B. Saunders Company, 1980. Used by permission.)

be complicated by the effects of increasing intracranial pressure.

Brain Tumors Brain tumors can be defined as abnormal tissue growths within the cranium. Whether benign or malignant, they cause increasing intracranial pressure. In cases of malignancy, the clinical picture may be further aggravated by a characteristic development of edema at the tumor site.

Brain tumors can generally be classified in a variety of ways. If categorized according to location, two major distinctions can be made:

1. *Growths occurring inside the brain —* Most typically, these tumors affect glial cells, which are found surrounding, supporting, and connecting neurons within the brain. *Gliomas,* in fact, account for approximately 40 to 50 per cent of all brain tumors.

2. *Growths occurring external to the brain, but within the cranium —* Most commonly, these tumors affect the meninges, which cover the brain surface. *Meningiomas* account for about 12 to 20 per cent of all brain tumors. A tabular summary of some major types of brain tumors is presented in Table 13.7.

Infectious Disorders When pathogenic microorganisms invade the central nervous system, a variety of diseases can result. Meningitis and encephalitis are classic examples of infectious neural disorders. In both cases, pathological findings are frequently characterized by the development of inflammatory

TABLE 13.7 **Some Major Types of Brain Tumors**

Classification of Tumor	Site of Neoplastic Growth	Incidence (%)
Glioma:	Neuroglial cells: support and shelter neurons within the CNS	40–50
Astrocytoma	Astrocytes: star-shaped cells that help to insulate neurons	27–35
Oligodendroglioma	Oligodendroglia: cells with fewer processes than astrocytes; believed to function in the production of myelin within the CNS	1–4
Ependyoma	Ependyma: epithelial cells that line the ventricles and aqueduct of the brain	1–3
Medulloblastoma	Primitive cells that may ultimately develop into either neurons or neuroglia; tumors frequently arise in cerebellum	3–5
Cerebral neuroblastoma	Cells that are precursors to neurons; tumors usually arise in the cerebral hemispheres	Very rare
Meningioma	Primary components of the meninges, including arachnoid cells, fibroblasts, and/or blood vessels	12–20

edema, with a subsequent increase in intracranial pressure. Associated vascular changes may additionally lead to thrombus formation, necrosis, and the ultimate development of localized infarctions.

Although certain aspects of underlying pathophysiology are the same for meningitis and encephalitis, the diseases do differ in a number of ways.

Meningitis, for example, is most frequently caused by meningococcal, staphylococcal, streptococcal, or pneumococcal bacteria that enter the body through the respiratory tract. The pathogens directly affect the pia and arachnoid membranes that cover the central nervous system, and cause symptoms of headache, high fever, seizures, alterations in consciousness, and stiffness of the neck (nuchal rigidity).

Encephalitis is primarily a viral disorder. The disease can be transmitted by mosquitoes from an intermediate host (such as a horse) or can evolve secondary to a viral infection such as measles, mumps, or chickenpox. Pathogens typically invade the glial cells of the brain, causing destruction of the cortex, basal ganglia, and brain stem. Characteristic symptoms include drowsiness, fever, chills, and vomiting, with head and neck stiffness and seizures being noted if the meninges become involved in the infectious process.

MANIFESTATIONS OF INCREASING INTRACRANIAL PRESSURE As tissue or fluid or both accumulate within the cranium, compensatory mechanisms can be called into play to offset the effects of increasing intracranial pressure. Frequently, a decrease in cerebral blood flow and a shunting of cerebrospinal fluid from the subarachnoid space surrounding the brain to the space surrounding the cord will alleviate pathological findings.

If pressure elevation is sudden or excessive, however, compensation attempts will often fail to relieve the effects of compression. In these cases, dysfunction generally occurs as a result of three primary processes:

1. Focal and localized destruction of neurons due to the direct effects of pressure increases.

2. More generalized neural degeneration as increased intracranial pressure causes diffuse compression of blood vessels, with resulting ischemia.

3. Extensive neural involvement as increases in pressure cause displacement of brain tissue, with subsequent herniation through the tentorium, falx cerebelli, or foramen magnum.

These mechanisms are summarized diagrammatically in Figure 13.44.

Generalized manifestations of increasing intracranial pressure include alterations in the

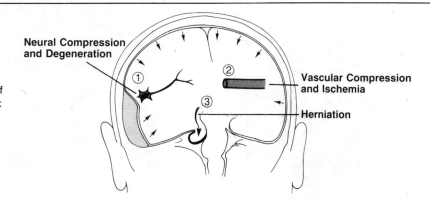

Figure 13.44 The effects of increasing intracranial pressure: a schematic presentation.

level of consciousness, increasing lethargy, irritability, and lack of orientation.

A number of more specific clinical symptoms often reflect the extent and location of neural damage. If the motor centers of the cerebrum are affected, contralateral loss of muscular contractility and coordination is frequently noted. Damage to the excitatory center of the reticular formation, results in muscular flaccidity, whereas dysfunction of the inhibitory center causes rigidity.

If pressure elevations are localized in more inferior structures, such as the brain stem or the cranial nerves, a number of additional symptoms will characteristically develop. Compression of the medulla, for example, can often initiate a broad range of physiological dysfunction, affecting the gastrointestinal, respiratory, and cardiovascular systems. Some

clinical manifestations resulting from increased cranial pressure are summarized in Table 13.8.

In cases in which the cranial nerves are affected, compression frequently triggers ocular changes. Two primary indications of cranial nerve involvement are:

1. *Papilledema* — or inflammation and swelling of the optic nerve at the point where it enters the eye. The optic nerve, which is surrounded by meninges, is considerably affected by increases in cerebrospinal fluid pressure. The head of the nerve (or optic disc) is often misplaced under these circumstances and is pushed above the retina, as illustrated in Figure 13.45.

2. *Dilation and fixation of the pupil* — or enlargement of the pupil, with lack of normal responsiveness. Pupillary changes are believed to be caused by pressure against the brain stem, with subsequent compression of the third cranial (oculomotor) nerve.

In summary, increasing intracranial pressure frequently initiates a wide variety of functional changes in the body. Although symptoms often correlate with the site of neural damage, clinical manifestations may also reflect the nature of causative pathology. A brief synopsis of some changes characteristically associated with specific neural disorders is presented in Table 13.9.

Pathology of the Spinal Cord

The spinal cord, as described earlier, provides a vital link between peripheral nerves and the brain, while simultaneously serving as a center for many reflex responses. Damage to the cord can thus result in diffuse dysfunc-

TABLE 13.8 **Clinical Manifestations of Increasing Intracranial Pressure**

Locus of Increased Pressure	Clinical Manifestations
Reticular formation; diencephalon	Drowziness; coma
Facilitory center of the reticular formation (in the brain stem)	Contralateral muscular flaccidity
Inhibitory center of the reticular formation (in the brain stem)	Contralateral muscular spasticity
Vomiting reflex center in the medulla	Anorexia, nausea, and vomiting
Respiratory center of the medulla	Hypoventilation, with secondary development of respiratory acidosis
Vasomotor center of the medulla	Rise in blood pressure, with reflex decrease in cardiac rate

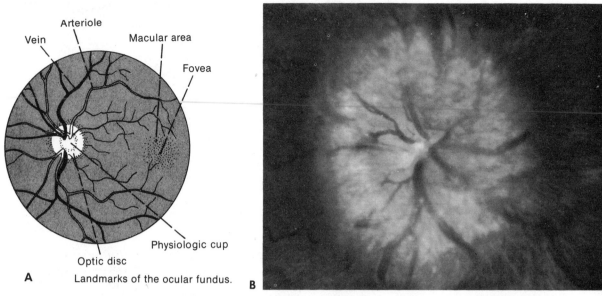

A Landmarks of the ocular fundus. **B**

Figure 13.45 Papilledema. Compare the normal ocular fundus (*A*) with pathology initiated by increasing intracranial pressure (*B*). Note the heightened redness and blurred shape of the optic disc in papilledema. This is due, in part, to congestive pressure developing in the retinal veins. (*A* from Luckmann, J., and Sorensen, K. C.: Medical Surgical Nursing: A Psychophysiological Approach, 2nd ed. Philadelphia, W. B. Saunders Company, 1980. *B* from Peyman, G. A., et al.: Principles and Practice of Ophthalmology, Vol. III. Philadelphia, W. B. Saunders Company, 1980. Used by permission.)

TABLE 13.9 **Some Changes Associated with Increases in Intracranial Pressure**

Causative Condition	Some Clinical Manifestations	Underlying Pathophysiology
Epidural hematoma	Short period of unconsciousness, followed by lucid interval	Herniation of brain stem ⟶ compression of midbrain and diencephalon ⟶ interruption of simulatory impulses from reticular activating system
	Unconsciousness	Herniation through the tentorium ⟶ pressure on the reticular formation
	Dilation of the pupil	Compression of the third cranial nerve
	Weakness of motor response	Compression of corticospinal tract
	Disturbance of vital signs and respiratory pattern	Compression of brain stem
Subdural hematoma		
Acute: symptoms evident in 24–48 hours	Similar to epidural hematoma (above)	Similar to epidural hematoma (above) — but may evolve more slowly if bleeding is of venous origin
Subacute: symptoms evident within 48 hours to 2 weeks after injury	Initial unconsciousness followed by seeming improvement; later loss of consciousness	Slow venous bleeding may result in gradual clot formation, with ultimate compression of vital cerebral tissue
	Dilation of pupil	Compression of third cranial nerve
Tumors	Headache	Displacement of pain-sensitive structures within the cranium
	Nausea and vomiting	Compression of the brain stem
	Seizures	Compression of the motor cortex
	Visual disturbances	Compression of optic nerve/occipital lobe
	Double vision	Compression of one or both of the sixth cranial nerves

tion, with symptoms reflecting the site and extent of causative trauma. In the following pages, some major causes and manifestations of spinal cord pathology are elucidated.

CAUSES OF SPINAL CORD PATHOLOGY

In the majority of cases, spinal cord pathology is characterized by some degree of neural ischemia, degeneration, or compression. Although dysfunction can be initiated by a wide range of disorders, it is most commonly associated with:

1. Accidental trauma.
2. Intervertebral disc extrusion.
3. Spinal tumors.
4. Infectious disorders.
5. Degenerative disorders.

It is important to realize that in many cases of spinal cord pathology dysfunction is not limited to the cord alone. In a number of infectious and degenerative disorders, the disease process frequently extends to include other aspects of the central or peripheral nervous system. Although, throughout the following pages, emphasis is placed upon disorders originating in the spinal cord, it must be remembered that clinical reality frequently defies arbitrary categorization. Symptoms therefore often reflect a more diffuse disease pattern and cannot always be strictly related to dysfunction of the spinal cord.

ACCIDENTAL TRAUMA Every year, approximately 2.5 of every 100,000 Americans will be affected by accidental spinal cord injury. Such trauma commonly results from sports or automobile accidents and is usually caused by compression or transection of the cord, with or without vertebral fracture. Most frequently, accidental injury affects the spine in one of three primary sites: (1) between the lower cervical and upper thoracic vertebrae, (2) between the lower thoracic and upper lumbar vertebrae, or (3) between the lower lumbar and sacral vertebrae.

In all cases, the majority of damage usually occurs at the time of initial injury. Secondary trauma can develop, however, from subsequent compression or laceration by bony fragments.

Immediately following spinal trauma, dysfunction is typically triggered by ischemia.

Decreased blood flow to the spinal cord results in hypoxia, edema, and small hemorrhages. Neural disruption follows and results in a state described as *"spinal shock."* During this time, impulses will not, at first, be transmitted through the damaged area. This phenomenon is characterized by an initial paralysis of the urinary bladder, areflexia, and flaccid paralysis. After a period of time (possibly as long as several months) autonomic reflexes may return, accompanied by hyperreflexia and spastic paralysis. The underlying physiological disruptions associated with spinal shock are summarized in Figure 13.46 and Table 13.10.

INTERVERTEBRAL DISC EXTRUSION Normally, the vertebrae surrounding the spinal cord are separated from one another by intervertebral discs. These discs are composed of fibrocartilage with a soft center called the *nucleus pulposus.*

Under certain circumstances, compression can result in the expulsion of the nucleus pulposus into the spinal cavity, where it exerts pressure upon the spinal cord, associated spinal nerve roots, or both. This condition, frequently initiated by trauma or vertebral degeneration, is illustrated in Figure 13.47. Although manifested most commonly in the lower lumbar area (particularly between L4 and L5, and L5 and the sacrum), disc extrusion can also occur in the cervical spine. Pain is the most predictable symptom, arising as a result of pressure upon the cord or adjacent spinal nerves. Discomfort is frequently escalated, however, by spastic contraction of paraspinal skeletal muscles.

SPINAL CORD TUMORS Spinal cord tumors can generally be defined as abnormal growths of tissue within the vertebral cavity. The majority of these neoplasms are benign and usually occur less frequently than brain tumors. If categorized according to location, they can be described as:

1. *Extradural* — when located external to the dura mater.
2. *Intradural* — when growing within the dura mater. Intradural tumors, moreover, can be more specifically identified as *extramedullary*, if found external to the cord, or *intramedullary*, if located inside the cord.

Approximately 90 per cent of the time extradural tumors are malignant. Having

Physiological Disruption	Functional Result
Trauma of the ascending spinal tracts	Lack of somatic and visceral sensation below the level of trauma
Trauma of descending spinal tracts	Loss of muscular tone, contractility, and reflex response below the level of trauma

A

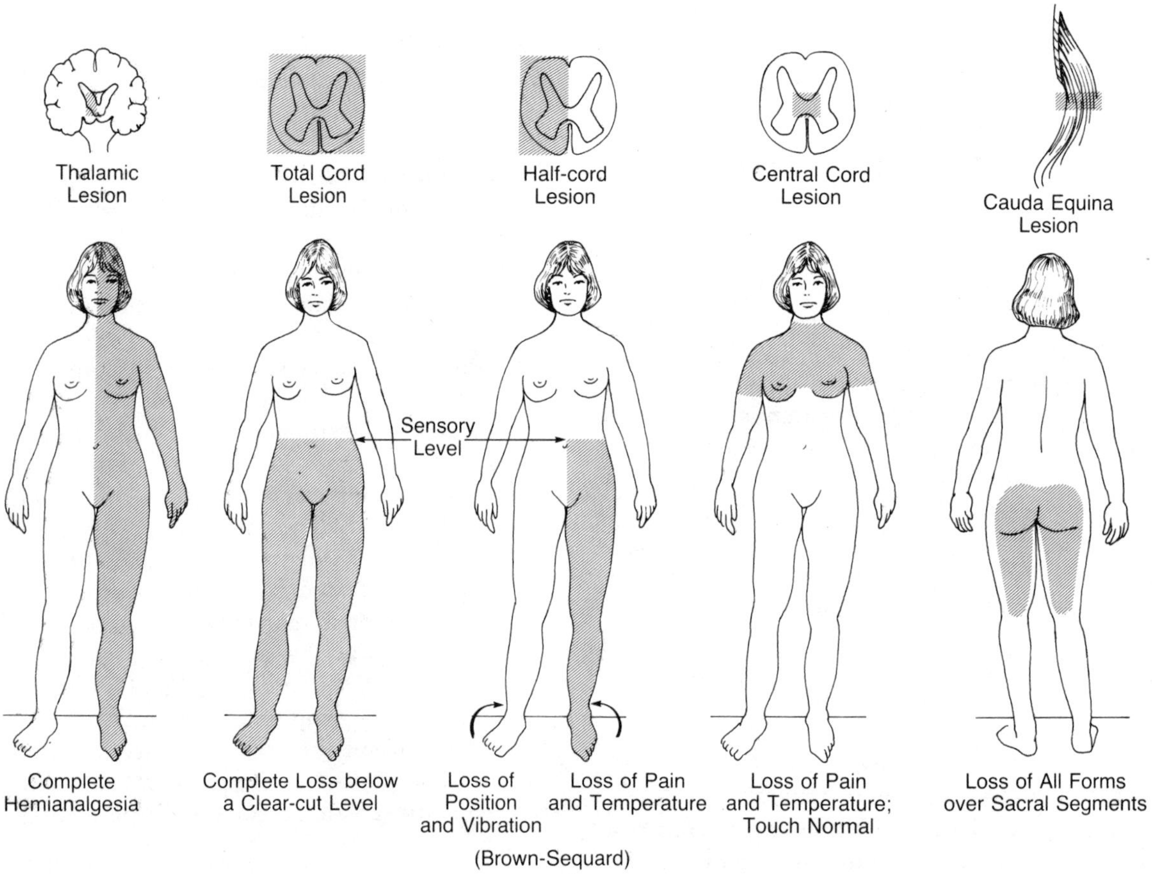

Thalamic Lesion	Total Cord Lesion	Half-cord Lesion	Central Cord Lesion	Cauda Equina Lesion

Sensory Level

Complete Hemianalgesia	Complete Loss below a Clear-cut Level	Loss of Position and Vibration	Loss of Pain and Temperature	Loss of Pain and Temperature; Touch Normal	Loss of All Forms over Sacral Segments

(Brown-Sequard)

B

Figure 13.46 Spinal shock: initial stages. *A*, Physiological disruptions and functional results of spinal shock. *B*, Common patterns of sensory abnormality. Upper diagrams show site of lesion; lower diagrams show distribution of corresponding sensory loss.

spread to the central nervous system from other areas of the body (such as the lung, breast, kidney, or prostate gland), they characteristically cause compression of the spinal cord and associated nerve roots. Pain typically results, accompanied by some degree of sensory or motor loss below the level of the lesion.

Intradural tumors, on the other hand, are usually benign. Whereas growths external to the spinal cord are most frequently thoracic meningiomas, 95 per cent of neoplasms developing within the cord are gliomas. Symptoms, in either case, depend upon the location and extent of neural involvement.

INFECTIOUS DISORDERS Whereas trauma, disc pathology, and tumors typically cause some degree of external pressure or stress upon the spinal cord, infectious disorders are characterized by an internal inflammatory response to a foreign protein.

TABLE 13.10 **Muscle Function after Spinal Cord Injury***

Spinal Cord Injury	Muscle Function Remaining	Muscle Function Lost
Cervical		
Above C4	None	All, including respiration
C5	Neck Scapular elevation	Arms Chest All below chest
C6–C7	Neck Some chest movement Some arm movement	Some arm, fingers Some chest All below chest
Thoracic	Neck Arms (full) Some chest	Trunk All below chest
Lumbosacral	Neck Arms Chest Trunk	Legs

*From Phipps, W. J., Long, B. C., and Woods, M. F. (eds.): Medical-Surgical Nursing: Concepts and Clinical Practice. St. Louis, The C. V. Mosby Company, 1979, p. 718.

Although a number of bacterial and viral diseases can affect the spinal cord, it is beyond the scope of this text to detail all causative infectious disorders. Instead, a few select examples will serve as a model upon which to build a better understanding of neural pathology due to infection.

Tetanus Tetanus is an infectious disorder caused by the rod-shaped *Clostridium tetani* bacterium. This pathogen is found widely distributed in soil contaminated by animal or human feces and typically exists in a highly resistant spore form, which can survive adverse environmental conditions for long periods of time.

The tetanus bacterium is frequently introduced into the body through an open wound and acts by releasing a harmful chemical into the blood. This poisonous substance is believed to act directly upon the spinal cord and brain stem, and its effects extend up the spinal cord along trunks of motor nerves.

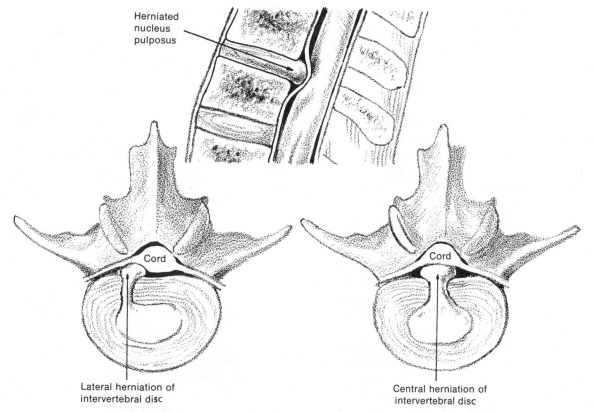

Forms of vertebral herniation.

Figure 13.47 Forms of vertebral herniation. (From Luckmann, J., and Sorensen, K. C.: Medical Surgical Nursing: A Psychophysiological Approach, 1st ed. Philadelphia, W. B. Saunders Company, 1974. Used by permission.)

Interference with the transmission of inhibitory motor impulses results in characteristically severe muscular spasms.

Depending upon the degree of neural involvement, a wide range of symptoms is possible. In mild cases, muscular rigidity and stiffness typically affect the jaw and facial muscles, with resulting alteration in expression and facial mobility. As the disease progresses, skeletal muscle spasms become more severe. The ability to swallow is affected, and the jaw can become locked into a closed position. Ventilation may be affected to the extent that respiratory muscles become involved; whereas hyperactivity of the sympathetic nervous system can cause blood pressure elevations and cardiac arrhythmias.

Fortunately, the incidence of tetanus is reduced considerably by the availability of an effective antitoxin vaccine. Although a full immunization program can provide protection for 12 to 20 years, more immediately acting passive immunity is available to those individuals who have not been adequately protected previously.

Polio   Like tetanus, polio is now relatively infrequent, thanks to the discovery of a highly effective immunization vaccine in the 1950's. Polio is caused by a virus that normally enters the body through the gastrointestinal tract, and the most serious forms are characterized by paralysis resulting from disruption of the somatic motor and autonomic neurons of the spinal cord and brain stem.

Most frequently, the polio virus attacks the anterior horns of the gray matter in the cord, causing redness, swelling, and congestion. Flaccid paralysis of the lower trunk and lower extremities results, with loss of stretch reflex response but with only minimal sensory deficit.

At times, the cranial nerves and lower brain centers become involved in a variant of polio specifically referred to as bulbar poliomyelitis. In these cases, cranial nerve pathology may result in some combination of facial paralysis, paralysis of the jaw, or paralysis of swallowing. Disruption of the autonomic nervous system, on the other hand, often causes severe hypertension, respiratory failure, and cardiac arrhythmias.

Syphilis   Syphilis is a venereal disease caused by a corkscrew-shaped bacterium called *Trepenoma pallidum*. Syphilis is transmitted, in most cases, by sexual contact and normally evolves in three stages:

1. *The primary stage* is characterized by the appearance of ulcerated skin lesions called chancres. Usually noted at the site of bacterial invasion, these sores typically appear approximately five to eight days after initial exposure.

2. *The secondary stage* usually evolves about two to four weeks after the primary stage. A characteristic syphilitic rash is frequently accompanied by symptoms of fever, malaise, headache, and sore throat.

3. *The tertiary stage* develops in only 30 per cent of syphilitic patients. Following a spontaneous clearing of the secondary stage, a long asymptomatic latent period can terminate in tertiary syphilis, which is characterized by cardiovascular and neural involvement. Damage occurring during this stage is frequently critical and irreversible.

The symptoms accompanying neurosyphilis typically result from two major types of pathological changes. In the first type, inflammation and thickening of the meninges with progressive degeneration of the cerebral cortex are frequently noted from 10 to 20 years after the initial onset of infection. Associated symptoms include irritability, tiredness, confusion, depression, and possibly seizures or paralysis. The second type involves degeneration of the posterior columns and roots of the spinal cord, which is specifically referred to as *tabes dorsalis*. Charasterstically developing 20 to 30 years after initial exposure, it is typically associated with loss of peripheral reflexes and sharp visceral pain.

DEGENERATIVE   DISORDERS   Although infection can be a cause of degenerative changes, neural degeneration will also occur for other reasons. In cases of *multiple sclerosis*, for example, characteristic demyelinization of neurons in the spinal cord and brain is believed to be due to a hypersensitivity reaction to specific viruses.

Multiple sclerosis most commonly affects young adults in the 20- to 45-year-old age group and is associated with lesions in the pyramidal tracts and posterior columns of the spinal cord, around the ventricles of the brain, and in the area of the optic nerves, pons,

TABLE 13.11 **Physical Findings in Multiple Sclerosis***

Visual
  Temporal pallor of the discs
  Abnormal fields of vision
  Abnormal ocular motor function (strabismus)
  Nystagmus
Motor findings
  Motor weakness or paralysis of extremities
  Scanning speech
  Ataxia
  Muscular atrophy in late stages
  Manual dysmetria
Sensory alterations
  Decreased perception to pain, touch, temperature
  Decrease or absence of positional sense
  Decrease or absence of vibration sense
Lhermitte's sign (an "electric sensation" or "shock" down the back following passive flexion of the neck)
Reflex findings
  Exaggerated tendon reflexes
  Absent or diminished abdominal skin reflexes
  Absent or diminished cremasteric reflexes
  Babinski's sign
  Hoffmann's sign
Charcot's triad (nystagmus, intention tremor, scanning speech)
Possible mental changes
  Early
    Apathy
    Euphoria
    Inattentiveness
  Late
    Depression
    Confusion
    Disorientation
    Memory defect

*From Clinical Highlights: Physical findings in multiple sclerosis. Hosp. Med. *13*:108, Sept., 1977.

medulla, and cerebellum. Specific symptoms vary with the location and extent of neural involvement and are summarized in Table 13.11.

MANIFESTATIONS OF SPINAL CORD PATHOLOGY

To understand the manifestations of spinal cord pathology, it is necessary to comprehend the intricate neural pathways and interconnections existing within the cord.

Ultimately, spinal cord dysfunction will result in some combination of sensory, motor, or reflex deficit. Since symptoms specifically reflect the function and location of involved neurons, it is particularly important to be aware of the type of cells that are affected.

When afferent nerve roots or neurons in the ascending tracts of the cord are involved, one could predictably expect some degree of sensory deficit. The areas affected would, of course, vary with the site of injury, as indicated in Figure 13.46B.

Interference with the transmission of efferent impulses through the cord is a more complicated phenomenon. Since the mediation of motor responses is considerably influenced by centers in the brain, symptoms often reflect the effect of pathological changes upon brain–cord linkages.

Under normal circumstances, impulses that affect the tone and contractility of skeletal muscle travel from the brain through descending tracts in the spinal cord via nerve cells referred to as upper motor neurons (UMN's). Information is subsequently conveyed to lower motor neurons (LMN's), which exit from the gray matter of the cord through peripheral spinal nerves and ultimately trigger muscular response. This conduction pathway is illustrated diagrammatically in Figure 13.25.

To the extent that LMN's become dysfunctional, it can be seen that paralysis would inevitably result. If spinal nerves are unable to transmit messages between the central nervous system and the periphery, neither voluntary nor reflex reactions can be mediated. As a result, skeletal muscle becomes flaccid and nonresponsive, atrophying from lack of neural stimulation.

Whereas LMN's are most directly functional in triggering effector responses, UMN's will often affect or modify the neural message that emerges from the spinal cord. Muscular contraction is facilitated by UMN impulses that originate in special centers of the brain's reticular activating system and travel through the cord in descending *pyramidal* (or *corticospinal*) tracts. Inhibition, on the other hand, is frequently mediated by impulses descending through *extrapyramidal* tracts from the basal ganglia and bulboreticular system of the lower brain stem.

In most cases, UMN lesions ultimately cause heightened muscular tone, spasticity, and hyperreflexia. Since pathological changes frequently originate in the extrapyramidal tracts or inhibitory centers of the brain, impulses that normally suppress muscular con-

---

TABLE 13.12 **Clinical Syndromes of Upper Motor Neuron (UMN) and Lower Motor Neuron (LMN) Lesions***

Motor Component	UMN Characteristics	LMN Characteristics
Reflex	Hyperreflexia, extensor toe sign (Babinski's sign)	Hyporeflexia or areflexia
Muscle tonus	Hypertonia, clasp-knife spasticity, clonus	Hypotonia, flaccidity
Muscle movement	Paralysis or paresis of movements in hemiplegic distribution, etc.	Paralysis or paresis of individual muscles in peripheral nerve distribution
Muscle wasting	Late atrophy from disuse	Early atrophy of denervation
Muscle fasciculations	Not present	Present

*From Phipps, W. J., Long, B. C., and Woods, N. F. (eds.): Medical-Surgical Nursing: Concepts and Clinical Practice. St. Louis, The C. V. Mosby Company, 1979, p. 678.

tractility are disrupted. Even when causative lesions are focused in the facilitative corticospinal tracts, there is usually some associated loss of inhibitory messages. Under these circumstances, hyperexcitability will prevail as long as only a few stimulatory conduction pathways remain intact.

In considering the effects of neural pathology, it is important to remember that many systemic responses are, in fact, coordinated, regulated, and initiated by the spinal cord. Primary among these are the mechanisms responsible for urination and defecation.

It has been determined that both urination and defecation are normally controlled by neurons emerging from the S2–S4 segments of the spinal cord. As long as the spinal cord remains intact and functional, elimination occurs appropriately and can be voluntarily regulated. Even if a lesion evolves above the

TABLE 13.13 **Spinal Cord Pathology**

Type of Pathology	Location	Clinical Manifestations
Herniated disc	Cervical	Stiff neck; shoulder pain radiating down into the hand; sensory disturbances of the hand
	Lumbar	Low back pain radiating down the posterior thigh; pain aggrevated by coughing, defecation, bending, and lifting
Tumors	Foramen magnum	Suboccipital pain, with sensory and motor weakness in the occipital region and neck; possible cerebellar dysfunction; compression of associated cranial nerves
	Cervical	Motor and sensory signs in the shoulders, arms, and hands; weakness and atrophy in the shoulder girdle and arms; lower tumors (C5–C7) may cause loss of tendon reflexes in the biceps, triceps, and brachioradialis muscles
	Thoracic	Tight feeling across chest and abdomen; spastic weakness of lower extremities; possible loss of lower abdominal reflexes in lower lesions
	Lumbosacral	Upper compression causes weakness of hip flexion and spasticity in the lower legs, loss of knee jerk reflex, and a bilateral positive Babinski's sign. Lower compression leads to weakness and atrophy of the perineum, calf, and foot; loss of perineal sensation; and impaired elimination from the bowel and bladder
Traumatic injury	above C4 / C5	Loss of all skeletal muscle function / Loss of skeletal muscle activity in the arms, chest; and below chest
	C6–C7	Loss of some skeletal muscle function in the arms, fingers, and chest; total lack of muscular activity below the chest
	Thoracic	Function remaining in the neck and arms; loss of some muscular activity in the chest; loss of all function below the chest
	Lumbosacral	Loss of muscular function in the legs; S2–S4 lesion leads to flaccid bladder and external anal sphincter muscles with associated retention of urine and feces

S2–S4 level, reflex elimination of wastes through the urethra and anus is still possible. In these cases (specifically described as an UMN bladder or bowel), exit of urine or feces is frequently triggered by a variety of inappropriate stimuli. Leg spasticity, sensory stimulation of the perineum or thigh, and defecation, will thus often initiate micturition under these circumstances.

In the event that a spinal lesion develops within segments S2–S4 of the cord, the reflex pathway itself becomes functionally disrupted. In these cases, peripheral motor nerves are no longer able to trigger sphincter relaxation, and elimination becomes difficult, if not impossible. This condition, described as a LMN bladder or bowel, is characterized by urinary and fecal retention.

In assessing the manifestation of spinal cord pathology, an understanding of the distinction between UMN and LMN lesions is obviously invaluable. As summarized in tabular form in Table 13.12, the information provides a conceptual framework within which to better evaluate dysfunction of diverse origin.

Regardless of the type of neural dysfunction generated, specific symptoms can also reflect the location and nature of injury or damage. When pathological changes evolve in particular areas of the cord, the clinical picture often closely mirrors both the origin and site of the causative lesion. Whereas herniation of a cervical disc characteristically results in a stiff neck and shoulder pain, lumbosacral tumors commonly cause weak hip flexion and spasticity in the lower legs. A summary of some major disorders and their clinical manifestations is presented in Table 13.13.

NEURAL PATHOLOGY: DISRUPTION OF CELLULAR NEEDS

Because the nervous system plays such a significant role in regulating and integrating organic response, neural pathology will frequently trigger multisystemic dysfunction. When functional activity of the nervous system is disrupted, a wide variety of peripheral disorders can result. To the extent that the cardiovascular, respiratory, renal or gastrointestinal system is affected, cellular needs will inevitably be compromised. Some major ways in which neural pathology can lead to cellular disequilibrium are summarized in Table 13.14.

TABLE 13.14   **Disruption of Homeostasis Associated with Neural Pathology**

Cellular Need Being Disrupted	Underlying Pathophysiological Mechanism	Causative Clinical Disorders
Oxygen	Compression of the midbrain $\longrightarrow$ hypoventilation $\longrightarrow$ possible $\downarrow$ pO_2	Intracerebral hematoma Subdural or epidural hematoma Cerebral tumor
	Transection of the cervical spinal cord $\longrightarrow$ loss of respiratory muscle function $\longrightarrow$ disrupted ventilation	Traumatic injury
Nutrients	Compression of the midbrain $\longrightarrow$ anorexia, nausea, and vomiting	Subdural or epidural hematoma Cerebral tumor Intracerebral hematoma
	CVA $\longrightarrow$ skeletal muscular weakness $\longrightarrow$ possible disruption of ingestion/swallowing	Cerebral ischemia
Elimination	Lesion of the spinal cord at S2–S4 level $\longrightarrow$ flaccidity of the bladder and external anal sphincter $\longrightarrow$ retention of urine and feces	Traumatic injury
Fluid/electrolyte and acid/base balance	Compression of the midbrain $\longrightarrow$ hypoventilation $\longrightarrow$ respiratory acidosis	Subdural or epidural hematoma Intracerebral hematoma Cerebral tumor
	Compression of the midbrain $\longrightarrow$ nausea and vomiting $\longrightarrow$ possible hypovolemia and metabolic alkalosis	

STUDY QUESTIONS

1. Define or describe the following terms:
   a. Dermatome
   b. Neuroglia
   c. Falx cerebri
   d. Reticular formation
   e. Synapse
   f. Ganglia
   g. Brain stem
   h. Decussation
   i. Myelin
   j. Meninges
   k. Hypothalamus
   l. Neurotransmitter
   m. Ascending spinal tracts
   n. Sympathetic nerves
   o. Plexus
   p. Visceral efferent nerves
   q. Ventricles of the brain
   r. Vagus nerve

2. Fainting is often caused by a sudden decrease in cerebral circulation. What mechanism normally functions to guard against the development of cerebral ischemia?

3. Mr. Vox is being evaluated for suspected cerebrovascular occlusion. Angiography (introduction of visible contrast dye into the cerebral blood vessels) is performed. If obstruction is noted in any of the following arteries, identify the area of the cerebrum that would predictably be deprived of oxygen and nutrients:
   a. Basilar artery
   b. Anterior cerebral artery
   c. Middle cerebral artery
   d. Posterior cerebral artery

4. A medical history can often be quite helpful in determining the nature of an existing cerebrovascular occlusion. In each of the following cases, predict whether obstruction is most likely to have been caused by (1) a thrombus, or (2) an embolus:
   a. A 57-year-old male with endocarditis
   b. A 45-year-old male with diabetes mellitus of early onset
   c. A 62-year-old female with sinus bradycardia and polycythemia
   d. A 48-year-old female with a history of angina and coronary insufficiency

5. Briefly describe how and why each of the following conditions could deprive cerebral cells of oxygen and/or nutrients:
   a. Vasogenic shock
   b. Rheumatic fever
   c. Anemia
   d. Congestive heart failure (CHF)
   e. Diabetes mellitus
   f. Myasthenia gravis
   g. Hypertension

6. A patient is admitted for observation and testing after having experienced two TIA episodes within three successive days. He is afraid he has had a stroke. Explain to him the difference between his disorder and a full-blown CVA.

7. Mrs. Saffer suffered a stroke several weeks ago and is now showing evidence of muscular rigidity on the affected side. The family wonders why there is an increase of tone in her originally flaccid limb. Explain the symptom to them.

8. Why will ischemia on the right side of the brain typically cause disruption of motor response on the left side of the body?

9. Billy Taylor fell from a tree while he was playing in his backyard. He lost consciousness briefly and complained of dizziness and severe headache upon arousal. A medical examination revealed no skull fracture and normal reflex responses. Why did the physician suggest that he be kept relatively quiet for 24 hours and watched for any indication of drowziness, disorientation, or lethargy?

10. Mr. Spaulding is admitted to the hospital for observation and evelution. His wife states that he has been complaining of severe headache for the past week and has become progressively more drowsy and disoriented. Nausea and vomiting began 24 hours before admission. Initial examination revealed hypoventilation, elevated blood pressure, respiratory acidosis, and fixed, dilated pupils. List two possible causes for these findings and briefly describe the development of dysfunction in each case.

11. A "slipped disc" is a frequent cause of lower back pain in the United States. What exactly is a "slipped disc" and how does it trigger so much pain and suffering?

12. Standard childhood immunization provides protection against tetanus. Briefly describe the cause and development of this infectious disorder.

13. Explain how or why each of the following disorders might cause alterations in the structure and/or function of the spinal cord:
    a. Multiple sclerosis
    b. Syphilis
    c. Spinal cord trauma secondary to a sports accident

14. Explain the predictable effects of a lesion in the extrapyramidal tracts of the spinal cord.

15. The existence of an intramedullary tumor in the L4–S4 segments of the spinal cord is confirmed. What effect would this neoplasm have upon urination and defecation?

16. What effect would severe compression and trauma of the upper lumbar cord have upon urination?

17. For each of the following specified sets of clinical symptoms, identify the area of the spinal cord where the causative lesion would most likely originate:
    a. Pain in the lower back, radiating down the posterior thigh
    b. Tight feeling across the chest and abdomen; spastic weakness of the lower extremities
    c. Loss of skeletal muscle activity in the arms, chest, and below the chest
    d. Fecal and urinary retention

Suggested Readings

Books

Aguayo, A. J.: Mechanical lesions of the nerve roots and spinal cord. *In* Beeson, P. B., McDermott, W., and Wyngaarden, J. B. (eds.): Cecil Textbook of Medicine, 15th ed. Philadelphia, W. B. Saunders Company, 1979, p. 889.

Anderson, W. A. D., and Scotti, T. M.: Synopsis of Pathology, 10th ed. St. Louis, The C. V. Mosby Company, 1980, pp. 730–763.

Barr, M. L.: The Human Nervous System, 2nd ed. Hagerstown, Md., Harper & Row Publishers, 1974.

Berry, M. A.: Normal structure and function of the nervous system. *In* Hudak, C. M., Lohr, T., and Gallo, B. M. (eds.): Critical Care Nursing, 2nd ed. Philadelphia, J. B. Lippincott Company, 1977, p. 387.

Crowley, W. J.: Neural control of skeletal muscle. *In* Frohlich, E. D. (ed.): Pathophysiology, Altered Regulatory Mechanisms in Disease, 2nd ed. Philadelphia, J. B. Lippincott Company, 1976, p. 735.

Dunbar, C. F., and Mahoney, P. E.: The concepts of perception and coordination. *In* Jones, D. A., Dunbar, C. F., and Jirovec, M. M. (eds.): Medical-Surgical Nursing: A Conceptual Approach. New York, McGraw-Hill Book Company, 1978, p. 1065.

Escourolle, R., and Poirier, J.: Manual of Basic Neurology. Philadelphia, W. B. Saunders Company, 1973.

Fishman, R. A.: Intracranial tumors and states causing increased intracranial pressure. *In* Beeson, P. B., McDermott, W., and Wyngaarden, J. B. (eds.): Cecil Textbook of Medicine, 15th ed. Philadelphia, W. B. Saunders Company, 1979, p. 863.

Freeman, A. R.: The central nervous system. In Selkurt, E. E. (ed.): Basic Physiology for the Health Sciences. Boston, Little, Brown and Company, 1975, p. 89.

Freeman, A. R.: Physiology of intercellular communication, neuronal interaction, and the reflex. In Selkurt, E. E. (ed.): Basic Physiology for the Health Sciences. Boston, Little, Brown and Company, 1975, p. 55.

Guttman, L.: Spinal Cord Injuries. Philadelphia, J. B. Lippincott Company, 1973.

Guyton, A. C.: Textbook of Medical Physiology, 5th ed. Philadelphia, W. B. Saunders Company, 1976, pp. 608–625; 649–661; 678–780.

Hass, W. K.: Acute ischemic cerebrovascular disease. *In* Conn, H. F. (ed.): Current Therapy 1978. Philadelphia, W. B. Saunders Company, 1978.

Hendee, R. M., McCracken, M. L., and Washburn, M. J.: Pathophysiology of the central nervous system. In Hudak, C. M., Lohr, T., and Gallo, B. M. (eds.): Critical Care Nursing, 2nd ed. Philadelphia, J. B. Lippincott Company, 1977, p. 397.

Hinkhouse, A. E., and Kirby, N. A.: Traumatic disturbances in perception and coordination. *In* Jones, D. A., Dunbar, C. F., and Jirovec, M. M. (eds.): Medical-Surgical Nursing: A Conceptual Approach. New York, McGraw-Hill Book Company, 1978, p. 1116.

Hoff, J. T.: Intracerebral hemorrhage. *In* Conn. H. F. (ed.): Current Therapy 1978. Philadelphia, W. B. Saunders Company, 1978.

Hole, J. W.: Human Anatomy and Physiology. Dubuque, Miss., Wm. C. Brown Company Publishers, 1978, pp. 262–312.

Hunt, W. E., and Goodman, J. E.: Acute head injuries. *In* Conn, H. F. (ed): Current Therapy 1978, Philadelphia, W. B. Saunders Company, 1978.

Judy, W. V., and Freeman, A. R.: The autonomic nervous system. *In* Selkurt, E. E. (ed.): Basic Physiology for the Health Sciences. Boston, Little, Brown and Company, 1975, p. 115.

Kent, T. H., Hart, M. N., and Shires, T. K.: Introduction to Human Disease. New York, Appleton-Century-Crofts, 1979, pp. 293–311.

Kinney, M.: Management of the person with common neurologic manifestations. *In* Phipps, W. J., Long, B. C., and Woods, N. F. (eds.): Medical-Surgical Nursing: Concepts and Clinical Practice. St. Louis, The C. V. Mosby Company, 1979, p. 656.

Kinney, M.: Neurologic assessment. *In* Phipps, W. J., Long B. C., and Woods, N. F. (eds.): Medical-Surgical Nursing: Concepts and Clinical Practice. St. Louis, The C. V. Mosby Company, 1979, p. 626.

Kinney, M.: Problems of the nervous system. *In* Phipps, W. J., Long, B. C., and Woods, N. F. (eds.): Medical-Surgical Nursing: Concepts and Clinical Practice. St. Louis, The C. V. Mosby Company, 1979, p. 695.

Kraut, R.: Inflammatory disturbances in perception and coordination. *In* Jones, D. A., Dunbar, C. F., and Jirovec, M. M. (eds.): Medical-Surgical Nursing: A Conceptual Approach. New York, McGraw-Hill Book Company, 1978, p. 1218.

Luckmann, J., and Sorensen, K. C.: Medical-Surgical Nursing: A Pathophysiologic Approach, 2nd ed. Philadelphia, W. B. Saunders Company, 1980, pp. 485–681.

McDowell, F. H.: Cerebrovascular diseases. *In* Beeson, P. B., McDermott, W., and Wyngaarden, J. B. (eds.): Cecil Textbook of Medicine, 15th ed. Philadelphia, W. B. Saunders Company, 1979, p. 777.

Meyers, E. A.: Microorganisms and Human Disease. New York, Appleton-Century-Crofts, 1974, pp. 107–110; 141–142; 180–184; 256–261.

Mumenthaler, M.: Neurology Yearbook. Chicago, Yearbook Medical Publishers, Inc., 1977.

Patterson, R. H., Jr.: Injuries of the head and spine. *In* Beeson, P. B., McDermott, W., and Wyngaarden, J. B. (eds.): Cecil Textbook of Medicine, 15th ed. Philadelphia, W. B. Saunders Company, 1979, p. 879.

Purtillo, D. T.: A Survey of Human Diseases. Menlo Park, Cal., Addison-Wesley Publishing Company, 1978, pp. 415–442.

Schoene, W. C.: The nervous system. *In* Robbins, S. L., and Cotran, R. S. (eds.): Pathologic Basis of Disease, 2nd ed. Philadelphia, W. B. Saunders Company, 1979, p. 1530.

Sexton, D. L.: Vascular disturbances in perception. *In* Jones, D. A., Dunbar, C. F., and Jirovec, M. M. (eds.): Medical-Surgical Nursing: A Conceptual Approach. New York, McGraw-Hill Book Company, 1978, p. 1173.

Tortora, G. H., and Anagnostakos, N. P.: Principles of Anatomy and Physiology, 2nd ed. San Francisco, Canfield Press, 1978, pp. 268–364.

Walter, J. B.: An Introduction to the Principles of Disease. Philadelphia, W. B. Saunders Company, 1977, pp. 685–699.

Williams, P. L., and Warwick. R.: Functional Neuroanatomy of Man. Philadelphia, W. B. Saunders Company, 1975.

Articles

Axelrod, J.: Neurotransmitters. Sci. Am., *230*:59, 1974.

Brooks, V. B., and Stoney, S. D., Jr.: Motor mechanisms: the role of the pyramidal system in motor control. Ann. Rev. Physiol., *33*:337, 1971.

Burch, G. E., and De Pasquale, N. P.: Axioms on cerebrovascular disease. Hosp. Med., *11*:8, 1975.

Dohrmann, G. J., and Wick, K. M.: Research in experimental cord trauma: past and present, a brief review. J. Neurol. Nurs., *4*:115, 1972.

Easton, T. A.: On the normal use of reflexes. Am. Sci., *60*:591, 1972.

Evarts, E. V.: Brain mechanisms in movement. Sci. Am., *229*:96, 1973.

Fishman, R. A.: Brain edema. New Engl. J. Med., *293*:706, 1975.

Haas, W. K.: Occlusive cerebrovascular disease. Med. Clin. North Am., *56*:1281, 1972.

Hinkhouse, A.: Craniocerebral trauma. Am. J. Nurs., *73*:1719, 1973.

Jacobansky, A. M.: Stroke. Am. J. Nurs., *72*:1260, 1972.

Javid, M.: Current concepts: Head injuries. New Eng. J. Med., *291*:890, 1974.

Jimm, L. R.: Nursing assessment of patients for increased intracranial pressure. Nurs. Digest, *3*:5, 1976.

Katzman, R., et al; Brain edema in stroke. Stroke, *8*:512, 1977.

Keller, M. R., and Truscott, B. L.: Transient ischemic attacks. Am. J. Nurs., *73*:1331, 1973.

Krasney, J. A., and Koehler, R. C.: Heart rate and
rhythm and intracranial pressure. Am. J. Physiol., *230*:1695, 1976.

Kuller, L. H.: The transient ischemic attack. Cur.
Concepts Cerebrovasc. Dis. — Stroke, *9*:23,
1974.

Kunkel, J., and Wiley, J. K.: Acute head injury;
What to do when . . . and why. Nursing 79,
9:23, March 1979.

Lowry, T.: What happens in spinal cord injury.
Nursing 78, *8*:74, Oct. 1978.

Mack, E. W., and Dawson, W. N., Jr.: Injury to the
spine and spinal cord. Hosp. Med., *12*:23, July
1976.

Maddox, M.: Subarachnoid hemorrhage. Am. J.
Nurs., *74*:2199, 1974.

Mancall, E.: The stroke: a review of current diagnostic and therapeutic considerations. Hosp.
Med., *11*:8, 1975.

McLaurin, R.: Answers to questions on head injuries. Hosp. Med., *5*:54, 1969.

Merton, P. A.: How we control the contraction of
our muscles. Sci. Am., *60*:591, 1972.

Michael, J. A.: Physiology of the nervous system:
from the molecular to the behavioral. Nursing
Dig., *4*:20, 1976.

Mitchell, P. H., and Mauss, N.: Intracranial pressure: fact and fancy. Nursing 76, *6*:53, June
1976.

Rudy, E.: Early omens of cerebral disaster. Nursing 77, *7*:58, Feb. 1977.

Tindall, G. T., and Fleisher, A. S.: Head injury.
Hosp. Med., *12*:89, May 1976.

Whisnant, J. P.: Epidemiology of stroke. Emphasis on transient cerebral ischemic attacks and
hypertension. Stroke, *5*:68, Jan–Feb. 1974.

Wiebe, R. A.: Bacterial meningitis. Hosp. Med.,
12:66, July 1976.

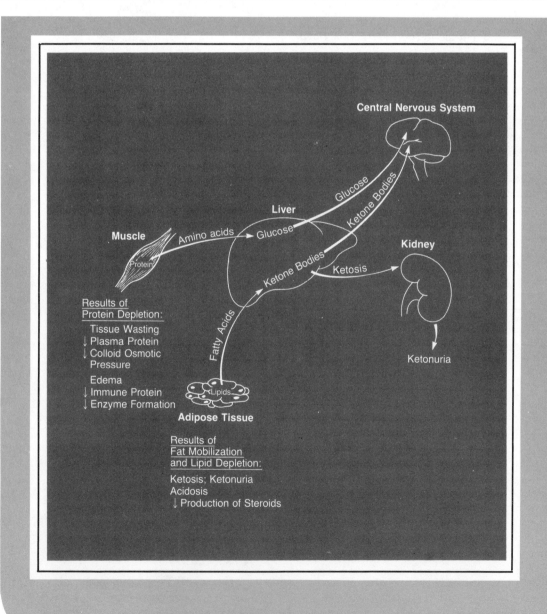

Pathology and Cellular Needs

Throughout this text, it has been shown that pathophysiology is characterized by the disruption of homeostasis. Thus far, emphasis has been placed upon systemic dysfunction and associated cellular disequilibrium. Of particular conceptual significance is the way in which a specific disorder may interfere with more than one cellular survival need. In cases of COPD, for example, cellular oxygen supply, nutrient utilization, carbon dioxide elimination, and fluid and electrolyte balance will all be compromised.

In order to fully understand pathophysiology, it is important to realize that any given cellular need may be disrupted by dysfunction within many different systems. Oxygen supply, for example, can be reduced by disorders of respiratory, cardiovascular, neural, and hematopoietic origin.

It is the purpose of Unit 4 to deal with pathophysiology from a nonsystemic conceptual perspective. Whereas diseases were previously classified as cardiovascular, respiratory, renal, gastrointestinal, or neural, they will be categorized in the following pages according to the cellular need they disrupt. In this way, it can be shown how disorders of diverse origin can often cause the onset of similar clinical symptoms.

Although the approach utilized in this Unit might seem to be somewhat redundant, experience has indicated that this type of reinforcement considerably enhances comprehension. Since most students find it particularly difficult to organize and correlate new information, they often avoid the challenge of conceptual integration. As a result, a very important aspect of the learning process is sacrificed, and comprehension is inevitably diluted.

In Chapters 14 through 17, diseases that have been previously elucidated are examined within the unifying framework of a cellular needs model. Owing to the integrative nature of this unit, a minimal amount of new material is introduced. Because it is assumed that the reader is thoroughly familiar with the information presented earlier in the text, charts and diagrams are used extensively to clarify and summarize major concepts.

Chapter Outline

chapter 14

Diseases Affecting The Cellular Need for Oxygen

Chapter Objectives

At the completion of this chapter, the student will be able to:

1. Identify and define the three major mechanisms responsible for maintaining cellular oxygen supply.
2. Differentiate between disruption of inspiration and disruption of diffusion, with respect to underlying pathological mechanisms and causative disorders.
3. Trace the evolution of a red blood cell from an undifferentiated stem cell and describe the significance of vitamin B_{12}, folic acid, iron, and erythropoietin in erythrocyte production.
4. Describe the clinical significance of the oxyhemoglobin dissociation curve.
5. Identify five laboratory measures commonly employed to evaluate the status of the red blood cell in the body.
6. Differentiate between anemias caused by blood loss, excessive hemolysis, and disruption in erythrocyte production, with respect to cause, development, and characteristic features.
7. Tell why cardiovascular disorders might disrupt cellular oxygen supply and identify eight causative disorders.
8. List and describe the clinical manifestations of cellular hypoxia.

INTRODUCTION

In order for cells to survive, oxygen must be continuously available to support the metabolic machinery. Three major functional processes are generally responsible for maintaining cellular oxygen supply:

1. *Inspiration* — or the passage of air from the environment, through the respiratory tract, into the alveoli.

2. *Diffusion* — or the transport of oxygen from the alveoli into the pulmonary capillaries.

3. *Transport* — or the circulation of oxygen from the alveoli, through the bloodstream, to the cells.

If inspiration, diffusion, or transport is disrupted, tissue hypoxia will frequently result. In the following pages, an elucidation of disorders that characteristically decrease cellular oxygen supply is followed by a clarification of associated clinical manifestations.

DISORDERS THAT DISRUPT INSPIRATION

In order to effectively inspire air, the ribs and diaphragm must work together to increase the volume of the thoracic cavity. As illustrated in Figure 14.1, pulmonary expansion causes a decrease in intrapulmonic pressure, and gases subsequently move from where they are under greater pressure (in the atmosphere) to where they are under lesser pressure (in the lungs). The intake of air is most commonly disrupted by two types of disorders: (1) those disorders that interfere with the rate or rhythm of ventilation, and (2) those disorders that increase the work of ventilation.

Although pathological conditions associated with inspiratory dysfunction have been discussed in considerable detail in Chapter 10, an overview of primary causative disorders is presented in Table 14.1. Studying of this chart reveals that diseases originating in a variety of systems can theoretically disrupt the intake of air.

DISORDERS THAT DISRUPT DIFFUSION

Diffusion generally refers to the exchange of gases that occurs between pulmonary capillaries and the alveoli of the lungs. Although both oxygen and carbon dioxide are involved in the diffusion process, emphasis in this chapter is focused upon disorders that decrease plasma oxygen levels. Related or associated alterations in carbon dioxide diffusion will be discussed in Chapter 16.

As outlined in Chapter 10, diffusion of respiratory gases can be disrupted in a number of ways. Most commonly, dysfunction is associated with one of four major phenomena: (1) disorders of alveolar ventilation, (2) disorders of alveolar perfusion, (3) ventilation-perfusion imbalances, or (4) diseases affecting the "respiratory membrane."

In Table 14.2, primary causative disorders are summarized, with specific emphasis upon the multisystemic nature of the pathological conditions.

DISORDERS THAT DISRUPT OXYGEN TRANSPORT

Once oxygen has been delivered into the bloodstream, its circulation throughout the

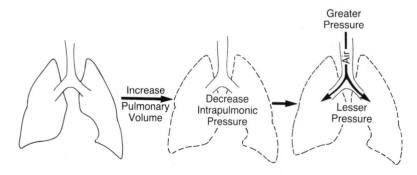

Figure 14.1 Inspiration. Note that when atmospheric pressure is greater than intrapulmonic pressure, air will enter the lungs.

TABLE 14.1 **Disorders That Disrupt Inspiration**

Pathological Mechanism	Causative Disorders	System of Origin
ALTERATION OF THE RATE OR RHYTHM OF VENTILATION		
Increased intracranial pressure affecting the respiratory center of the brain	Cerebral contusion Subdural or epidural hematoma Cerebrovascular occlusion or hemorrhage, if accompanied by edema Brain tumors Meningitis Encephalitis Overdose of anesthetics or narcotics	Nervous system
Interference with the neural stimulation of respiratory muscles	Poliomyelitis Guillain-Barré syndrome Myasthenia gravis Tetanus Botulism	Nervous system
INCREASES IN THE WORK OF VENTILATION		
Decreased compliance of the lungs or thorax	Scoliosis Kyphosis Extensive rib fractures Abdominal pain or distention	Skeletal system Digestive system
Increased gas or fluid pressure within the thoracic cavity	Left heart failure Inflammation or malignancy of the pleura	Cardiovascular system Respiratory system
Pulmonary fibrosis	COPD Pneumoconioses Pneumonia Tuberculosis	Respiratory system
Resistance to the transport of air through the respiratory tree	COPD Cystic fibrosis Bronchiectasis Lung cancer	Respiratory system

TABLE 14.2 **Some Primary Disorders That Disrupt Diffusion**

Pathological Mechanism	Causative Disorders	System of Origin
Disruption of alveolar ventilation	Alveolar ventilation may ultimately be disrupted by all disorders that interfere with inspiration. The reader is referred to Table 14.1 for a summary of diseases associated with ventilation disorders.	
Interference with the circulation of blood through the pulmonary vessels	Pulmonary emboli or thrombi Right-left shunt	Cardiovascular system
Ventilation-perfusion imbalances	Any isolated decrease in ventilation or perfusion could lead to ventilation-perfusion imbalances. Dysfunctions of this type are thus frequently associated with disruption of alveolar ventilation or depression of pulmonary circulation.	
Disease of the respiratory membrane Altered structure	Bronchiectasis COPD Pneumonia Tuberculosis Pneumoconioses	Respiratory system
Altered function, associated primarily with pulmonary edema	Left heart failure Inhalation of respiratory irritants } Pleural inflammation	Cardiovascular system Respiratory system

body depends upon the existence of: (1) an erythrocyte population of adequate quantity and quality, and (2) a functional cardiovascular system. If either of these factors is disrupted, some degree of tissue hypoxia will result.

Alterations in the Quantity or Quality of Erythrocytes

In order for oxygen to be effectively transported to metabolizing cells, a sufficient quantity of hemoglobin must be present in whole blood. Although approximately 1 per cent of available oxygen may be carried through plasma in simple solution, this amount is not nearly enough to support cellular health. The majority of oxygen is transported in chemical combination with hemoglobin, as follows: $Hb + O_2 \rightleftharpoons HbO_2$. The reversibility of this reaction allows for dissociation of oxyhemoglobin at the cellular level and ultimate release of free oxygen to service cellular needs.

Since hemoglobin is found packaged within red blood cells, any alteration in the quantity or structure of erythrocytes can significantly affect cellular oxygenation. In subsequent pages, a brief review of the factors affecting red blood cell production and function is followed by an explanation of the mechanism causing erythrocyte deficiency.

RED BLOOD CELL PRODUCTION

Red blood cells are normally produced in the bone marrow from undifferentiated stem cells. As illustrated in Figure 14.2, these precursor cells undergo a series of progressive structural alterations and ultimately evolve into mature red blood cells. Between the initial hemocytoblast stage and the terminal erythrocyte, a number of significant changes occur. Hemoglobin synthesis typically begins in the basophil erythroblast and continues until a pigment concentration level of approximately 34 per cent is reached. At this point, described as the normoblast stage, the nucleus is characteristically extruded. Water, hemoglobin, some ions and enzymes, and small amounts of endoplasmic reticulum remain as the primary cytoplasmic constituents. Cells containing reticular fragments are specifically labeled as reticulocytes. They typically evolve

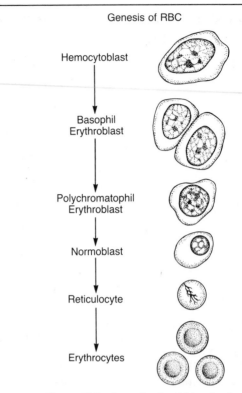

Genesis of RBC

Hemocytoblast

Basophil Erythroblast

Polychromatophil Erythroblast

Normoblast

Reticulocyte

Erythrocytes

Figure 14.2   Genesis of red blood cells.

into mature erythrocytes by losing reticulum and thus constitute a very small percentage of the circulating red blood cell population. When erythrocytes are produced at an extremely rapid rate, however, increasing numbers of immature cells may be released into the bloodstream. Under these circumstances, reticulocytes can account for as much as 30 to 50 per cent of total red cell volume.

A number of factors play a significant role in promoting and supporting the erythrocyte maturation process. As discussed in Chapter 2, they include: (1) vitamin B_{12} and folic acid, (2) iron, and (3) erythropoietin.

VITAMIN B_{12} AND FOLIC ACID   Both vitamin B_{12} and folic acid are needed to facilitate the ongoing production of erythrocytes by the bone marrow. Involved directly in the formation of DNA, these substances are essential to red blood cell maturation. While folic acid can be manufactured by colonic bacteria, it is also found in certain foods, such as green leafy vegetables and liver.

Although Vitamin B_{12} may also be ingested through dietary sources such as liver, kidney, and fresh muscle meat, its utilization is

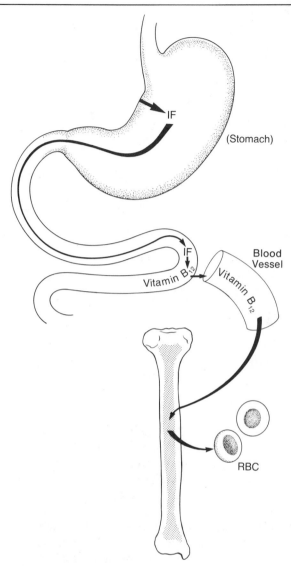

Figure 14.3 The function of intrinsic factor (IF) in promoting red blood cell production. Note that intrinsic factor produced by the gastric mucosa is needed to facilitate absorption of vitamin B_{12}.

ultimately dependent upon the existence of a functional gastric mucosa. As illustrated in Figure 14.3, the intrinsic factor generated by specialized cells lining the stomach is largely responsible for facilitating the absorption of vitamin B_{12} out of the gastrointestinal tract. If vitamin B_{12} is unable to pass into the bloodstream, erythrocyte maturation can be considerably disrupted.

IRON For red blood cells to function adequately in oxygen transport, they must contain sufficient quantities of viable hemo-

globin. Since iron is such a significant functional constituent of hemoglobin, iron deficiency can cause varying degrees of cellular hypoxia.

Normally, the iron required for hemoglobin synthesis is derived from two primary sources: (1) ingestion of foods such as liver, meats, molasses, beans, and leafy vegetables, and (2) recycling of iron from old red blood cells.

Assuming adequate dietary intake, ingested iron is normally absorbed from the small intestine by an active transport mechanism that is responsive to cellular needs. Rate and quantity of absorption vary with the amount of available iron in the body and can increase considerably at times of iron deficiency. Once absorbed, iron is normally carried throughout the bloodstream in loose combination with the globulin *transferrin*. Approximately 60 per cent of any excess iron is stored in liver cells, where it combines with the protein *apoferritin* to form the storage compound *ferritin*.

An alternate source of iron is provided by old red blood cells, which are characteristically broken down by reticuloendothelial tissue within the spleen and liver. The hemoglobin released from fragmented erythrocytes is subsequently split into a heme and a globin fragment, with iron being specifically released from the heme fraction of the molecule. As free iron enters the bloodstream, it is carried by transferrin to one of two major areas:

1. Some iron is transported to the bone marrow, where it is utilized in the production of hemoglobin.

2. Some iron is transported to the liver, where it is stored in the form of ferritin.

Some primary aspects of iron transport and metabolism are summarized diagrammatically in Figure 14.4.

ERYTHROPOIETIN While vitamin B_{12}, folic acid, and iron are needed to ensure normal erythrocyte maturation and hemoglobin generation, erythropoietin serves as an overall stimulant to red blood cell production. Believed to be released by the kidneys in reponse to hypoxia, it acts upon the bone marrow to trigger the manufacture of erythrocytes. Because of the erythropoietin mechanism, the rate of red blood cell production is

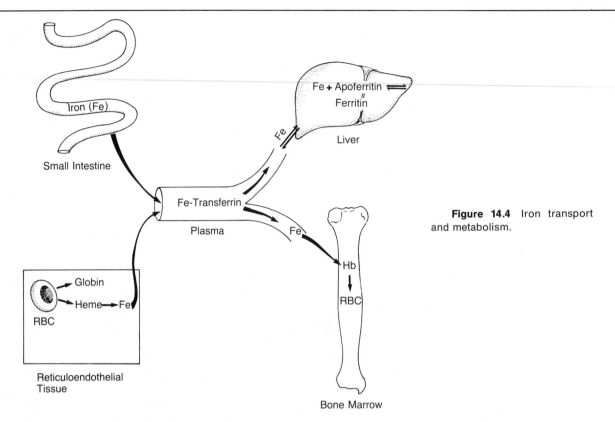

Figure 14.4 Iron transport and metabolism.

generally quite responsive to fluctuating cellular needs. Whereas in the absence of erythropoietin, few red blood cells can be formed, excessive secretion by renal tissue may cause erythrocyte production to increase by a factor of 800 to 1000 per cent.

RED BLOOD CELL FUNCTION

Even with normal production of red blood cells by the bone marrow, adequate cellular oxygenation will not necessarily result. Since the majority of oxygen is carried in chemical combination with hemoglobin ($Hb + O_2 \rightleftarrows HbO_2$), it is necessary to carefully consider those factors that may affect oxygen-hemoglobin affinity. In cases of carbon monoxide poisoning, for example, tissue hypoxia will characteristically develop as carbon monoxide displaces oxygen in the red blood cell. Cellular oxygen deprivation thus results, in spite of the existence of a normal erythrocyte population.

As described in Chapter 10, the combination of oxygen with hemoglobin is a characteristically reversible reaction, which can proceed in either direction depending upon

circumstances. Normally, the formation of bright red oxyhemoglobin increases considerably as pO_2 moves from 0 to 50 mm. Hg. Above 50 mm. Hg, the effect of increasing oxygen tension is relatively less significant. In fact, when pO_2 approaches 80 mm. Hg, additional oxygen will not combine with hemoglobin to any great extent. The relationship between pO_2 and oxyhemoglobin formation is traditionally plotted on an oxyhemoglobin dissociation curve, as illustrated in Figure 14.5

In considering the oxyhemoglobin dissociation curve, it is significant to realize that a number of factors can alter or modify the normal relationship between oxygen and hemoglobin. Primary among these are pH, pCO_2, temperature, and the concentration of the organic phosphate 2,3 diphosphoglycerate (2,3-DPG) within the red blood cell.

Characteristically, the affinity of hemoglobin for oxygen is depressed as pH decreases, pCO_2 increases, temperature increases, or 2,3-DPG increases. As a result, oxyhemoglobin dissociates more readily to release free oxygen for cellular use, and the oxyhemoglobin dissociation curve is shifted

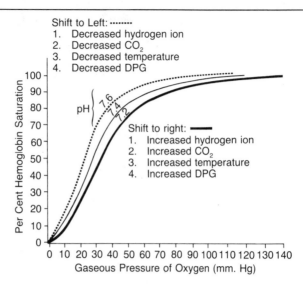

Figure 14.5 The oxyhemoglobin dissociation curve.

to the right. Chemically, this phenomenon can be summarized as follows:

$$Hb + O_2 \xrightleftharpoons[\downarrow pH, \uparrow pCO_2, \uparrow temperature, \uparrow 2,3\text{-}DPG]{} HbO_2.$$

Alternatively, the oxygen-hemoglobin combining capacity is enhanced by pH increases, pCO_2 decreases, temperature decreases, or decreases in the concentration of 2,3-DPG. Under these circumstances, the affinity of hemoglobin for oxygen is increased, but oxyhemoglobin dissociation is depressed. Free oxygen is thus less available for cellular use, and hypoxia may develop. The shift of the oxyhemoglobin dissociation curve to the left can be summarized as follows:

$$Hb + O_2 \xrightleftharpoons[\quad]{\uparrow pH, \downarrow pCO_2, \downarrow temperature, \downarrow 2,3\text{-}DPG} HbO_2.$$

Because of these variables, which modify oxygen transport by the erythrocyte, cellular oxygen supply may be disrupted even when inspiration, diffusion, and RBC production are optimally functional. In considering the evolution of hypoxia, it is therefore necessary to take into account the effects of all factors that may alter the relationship between oxygen and hemoglobin. Some of these variables are summarized in Table 14.3.

ERYTHROCYTE DEFICIENCY

When erythrocytes are deficient in number or concentration of functional hemoglobin, a condition of anemia is said to exist. In order to understand red blood cell abnormalities, it is helpful to have some idea of the measures commonly employed to determine erythrocyte status. In the laboratory, the following factors are frequently evaluated:

1. *Red cell count* — the number of red blood cells in 1 cubic millimeter of blood. Norms range from 4.7 to 6.1 million in the male and from 4.2 to 5.2 million in the female.

2. *Hemoglobin concentration* — the amount of hemoglobin in a given volume of blood, expressed as gm. per cent. Male norms are 13.4 to 17.6; female averages range from 12.0 to 15.4.

3. *Hematocrit* — the percentage of blood that is composed of red blood cells, expressed as volume per cent. Norms are 42 to 53 in the male and 38 to 46 in the female.

4. *Mean corpuscular volume (MCV)* — the volume of a single red blood cell in cubic micrometers. Determined by dividing hematocrit by the red blood cell count, the norms range from 81 to 96.

5. *Mean corpuscular Hb concentration (MCHC)* — the amount of hemoglobin in each red blood cell, expressed as gm. Hb per 100 ml. of erythrocytes. Determined by dividing hemoglobin concentration by hematocrit, the norms are between 30 and 36.

Anemia is frequently characterized by deviations from some of these norms. Often, classification is based on the nature of the red blood cell, with respect to size and color. Whereas healthy cells are described as *normocytic* (normal size) and *normochromic* (normal color), anemic cells are frequently macrocytic (large) or microcytic (small) and hypochromic

TABLE 14.3 **Factors That Affect The Affinity Between Oxygen And Hemoglobin**

When Affinity Between Oxygen And Hb Is	Causative Mechanisms Include	And Are Associated With Disorders Such As
Increased	Increased pH	Hyperventilation Gastric vomiting
	Decreased pCO_2	Hyperventilation
	Decreased temperature	Hypothermia
	Decreased 2,3-DPG	Acidosis Excessive storage of blood Phosphate deficit Inhibition of glycolysis
	Decreased binding of 2,3-DPG to reduced Hb	Excessive concentration of fetal hemoglobin Diabetes mellitus
	Hemoglobin abnormalities	Carbon monoxide poisoning Genetic hemoglobinopathies
Decreased	Decreased pH	Hypoventilation COPD Diarrhea Renal failure
	Increased pCO_2	Hypoventilation COPD
	Increased temperature	Infection Inflammation Burns Heat stroke
	Increased 2,3-DPG	Alkalosis Hypoxemia Anemia
	Hemoglobin abnormalities	Select genetic hemoglobinopathies

(pale). Cells that are structurally immature are termed *megaloblastic*.

Since a specific change in the morphology of erythrocytes can often be induced in a variety of ways, it is also possible to categorize anemias according to underlying causative mechanisms. Because this approach promotes a better understanding of pathogenesis, anemias will be classified in this chapter as follows: (1) anemias caused by blood loss, (2) anemias caused by excessive hemolysis of red blood cells, and (3) anemias caused by disruptions in erythrocyte production.

ANEMIAS CAUSED BY BLOOD LOSS The reaction of the body to blood loss varies with the extent and severity of deple-

tion. In cases of acute hemorrhage, for example, the effects of declining plasma volume are often clinically more significant than the decrease in hemoglobin. Cardiovascular shock may result, as described in Chapter 9. If the patient survives, initial adaptation involves the shift of fluid out of the interstitial compartment back into the vascular tree. Under these circumstances, the erythrocytes remaining in plasma may be considerably diluted, causing a decrease in red cell count, hemoglobin concentration, and hematocrit.

To the extent that blood is lost externally, recovery may be hampered by associated iron deficiency, which interferes with the generation of new red blood cells. In cases of internal bleeding, on the other hand, hemoglobin can

TABLE 14.4   **Acute and Chronic Hemorrhagic Anemia**

	Acute Hemorrhagic Anemia	Chronic Hemorrhagic Anemia
Definition	Anemia that develops secondary to the rapid loss of a large volume of blood	Anemia that develops secondary to slow, chronic blood loss
Causative pathological conditions	Trauma $\longrightarrow$ severing of a blood vessel Aneurysm $\longrightarrow$ rupture of a blood vessel Arterial malignancy or ulceration $\longrightarrow$ hemorrhage	Bleeding peptic ulcers Prolonged or excessive menstrual bleeding Bleeding from hemorrhoids or diverticuli Ulcerative colitis Salicylate poisoning
Evolution	Initial loss of blood $\longrightarrow$ compensatory vasoconstriction Fluid shift into plasma compartment within 24 to 48 hours $\longrightarrow$ hemodilution Regeneration of RBC's begins within 4 to 5 days after hemorrhage has stopped and is usually complete within 4 to 6 weeks.	Long-term depletion of RBC's $\longrightarrow$ iron deficiency anemia

Clinical manifestations	Initial depletion of blood volume $\longrightarrow$ shock symptoms, including
	    dizziness
	    restlessness
	    sweating
	    hypotension
	    rapid, thready pulse
	    headache
	    disorientation
	
	If bleeding is internal, associated manifestations of fever and pain may be evident.
	
	Until recovery is complete, depleted Hb levels may $\longrightarrow$ varying degrees of
	    dyspnea after exercise
	    palpitations after exercise
	    fatigue
	    weakness
	    pallor
	    sensitivity to cold
	    anorexia
		In mild cases, patient may be asymptomatic.
		
		When iron stores are sufficiently depleted $\longrightarrow$
		    dyspnea after exercise
		    palpitations after exercise
		    fatigue
		    weakness
		    pallor
		    sensitivity to cold
		    anorexia
		
		During later stages, manifestations may include
		    brittle hair and nails
		    dysphagia
		    inflammation of mucosa of the mouth
		    inflammation of the tongue

Characteristics of blood	As a result of hemodilution, there is a decrease in the concentration of RBC's, with associated depression in red cell count, Hb concentration, and hematocrit. Since individual erythrocytes are normocytic and normochromic, MCV and MCHC are within normal limits.	As a result of iron deficiency, individual erythrocytes are microcytic and hypochromic; MCV and MCHC are depressed. Hemoglobin concentration may fall as low as 3.6 gm. percent of whole blood.

be recovered rather easily from erythrocytes that have escaped from the vascular tree but remain within the confines of the body. Under these circumstances, recycled iron is readily available to facilitate the generation of new red blood cells.

While iron deficiency is a possible complication of acute hemorrhage, it constitutes the primary physiological disruption in cases of slow, chronic blood loss. Characteristic symptoms are similar to those caused by nutritional iron deficiency (as described subsequently in this chapter). Some primary differences between acute and chronic hemorrhagic anemia are summarized in Table 14.4.

ANEMIAS CAUSED BY EXCESSIVE HE-MOLYSIS Excessive hemolysis (the excessive breakdown of red blood cells) usually takes place in one of two major areas: (1) within the vascular tree, or (2) within the spleen.

In cases of intravascular hemolysis, common causative mechanisms include mechanical stress and antigen-antibody reactions. Erythrocytes sheared within narrowed atherosclerotic vessels, or victimized by complement-mediated transfusion reactions, are thus particularly prone to excessive intravascular breakdown. Jaundice evolves secondarily as hemoglobin, released into plasma by ruptured red blood cells, is extracted by reticuloendothelial cells and converted into unconjugated bilirubin.

When hemolysis occurs within the spleen, on the other hand, lack of erythrocyte flexibility is a primary causative factor. Splenic enlargement results, as the spleen traps and hemolyzes excessive numbers of rigid or fragile red blood cells. Jaundice commonly reflects the release of unconjugated bilirubin into plasma. Some typical causative disorders are summarized in Table 14.5

In all cases of hemolytic anemia, tissue hypoxia characteristically triggers the release of erythropoietin. Resulting increases in the rate of red blood cell production cause an elevation in the volume of circulating reticulocytes. Secondary increases in the formation of gallstones may also be noted as elevated plasma bilirubin causes alterations in the composition of bile. A tabular summary of the hemolytic anemias is presented in Table 14.6.

ANEMIAS CAUSED BY DEFICIENT PRODUCTION OF RED BLOOD CELLS A deficiency in the production of erythrocytes may be induced by a number of phenomena, including: (1) iron deficiency, (2) vitamin B_{12} or folic acid deficiency, (3) erythropoietin deficiency, or (4) bone marrow failure.

Iron Deficiency In cases of iron deficiency anemia, dysfunction may be caused by a lack of nutritional intake, absorption failures, excessive or chronic blood loss (as described previously), or increases in iron requirements (as noted during pregnancy, infancy, lactation, and puberty).

Regardless of the pathogenesis, iron deficiency generally evolves in a progressive, se-

TABLE 14.5 **Some Causes of Erythrocyte Rigidity/Fragility**

Causative Disorder	Characteristic Features
Hereditary spherocytosis (HS)	Genetic disorder characterized by the formation of relatively inflexible, spheroid red blood cells
Glucose-6-phosphate dehydrogenase (G6PD) deficiency	Genetic disorder characterized by deficiency of the red blood cell enzyme G6PD. Erythrocytes are rendered more susceptible to hemolysis following exposure to chemical oxidants, phenacetin, sulfonamides, chloramphenicol, and the thiazide diuretics.
Sickle cell anemia	Genetic disorder characterized by crystallization of abnormal hemoglobin and subsequent deformity of the red blood cell. Disease is most often triggered by depression of pO_2.
Thalassemia syndromes	Genetic disorders characterized by abnormal synthesis of the globin component of hemoglobin; results in the formation of unstable hemoglobins that are vulnerable to hemolysis.

TABLE 14.6 **The Hemolytic Anemias**

Primary Site of Hemolysis	Causative Disorders	Clinical Manifestations
Within the vascular tree	Atherosclerosis Transfusion reactions Disseminated intravascular coagulation (DIC)	Accumulation of free Hb and oxidized methemoglobin in the plasma Elimination of Hb and methemoglobin in the urine Jaundice Elevated reticulocyte count Possible formation of gallstones
Within the spleen	Hereditary spherocytosis G6PD deficiency Sickle cell anemia Thalassemia syndromes	Enlargement of the spleen Jaundice Elevated reticulocyte count Possible formation of gallstones

quential manner. Clinical symptoms do not typically appear until the body is depleted of all reserve iron stores. At this point, red blood cells become characteristically microcytic and hypochromic. Decreases are noted in hemoglobin concentration, hematocrit, MCV, and MCHC.

Since iron is also an important constituent of certain intracellular enzymes throughout the body, deficit of this mineral may trigger metabolic disruptions that occur independently of erythrocyte abnormalities. The fatigue characteristically associated with iron deficiency anemia, for example, is believed to be considerably exacerbated by the depletion of critical iron-containing intracellular enzymes. When severe deficiency exists, changing patterns of energy generation may also be responsible for cellular growth disturbances. In these cases the disorder is indicated by the onset of baldness (alopecia), atrophic changes of the tongue and gastric mucosa, and malabsorption.

Vitamin B_{12} or Folic Acid Deficiency When vitamin B_{12} or folic acid is deficient, the maturation of red blood cells is disrupted. In these cases, the production of erythrocytes is believed to be affected at early developmental stages in the bone marrow. Failure to progress from the erythroblast stage to the normoblast-reticulocyte cellular forms charac-

teristically results in the generation of megaloblastic, macrocytic red blood cells. The reticulocyte population is depressed in spite of increased stimulation by erythropoietin, and erythrocytes are typically fragile and prone to hemolysis.

While deficiency of either folic acid or vitamin B_{12} may arise secondary to decreased ingestion or absorption, vitamin B_{12} utilization is specifically dependent upon the presence of intrinsic factor generated by the gastric mucosa. For this reason, disorders involving the gastric lining may cause depression of vitamin B_{12} absorption, as typically occurs in cases of pernicious anemia. Since deficiency of vitamin B_{12} also causes degeneration of myelin in the central nervous system, neural symptoms frequently accompany disruptions in oxygen transport.

Erythropoietin Deficiency If erythropoietin is not released by renal cells, anemia will result. Disease of the kidneys is thus often characterized by a disruption in the normal production of red blood cells. The effects of uremia often complicate the disorder and are believed to be responsible for decreasing the life span of circulating erythrocytes.

It is significant to note that erythropoietin deficiency has recently been cited as a possible cause of the anemia that is characteristically associated with chronic disease. Although ev-

TABLE 14.7   **Some Major Causes of Aplastic Anemia**

Agents that *always* cause marrow damage (in sufficient dosage)	Radiant energy
	   x-rays
	   radium
	   radioactive isotopes
	Benzene
	Alkylating agents
	Antimetabolites

Agents that *occasionally* cause marrow damage	Chloromycetin Sulfonamides Quinacrine Phenylbutazone Diphenylhydantoin Mephenytoin Gold compounds
Agents that cause marrow damage in *only a few cases*	Streptomycin Tripelennamine DDT Meprobamate Hair dyes Carbon tetrachloride

idence is not conclusive, erythropoietin decreases may account for the normocytic, normochromic anemia that often accompanies disorders such as tuberculosis, osteomyelitis, rheumatoid arthritis, lymphomas, and widespread carcinomas.

Bone Marrow Failure When the bone marrow is unable to produce an adequate number of erythrocytes, a condition described as aplastic anemia is said to exist. In these cases, red blood cells are typically normocytic and normochromic, and associated decreases in the production of white blood cells and platelets are frequently noted.

Although aplastic anemia may arise spontaneously for unknown reasons (approximately 50 per cent of the time), it is also induced by exposure to whole-body irradiation or triggered by the presence of certain drugs, chemicals, or pathogenic microbes in the body. A

TABLE 14.8   **Types of Anemia: A Comparative Summary**

Anemias Characterized by	Some Causative Disorders	Clinical Manifestations
EXCESSIVE BLOOD LOSS Acute hemorrhage	Trauma Aneurysm Arterial malignancy or ulceration	Shock symptoms Dyspnea and palpitation after exercise Fatigue and weakness Pallor Sensitivity to cold Depressed RBC count, Hb concentration, and hematocrit Normal MCV and MCHC

Chronic hemorrhage	Bleeding peptic ulcer
	Excessive menstrual bleeding
	Ulcerative colitis
	Bleeding from hemorrhoids or diverticuli
	Salicylate poisoning
		Dyspnea and palpitation after exercise
		Fatigue and weakness
		Pallor
		Sensitivity to cold
		Symptoms associated with iron deficiency:
		   dysphagia
		   inflammation of the mucosa of the mouth and stomach
		   brittle hair and nails
		Depressed Hb concentration and hematocrit
		Depressed MCV and MCHC

EXCESSIVE HEMOLYSIS Within the vascular tree	Atherosclerosis Transfusion reactions DIC	Dyspnea and palpitation after exercise Fatigue and weakness Pallor Sensitivity to cold Hemoglobinemia and methemoglobinemia Hemoglobinuria and methemoglobinuria Jaundice Elevated reticulocyte count RBC's normochromic and normocytic or macrocytic

list of some primary causative agents is presented in Table 14.7.

ANEMIAS: A SUMMARY It can be said that anemias of diverse origin will ultimately disrupt the transport of oxygen between alveoli and metabolizing cells. Although causative mechanisms are varied and characteristic laboratory values are not necessarily similar, tissue hypoxia inevitably results. A tabular comparative summary of the primary types of anemia is presented in Table 14.8.

Cardiovascular Pathology

Disruptions in oxygen transport are not caused only by anemias. Adequate cellular oxygenation is also dependent upon the existence of a functional cardiovascular system. If the heart and blood vessels are unable to transport a sufficient quantity of blood to the cells, tissue hypoxia will result.

As elucidated in Chapter 9, cardiovascular disease may evolve through a variety of mechanisms. Some major examples are summarized in Table 14.9.

CLINICAL MANIFESTATIONS OF CELLULAR HYPOXIA

When cells are deprived of oxygen, metabolism generally shifts to favor anaerobic glycolysis, as illustrated in Figure 14.6. It can be seen that in the absence of oxygen, pyruvic acid will not enter the citric acid cycle. Instead, it is converted into lactic acid until a supportive oxygen environment can be reestablished. Under these circumstances, systemic accumulation of lactic acid may lead to

TABLE 14.8 **Types of Anemia: A Comparative Summary** *(Continued)*

Anemias Characterized by	Some Causative Disorders	Clinical Manifestations
EXCESSIVE HEMOLYSIS *(Continued)*		
Within the spleen	Hereditary spherocytosis G6PD deficiency Sickle cell anemia Thalassemia	Dyspnea and palpitation after exercise Fatigue and weakness Pallor Sensitivity to cold Enlargement of the spleen Jaundice Elevated reticulocyte count RBC's normochromic and normocytic or macrocytic
DEFICIENT PRODUCTION OF ERYTHROCYTES		Dyspnea and palpitation after exercise Fatigue and weakness Pallor Sensitivity to cold

Iron deficiency	Deficient intake
	Malabsorption
	Chronic hemorrhage
	Increase in iron requirements
		Alopecia
		Atrophic changes of the tongue
		  and gastric mucosa
		Dysphagia
		Malabsorption
		RBC's microcytic and hypochromic
		Depressed Hb concentration,
		  'hematocrit, MCV, and MCHC

Vitamin B_{12} or folic acid
  deficiency
	Deficient intake
	Malabsorption
	Pernicious anemia (in cases of
	  vitamin B_{12} deficiency)
		Depressed RBC count
		Erythrocytes are macrocytic and
		  megaloblastic

Erythropoietin deficiency	Renal failure	Depressed RBC count Erythrocytes are normocytic and normochromic
Bone marrow failure	Exposure to radiation	Depressed RBC count

	Exposure to select drugs and
	  chemicals
		Erythrocytes normocytic and
		  normochromic

TABLE 14.9   **Cardiovascular Pathology**

Primary Origin of Pathological Condition	Pathological Mechanism	Examples of Associated Disorders
Heart	Ischemia	Angina pectoris Myocardial infarction
	Infection	Rheumatic fever
	Arrhythmias	Premature atrial contractions Atrial tachycardia First-, second-, and third-degree heart blocks Premature ventricular contractions Ventricular fibrillation
	Congenital defects	Septal defects Tetralogy of Fallot
	Restrictive defects	Pericarditis Pericardial effusion Cardiac tamponade
	Decompensation	Congestive heart failure
Blood vessels	Vascular occlusion	Arteriosclerosis Atherosclerosis Thrombophlebitis
	Inappropriate vascular constriction/ dilation	Pheochromocytoma Septic shock

metabolic acidosis, while deficient energy production frequently causes tiredness, weakness, and lassitude.

In considering the specific effects of hypoxia upon the body, it is significant to distinguish between two related response patterns. On the one hand, oxygen deprivation will induce *organic dysfunction* in a variety of critical structures by altering normal metabolic reactions. Alternatively, hypoxia will trigger *compensatory systemic responses* that are designed to maximize cellular oxygenation and facilitate return to equilibrium.

Organic Dysfunction

Because oxygen is critical to cellular survival, hypoxia can cause considerable dysfunction throughout the body. Since various structures react differently to oxygen deprivation, it is beneficial to look more specifically at particular organs and the way in which they are affected by hypoxia.

In the blood, for example, lack of available oxygen may shift the equilibrium that exists between oxygenated and nonoxygenated (or reduced) hemoglobin. Normally, the amount of reduced hemoglobin in the vascular tree does not exceed 2.5 gm. per cent. Under conditions of oxygen deprivation, the concentration of reduced hemoglobin can increase considerably. When values reach 5 gm. per cent, elevated levels of bluish, nonoxygenated hemoglobin may cause the skin to take on a dusky, purplish hue. This condition, referred to as *cyanosis*, is often associated with chronic obstructive pulmonary disease or right-to-left shunts in congenital heart disease. Since cyanosis is due primarily to depressions in hemoglobin-oxygen saturation, it is rarely noted in the anemic patient. This is because the hemoglobin available in anemic erythrocytes is typically combined with oxygen in optimal proportions.

In addition to affecting the status of the blood, hypoxia is also responsible for widespread alteration of organic function. Depression in cellular oxygen supply, for example, is believed to directly increase the irritability of cardiac muscle. Tachycardia results and may be associated with aspects of heart failure, as described in Chapter 9. To the extent that the myocardium does not receive sufficient quantities of oxygen, ischemia can also lead to a considerable decline in cardiac output. Under these circumstances, systemic hypoxia may be significantly exacerbated.

Cardiac dysfunction, during times of low-oxygen stress, is often aggravated by increased resistance to right ventricular output. For unknown reasons, hypoxia in the lung is known to trigger vasoconstriction, thereby promoting the accumulation of blood in pulmonary arterial vessels. The right ventricle of the heart is thus forced to work harder in order to pump sufficient quantities of blood into pulmonary tissue.

Depressions in cellular oxygen supply may also lead to renal or hepatic dysfunction. Both the nephrons and the central lobules of the liver are particularly sensitive to hypoxia. Disruption of renal tubular activity and hepatic fibrosis are thus frequently noted complications in cases of oxygen deprivation.

Since cerebral cells normally consume approximately 20 per cent of available circulating

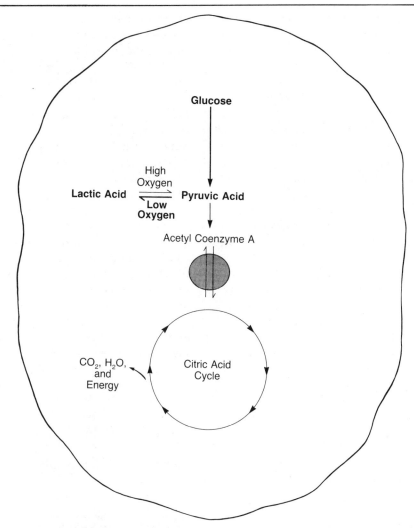

Figure 14.6 Anaerobic glycolysis. The sequence marked in bold face type indicates the pathway of intracellular glucose catabolism under anaerobic conditions. Note the inability of pyruvic acid to enter the citric acid cycle.

oxygen to support ongoing metabolism, they are significantly affected by hypoxia. Symptoms of dizziness, restlessness, poor concentration, and altered states of consciousness are often aggravated by cerebral edema. The accumulation of interstitial fluid within the brain is specifically triggered by oxygen deficit and caused by increases in cerebral capillary permeability.

Compensatory Systemic Responses

As hypoxia evolves, the body attempts to compensate for oxygen deficit in a variety of ways. Some of the primary adaptation mechanisms mediated by the bone marrow, cardiovascular system, respiratory system, and nervous systems are elucidated in the following pages.

BONE MARROW

When cellular oxygen supply is depressed, the bone marrow is stimulated by erythropoietin to increase the rate of red blood cell production. *Secondary polycythemia* results and is characterized by an increase in the concentration of erythrocytes. Although not present in all cases of hypoxia, secondary polycythemia is frequently associated with high-altitude oxygen deficit, alveolar hypoventilation, and right-to-left shunt congenital heart disease.

CARDIOVASCULAR SYSTEM

When hypoxia exists, the cardiovascular system attempts to compensate in two primary ways: (1) Cardiac output is increased, so that oxygenated blood may circulate more rapidly through the body; and (2) the distribution of blood flow is selectively modified, so that critical organs may be serviced by a relatively larger proportion of circulating erythrocytes.

Changes in cardiac output are controlled primarily through the central nervous system. As illustrated in Figure 14.7, chemoreceptors in the carotid and aortic bodies are particularly sensitive to alterations in the concentration of respiratory gases. As oxygen levels decline, neural messages are sent to the medulla, which, in turn, triggers sympathetic stimulation of the heart. As a result of this mechanism, the rate and strength of cardiac contraction increase.

Variations in the distribution of circulating blood occur primarily through adaptive alterations in vascular diameter. For reasons not completely understood, hypoxia is known to directly trigger localized vasodilation. This mechanism functions primarily in organs that are critically sensitive to oxygen deficit, such as the heart, brain, and gastrointestinal tract as well as skeletal muscle. It tends to take precedence over the effects of autonomic neural stimulation and plays a significant role in the maintenance of homeostasis. It is important to realize that localized vasodilation is relatively less effective as a compensatory mechanism in areas such as the kidneys (where normal blood flow is usually sufficient to provide an emergency reserve in cases of hypoxia) and the skin (where blood flow is regulated primarily by neural mechanisms, that respond to changes in internal body temperature).

In cases in which hypoxia is sustained and chronic, additional vascular modifications may occur. When a specific area is deprived of circulation or oxygen over an extended period of time, collateral circulation may develop. This phenomenon, characterized by increased vascularity of oxygen-deprived tissue, is frequently noted in the myocardium as a response to ischemia. It is also believed to be at least partially responsible for the digital club-

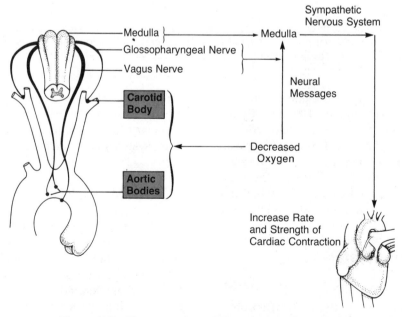

Figure 14.7 Chemoreceptors: Effect upon cardiac output.

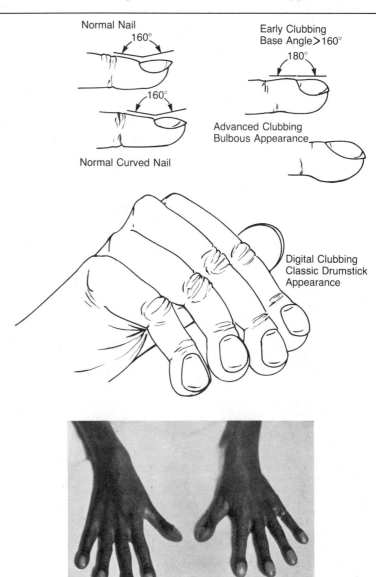

Normal Nail
160°

160°

Normal Curved Nail

Early Clubbing
Base Angle > 160°
180°

Advanced Clubbing
Bulbous Appearance

Digital Clubbing
Classic Drumstick
Appearance

Figure 14.8 Digital clubbing. (Photograph reprinted with permission of Delp, M. H., and Manning, R. T.: Major's Physical Diagnosis, 9th ed. Philadelphia, W. B. Saunders Company, 1981.)

bing that is often associated with pulmonary disease. The characteristic bulbous changes in the terminal digits of the fingers are illustrated in Figure 14.8.

RESPIRATORY SYSTEM

As hypoxia evolves, the rate and depth of ventilation are increased to help compensate for deficient cellular oxygen supplies. Chemoreceptors located in the carotid and aortic bodies are most directly instrumental in mediating this adaptive response. As oxygen levels fall, neural messages are sent to the medulla, which, in this case, triggers appropriate changes in ventilation.

Although hypoxia can thus modify respiratory activity, ventilation is more directly influenced by plasma pCO_2 levels. When carbon dioxide concentration increases, the medulla is directly stimulated to increase the rate and depth of ventilation. Only in cases of chronic hypercapnia, (characterized by desensitization of the medulla to the effects of carbon dioxide) will the hypoxic mechanism take precedence.

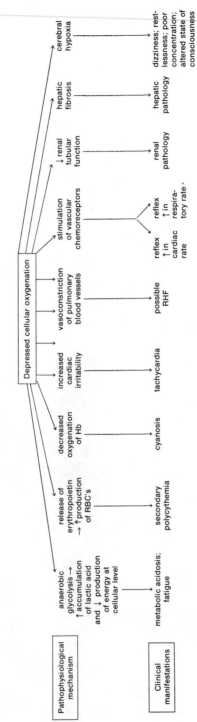

Figure 14.9 Clinical manifestations of cellular hypoxia

NERVOUS SYSTEM

The nervous system is primarily influential in determining cardiac and respiratory changes, as previously described. Peripheral chemoreceptors keep the central nervous system continually apprised of alterations in systemic oxygen status. Neural messages can thus be directed to initiate adaptive organic responses and facilitate a return to homeostasis.

Clinical Manifestations of Cellular Hypoxia: A Summary

Clearly, the effects of cellular hypoxia are widespread and multisystemic in nature. While organic dysfunction may be a direct result of oxygen deprivation, compensatory response mechanisms will also lead to functional changes throughout the body. A summary of some primary manifestations of cellular hypoxia is presented in Figure 14.9.

STUDY QUESTIONS

1. In each of the following cases, briefly describe how or why cellular hypoxia could develop:
   a. overdose of anesthetic
   b. left heart failure
   c. COPD
   d. abdominal distention
   e. pneumoconioses
   f. cystic fibrosis
   g. carbon monoxide poisoning
   h. renal failure
   i. metabolic alkalosis
   j. total gastrectomy
   k. iron deficiency

2. Explain how each of the following disorders could affect the size, shape, number, or hemoglobin concentration of the red blood cell:
   a. acute hemorrhage
   b. long-term bleeding associated with peptic ulcer
   c. sickle cell anemia
   d. extensive degeneration of gastric mucosa
   e. radiation poisoning

3. Mild cyanosis is noted in a patient being treated for congestive heart failure. Identify two factors that could be contributing to the cyanotic condition and explain how or why they would do so.

4. Mrs. Linwood has relocated from the East Coast to the Colorado Rockies. A blood test several months after the move reveals the existence of polycythemia. Explain.

5. Mr. Eaton is admitted into the hospital in respiratory failure. Initial examination reveals cyanosis, tachycardia, dizziness, restlessness, and hyperventilation. Laboratory tests indicate the existence of metabolic acidosis. Explain the pathogenesis of each of these symptoms.

Suggested Readings

Books

Anderson, W. A. D., and Scotti, T. M.: Synopsis of Pathology, 10th ed. St. Louis, The C.V. Mosby Company, 1980, pp. 496–510.

Balarzak, S., and Munsey, E.: Disorders of iron metabolism. In Mengel, C. E. (ed.): Hematology: Principles and Practice. Chicago, Year Book Medical Publishers, Inc., 1971, pp. 43–65.

Brain, M. C.: Aplastic anemia. In Beeson, P. B., McDermott, W., and Wyngaarden, J. B. (eds.): Cecil Textbook of Medicine, 15th ed. Philadelphia, W. B. Saunders Company, 1979, p. 1733.

Brown, E. B.: Acute hemorrhagic anemia. In Beeson, P. B., McDermott, W., and Wyngaarden, J. B. (eds.): Cecil Textbook of Medicine, 15th ed. Philadelphia, W. B. Saunder Company, 1979, p. 1729.

Brown, E. B.: Anemias associated with infection and chronic systemic diseases. In Beeson, P. B., McDermott, W., and Wyngaarden, J. B. (eds.): Cecil Textbook of Medicine, 15th ed. Philadelphia, W. B. Saunders Company, 1979, p. 1731.

Brown, E. B.: Iron deficiency anemia. In Beeson, P. B., McDermott, W., and Wyngaarden, J. B. (eds.): Cecil Textbook of Medicine, 15th ed. Philadelphia, W. B. Saunders Company, 1979, p. 1743.

Conley, C. L.: Hemoglobin, hemoglobinopathies,

and the thalassemias. *In* Beeson, P. B., McDermott, W., and Wyngaarden, J. B. (eds.): Cecil Textbook of Medicine, 15th ed. Philadelphia, W. B. Saunders Company, 1979, p. 1771.

Cook, J. D.: Anemia due to iron deficiency. *In* Conn, H. F. (ed.): Current Therapy 1980. Philadelphia, W. B. Saunders Company, 1980, p. 241.

Edwards, V., and Murphy, M.: Disruptions in the oxygen-carbon dioxide exchange mechanism. *In* Jones, D. A., Dunbar, C. F., and Jirovec, M. M.: Medical-Surgical Nursing, A Conceptual Approach. New York, McGraw-Hill Book Company, 1978, p. 1009.

Erslev, A. J., and Gabuzda, T. G.: Pathophysiology of Blood. Philadelphia, W. B. Saunders Company, 1975.

Erslev, A. J., and Gabuzda, T. G.: Pathophysiology of hematologic disorders. *In* Sodeman, W. A., and Sodeman, T. M.: Pathologic Physiology, Mechanisms of Disease, 6th ed. Philadelphia, W. B. Saunders Company, 1979, p. 587.

Guyton, A. C.: Textbook of Medical Physiology, 5th ed. Philadelphia, W. B. Saunders Company, 1976, pp. 56–65; 543–556.

Herbert, V.: Megaloblastic anemias. *In* Beeson, P. B., McDermott, W., and Wyngaarden, J. B. (eds.): Cecil Textbook of Medicine, 15th ed. Philadelphia, W. B. Saunders Company, 1979, p. 1719.

Hillman, R. S., and Finch, C. A.: Red Cell Manual, 4th ed. Philadelphia, F. A. Davis Company, 1974.

Hole, J. W.: Human Anatomy and Physiology. Dubuque, Wm. C. Brown Company, 1978, pp. 536–562.

Jones, D. A., and Martin, J. S.: The concept of oxygenation. *In* Jones, D. A., Dunbar, C. F., and Jirovec, M. M.: Medical-Surgical Nursing, A Conceptual Approach. New York, McGraw-Hill Book Company, 1978, p. 743.

Kent, T. H., Hart, M. N., and Shires, T. K.: Introduction to Human Disease. New York, Appleton-Century-Crofts, 1979, pp. 106–123.

Luckmann, J., and Sorensen, K. C.: Medical-Surgical Nursing, A Pathophysiologic Approach, 2nd ed. Philadelphia, W. B. Saunders Company, 1980. pp. 1022–1055.

McFarlane, J. M.: Disturbances in the oxygen-carrying mechanism. *In* Jones, D. A., Dunbar, C. F., and Jirovec, M. M.: Medical-Surgical Nursing Conceptual Approach. New York, McGraw-Hill Book Company, 1978, p. 779.

Medal, L. S.: Aplastic anemia. *In* Conn, H. F. (ed.): Current Therapy 1980. Philadelphia, W. B. Saunders Company, 1980, p. 239.

Pflanzer, R. G.: The blood. *In* Selkurt, E. E. (ed.): Basic Physiology for the Health Sciences. Boston, Little, Brown & Company, 1975, p. 325.

Purtillo, D. T.: A Survey of Human Diseases. Menlo Park, Addison-Wesley Publishing Company, 1978, pp. 209–222.

Robbins, S. L., and Cotran, R. S.: Pathologic Basis of Disease, 2nd ed. Philadelphia, W. B. Saunders Company, 1979, pp. 712–745.

Sheehy, T. W.: Pernicious anemia and other megaloblastic anemias. *In* Conn, H. F. (ed.): Current Therapy 1980. Philadelphia, W. B. Saunders Company, 1980, p. 250.

Surgenor, D. M.: The Red Blood Cell, 2nd ed., Vol. 21. New York, Academic Press, 1975.

Tortora, G. H., and Anagnostakos, N. P.: Principles of Anatomy and Physiology, 2nd ed. San Francisco, Canfield Press, 1978, pp. 424–428.

Xistris, D. M.: Problems of the blood and blood-forming organs. *In* Phipps, W. J., Long, B. C., and Woods, N. F. (eds.): Medical-Surgical Nursing, Concepts and Clinical Practice. St. Louis, The C. V. Mosby Company, 1979, p. 1058.

Articles

Adamson, J. W., and Finch, C. A.: Hemoglobin function oxygen affinity, and erythropoietin. Ann. Rev. Physiol., *37*:351, 1975.

Bonnett, J. D.: Normocytic normochromic anemia. Postgrad. Med., *61*:139, 1977.

Byrne, J.: Hematology studies: Part VI. A review of mean corpuscular values and red cell indices. Nursing 77, 7:10, 1977.

Carmel, R.: Iron-related anemias: Look for more than deficiency. Consultant, *19*:135, 1979.

Finch, C. A.: Anemia of chronic disease. Postgrad. Med., *64*:107, 1978.

Finch, C. A., and Lenfant, C.: Oxygen transport in man. N. Engl. J. Med., *286*:407, 1972.

Foster, S.: Sickle cell anemia: Closing the gap between theory and therapy. Am. J. Nurs., *71*:1952, 1971.

Garby, L.: Iron deficiency: Definition and prevalence. Clin. Hematol., 2:245, 1973.

Green, J. B.: Macrocytic anemias. Postgrad. Med., *61*:155, 1977.

Hillman, R. S.: Blood loss anemia. Postgrad. Med., *64*:88, 1978.

Linman, J.: Physiologic and pathophysiologic effects of anemia. N. Engl. J. Med., *279*:812, 1968.

McCurdy, P. R.: Microcytic hypochromic anemias. Postgrad. Med., *61*:147, 1977.

Nathan, D. G.: Regulation of erythropoiesis. N. Engl. J. Med., *296*:685, 1977.

Schade, S. G.: Iron metabolism. Postgrad. Med., *55*:119, 1974.

Vaz, D.: The common anemias: Nursing approaches. Nurs. Clin. North Am., *7*:711, 1972.

Ward, P. C. J.: Investigation of macrocytic anemia. Postgrad. Med., *65*:203, 1979.

Ward, P. C. J.: Investigation of microcytic anemia: Postgrad. Med., *65*:235, 1979.

Ward, P. C. J.: Red cell indices revised: Review with test cases. Postgrad. Med., *65*:282, 1979.

Wilson, P.:Iron-deficiency anemia. Am. J. Nurs., *72*:502, 1972.

Chapter Outline

chapter **15**

Diseases Affecting the Cellular Need for Nutrients

Chapter Objectives

At the completion of this chapter, the student will be able to:

1. Identify the four major mechanisms responsible for maintaining cellular nutrient supply.
2. List five major disorders that interfere with nutrient ingestion and identify the system within which they originate.
3. List ten major disorders that interfere with digestion or absorption and identify the associated pathological mechanism in each case.
4. List eight major disorders that interfere with nutrient transport and indicate whether they are characterized by: (1) a decrease in cardiac output, or (2) a disruption in the circulation of blood.
5. Describe five metabolic disturbances associated with hepatocellular disease and identify characteristic clinical manifestations in each case.
6. Identify three endocrine disturbances that affect metabolic activity within the liver and describe associated clinical manifestations.
7. Describe the function of insulin and the metabolic disturbances associated with diabetes mellitus.
8. Briefly describe the effect of each of the following upon intracellular metabolism: vitamin B_1, vitamin B_2, pyrodoxine, pantothenic acid and biotin, male sex hormones, epinephrine, thyroxine, growth hormone, fever, muscular exercise, and aging.
9. Differentiate between phenylketonuria, galactosemia, and gout, with respect to causative deficit and clinical manifestations.
10. Describe the clinical manifestations of cellular nutrient deficit.

INTRODUCTION

In considering the cellular need for metabolic fuel, it is important to distinguish between the supply and the utilization of nutrients. Cells are generally supplied with nutrients by cooperation between the processes of ingestion, digestion, absorption, and transport. For maximal benefits to be derived from these nutrients, however, they must ultimately be catabolized intracellularly, in the presence of oxygen, to yield energy.

In the following pages, a description of some disorders that characteristically depress nutrient supply or utilization is followed by a clarification of their clinical manifestations.

DISORDERS THAT DISRUPT INGESTION

For our purposes, ingestion will be defined as the intake of nutrients from the environment into the gastrointestinal tract. As such, it generally involves the integrated and coordinated manipulation of muscles in the arms, hands, and face, so as to facilitate the introduction of food into the mouth. Perceptual and neuromuscular skills are thus of primary significance in ensuring optimal ingestion.

The intake of food is also influenced by variables that affect the desire to eat. Ideally, the hypothalamus helps to establish a balance between feelings of hunger and satiety (satisfaction). Under normal circumstances, for example, intake does not continue indiscriminately because sensations of fullness tend to inhibit superfluous ingestion.

In many individuals, however, psychoemotional factors may take precedence and disrupt the normal control mechanisms. In these cases, caloric intake may be excessive (as in obesity) or deficient (as in anorexia nervosa).

The desire to eat is also influenced by one's general state of health. Even a mild viral cold can considerably suppress appetite; and anorexia is characteristically associated with a wide range of disorders, including advanced renal disease, congestive heart failure, alcoholism, depression, peptic ulcers, hepatitis, cirrhosis, and gastrointestinal cancers.

Assuming a normal appetite, however, the majority of ingestive disorders are primarily neuromuscular in origin. Examples of some causative disorders are presented in Table 15.1.

DISORDERS THAT DISRUPT DIGESTION OR ABSORPTION

In order for nutrients to play a functional role in cellular metabolism, they must first be broken down within the gastrointestinal tract and then absorbed into the bloodstream.

Most predictably, gastrointestinal disease is a primary cause of digestive-absorptive disruption, as summarized in Table 15.2.

TABLE 15.1   **Some Disorders That May Interfere With Ingestion**

Pathological Mechanism	Causative Disorders	System of Origin
Interference with the neural stimulation of muscles associated with ingestion	CVA Parkinson's disease Poliomyelitis Myasthenia gravis Tetanus Guillain-Barré syndrome Multiple sclerosis Spinal cord transection	Nervous system
Degeneration of the muscles associated with ingestion	Muscular dystrophies	Muscular system

TABLE 15.2   Disruption of Digestion/Absorption

Pathological Mechanism	Causative Disorder
Inflammation of gastro-intestinal mucosa	Gastritis Peptic ulcer Diverticulitis Ulcerative colitis Enteritis Irritable colon
Malabsorption	Celiac disease Crohn's disease
Obstruction/disruption of peristalsis	Pyloric stenosis Gastrointestinal cancer Crohn's disease Strangulated hernia Postoperative adhesions Volvulus Intussusception Paralytic ileus
Functional disruption of accessory organs of the digestive system	Pancreatitis Cholelithiasis Hepatitis Cirrhosis

TABLE 15.3   Disorders That Disrupt Nutrient Transport

Pathological Mechanism	Causative Disorder
Decrease in cardiac output	Myocardial infarction Valvular disease Cardiac arrhythmias Cardiac tamponade Congestive heart failure Hypovolemia
Disruption in the circulation of blood	Atherosclerosis Arteriosclerosis Thrombi Emboli Septic shock Neurogenic shock

DISORDERS THAT DISRUPT NUTRIENT TRANSPORT

As indicated in Figure 15.1, gastrointestinal absorption is a somewhat selective process. While fats pass into small lymph vessels called lacteals, carbohydrates and proteins are absorbed directly into the bloodstream. As a result, initial circulatory patterns will vary as a function of the nutrient involved.

Lymph rich in digested fats, for example, is transported to a large collecting vessel, called the thoracic duct, before being emptied into the left subclavian vein (in the region of the left shoulder). Blood containing digested carbohydrates and proteins, on the other hand, is transported to the liver through the portal vein and subsequently through the hepatic vein into the inferior vena cava. In spite of this differential transport route, however, all nutrients are ultimately carried to metabolizing cells via the bloodstream.

Optimal nutrient distribution is, therefore, dependent upon a functional cardiovascular system. If the volume of circulating blood is substantially reduced, considerable cellular nutrient deficit may occur. Some disorders characterized by depressed cardiac output or vascular dysfunction are summarized in Table 15.3.

DISORDERS THAT DISRUPT METABOLISM

The complex chemical reactions that enable cells to utilize nutrients for the maintenance of growth, repair, and functional activity are collectively referred to as metabolism. Metabolism, which is described thoroughly in

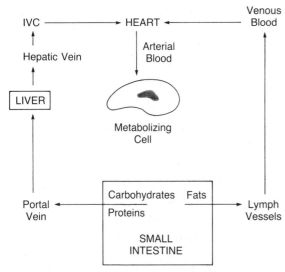

Figure 15.1 The absorption and circulation of digested nutrients: a schematic presentation.

Chapter 2, is essentially a two-step process that can be summarized as follows:

1. Initially, nutrients are processed by the liver. In this way, carbohydrate, fat, and protein molecules can be stored or modified to facilitate optimal cellular utilization.

2. Ultimately, nutrient particles are used intracellularly in the creation of new substances and the generation of energy.

Because of the dual nature of the metabolic process, disorders can be caused by disruption of either the hepatic or the intracellular aspect of nutrient utilization. Some primary metabolic disorders are discussed in the following pages.

Disorders that Disrupt the Hepatic Aspect of Metabolism

For a review of the role played by the liver in the metabolic process, the reader is referred to Chapter 2. In brief, it can be said that the liver provides cells throughout the body with an optimal mix of utilizable nutrients.

For example, when caloric intake is excessive, the liver functions to convert superfluous nutrient particles into glycogen or fat through the processes of glycogenesis and lipogenesis, respectively. Cellular nutrient demand, on the other hand, is often met by converting stored lipids or proteins into glucose, via gluconeogenesis, or glycogen into glucose, via glycogenolysis.

In considering metabolic activity within the liver, it is important to remember that the endocrine system plays a critical regulatory role. As indicated in Table 15.4, hepatic functional activity is influenced by hormones in a variety of ways. Endocrine imbalances may, therefore, trigger metabolic disturbances by altering the way in which the liver prepares nutrients for cellular utilization.

Whenever hepatic aspects of metabolism are disrupted, cells throughout the body may ultimately suffer from some form of malnutrition. Pathogenesis is most commonly characterized by one of two major mechanisms: (1) hepatocellular disease, or (2) endocrine dysfunction.

TABLE 15.4 **Some Hormones Affecting Hepatic Metabolic Activity**

Hormone	Site of Release	Effect on Metabolic Activity in the Liver
Glucagon	Alpha cells of pancreas	Promotes glycogenolysis and gluconeogenesis Promotes lipolysis
Insulin	Beta cells of pancreas	Stimulates glycogenesis Promotes lipogenesis
Epinephrine and norepinephrine	Adrenal medulla	Promotes glycogenolysis and gluconeogenesis Promotes lipolysis
Glucocorticoids	Adrenal cortex	Promotes lipolysis Promotes gluconeogenesis of amino acids Promotes glycogenolysis
ACTH	Anterior pituitary	Stimulates release of glucocorticoids, thereby promoting lipolysis and gluconeogenesis
Growth hormone (GH)	Anterior pituitary	Promotes mobilization of fats Promotes lipolysis
Thyroxine	Thyroid gland	Promotes gluconeogenesis of amino acids Promotes lipolysis Promotes use of protein for energy if carbohydrate or fat unavailable (liver must first deaminate the amino acids)

TABLE 15.5 **Metabolic Disturbances Associated With Hepatocellular Disease***

Metabolic Imbalance	Manifestation
Decreased glycogenesis, glyco-genolysis, gluconeogenesis, and fatty acid oxidation	Weight loss
	Fatigue
Possible hypoglycemia	Ketoacidosis
Possible hyperglycemia	Glycosuria
Decreased lipogenesis	Decreased serum cholesterol
Decreased extraction and metabolism of plasma amino acids	Elevation in plasma amino acids, aminoaciduria, and negative nitrogen balance
Decreased production of albumin and prothrombin	↓ Albumin → ↓ COP → edema ↓ Prothrombin → possible ↑ bleeding time

*Adapted from Jones, D. A., Dunbar, C. F., and Jirovec, M. M.: Medical-Surgical Nursing, A Conceptual Approach. New York, McGraw-Hill Book Company, 1978, p. 640.

HEPATOCELLULAR DISEASE

Since the cells of the liver play such a central role in the metabolic processing of nutrients, it stands to reason that hepatic disease will cause some degree of physiological imbalance. Although disruptions are not always predictable, a variety of potential changes can be identified.

In cases of hepatocellular disease, decreases in glycogenesis, glycogenolysis, gluconeogenesis, lipogenesis, and fatty acid oxidation are characteristically noted. As liver cells fail to extract and metabolize plasma amino acids, they accumulate in the bloodstream and trigger the release of glucagon from the pancreas. Subsequent stimulation of gluconeogenesis by glucagon will promote insulin secretion, and hyper- or hypoglycemia may develop, depending upon which of the pancreatic hormones takes precedence.

Manifestations of metabolic dysfunction are varied and reflect the specific nature of chemical imbalance. In cases of hypoglycemia, increased secondary mobilization of fats and proteins will cause the development of keto-acidosis. Depression of lipogenesis, on the other hand, is often reflected by a decrease in

serum cholesterol levels, while impaired protein metabolism will frequently result in decreased production of albumin and prothrombin. Some major metabolic disturbances associated with hepatocellular disease are summarized in Table 15.5.

ENDOCRINE DYSFUNCTION

Since the endocrine system is instrumental in regulating metabolic activity within the liver, various hormonal imbalances may cause secondary disruptions in nutrient utilization.

Cushing's syndrome provides a primary example of endocrine-induced metabolic disease. Characterized by elevated secretion of glucocorticoids by the adrenal cortex, it can result from an adrenocortical tumor or from excessive stimulation of the adrenal gland by pituitary-mediated ACTH hormone. In either case, dysfunction is characterized by a variety of metabolically based symptoms:

1. Hyperglycemia is often noted, secondary to excessive gluconeogenesis.

2. Atrophy of the skin, muscle weakness, and poor wound healing frequently result from the combined effects of suppressed protein synthesis and increased utilization of amino acids in the production of glucose.

3. Redistribution of adipose tissue, with accumulation of fat in the trunk, neck, and face ("moon face"), is a common symptom. The mechanism responsible for this has not as yet been elucidated.

It can be seen that many manifestations of Cushing's syndrome reflect underlying metabolic disturbances. Other hormonal imbalances that may disrupt functional activity within the liver include hypo- and hyperthyroidism and Addison's disease. Some characteristic manifestations of these disorders are summarized in Table 15.6.

Disorders that Disrupt the Intracellular Aspect of Metabolism

Ultimately, cellular survival depends upon the ability of cells to utilize available nutrients for growth, repair, and energy generation. The reader is referred to Chapter 2 for

TABLE 15.6 **Some Endocrine Imbalances That Disrupt Functional Activity Within the Liver**

Hormonal Imbalance	Effect upon Hepatic Metabolism	Manifestations
Cushing's syndrome (elevated secretion of glucocorticoids)	Stimulates gluconeogenesis	Hyperlgycemia
	Suppresses protein synthesis	Muscular weakness; poor wound healing
	Redistribution of adipose tissue	Fat deposit in trunk, neck, and face "Moon face"
Addison's disease (adrenocortical insufficiency)	Depresses gluconeogenesis	Hypoglycemia
		Muscular weakness
		Mental and emotional changes
	May deplete liver glycogen in attempt to counteract hypoglycemia	
Hypothyroidism	Depresses protein synthesis	Possible decrease in colloid osmotic pressure
		Possible disruption of immune mechanism
	Disruption of cholesterol metabolism	Increase in serum cholesterol levels
		Associated atherosclerotic changes
Hyperthyroidism	Stimulates lipolysis	Weight loss
	Promotes conversion of cholesterol to bile acids	Decrease in serum cholesterol levels

a detailed elucidation of intracellular metabolism. In general, it can be said that intracellular metabolic dysfunction stems primarily from two kinds of disorders: (1) those characterized by interference with the transport of nutrients from interstitial into intracellular fluid, and (2) those characterized by deficit of enzymes or other factors essential to intracellular chemical reactions.

DISRUPTION OF INTRACELLULAR TRANSPORT

The transport of glucose (the preferred metabolic fuel) into body cells is facilitated most directly by the action of insulin, a hormone secreted by the beta cells of the pancreas. When insufficient insulin is produced, a condition known as diabetes mellitus occurs. To fully understand the nature of this disease, it is necessary to take a closer look at the metabolic process itself.

Normally, plasma glucose levels range between 80 and 100 mg. per cent. Immediately after eating, of course, carbohydrate absorption causes these values to increase. In the healthy individual, maintenance of homeostasis is promoted by two mechanisms: (1) the extraction of excess glucose from the portal vein by hepatic cells, and (2) the transport of glucose into adipose and muscle cells, as facilitated by insulin. If insulin levels are deficient, excessive quantities of glucose will accumulate in the bloodstream, resulting in a condition described as hyperglycemia.

When glucose is unable to pass into the intracellular fluid compartment, the cells are forced to draw upon other nutrients as a source of metabolic fuel. Lipids are often mobilized first and broken down into fatty acids and glycerol through a process known as lipolysis. Whereas glycerol can be converted into glucose, via gluconeogenesis, fatty acids are typically changed into ketone bodies. To the extent that fats are being excessively mobilized, increases in the generation of acidic ketone bodies will cause the development of ketosis and acidosis.

Further complicating these metabolic imbalances are fluid and electrolyte disturbances that arise secondarily. As glucose and ketones increase in concentration, they filter into the nephron in excessive quantities. Since both glucose and ketone bodies osmotically attract water, they draw a large volume of fluid into the urine. Resulting hypovolemia may lead to shock, if the depletion is of significant magnitude.

Vascular changes are also characteristically associated with diabetes mellitus. Alterations in the structure of small blood vessels most commonly leads to retinal dysfunction, and occlusion of larger vessels can cause cerebral or myocardial ischemia.

The nervous system also may be affected, as peripheral neurons exhibit a loss of myelin. Resulting clinical symptoms include pain, motor weakness, muscular atrophy, nocturnal diarrhea, and impotence. In later stages of the disease, characteristic renal dysfunction frequently causes manifestations of proteinuria and hypertension.

DISRUPTION OF INTRACELLULAR ENZYMES

In order to effectively utilize nutrients as metabolic fuel, a large number of intracellular enzymes are needed to catalyze the chemical reactions involved in glycolysis and the citric acid cycle. In the absence of these enzymes, a substantial reduction in cellular energy generation can result.

Most commonly, metabolism is facilitated by the presence of vitamins and minerals that function primarily as intracellular enzymes or coenzymes. A summary of some of the major substances essential to metabolism is presented in Table 15.7. Nutritional deficiency of any one of these factors could considerably alter the nature of intracellular chemical reactions.

Lack of vitamin B_1, for example, causes a defect in carbohydrate metabolism, which is characterized by an inability to utilize pyruvic acid. Increased levels of pyruvate in the plasma are believed to be responsible for the clinical symptoms of peripheral neuritis and cardiac failure.

Vitamin B_2 and niacin both function as cofactors for enzymes that catalyze intracellular oxidation. Whereas riboflavin deficiency typically results in a depression of metabolic

TABLE 15.7 **Some Vitamins and Minerals Essential to Cellular Metabolism**

Substance	Metabolic Significance
Vitamin B_1 (thiamine)	Serves as coenzyme for 24 different enzymes of the Krebs cycle.
Vitamin B_2 (riboflavin)	Component of certain coenzymes involved in carbohydrate and protein metabolism.
Niacin (nicotinamide)	Component of certain coenzymes involved in cellular energy generation.
Vitamin B_6 (pyridoxine)	Coenzyme in amino acid metabolism.
Panthothenic acid	Essential for conversion of pyruvic acid into acetyl COA; gluconeogenesis of amino acids and lipids.
Biotin	Serves as one coenzyme in breakdown of pyruvic acid via Krebs cycle.
Phosphorus	Component of ATP and ADP; essential to energy storage.
Iron	Component of cytochromes; involved in electron transfer and energy generation via Krebs cycle.
Iodine	Component of hormone thyroxin, which helps to regulate metabolic rate.
Magnesium	Critical constituent of some coenzymes.

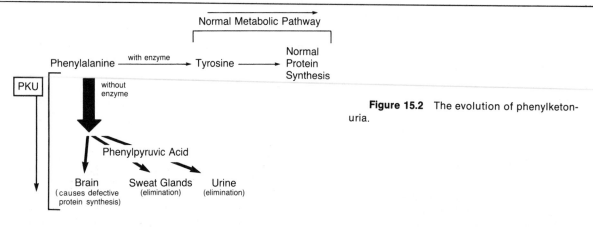

Figure 15.2 The evolution of phenylketon-uria.

rate, lack of niacin causes the development of characteristic lesions on the skin and mucous membranes.

The metabolism of amino acids is specifically facilitated by the presence of pyridoxine. Deficiency can lead to skin lesions around the eyes, nose, mouth, and tongue as well as hypochromic, microcytic anemia and, in severe cases, convulsions caused by damage to the central nervous system.

Pantothenic acid and biotin serve as coenzymes in the metabolism of fat. Since these substances are usually widely available, clinical deficit is not commonly noted.

In considering the effect of enzymes upon intracellular metabolism, it is important to realize that deficits are not always caused by nutritional imbalances. Since genes dictate protein formation, and enzymes are protein molecules, genetic defects may also be responsible for enzyme lack. Phenylketonuria (PKU), galactosemia, and gout are primary examples of genetically induced metabolic dysfunction.

Phenylketonuria is a disorder caused by the lack of an enzyme needed to convert the amino acid phenylalanine into tyrosine. As illustrated in Figure 15.2, phenylalanine and its keto derivatives subsequently accumulate in the bloodstream, causing disruption of neural myelinization and cerebral maturation. Mental retardation will result unless the newborn is placed on a phenylalanine-restricted diet.

In cases of galactosemia, the enzyme needed to convert the milk sugar galactose into glucose is lacking. Galactose and its de-rivatives thus accumulate in plasma, and interfere with the development of the brain, the eyes, and the liver. Retardation, cataracts, and cirrhosis will result unless lactose is eliminated from the diet.

Gout is a disorder characterized by elevations in the plasma levels of uric acid. Normally, uric acid is generated as an end product of purine metabolism and eliminated in the urine. Primary gout develops when genetically induced metabolic errors cause an increase in formation or a decrease in excretion of uric acid. Although the exact nature of the causative defect has not as yet been established, the result is the deposit of urate salts in joints and connective tissue. Ultimately, the disease can lead to chronic painful arthritis in all four limbs and renal failure (if urate stones deposit in the kidneys).

It can be seen that when intracellular enzymes are lacking or deficient, metabolism can be seriously disrupted. It is also important to realize that even when these enzymes are present, their functional activity is largely regulated by endocrine secretions and neuro-transmitters.

The male sex hormone, growth hormone, epinephrine and norepinephrine (released by the adrenal medulla), and thyroxine are all known to stimulate the rate of intracellular chemical reactions. Since thyroxine production is dependent upon the presence of sufficient quantities of iodine, lack of this mineral can secondarily disrupt the metabolic process.

The sympathetic nervous system also plays a significant role in modifying the meta-

TABLE 15.8 **Factors That Modify Metabolic Rate**

Promote Increase in Metabolic Rate	Promote Decrease in Metabolic Rate
Sympathetic neural stimulation	Depressed thyroxine secretion
Hormones	Sleep
Male sex hormone	Prolonged malnutrition
Norepinephrine	Tropical climate
Thyroxine	Old age
Growth hormone	
Fever	
Muscular exercise	
Cold climate	

bolic rate. Release of norepinephrine by postganglionic sympathetic neurons stimulates chemical activity in most body tissues. A summary of some of the primary factors that affect the functional activity of intracellular enzymes is presented in Table 15.8.

CLINICAL MANIFESTATIONS OF CELLULAR NUTRIENT DEFICIT

When cellular nutrient supply or utilization is inadequate, both anabolism and catabolism will be disrupted. Deficient growth, repair, and energy generation will predictably cause weakness and tissue wasting. At the extreme, metabolic rate may drop by as much as 20 to 30 per cent.

In cases of cellular nutrient deficit, specific symptoms often reflect the particular nature of the causative disorder. When deprivation is characterized by decreased availability of proteins, for example, changes are noted in the formation of structural tissue, enzymes, certain acid-base buffers, and immune factors. Since proteins are largely responsible for the maintenance of plasma colloid osmotic pressure, deficit can also affect intercompartmental fluid distribution within the body. Typically, a drop in colloid osmotic pressure will promote the evolution of edema, as fluid accumulates excessively within the interstitial compartment.

Kwashiorkor is a disease of young children that provides a classic example of the effects of protein malnutrition. Characteristically noted in economically deprived, underdeveloped countries, it is usually associated with a high-carbohydrate, low-protein diet. As illustrated in Figure 15.3, afflicted youngsters show symptoms of muscle wasting, growth retardation, edema, and ascites. Loss of surface skin, diarrhea, and anemia may further complicate the clinical picture.

Whereas proteins function significantly in tissue formation, enzymatic activity, buffering, immunity, and fluid distribution, fats are utilized primarily for energy generation, myelinization of neurons, production of bile salts, and manufacture of certain lipid-derived hormones in the body. Of greatest clinical relevance is the metabolic role played by fats in the absence of readily available carbohydrates. It has been found that fatty acids and ketone bodies are the preferred cellular fuels in cases of monosaccharide deficit. As a result, amino acids and proteins can be spared during early stages of starvation and utilized only minimally in the process of catabolism. At the extremes of nutrient deficit, however, lipid reserves may become totally depleted. In these cases, proteins will be rapidly mobilized from body tissue, causing severe structural disequilibrium. Death will usually result within 24 hours.

The effect of starvation upon food stores in the body is illustrated in Figure 15.4. It can be seen that caloric deprivation triggers the immediate depletion of carbohydrate reserves. Under these conditions, proteins and fats remain as the sole sources of metabolic fuel. Initially, both of these nutrients are utilized in the generation of cellular energy. While proteins are converted into glucose by hepatic cells, lipids are used in the production of acidic ketone bodies. After a short time, these ketone bodies become the primary cellular fuel and are fed into the citric acid cycle to service metabolic needs. In this way, amino acids can be spared further depletion and are utilized only during the terminal stages of starvation, when lipid reserves have been totally exhausted. Some primary manifestations of cellular nutrient deficit are elucidated in Figure 15.5.

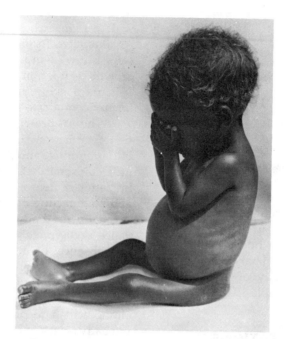

Figure 15.3 *A,* An African child suffering from kwashiorkor, the regional name for protein malnutrition. Note uncurled, graying hair, edema and skin lesions. The condition is common in areas where diets are high in starchy foods and low in protein and can be cured by protein-rich foods or by skim milk. (Courtesy Food and Agriculture Organization of the United Nations. Photo by M. Autret).

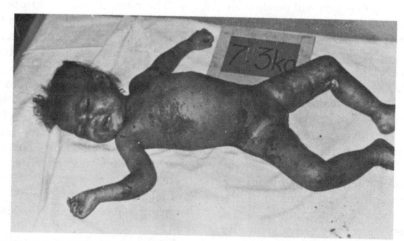

Figure 15.3 *B,* Dermatosis of kwashiorkor. (From: McLaren, D. S., and Burman, D.: Textbook of Paediatric Nutrition. New York, Longman, 1976, p. 123. © 1976 by Longman Group Ltd.)

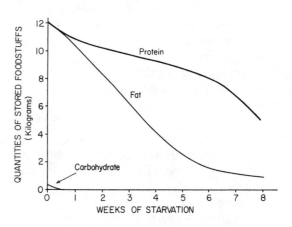

Figure 15.4 The effect of starvation upon food stores in the body. (From Guyton, A. C.: Textbook of Medical Physiology, 6th ed. Philadelphia, W. B. Saunders Company, 1978. Used by permission.)

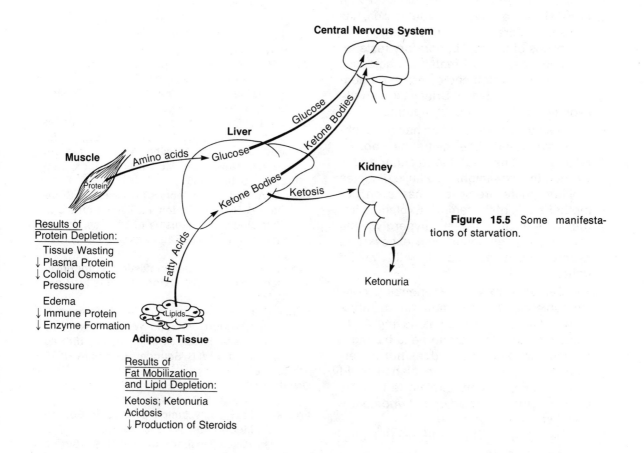

Figure 15.5 Some manifestations of starvation.

Study Questions

1. The following disorders may interfere with nutrient ingestion. In each case, determine whether dysfunction originates in (a) the nervous system, or (b) the muscular system:
   a. multiple sclerosis
   b. myasthenia gravis
   c. muscular dystrophy
   d. tetanus
   e. CVA

2. Briefly describe how or why each of the following disorders could disrupt cellular nutrient supply:
   a. peptic ulcer
   b. vasogenic shock
   c. celiac disease
   d. myocardial infarction
   e. pancreatitis
   f. spinal cord transection

3. A patient is admitted to the hospital with cirrhosis of the liver. He is edematous, has lost a considerable amount of weight, and complains of fatigue. Laboratory tests reveal the existence of metabolic acidosis, decreases in serum cholesterol, and negative nitrogen balance. Briefly explain the evolution of his clinical symptoms.

4. Mrs. Fagan is diagnosed as having Cushing's syndrome. She hears her doctor talking about her high blood sugar and is worried that she might also have diabetes mellitus (there are several cases on her mother's side of the family). Explain to her the difference between hyperglycemia secondary to glucocorticoid excess and hyperglycemia associated with insulin deficit.

5. Mr. Parker, who was experiencing considerable mental and emotional instability, was finally diagnosed as having Addison's disease. He is afraid he is having a nervous breakdown and does not understand how an endocrine imbalance could cause his depression. Explain to him the effect of glucocorticoid deficit upon emotional stability.

6. Why is a patient with unregulated diabetes mellitus susceptible to the development of metabolic acidosis?

7. Mr. Hoffman, who is 68 years old, is being examined for general fatigue and malaise. His doctor recommends a multivitamin capsule to supplement his rather limited diet. He thinks that "all those pills" don't have any real value; they're just like taking a "sugar capsule." Explain the significance of vitamins to the nutritional status of the body, giving specific examples.

8. Baby Tillis is diagnosed as having PKU. What causes this disorder, and what is the prognosis?

9. Why will starvation predictably cause ketonuria?

Suggested Readings

Books

Alyn, I. B.: Disturbances in hepatic function. *In* Jones, D. A., Dunbar, C. F., and Jirovec, M. M.: Medical-Surgical Nursing, A Conceptual Approach. New York, McGraw-Hill Book Company, 1978, p. 639.

Bacchus, H.: Essentials of Metabolic Diseases and Endocrinology. Baltimore, University Park Press, 1976.

Beck, R. R.: Hormonal regulation of intermediary metabolism. *In* Selkurt, E. E. (ed.): Basic Physiology for the Health Sciences. Boston, Little, Brown & Company, 1975, p. 293.

Braden, B.: Disturbances in ingestion. *In* Jones, D. A., Dunbar, C. F., and Jirovec, M. M.: Medical-Surgical Nursing, A Conceptual Approach. New York, McGraw-Hill Book Company, 1978, p. 555.

Bray, G. A.: Nutritional factors in disease. *In* Sodeman, W. A., and Sodeman, T. M.: Pathologic Physiology, Mechanisms of Disease, 6th ed. Philadelphia, W. B. Saunders Company, 1979, p. 971.

Brooks, F. P. (ed.): Gastrointestinal Pathophysiology. New York, Oxford University Press, 1974.

Cahill, G. F., Jr.: Diabetes mellitus. *In* Beeson, P. B., McDermott, W., and Wyngaarden, J. B. (eds.): Cecil Textbook of Medicine, 15th ed. Philadelphia, W. B. Saunders Company, 1979, p. 1969.

Davidson, C. S.: Liver Pathophysiology. Boston, Little, Brown & Company, 1970.

Freinkel, N.: Hypoglycemic disorders. *In* Beeson, P. B., McDermott, W., and Wyngaarden, J. B. (eds.): Cecil Textbook of Medicine, 15th ed. Philadelphia, W. B. Saunders Company, 1979, p. 1989.

Grieg, J. L.: Dysfunction of liver and related

structures. *In* Phipps, W. J., Long, B. C., and Woods, N. F. (eds.): Medical-Surgical Nursing, Concepts and Clinical Practice. St. Louis, The C. V. Mosby Company, 1979, p. 626.

Guyton, A. C.: Textbook of Medical Physiology, 5th ed. Philadelphia, W. B. Saunders Company, 1976, pp. 893–901; 936–944; 970–986; 1019–1051.

Hole, J. W.: Human Anatomy and Physiology. Dubuque, Wm. C. Brown Company, 1978, pp. 451–485.

Iber, F. L.: Normal and pathologic physiology of the liver. *In* Sodeman, W. A., and Sodeman, T. M.: Pathologic Physiology, Mechanisms of Disease, 6th ed. Philadelphia, W. B. Saunders Company, 1979, p. 885.

Jeffries, G. H.: Diseases of the Liver. *In* Beeson, P. B., McDermott, W., and Wyngaarden, J. B. (eds.): Cecil Textbook of Medicine, 15th ed. Philadelphia, W. B. Saunders Company, 1979, p. 1637.

Kent, T. H., Hart, M. N., and Shires, T. K.: Introduction to Human Disease. New York, Appleton-Century-Crofts, 1979, pp. 151–188; 436–442.

Levine, R., and Laft, R. (eds.): Advances in Metabolic Disorders, Vol. 7. New York, Academic Press, 1974.

Liddle, G. W.: Adrenal cortex. *In* Beeson, P. B., McDermott, W., and Wyngaarden, J. B. (eds.): Cecil Textbook of Medicine, 15th ed. Philadelphia, W. B. Saunders Company, 1979, p. 2144.

Luckmann, J., and Sorensen, K. C.: Medical-Surgical Nursing, A Pathophysiologic Approach, 2nd ed. Philadelphia, W. B. Saunders Company, 1980, pp. 1385–1464; 1469–1487; 1495–1512; 1542–1577; 1599–1621.

Mitten, C. J., and Phipps, W. J.: Endocrine dysfunction. *In* Phipps, W. J., Long, B. C., and Woods, N. F. (eds.): Medical-Surgical Nursing, Concepts and Clinical Practice. St. Louis, The C. V. Mosby Company, 1979, p. 568.

Mulrow, P. J.: Adrenal cortical insufficiency. *In* Conn, H. F. (ed.): Current Therapy 1980. Philadelphia, W. B. Saunders Company, 1980, p. 480.

Purtiilo, D. T.: A Survey of Human Diseases. Menlo Park, Addison-Wesley Publishing Company, 1978, pp. 242–258; 309–335.

Safer, N. G.: Disturbances in digestion. *In* Jones, D. A., Dunbar, C. F., and Jirovec, M. M.: Medical-Surgical Nursing, A Conceptual Approach. New York, McGraw-Hill Book Company, 1978, p. 583.

Schiff, L. (ed.): Diseases of the Liver, 4th ed. Philadelphia, J. B. Lippincott Company, 1975.

Schumann, D.: Disturbances in glucose metabo-

lism. *In* Jones, D. A., Dunbar, C. F., and Jirovec, M. M.: Medical-Surgical Nursing, A Conceptual Approach. New York, McGraw-Hill Book Company, 1978, p. 665.

Scrimshaw, N. S.: Deficiencies of individual nutrients: vitamin diseases. *In* Beeson, P. B., McDermott, W., and Wyngaarden, J. B. (eds.): Cecil Textbook of Medicine, 15th ed. Philadelphia, W. B. Saunders Company, 1979, p. 1684.

Scrimshaw, N. S.: Undernutrition, starvation, and hunger edema. *In* Beeson, P. B., McDermott, W., and Wyngaarden, J. B. (eds.): Cecil Textbook of Medicine, 15th ed. Philadelphia, W. B. Saunders Company, 1979, p. 1684.

Taylor, A. G., and Hamory, A. Z.: Hormonal disturbances and their effects upon metabolism. *In* Jones, D. A., Dunbar, C. F., and Jirovec, M. M.: Medical-Surgical Nursing, A Conceptual Approach. New York, McGraw-Hill Book Company, 1978, p. 697.

Tortora, G. H., and Anagnostakos, N. P.: Principles of Anatomy and Physiology, 2nd ed. San Francisco, Canfield Press, 1978, pp. 578–595.

Travis, R. H.: Cushing's syndrome. *In* Conn, H. F. (ed.): Current Therapy 1980. Philadelphia, W. B. Saunders Company, 1980, p. 481.

Articles

Blount, M., and Kinney, A. B.: Chronic steroid therapy. Am. J. Nurs., *74*:1626, 1974.

Carozza, V.: Ketoacidotic crisis: Mechanism and management, Nursing '73, *3*:13, 1973.

Cherner, R.: Ten pitfalls to avoid in managing diabetic ketoacidosis. Consultant, *17*:21, 1977.

DeJong, N.: CNS manifestations of diabetes mellitus. Postgrad. Med., *61*:101, 1977.

Diabetic ketoacidosis. Emergency Med., *5*:103, 1973.

Fredlund, P. N., and Mecklenburg, R. S.: Acute adrenal insufficiency: Diagnosis and management. Hosp. Med., *15*:28, 1979.

Kissebah, A. N.: Management of hyperlipidemia in diabetes. Am. Fam. Physician, *19*:144, 1979.

Kozak, G. P.: Primary adrenocortical insufficiency (Addison's disease). Am. Fam. Physician, *15*:124, 1977.

Martin, P.: It is ketoacidosis. J. Emergency Med., *3*:11, 1977.

McKenna, T. J.: Acute adrenal insufficiency. Hosp. Med., *12*:77, 1976.

Metabolic effects of glucocorticoids in man. Nutr. Rev., *32*:301, 1974.

Newton, D. W., et al.: Corticosteroids. Nursing '77, *7*:26, 1977.

Walesky, M. E.: Diabetic ketoacidosis. Am. J. Nurs., *78*:872, 1978.

Chapter Outline

chapter **16**

Diseases Affecting the Cellular Need for Elimination

Chapter Objectives

At the completion of this chapter, the student will be able to:

1. Differentiate between nondigestible and metabolic wastes.
2. Identify two pathological mechanisms that may disrupt the elimination of nondigestible wastes, and give examples of causative disorders.
3. Briefly describe the way in which lipids and amino acids are processed in the liver for utilization as metabolic fuels.
4. Identify two major pathological mechanisms that may disrupt the transport of carbon dioxide from metabolizing cells to the lungs, and give examples of causative disorders.
5. Identify four major pathological mechanisms that may disrupt the diffu-

sion of carbon dioxide from pulmonary capillaries into alveoli, and give examples of causative disorders.
6. Identify and describe two major pathological mechanisms that may interfere with the expiration of carbon dioxide and give examples of causative disorders.
7. Identify ten disorders that may interfere with the elimination of ketone bodies and urea.
8. Describe the clinical manifestations of (a) constipation, (b) hypercapnia, (c) ketosis, and (d) uremia.
9. Describe the way in which waste accumulation may cause disruption of cellular (a) oxygen supply, (b) nutrient supply, and (c) fluid/electrolyte and acid/base balance.

INTRODUCTION

In the process of providing for cellular needs, a number of waste products are formed that must be eliminated if homeostasis is to be maintained. Primary among these are:

1. Nondigestible wastes — which cannot be totally broken down and absorbed through the gastrointestinal tract. These products are normally excreted as feces.

2. Metabolic wastes — which are produced as the by-products of intracellular chemical reactions. Primary examples include carbon dioxide, nitrogenous wastes, and water.

To the extent that waste products are unable to be eliminated, physiological disequilibrium results. In subsequent pages, an elucidation of some major disorders that disrupt elimination is followed by an analysis of the clinical manifestations of imbalance.

DISORDERS THAT DISRUPT THE ELIMINATION OF NONDIGESTIBLE WASTES

The majority of ingested nutrients are destined to be broken down within the gastrointestinal tract and absorbed into the bloodstream. In this way, they are able to support metabolism and facilitate cellular growth, repair, and energy generation.

Materials that cannot be sufficiently degraded within the intestinal lumen form the primary constituents of feces. Typically, they are processed in the large intestine and are propelled into the rectum by a series of mass peristaltic waves. Ultimately, elimination occurs when the internal and external anal sphincter muscles relax.

Fecal retention develops most frequently as a consequence of gastrointestinal obstruction and/or motility failure. A summary of some major causes of impaired elimination of nondigestible wastes is presented in Table 16.1.

DISORDERS THAT DISRUPT THE ELIMINATION OF METABOLIC WASTES

To facilitate better understanding of metabolic waste elimination it is helpful to briefly review some of the basic mechanisms that govern nutrient utilization.

Carbohydrates are the preferred metabolic fuels for generation of cellular energy. Normally, absorbed monosaccharides are initially transported to the liver, where they are converted into glucose. Glucose, in turn, is circulated by the bloodstream to cells throughout the body. Glucose crosses the membrane into the intracellular fluid compartment and is ultimately broken down into carbon dioxide and

---

TABLE 16.1   **Disorders that Disrupt the Elimination of Nondigestible Wastes**

Pathological Mechanism	Causative Disorders	System Within Which Pathology Originates
Obstruction	Pyloric stenosis	Digestive
	Hernias	Digestive/skeletomuscular
	Inflammatory hyperplasia (Crohn's disease)	Digestive
	Adhesions	Digestive
	Volvulus	Digestive
	Intussusception	Digestive
	Paralytic ileus	Digestive
	Intraluminal neoplasm	Digestive
	Mesenteric ischemia	Cardiovascular
Motility failure	Atonic colon	Digestive/neural
	Megacolon	Neural
	Sacral cord trauma	Neural

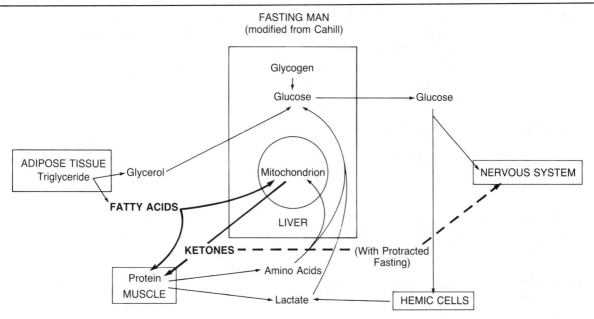

Figure 16.1 Metabolism during fasting in man. (Reprinted by permission of the New England Journal of Medicine *282*:668, 1970.)

water, with the associated release of utilizable energy.

In the event that carbohydrates are not available, fats and proteins can serve as alternative sources of fuel. To be optimally effective, however, these nutrients must first be processed by the liver into products that can be fed directly into the citric acid cycle.

As illustrated in Figure 16.1, lipids are characteristically mobilized and split into fatty acids and glycerol. In the process of readying fats for metabolic use, many fatty acids are typically converted into acidic ketone bodies. These substances frequently accumulate in plasma as by-products of lipid catabolism and are subsequently eliminated in the urine.

Amino acids, on the other hand, are normally carried to the liver, where the amino group (NH_2) is removed from the rest of the molecule. Although the deaminated amino acid can be utilized metabolically, the liberated amino component is converted by hepatic cells first into ammonia and then into urea. These chemical changes are summarized diagrammatically in Figure 16.2.

In summary, it can be said that water, carbon dioxide, ketone bodies, and urea are among the primary metabolic by-products in the body. Since excess or deficit of water can cause fluid and electrolyte imbalance, disor-

ders causing hyper- and hypovolemia will be discussed in Chapter 17. In the following pages, the disruption of carbon dioxide, ketone, and urea elimination will be emphasized.

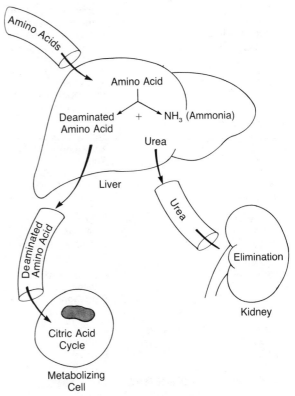

Figure 16.2 Protein metabolism.

TABLE 16.2   Disorders that Disrupt the Transport of Metabolic Wastes

Pathological Mechanism	Causative Disorders
Decrease in cardiac output	Myocardial infarction Valvular pathologies Cardiac arrhythmias Cardiac tamponade Congestive heart failure Hypovolemia
Disruption in the circulation of blood	Atherosclerosis Arteriosclerosis Thrombi Emboli Septic shock Neurogenic shock

Disorders that Disrupt the Elimination of Carbon Dioxide

The elimination of carbon dioxide from the body is dependent upon three major functional processes:

1. Transport — or the circulation of carbon dioxide from metabolizing cells, through the bloodstream, to the lungs.

2. Diffusion — or the transport of carbon dioxide from pulmonary capillaries into alveoli.

3. Expiration — or the passage of gases from the air sacs of the lungs, through the respiratory tree, out into the atmosphere. To the extent that any of these mechanisms is disrupted, carbon dioxide retention may result.

TABLE 16.3   Disorders that Disrupt Expiration

Pathological Mechanism	Causative Disorders	System Within Which Pathology Originates
ALTERATION OF THE RATE AND/OR RHYTHM OF VENTILATION		
Increased intracranial pressure affecting the respiratory center of the brain	Cerebral contusion Subdural or epidural hematoma Cerebrovascular occlusion or hemorrhage accompanied by edema Brain tumors Meningitis Encephalitis Overdose of anesthetics or narcotics	Nervous system
Interference with the neural stimulation of respiratory muscles	Poliomyelitis Guillain-Barré syndrome Myasthenia gravis Tetanus Botulism	Nervous system
INCREASES IN THE WORK OF VENTILATION		
Decreased compliance of the lungs and/or thorax	Scoliosis Kyphosis Extensive rib fractures	Skeletal system
	Abdominal pain or distention	Digestive system
Pulmonary fibrosis	Chronic obstructive pulmonary disease (COPD) Pneumonia Tuberculosis	Respiratory system
Resistance to the transport of air through the respiratory tree	COPD Cystic fibrosis Bronchiectasis Lung cancer	Respiratory system

Since transport is primarily mediated by a functional cardiovascular system, carbon dioxide elimination may be disrupted if the heart and/or blood vessels are unable to supply the cells with an adequate quantity of circulating blood. Pathological changes can be triggered by a variety of disorders, as outlined in Table 16.2.

Diffusion disorders, on the other hand, are most commonly associated with four major phenomena:

1. Disruption of alveolar ventilation.
2. Disruption of alveolar perfusion.
3. Ventilation/perfusion imbalances.
4. Diseases affecting the "respiratory membrane."

A number of causative disorders are elucidated in Chapter 14 (see Table 14.2).

Expiration normally constitutes the final step in the elimination of carbon dioxide. As thoracic volume decreases, resulting intrapulmonic compression forces gases to move from where they are under greater pressure (in the lungs) to where they are under lesser pressure (in the atmosphere). Ventilation pathology, as outlined in Table 16.3, thus frequently results in hypercapnia.

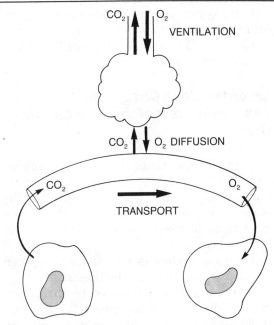

Figure 16.3 Respiratory gas disequilibrium: a schematic presentation.

In considering disorders associated with carbon dioxide retention, it is important to note that causative mechanisms simultaneously play a central role in the disruption of

TABLE 16.4 **Renal Pathology**

Type of Renal Failure	Nature of Pathology	Examples of Causative Disorders
ACUTE RENAL FAILURE	Prerenal	Cardiovascular pathology
	Intrarenal	Acute poststreptococcal glomerulonephritis Acute pyelonephritis Renal poisoning Transfusion reaction
	Postrenal	Prostatic enlargement Neoplasms Ureteral/urethral obstruction
CHRONIC RENAL FAILURE	Glomerular pathology	Systemic lupus erythematosus (SLE) Acute poststreptococcal glomerulonephritis Antiglomerular basement membrane nephritis Serum sickness nephritis Diabetic glomerulosclerosis
	Tubular/interstitial pathology	Nephrosclerosis Chronic pyelonephritis Chronic analgesic nephritis Ureteral/urethral obstruction

cellular oxygen supply. Disorders of transport, diffusion, and/or ventilation may, therefore, cause disequilibrium on several different levels, as illustrated in Figure 16.3.

Disorders that Disrupt the Elimination of Ketone Bodies and Urea

Both ketone bodies and urea are eliminated primarily through the kidneys. They are transported to the nephrons through the bloodstream and are initially filtered from the glomerulus into Bowman's capsule. Ultimately, as constituents of urine, they are carried through the ureters to the bladder and then out of the body through the urethra.

Any disease characterized by disruption of renal filtration and/or depressed micturition could lead to ketosis and uremia. A summary of some disorders causing renal pathology is presented in Table 16.4.

CLINICAL MANIFESTATIONS OF WASTE ACCUMULATION

Waste accumulation can initiate many different pathological responses in the body. To a large extent, specific manifestations vary according to the substances being retained. It is, thus, helpful to look separately at the effects of (1) constipation, (2) hypercapnia, (3) ketosis, and (4) uremia upon physiological equilibrium.

Constipation

Since constipation is often a reflection of a more serious problem, associated manifestations will vary according to the cause.

Assuming normal dietary and bowel habits, sustained inability to eliminate feces may frequently be caused by an obstructive or paralytic disorder. If dysfunction originates in the small intestine, waste retention may be accompanied by a variety of secondary changes, including:

1. The excessive accumulation of fluid within the intestinal lumen, as secretion exceeds absorption.
2. The shift of fluid and bacteria from the intestinal lumen into the abdominopelvic cavity, as inflammatory changes promote increases in permeability.
3. The vomiting of intestinal contents, as ingested nutrients accumulate and are unable to be expelled as feces.

Because of fluid shifts and losses, hypotension and shock frequently occur. A drop in blood pressure is also caused by intestinal bacteria, as the toxins they release into the plasma promote systemic vasodilation.

Regardless of the cause, occlusion and motility failure are generally associated with pain, distention, and vomiting.

Excess Carbon Dioxide

When carbon dioxide accumulates excessively in plasma, hypercapnia is said to exist. With elevations in pCO_2, there is a characteristic increase in the formation of carbonic acid, and respiratory acidosis develops.

Generally, acidosis will cause central nervous system depression, with associated symptoms of confusion, delirium, and possible coma. Hyperkalemia is frequently noted as excess hydrogen ions shift into the intracellular fluid and potassium ions move into the interstitial compartment to maintain electrical neutrality. Resulting increases in the concentration of plasma potassium will cause a variety of symptoms, including abdominal distention, vomiting, skeletal muscle weakness, shallow respirations, and cardiac arrhythmias.

Functional hypercalcemia may also develop, as acidosis causes the balance between protein-bound and ionized calcium to shift in favor of the latter. In these cases, additional manifestations of decreased muscular tone, weakness, lethargy, and cardiac stimulation will occur.

If the elevation in pCO_2 is a short-term phenomenon, stimulation of the respiratory center in the medulla typically triggers a compensatory increase in respiratory rate. To the extent that hypercapnia is chronic and sustained, however, the brain stem becomes desensitized to the effects of carbon dioxide, and hyperventilation is not characteristically noted.

Once respiratory acidosis has been established, a number of mechanisms help restore acid-base equilibrium. Primary among these is renal compensation, characterized by the secretion of hydrogen ions and retention of bicarbonate. The kidneys therefore play a significant role in bringing about a return to equilibrium.

Excess Ketone Bodies

Although ketosis can be exacerbated by renal failure, it is most frequently caused by metabolic imbalances that trigger excessive mobilization of fats. To the degree that the kidneys are unable to handle the elevated load of acidic ketone bodies, metabolic acidosis will develop.

As in cases of respiratory acidosis, general symptoms reflect functional disruptions of the central nervous system, potassium balance, and calcium balance. Compensation in these cases, however, is largely dependent upon respiratory mechanisms. Kussmaul respirations facilitate carbon dioxide elimination and cause an associated decrease in plasma carbonic acid levels. With depletion in the total pool of extracellular fluid hydrogen ions, pH values shift back toward the normal range of 7.35 to 7.45.

Excess Urea

When renal failure causes retention of urea, a number of related nitrogenous waste products will also accumulate in the plasma. Characteristically, increases in urea are accompanied by elevations in creatinine, phe-

nols, and guanidines. The resulting condition is referred to as *azotemia*.

Associated physiological disequilibrium is often widespread and reflects the generally toxic nature of these protein derivatives. In the uremic environment, red blood cells are believed to hemolyze more readily, thereby promoting the development of anemia. There is also an increased predisposition toward the formation of gastrointestinal ulcers. If bleeding from these lesions is extensive, hypovolemia and shock can develop. Changes in appearance are noted, as abnormal deposits of urinary pigment cause the skin to take on a waxy yellow to ashen gray hue. At the extreme, fine white urea crystals may be found on the skin surface. This occurs when the sweat glands attempt to compensate for renal failure by eliminating large quantities of nitrogenous wastes in perspiration.

Summary: Clinical Manifestations of Waste Accumulation

In summary, it can be said that failure to eliminate wastes from the body may trigger extensive disequilibrium. Ultimately, the physiological dysfunction caused by waste retention will interfere with the servicing of all cellular needs. Secondary deficits in oxygen and nutrient supply frequently develop, and fluid and electrolyte imbalances are common. A review of some major disruptions associated with waste accumulation is presented in Table 16.5.

TABLE 16.5   **The Retention of Wastes: Disruption of Cellular Equilibrium**

Cellular Need Disrupted	Pathological Mechanism
OXYGEN SUPPLY	Azotemia → Bleeding ulcers / Anemia } → Depression of O₂ transport to cells
NUTRIENT SUPPLY	Fecal retention → Vomiting → Decrease in available cellular nutrients CO₂ retention / Ketosis → Acidosis → Hyperkalemia → Vomiting → Decrease in available cellular nutrients
FLUID AND ELECTROLYTE BALANCE	Fecal retention → Vomiting → Hypovolemia; electrolyte and acid/base imbalances CO₂ retention → Respiratory acidosis Ketosis → Metabolic acidosis Azotemia → Possible gastrointestinal bleeding → Hypovolemia

STUDY QUESTIONS

1. Determine whether the following disorders would interfere most directly with the elimination of (a) nondigestible, or (b) metabolic wastes:
   a. Acute poststreptococcal glomerulonephritis
   b. Hernia
   c. Emphysema
   d. Pyloric stenosis
   e. Diabetic glomerulosclerosis
   f. Crohn's disease
   g. Hypovolemic shock
   h. Volvulus

2. Mrs. Zonet is admitted to the hospital with gastrointestinal discomfort associated with fecal retention. List five disorders that could be causative.

3. Mr. Wells is suffering from cirrhosis of the liver. Explain how or why hepatic pathology could interfere with the elimination of urea via the kidneys.

4. Briefly describe how or why the following disorders could interfere with the elimination of carbon dioxide from the body:
   a. Bronchiectasis
   b. Myocardial infarction (MI)
   c. Myasthenia gravis
   d. Chronic obstructive pulmonary disease (COPD)
   e. Pleural inflammation
   f. Cardiac tamponade
   g. Left heart failure
   h. Septic shock

5. In each of the following disorders, briefly describe how or why ketosis and acidosis would develop:
   a. Acute poststreptococcal glomerulonephritis
   b. Enlargement of the prostate gland
   c. Hypovolemia
   d. Chronic pyelonephritis

6. Failure to eliminate wastes may disrupt homeostasis in many different ways. In each of the following situations, trace the way in which cellular oxygen supply, cellular nutrient supply, and/or fluid and electrolyte balance may be disrupted. In each case, list some associated clinical manifestations of pathology.
   a. Paralytic ileus
   b. Chronic renal failure
   c. COPD

Suggested Readings

Books

Alfrey, A. C., and Butkus, D. E.: Renal failure: Pathophysiology and management. *In* Hudak, C. M., Lohr, T., and Gallo, B. M. (eds.): Critical Care Nursing, 2nd ed. Philadelphia, J. B. Lippincott Company, 1977, p. 319.

Bricker, N. S.: Acute renal failure. *In* Beeson, P. B., McDermott, W., and Wyngaarden, J. B. (eds.): Cecil Textbook of Medicine, 15th ed. Philadelphia, W. B. Saunders Company, 1979, p. 1367.

Broughton, J. O.: Pathophysiology of the respiratory system. *In* Hudak, C. M., Lohr, T., and Gallo, B. M. (eds.): Critical Care Nursing, 2nd ed. Philadelphia, J. B. Lippincott Company, 1977, p. 221.

Burgess, A.: The Nurse's Guide to Fluid and Electrolyte Balance, 2nd ed. New York, McGraw-Hill Book Company, 1979, pp. 146–182.

Busby, H. C.: Hepatic failure: ammonia intoxication. *In* Hudak, C. M., Lohr, T., and Gallo, B. M. (eds.): Critical Care Nursing, 2nd ed. Philadelphia, J. B. Lippincott Company, 1977, p. 503.

Daly, B. J., Phipps, W. J., and Brown, F. R.: Management of the person with impaired oxygen-carbon dioxide exchange. *In* Phipps, W. J., Long, B. C., and Woods, N. F. (eds.): Medical-Surgical Nursing: Concepts and Clinical Practice. St. Louis, The C. V. Mosby Company, 1979, p. 942.

Durham, N.: Assessment of gastrointestinal tract function. *In* Phipps, W. J., Long, B. C., and Woods, N. F. (eds.): Medical-Surgical Nursing: Concepts and Clinical Practice. St. Louis, The C. V. Mosby Company, 1979, p. 1218.

Edwards, V., and Murphy, M. A.: Disruptions in oxygen-carbon dioxide exchange mechanism. *In* Jones, D. A., Dunbar, C. F., and Jirovec, M. M. (eds.): Medical-Surgical Nursing: A Conceptual Approach. New York, McGraw-Hill Book Company, 1978, p. 1009.

Grant, M. M.: The kidney and fluid and electrolyte imbalances. *In* Jones, D. A., Dunbar, C. F., and Jirovec, M. M. (eds.): Medical-Surgical

Nursing: A Conceptual Approach. New York, McGraw-Hill Book Company, 1978, p. 493.

Guyton, A. C.: Textbook of Medical Physiology, 5th ed. Philadelphia, W. B. Saunders Company, 1976, pp. 501–513; 572–583; 893–901.

Hartman, C. E.: Disturbances in elimination. *In* Jones, D. A., Dunbar, C. F., and Jirovec, M. M. (eds.): Medical-Surgical Nursing: A Conceptual Approach, New York, McGraw-Hill Book Company, 1978, p. 611.

Kerr, D. N. S.: Chronic renal failure. *In* Beeson, P. B., McDermott, W., and Wyngaarden, J. B. (eds.): Cecil Textbook of Medicine, 15th ed. Philadelphia, W. B. Saunders Company, 1979, p. 1351.

Luckmann, J., and Sorensen, K. C.: Medical-Surgical Nursing: A Psychophysiologic Approach, 2nd ed. Philadelphia, W. B. Saunders Company, 1980, pp. 986–1012; 1200–1222; 1442–1458.

Miller, P. L.: Assessment of urinary function. *In* Phipps, W. J., Long, B. C., and Woods, N. F. (eds.): Medical-Surgical Nursing: Concepts and Clinical Practice. St. Louis, The C. V. Mosby Company, 1979, p. 1227.

Murray, J. F.: Respiratory failure. *In* Beeson, P. B., McDermott, W., and Wyngaarden, J. B. (eds.): Cecil Textbook of Medicine, 15th ed. Philadelphia, W. B. Saunders Company, 1979, p. 1021.

Nivinski, J., Durham, N., and Miller, P. L.: Management of the person with impaired elimination. *In* Phipps, W. J., Long, B. C., and Woods, N. F. (eds.): Medical-Surgical Nursing: Concepts and Clinical Practice. St. Louis, The C. V. Mosby Company, 1979, p. 1243.

Articles

Benson, J.: Simple chronic constipation. Postgrad. Med., *57*:55, Jan. 1975.

Biddle, T. L.: Acute pulmonary edema. Hosp. Med., *13*:56, Dec. 1977.

Cronin, R., et al.: Acute renal failure: Diagnosis, pathogenesis, and management. Hosp. Med., *12*:26, Aug. 1976.

Dack, S.: Acute pulmonary edema. Hosp. Med., *14*:112, Mar. 1978.

DelBueno, D. J.: A quick review on using blood-gas determinations. RN, *41*:68, Mar. 1978.

Ferguson, D. J.: Intestinal obstruction and paralytic ileus. Hosp. Med., *9*:8, Oct. 1973.

Flanagan, M.: Acute urinary retention. Hosp. Med., *12*:60, Sept. 1976.

Johnson, K., et al.: Nursing care of the patient with acute renal failure. Nursing Clin. North Am., *10*:421, 1975.

Kettel, L. J.: Acute respiratory acidosis. Hosp. Med., *12*:31, Feb. 1976.

Leman, J.: Acute renal failure. Am. Family Phys., *18*:146, Sept. 1978.

Mitchell, J.: Axioms on uremia. Hosp. Med., *14*:6, July 1978.

Simon, N., et al.: Chronic renal failure: Pathophysiology and medical management. Cardiovasc. Nurse, *12*:7, Mar./Apr. 1976.

Stahlgren, L. H., and Morris, N. W.: Intestinal obstruction. Am. J. Nursing, *77*:999, 1977.

Sweetwood, H.: Acute respiratory insufficiency: How to recognize this emergency . . . how to treat it. Nursing 77, *7*:24, Dec. 1977.

Wilson, R. F.: Acute respiratory failure and how to manage it. Consultant, *18*:25, May 1978.

Chapter Outline

INTRODUCTION

ENDOCRINE DISORDERS
    ADH
    The Corticosteroids
        ALDOSTERONE
        THE GLUCOCORTICOIDS
    Parathormone (PTH)
    Insulin

CARDIOVASCULAR DISORDERS

RESPIRATORY DISORDERS

RENAL DISORDERS

GASTROINTESTINAL DISORDERS

NEURAL DISORDERS

SUMMARY

Diseases Affecting the Cellular Need for Fluid-Electrolyte and Acid-Base Balance

Chapter Objectives

At the completion of this chapter, the student will be able to:

1. Describe the effects of ADH, corticosteroids, PTH, and insulin upon fluid-electrolyte and acid-base balance in the body.

2. Differentiate between aldosterone and the glucocorticoids, with respect to site of secretion, regulation of output, and causes of hypo- or hypersecretion.

3. Trace the evolution of fluid-electrolyte and acid-base imbalances initiated by cardiovascular pathology.

4. Describe why respiratory pathology frequently leads to: (a) metabolic acidosis, and (b) respiratory acidosis.

5. Identify the fluid and electrolyte imbalances characteristically associated with (a) prerenal pathology, (b) nephrotic syndrome, and (c) acute or chronic tubular pathology.

6. Differentiate between saliva, gastric juice, pancreatic juice, bile, and small intestinal juice with respect to pH and electrolyte composition.

7. Trace the evolution of fluid-electrolyte and acid-base imbalances secondary to (a) vomiting, (b) diarrhea, and (c) hepatic pathology.

8. Describe the way in which neural pathology may affect fluid-electrolyte and acid-base balance in the body.

INTRODUCTION

In earlier chapters, much attention was devoted to clarifying the mechanisms underlying fluid-electrolyte balance and imbalance. As understanding of pathophysiology grows, it is possible to integrate information and more specifically identify the way in which systemic dysfunction may affect cellular equilibrium. In the following pages, the relationship between disease and fluid-electrolyte/acid-base status will be elucidated. Causative disorders will be categorized systemically as endocrine, cardiovascular, respiratory, renal, gastrointestinal, or neural in origin.

ENDOCRINE DISORDERS

The endocrine glands in the body function significantly in the maintenance of homeostasis. The hormones specifically involved in the regulation of fluid-electrolyte and/or acid-base balance are ADH, corticosteroids, parathormone (PTH), and insulin.

ADH

ADH is produced by the hypothalamus and released from the posterior pituitary gland. Promoting reabsorption of water from the collecting ducts of the nephrons, ADH helps to regulate fluid balance. Normally, secretion of antidiuretic hormone is responsive to plasma solute concentration. Increases in plasma osmolarity trigger release of ADH, whereas decreasing solute concentrations inhibit ADH secretion. This regulatory feedback mechanism is illustrated in Figure 17.1.

When the body is unable to release sufficient quantities of antidiuretic hormone (as in cases of diabetes insipidus), urinary output will increase considerably. Since water is eliminated without proportional quantities of electrolytes, hypernatremia may result. Urine is characteristically dilute, and hypovolemia will ensue if fluid loss is not replaced.

Excessive release of ADH, on the other hand, causes water retention and hyponatremia. Urinary output decreases, and hypervolemia may result. Inappropriate secretion of ADH (SIADH) is known to be triggered by a number of factors, including anxiety, pain, surgical trauma, administration of certain barbiturates and anesthetics, and certain cerebral disorders.

The Corticosteroids

The cortex, or outer layer, of the adrenal glands secretes a number of hormones that are derived chemically from the steroid cholesterol. Described as corticosteroids, they differ with respect to site of production and functional activity. The *mineralocorticoids* (such as aldosterone) are released from the outermost zona glomerulosa of the cortex and act specifically to regulate renal reabsorption and secretion of water and select ions. The *glucocorticoids* (such as cortisol) function most significantly in modifying the metabolic utilization of carbohydrates, fats, and proteins but also play a role in fluid and electrolyte balance.

ALDOSTERONE

Whereas ADH directly regulates the renal reabsorption of water, aldosterone affects fluid volume only secondarily. The primary function of aldosterone is to promote the reab-

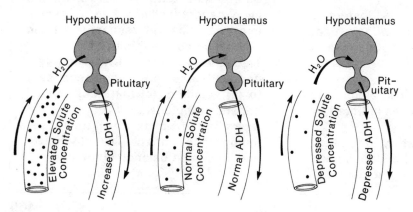

Figure 17.1 Regulation of ADH secretion.

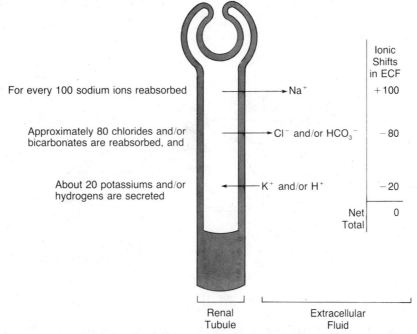

For every 100 sodium ions reabsorbed → Na⁺

Approximately 80 chlorides and/or bicarbonates are reabsorbed, and → Cl⁻ and/or HCO₃⁻

About 20 potassiums and/or hydrogens are secreted ← K⁺ and/or H⁺

Ionic Shifts in ECF

+100

−80

−20

Net Total | 0

Renal Tubule | Extracellular Fluid

Figure 17.2 Electrolyte exchanges associated with sodium reabsorption from the nephron.

sorption of sodium from the nephron into the plasma. Since water follows sodium passively into the extracellular fluid, the plasma concentration of sodium may remain relatively stable. Fluctuations in the secretion of aldosterone, however, can result in the development of hyper- or hypovolemia.

As illustrated in Figure 17.2, a number of electrolyte shifts are typically associated with sodium reabsorption. Designed to promote the maintenance of electrical neutrality and acid-base balance, they can be summarized as follows:

1. If electrical neutrality is to be maintained in the extracellular fluid, the reabsorption of a positively charged sodium ion must be balanced by the retention of an anion or the secretion of a cation.

2. Normally, for every 100 sodium ions reabsorbed, 80 chloride (Cl^-) and/or bicarbonate anions are retained, and a total of 20 potassium and/or hydrogen cations are eliminated.

3. The balance between hydrogen and potassium secretion is determined by the relative availability of these ions at any given time.

4. If potassium levels are depleted or hy-

drogen concentration is elevated, considerably more hydrogen than potassium will be eliminated.

5. Conversely, if hyperkalemia or alkalosis exists, potassium secretion will be favored.

6. As the kidneys compensate for acidosis or alkalosis, one must remember that bicarbonate (HCO_3^-) concentration will be indirectly affected.

7. The hydrogen ion secreted during acidosis is derived from carbonic acid as follows: $H_2CO_3 \rightarrow H^+ + HCO_3^-$.

8. A bicarbonate is thus released into plasma for every hydrogen ion eliminated. Under these circumstances, the negatively charged bicarbonate competes with chloride for affiliation with sodium, and chloride reabsorption declines.

9. Conversely, during alkalosis, relatively less hydrogen ion is secreted, less bicarbonate is generated, and more chloride is reabsorbed.

Normally, the secretion of aldosterone is most directly responsive to changing plasma potassium concentrations. It is additionally affected, however, by the renin-angiotensin mechanism (described in Chapter 5), plasma sodium levels, and the permissive effects of

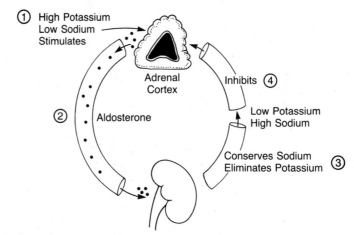

A, The release of aldosterone is directly responsive to the plasma concentration of potassium and sodium.

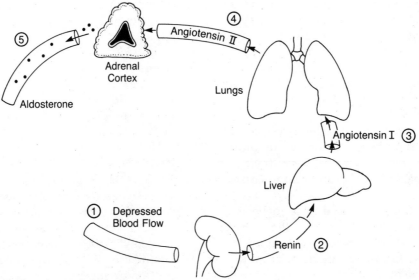

B, The release of aldosterone is also regulated by the renin-angiotensin mechanism.

Figure 17.3 Mechanisms governing the release of aldosterone.

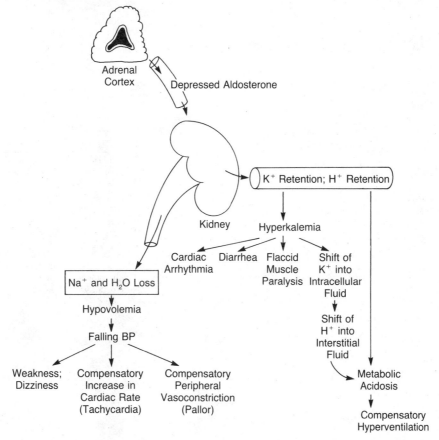

Figure 17.4 Symptoms associated with deficient aldosterone secretion (Addison's disease).

the anterior pituitary adrenocorticotropic hormone (ACTH). The feedback mechanisms governing the release of aldosterone are summarized in Figure 17.3.

Insufficient secretion of aldosterone is most typically associated with atrophy of the adrenal cortices. The accompanying clinical condition, Addison's disease, is characterized by fluid and electrolyte imbalance. Associated symptoms are summarized in Figure 17.4.

Hypersecretion of aldosterone, on the other hand, is usually caused by hyperplasia of the adrenal cortical cells that produce this hormone. If the pathological condition is triggered by an adrenal adenoma, it is referred to as primary aldosteronism. Associated clinical manifestations stem primarily from resulting hypervolemia, hypokalemia, or metabolic alkalosis, as illustrated in Figure 17.5.

THE GLUCOCORTICOIDS

Although most significant for their effects upon the metabolic utilization of carbohydrates, fats, and proteins, the glucocorticoids also affect fluid and electrolyte balance in the body. By mimicking the action of aldosterone upon the renal tubule, they influence the relative retention and elimination of water, sodium, potassium, chloride, and bicarbonate.

Unlike aldosterone, the secretion of glucocorticoids is primarily regulated by the corticotropic hormone of the anterior pituitary (see Figure 17.6). Whereas glucocorticoid deficit is commonly associated with Addison's disease, excesses can occur secondary to a number of different pathologies, as follows:

1. Increase in production caused by the

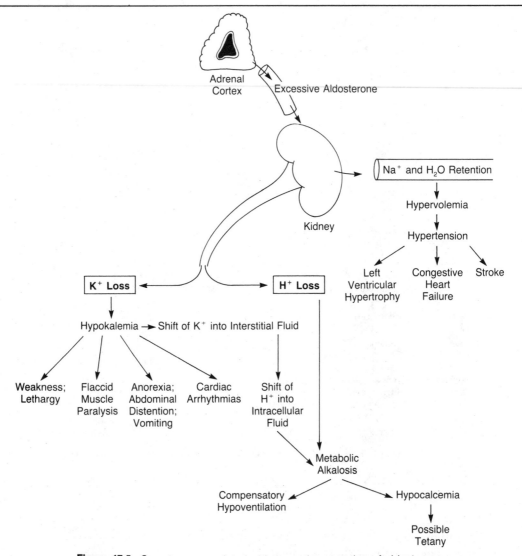

Figure 17.5 Symptoms associated with excessive secretion of aldosterone.

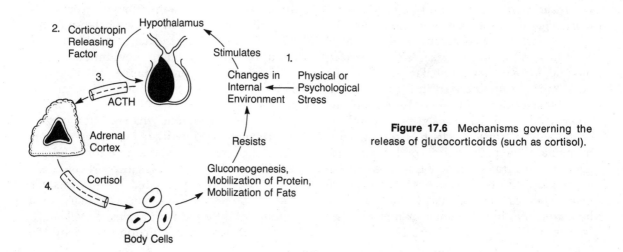

Figure 17.6 Mechanisms governing the release of glucocorticoids (such as cortisol).

TABLE 17.1 **Excessive Production of Glucocorticoids***

Condition	Responsible Lesion	Therapies	Remarks
Cushing's syndrome	Unilateral adrenal tumors (benign or malignant); bilateral adrenal tumors	*Adrenalectomy* (surgical excision of the adrenal gland containing the tumor); total bilateral adrenalectomy (surgical excision of both adrenal glands)	Adrenalectomy for a benign unilateral tumor usually curative Bilateral adrenalectomy must be followed by lifelong administration of *corticosteroids* to prevent Addison's disease
	Adrenal carcinoma with widespread metastases	Chemotherapy: *o,p'*-DDD, aminoglutethimide, and metyrapone used to promote remission in patients with inoperable cancer	Chemotherapy largely unsuccessful; drugs used highly toxic
Cushing's disease	Pituitary tumor (or unidentified lesion) that secretes excessive amounts of ACTH	Irradiation of the pituitary gland	Irradiation successful in 25% of cases; therapeutic effects not apparent for months following initiation of therapy
		Total bilateral adrenalectomy (corrects adrenal hyperplasia due to excessive ACTH stimulation)	Total bilateral adrenalectomy must be followed by lifelong replacement therapy with a glucocorticoid and mineralocorticoid
		Hypophysectomy or subtotal destruction of the pituitary by microsurgical resection, cryosurgery, yttrium implant, proton beam, or localized high-dosage irradiation	Hypophysectomy results in panhypopituitarism; all hormonal secretions dependent upon pituitary stimulation must be replaced for rest of patient's life (i.e., glucocorticoids, thyroid hormone, gonadal steroids, antidiuretic hormone)
Ectopic ACTH syndrome	Extra-adrenal malignant tumor	Surgical removal of the ectopic malignant tumor. Chemotherapy; used to control hypercorticism and promote remission in patients with inoperable cancer	Surgery rarely successful because metastasis usually occurs prior to diagnosis; chemotherapy purely palliative

*From Luckmann, J., and Sorensen, K. C.: Medical-Surgical Nursing: A Psychophysiologic Approach, 2nd ed. Philadelphia, W. B. Saunders Company, 1980. Used by permission.

existence of an adrenal tumor, in which case the disorder is referred to as *Cushing's syndrome.*

2. Increase in production secondary to the existence of a pituitary tumor, with associated hypersecretion of ACTH. In this case, the disorder is referred to as *Cushing's disease.*

3. Increase in production triggered by the release of excessive ACTH from malignant cells external to the pituitary. In these instances, the disorder is referred to as *ectopic ACTH syndrome.*

A comparative summary of these imbalances is presented in Table 17.1.

In considering the effects of hypo- or hypersecretion of the glucocorticoids upon fluid and electrolyte balance, it is important to remember that these hormones act like aldosterone upon the nephron. Thus, Addison's disease is associated with hypovolemia, hyperkalemia, and metabolic acidosis, whereas Cushing's syndrome and Cushing's disease are characterized by hypervolemia, hypokalemia, and metabolic alkalosis.

Parathormone (PTH)

PTH is produced and secreted by four small parathyroid glands that are embedded in the posterior thyroid. Released in direct response to hypocalcemia, it is responsible for increasing the concentration of calcium in

TABLE 17.2 **Signs and Symptoms of Calcium Deficit***

Signs and Symptoms	Causative Mechanisms
Painful tonic muscle spasms; facial spasms ("tetany facies"); grimacing; fatigue; laryngospasm; Trousseau's sign; positive Chvostek's sign; convulsions	Increased neuromuscular irritability producing hyper-reaction of motor and sensory nerves to stimuli
Tingling and numbness of fingers and circumoral region	Increased irritability of vascular smooth muscle and nerves
Definitive ECG tracing; palpitations; arrhythmias	Decreased cardiac contractility
Laboratory findings: Serum Ca^{++} decreased below 4.5 mEq./L.; serum phosphorus elevated; Sulkowitch urine test shows no precipitation. (For the Sulkowitch test, a 24-hour urine sample is collected and tested for Ca^{++} ions.)	Loss of Ca^{++} from serum; decreased Ca^{++} excretion

*From Luckmann, J., and Sorensen, K. C.: Medical-Surgical Nursing: A Psychophysiologic Approach, 2nd ed. Philadelphia, W. B. Saunders Company: 1980. Used by permission.

extracellular fluid through three major mechanisms:

1. PTH stimulates the osteoclastic reabsorption of bone, with subsequent release of calcium into the plasma.

2. PTH triggers the renal reabsorption of calcium.

3. PTH (in conjunction with vitamin D)

facilitates the absorption of calcium out of the gastrointestinal tract into the bloodstream.

Hyposecretion of PTH is frequently associated with accidental surgical removal of the parathyroid glands. Characteristic symptoms of hypocalcemia evolve, as summarized in Table 17.2.

Hypersecretion of PTH, on the other

TABLE 17.3 **Signs and Symptoms of Calcium Excess***

Signs and Symptoms	Causative Mechanisms
Bone pain; osteoporosis; osteomalacia (softening of bone); pathological fractures	Decalcification of bones (calcium moves from the bones into the blood)
Flank pain; kidney infection; kidney stones; polyuria; renal failure, which may result in death	Hypercalciuria due to increased Ca^{++} deposits in the renal pelvis and parenchyma; kidney loses its ability to concentrate urine
Diarrhea; constipation; atony of intestinal tract; peptic ulcer (in 8 per cent of patients); anorexia; nausea; vomiting	Gastrointestinal disorders due to an increase of Ca^{++} ions in sympathetic ganglia; this impedes transmission of afferent stimuli
Lethargy; exhaustion; mental confusion; loss of interest in surroundings; irritability, coma	Behavioral changes due to neurological hypofunction
Possible cardiac arrhythmia	Increased irritability of cardiac muscle
Laboratory findings: Plasma calcium levels above 5.8 mEq./L.; definitive ECG tracing; serum phosphorus decreased; Sulkowitch urine test shows increased Ca^{++} precipitation	Increased Ca^{++} in serum; increased Ca^{++} excretion; increased cardiac contractility

*Adapted from Luckmann, J., and Sorensen, K. C.: Medical-Surgical Nursing: A Psychophysiologic Approach; 2nd ed. Philadelphia, W. B. Saunders Company, 1980.

hand, is commonly caused by parathyroid tumors. The clinical manifestations of this disorder are summarized in Table 17.3.

Insulin

Insulin is manufactured by the beta cells of the pancreas and facilitates the cellular utilization of glucose. Although insulin is not directly involved in the maintenance of fluid-electrolyte/acid-base balance, hyposecretion will cause considerable disruption of homeostasis.

When insufficient quantities of insulin are produced, as in cases of diabetes mellitus, glucose accumulates in the extracellular fluid. In the event that plasma glucose concentration exceeds 180 mg. per 100 ml., large quantities of glucose may be eliminated in the urine. Hypovolemia develops as each gram of glucose osmotically draws approximately 10 to 20 ml. of water into the lumen of the nephron. Since diuresis inhibits the reabsorption of sodium and chloride, depletion of these electrolytes also occurs.

In the untreated diabetic, altered metabolic patterns further contribute to physiological imbalance. In the absence of available glucose, fats are mobilized to service cellular energy needs. Resulting ketoacidosis may cause hyperkalemia as hydrogen ions shift into the intracellular fluid, in exchange for a positively charged potassium ion. Acidosis also promotes hypercalcemia by shifting the equilibrium between protein-bound and freely ionized calcium to favor the latter.

As plasma pH declines, compensation mechanisms are activated. Acidic ketone bodies are buffered by plasma bicarbonate in the following manner: $H^+ + HCO_3^- \rightarrow H_2CO_3$. As a result, bicarbonate concentration declines, and increasing amounts of carbonic acid are formed. Carbonic acid, in turn, triggers an increase in the rate and depth of respirations (Kussmaul respirations). With the expulsion of carbon dioxide, the concentration of hydrogen ion in extracellular fluid decreases. Some characteristic fluid and electrolyte imbalances associated with diabetes mellitus are summarized in Figure 17.7.

CARDIOVASCULAR DISORDERS

The cardiovascular system is intimately involved with the maintenance of all aspects of homeostasis. Characteristically, disequilibrium occurs secondary to a decrease in cardiac output or vascular circulation or both. Some causative pathological mechanisms are summarized in Chapter 14.

When circulation is disrupted, for whatever reason, fluid-electrolyte or acid-base imbalances or both may result. As arterial blood

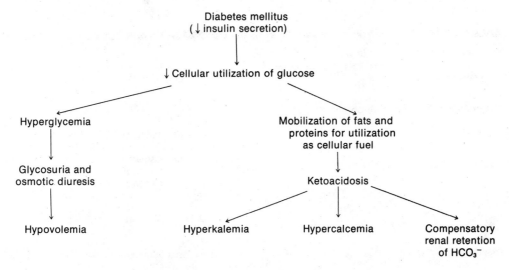

Figure 17.7 Some characteristic fluid and electrolyte imbalances associated with diabetes mellitus

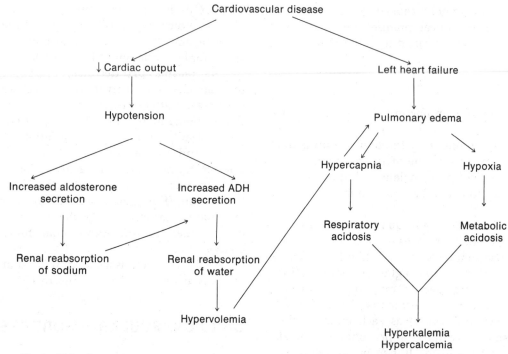

Figure 17.8 Some fluid and electrolyte imbalances that may be initiated by cardiovascular disease

pressure decreases, for example, compensatory increases in the secretion of ADH and aldosterone occur. Subsequent fluid retention may lead to hypervolemia, with associated shifts of fluid into the interstitial spaces.

To the extent that fluid retention or left heart failure causes pulmonary edema, interference with the diffusion of respiratory gases may additionally affect acid-base equilibrium. Whereas hypercapnia leads to respiratory acidosis, hypoxia promotes the excessive accumulation of lactic acid. Some of the imbalances initiated by cardiovascular disorders are illustrated in Figure 17.8.

RESPIRATORY DISORDERS

The respiratory system functions primarily to service the cellular needs for oxygen

---

TABLE 17.4 **Respiratory Acidosis**

Signs and Symptoms	Pathological Mechanism
Apathy; disorientation; weakness; stupor, coma	Central nervous system depression secondary to acidosis
Hyperventilation	Compensatory response to acidosis; pulmonary disorder often interferes with respiratory compensation mechanisms
Cardiac arrhythmias, tachycardia	Direct effect of increase in pCO_2; indirectly caused by secondary occurrence of hyperkalemia and hypercalcemia
Laboratory findings: Plasma pH below 7.35	Elevated $pCO_2 \longrightarrow$ increased generation of H_2CO_3.
Elevated plasma HCO_3^- Depressed urinary pH	Compensatory renal retention of HCO_3^- Compensatory renal elimination of hydrogen ions

TABLE 17.5 **Metabolic Acidosis**

Signs and Symptoms	Pathological Mechanism
Apathy; disorientation; weakness; stupor; coma	Central nervous system depression secondary to acidosis
Kussmaul respirations	Compensatory response to acidosis
Cardiac arrhythmias; tachycardia	Caused by secondary evolution of hyperkalemia and hypercalcemia
Laboratory findings:	
Plasma ph below 7.35	Excess of acid or loss of base
Depressed plasma HCO_3^-	Depletion of HCO_3^- as it is used to buffer excess acid; elimination of HCO_3^- secondary to dysfunction
Depressed urinary pH	Compensatory renal elimination of hydrogen ions

supply and carbon dioxide elimination. As elucidated in Chapter 10, respiratory dysfunction is generally characterized by disruption of the ventilation, diffusion, and/or perfusion processes. Regardless of the causative mechanisms, however, dysfunction frequently results in hypoxia or hypercapnia or both.

To the extent that cells are deprived of adequate oxygen supply, lactic acid accumulation will cause the development of metabolic acidosis. Carbon dioxide retention, on the other hand, is associated with the generation of carbonic acid and respiratory acidosis. Some clinical manifestations of these acid-base imbalances are summarized in Tables 17.4 and 17.5.

RENAL DISORDERS

The kidneys play a significant role in the maintenance of fluid-electrolyte and acid-base balance in the body. Normally, they function in the optimal elimination of water, sodium, potassium, chloride, calcium, and phosphate, while simultaneously regulating the relative proportion of hydrogen ion and bicarbonate in the extracellular fluid. Renal disorders can thus trigger considerable physiological disequilibrium.

As indicated in Table 17.6, dysfunction can arise secondary to a wide variety of disorders. Resulting functional imbalances, moreover, depend somewhat on the nature of the causative disease.

Prerenal disease, for example, is characterized by a depression in renal blood flow.

Resulting decreases in glomerular filtration will lead to oliguria, fluid retention, and elevations in the plasma concentration of nitrogenous wastes.

The nephrotic syndrome is associated with degenerative changes in the structure of the glomeruli. Increased glomerular permeability permits the filtration of large protein molecules into the nephron, resulting in hypoproteinemia and a decrease in plasma colloid osmotic pressure. Edema develops as fluid subsequently accumulates in the interstitial compartment.

To the extent that the tubular cells of the nephron are specifically affected by acute disease, dysfunction often progresses through three definable stages:

1. *Oliguria* — characterized by a decrease in urinary output to less than 400 ml. per day. Failure to eliminate fluids, electrolytes, metabolic acids, and the wastes of protein metabolism results in the evolution of hypervolemia, hyperkalemia, metabolic acidosis, and azotemia.

2. *Diuresis* — characterized by an increase in urinary output to greater than 400 ml. per day. During this stage, large volumes of fluids and electrolytes may be eliminated. Since tubular cells are not yet capable of responding adaptively to varying levels of hydration and electrolyte concentration, many substances may be inappropriately retained or excreted.

3. *Recovery* — characterized by healing and complete return to functional activity.

When renal disease is chronic and extensive, recovery may not be possible. In these

TABLE 17.6   **Renal Pathology**

Classification of Disease	Nature of Disease	Causative Disorders
ACUTE RENAL FAILURE		
Prerenal Disease	Sudden decline in renal function Caused by decrease of blood flow to the nephron	Myocardial infarction Neurogenic shock Hemorrhage Hypovolemia
Intrarenal Disease	Caused by primary destruction of renal tissue	APSGN (acute poststreptococcal glomerulonephritis) Acute pyelonephritis Renal poisoning Transfusion reaction Neoplasms
Postrenal Disease	Caused by urinary obstruction	Stones in the ureter or urethra Scarring of the ureter or urethra Enlargement of the prostate
CHRONIC RENAL FAILURE		
Glomerular Pathology	Progressive, irreversible destruction of renal tissue Characterized by glomerular degeneration	CGN (chronic glomerulonephritis) APSGN (acute poststreptococcal glomerulonephritis) SLE Antiglomerular basement nephritis Serum sickness nephritis Diabetic glomerulosclerosis Nephrosclerosis
Tubular-Interstitial Disease	Characterized by degeneration of the tubular cells of the nephron	Chronic pyelonephritis Chronic analgesic nephritis Urinary obstruction

cases, disequilibrium culminates in uremia or end-stage renal failure. As elucidated in Chapter 11, this phase of disease ultimately leads to hyperkalemia, sodium and water retention, metabolic acidosis, and azotemia. A summary of the imbalances associated with renal dysfunction is presented in Table 17.7.

GASTROINTESTINAL DISORDERS

In order to adequately service the cellular need for nutrients, ingested food must first be broken down and absorbed from the gastrointestinal tract into the bloodstream. Enzymes and chemicals that facilitate the digestive process are normally released into the gastrointestinal lumen in combination with large quantities of electrolyte-rich fluids. As indi-

cated in Table 17.8, glandular tissue generally produces approximately 8000 ml. of digestive secretions daily.

It can be seen that gastric juice contains relatively high concentrations of sodium, potassium, and hydrogen ion, whereas intestinal fluids are rich in sodium, potassium, and bicarbonate. Since the majority of intestinal secretions are reabsorbed from the ileum and proximal colon back into the bloodstream, only 150 ml. of relatively electrolyte-free fluid are normally eliminated from the lower digestive tract in a 24-hour period.

Because of the nature of gastrointestinal secretions, any depletion of luminal contents can considerably disrupt fluid-electrolyte and acid-base balance. Vomiting and diarrhea are perhaps the most common causes of digestive fluid loss. In both cases, hypovolemia may be accompanied by sodium and potassium deficit. Whereas the excessive elimination of acid-

TABLE 17.7 **Fluid and Electrolyte Imbalances Associated with Renal Pathology**

Type of Pathology	Causative Diseases	Associated Fluid and Electrolyte Imbalances
Prerenal disease	Myocardial infarction Neurogenic shock Septic shock Hemorrhage Hypovolemia	↓ glomerular filtration → oliguria fluid retention → hypervolemia electrolyte retention → hyperkalemia, metabolic acidosis nitrogenous waste retention → azotemia
Nephrotic syndrome	CGN (chronic glomerulo-nephritis) APSGN (acute poststreptococcal glomerulonephritis) SLE Serum sickness nephritis Diabetic glomerulosclerosis	filtration of protein into glomerulus → hypoproteinemia → decreased plasma colloid osmotic pressure → edema
Tubular disease	Nephrosclerosis Chronic pyelonephritis Chronic analgesic nephritis Urinary obstruction Renal poisoning Renal ischemia	**Initially** ↓ glomerular filtration → oliguria fluid retention → hypervolemia electrolyte retention → hyperkalemia, metabolic acidosis nitrogenous waste retention → azotemia **Later** excess diuresis → hypovolemia, electrolyte depletion

TABLE 17.8 **Gastrointestinal Secretions***

Secretion	Source of Production	Volume Secreted (ml./24 hours)	pH	Some Primary Electrolytes
Saliva	Salivary glands	1500	6–7	K^+
Gastric juice	Gastric mucosa	2500	1–3.5	Na^+, K^+, Cl^-, H^+
Pancreatic juice	Exocrine cells of pancreas	700	8.0–8.3	Na^+, K^+, Cl^-, HCO_3^-
Bile	Liver	500	7.8	Na^+, K^+, Cl^-, HCO_3^-
Small intestinal juice	Small intestinal mucosa	3000	7.8–8.0	Na^+, K^+, Cl^-, HCO_3^-

*Adapted from Metheny, M., and Snively, W.: Nurses' Handbook of Fluid Balance, 3rd ed. Philadelphia, J. B. Lippincott Company, 1979.

TABLE 17.9   **Loss of Fluid from the Gastrointestinal Lumen**

Causative Mechanisms	Associated Disorders
Vomiting	Pyloric stenosis Neoplasms Gastritis Peptic ulcer Obstruction Paralytic ileus
Diarrhea	Celiac disease Crohn's disease Ulcerative colitis Spastic colon Enteritis
Shifting of fluid out of the gastrointestinal lumen into the interstitial compartment	Obstruction Paralytic ileus Portal hypertension

TABLE 17.10   **Fluid and Electrolyte Changes Associated with Hepatic Disease**

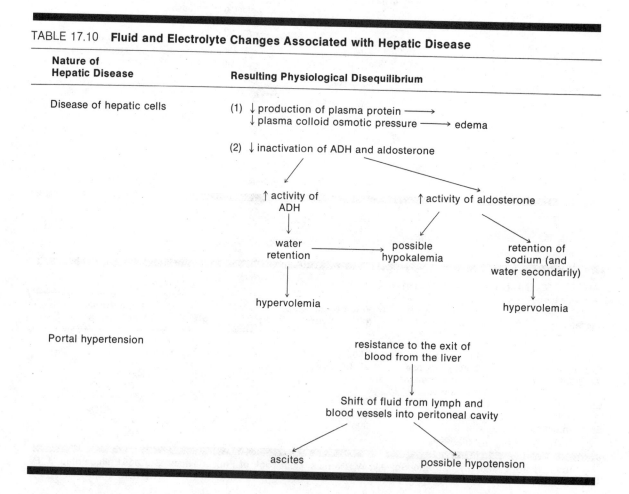

Nature of Hepatic Disease	Resulting Physiological Disequilibrium
Disease of hepatic cells	(1) ↓ production of plasma protein ⟶ ↓ plasma colloid osmotic pressure ⟶ edema (2) ↓ inactivation of ADH and aldosterone
Portal hypertension	

ic gastric juices can cause the evolution of metabolic alkalosis, diarrhea is associated with bicarbonate loss and metabolic acidosis. Examples of causative disorders are presented in Table 17.9.

Serious disequilibrium may also be induced by extensive liver disease. In cases of cirrhosis, for example, a variety of mechanisms are responsible for fluid-electrolyte and acid-base disturbances.

Failure of diseased hepatic cells to inactivate aldosterone and ADH causes plasma levels of these hormones to increase. Sodium and water are subsequently retained, and potassium is depleted. Since the liver plays a significant role in the production of plasma proteins, hepatic disease may also cause colloid osmotic pressure to decrease, leading to an accumulation of fluid in the interstitial compartment. To the extent that hepatic dysfunction is associated with portal hypertension, increases in capillary blood pressure within the abdominopelvic cavity will additionally lead to ascites, as fluid shifts into peritoneal spaces. The changes associated with hepatic disease are summarized in Table 17.10.

NEURAL DISORDERS

It is through the nervous system that many responses designed to maintain homeostasis are initiated and integrated. For example, fluid and electrolyte balance is specifically influenced by the hypothalamus, and acid-base equilibrium is particularly affected by the respiratory center of the medulla.

Normally, ADH is secreted adaptively by the hypothalamus in response to changing levels of plasma solute concentration. Inappropriate secretion of ADH (SIADH) may arise secondary to cerebral trauma, inflammation, or neoplasm and is characterized by the excessive reabsorption of water from the nephron into the bloodstream. This clinical phenomenon results in hypervolemia, hyponatremia, and the excretion of small quantities of concentrated urine.

Alternatively, depressed ADH secretion (diabetes insipidus) may be caused by brain tumors, cerebral trauma, or encephalitis. Deficit of antidiuretic hormone results in the elimination of large volumes of dilute urine. In-

creased thirst and excessive drinking partially compensate for the associated fluid loss.

While the hypothalamus acts to mediate changes in fluid volume and concentration, the medulla is more specifically involved with the regulation of acid-base balance. By modifying respiratory rate, the medulla indirectly controls the concentrations of carbon dioxide and carbonic acid in the extracellular fluid.

Whenever neural dysfunction triggers hyperventilation (as noted in cases of meningitis, encephalitis, and certain brain tumors), associated loss of volatile hydrogen causes the development of respiratory alkalosis. Conversely, hypoventilation promotes the retention of carbonic acid and the development of respiratory acidosis. Depression of respiratory rate is commonly caused by direct trauma to the medulla or compression of respiratory neurons secondary to tumor or hemorrhage.

SUMMARY

In considering fluid-electrolyte and acid-base imbalances, it is important to remember that a variety of unrelated disorders may ultimately trigger the same physiological disruption.

Hypovolemia, for example, often arises secondary to diabetes insipidus, excessive gastrointestinal losses, or extensive diaphoresis. In all cases, clinical manifestations will be similar, as falling blood pressure causes cerebral hypoxia and produces compensatory alterations in cardiac rate and vascular tone.

Similarly, acidosis may be initiated by a variety of pathological conditions including: (1) respiratory disorders, with secondary retention of carbon dioxide; (2) hypoxia, with associated generation of lactic acid; and (3) metabolic imbalances, with subsequent increases in the production of acidic ketone bodies.

Regardless of the causative mechanism, characteristic manifestations of acidosis include central nervous system depression, hyperventilation, and cardiac arrhythmias.

To aid in conceptualizing some of these complex interrelationships Table 17.11 presents an overview of some primary fluid-electrolyte imbalances and the diverse causative disorders that may trigger disequilibrium.

TABLE 17.11 **The Evolution of Some Primary Fluid-Electrolyte and Acid-Base Imbalances**

Imbalance	Some Underlying Pathological Mechanisms	Causative Disorders
Hypervolemia	SIADH ⟶ excessive and inappropriate secretion of ADH	Cerebral trauma Cerebral inflammation Cerebral neoplasm Pulmonary neoplasm
	↓ Volume of circulating blood ⟶ ↑ secretion of ADH and aldosterone	Heart failure Hypovolemia Neurogenic shock Septic shock
	Failure to inactivate ADH or aldosterone	Hepatitis Cirrhosis
Hypovolemia	Diabetes insipidus ⟶ excessive diuresis	Brain tumor Cerebral trauma Encephalitis
	Excessive vomiting or diarrhea	Colitis GI obstruction Enteritis Acute peptic ulcer
Sodium imbalance	Excessive vomiting or diarrhea ⟶ sodium depletion	Colitis GI obstruction Enteritis Acute peptic ulcer
	SIADH ⟶ sodium dilution	Cerebral trauma Cerebral inflammation Cerebral neoplasm Pulmonary neoplasm
	Diabetes insipidus ⟶ sodium concentration	Brain tumor Cerebral trauma Encephalitis
Potassium imbalance	Excessive vomiting or diarrhea ⟶ potassium depletion	Colitis GI obstruction Enteritis Acute peptic ulcer
	Failure to inactivate aldosterone ⟶ potassium depletion	Hepatitis Cirrhosis
	Excessive secretion of aldosterone ⟶ potassium depletion	Heart failure Hypovolemia Neurogenic shock Septic shock Excessive ACTH secretion Adrenal lesion
	Renal failure ⟶ potassium retention	Pyelonephritis Renal poisoning Renal ischemia Transfusion reaction Nephritis Nephrosclerosis Urinary obstruction

TABLE 17.11   The Evolution of Some Primary Fluid-Electrolyte and Acid-Base Imbalances *(Continued)*

Imbalance	Some Underlying Pathological Mechanisms	Causative Disorders
Potassium imbalance *(Continued)*	↓ Secretion of aldosterone ⟶ potassium retention	Addison's disease
	Acidosis ⟶ hyperkalemia	Hypercapnia Hypoxia Diarrhea Renal failure Diabetes mellitus Starvation
Calcium imbalance	↓ Secretion of PTH ⟶ hypocalcemia	Surgical removal of the parathyroid glands
	Depressed availability of vitamin D ⟶ ↓ GI absorption of calcium	Malabsorption Biliary duct obstruction Cirrhosis Renal failure
	Alkalosis ⟶ hypocalcemia	Hyperventilation Gastric vomiting
	↑ Secretion of PTH ⟶ hypercalcemia	Parathyroid tumor
	Acidosis ⟶ Hypercalcemia	Hypercapnia Hypoxia Diarrhea Renal failure Diabetes mellitus Starvation
Acidosis	Respiratory disorder ⟶ hypercapnia ⟶ respiratory acidosis	COPD Pulmonary fibrosis Pulmonary edema
	Hypoventilation ⟶ hypercapnia ⟶ respiratory acidosis	Cerebral tumor Cerebral hemorrhage
	Metabolic disruption ⟶ ↑ mobilization of fats and proteins as cellular fuel ⟶ ketosis ⟶ metabolic acidosis	Starvation Diabetes mellitus
	↓ Elimination of metabolic acids ⟶ metabolic acidosis	Renal failure
	Hypoxia ⟶ ↑ generation of lactic acid ⟶ metabolic acidosis	Respiratory disease Cardiovascular disease Severe anemia
	↑ Elimination of base ⟶ metabolic acidosis	Diarrhea
Alkalosis	Hyperventilation ⟶ hypocapnia ⟶ respiratory alkalosis	Meningitis Encephalitis Cerebral tumors Anxiety/hysteria
	Excessive elimination of metabolic acid ⟶ metabolic alkalosis	Gastric vomiting

STUDY QUESTIONS

1. Describe how and why acid-base imbalance might evolve in cases of (a) diabetes mellitus, and (b) primary aldosteronism.

2. A patient is admitted for evaluation and treatment of Addison's disease. Explain the nature of each of the following symptoms:
   a. low blood pressure
   b. cardiac arrhythmias
   c. hyperventilation

3. Why is a patient with Cushing's disease susceptible to the development of congestive heart failure?

4. During a thyroidectomy, the parathyroid glands are accidentally removed. Explain why postoperative symptoms might predictably include tonic muscle spasms, tingling and numbness of the fingers, and cardiac arrhythmias.

5. Why do hypervolemia and pulmonary edema frequently occur subsequent to a left ventricular myocardial infarction?

6. A patient with COPD is admitted to the hospital in extreme respiratory distress. He is weak, disoriented, and experiencing tachycardia. Laboratory tests reveal depressed plasma pH and elevated plasma HCO_3^-. Explain the development of his symptoms.

7. Explain why edema might be noted in each of the following cases of renal disease:
   a. acute pyelonephritis
   b. prerenal disease
   c. chronic glomerulonephritis

8. Mrs. Barker has an acute peptic ulcer that has caused considerable bleeding and vomiting. She is admitted for observation and treatment. What fluid-electrolyte and acid-base imbalances would be noted, and why?

9. Why are symptoms of hyperaldosteronism frequently noted in cases of extensive liver disease?

10. Mr. Brady is admitted to the hospital with a suspected brain tumor. Explain why each of the following imbalances could develop subsequent to increases in intracranial pressure:
   a. hypervolemia and hyponatremia
   b. hypovolemia and hypernatremia
   c. respiratory acidosis
   d. respiratory alkalosis

Suggested Readings

Books

Aurbach, G. D.: Parathyroid. In Beeson, P. B., McDermott, W., and Wyngaarden, J. B. (eds.): Cecil Textbook of Medicine, 15th ed. Philadelphia, W. B. Saunders Company, 1979, p. 2199.

Beck, R. R.: Hormonal control of water and electrolytes. In Selkurt, E. E. (ed.): Basic Physiology for the Health Sciences. Boston, Little, Brown & Company, 1975, p. 503.

Beck, R. R.: Hormonal regulation of calcium metabolism. In Selkurt, E. E. (ed.): Basic Physiology for the Health Sciences. Boston, Little, Brown & Company, 1975, p. 317.

Burgess, A.: The Nurse's Guide to Fluid and Electrolyte Balance, 2nd ed. New York, McGraw-Hill Book Company, 1979.

Burke, S. R.: The Composition and Function of Body Fluids, 2nd ed. St. Louis, The C.V. Mosby Company, 1976.

Cahill, G. F., Jr.: Diabetes mellitus. In Beeson, P. B., McDermott, W., and Wyngaarden, J. B. (eds.): Cecil Textbook of Medicine, 15th ed. Philadelphia, W. B. Saunders Company, 1979, p. 1969.

Goldberger, E.: A Primer of Water, Electrolytes, and Acid-Base Syndromes, 5th ed. Philadelphia, Lea & Febiger, 1975.

Grant, M. M.: The kidney and fluid and electrolyte balance. In Jones, D. A., Dunbar, C. F., and Jirovec, M. M.: Medical-Surgical Nursing, A Conceptual Approach. New York, McGraw-Hill Book Company, 1978, p. 493.

Guyton, A. C.: Textbook of Medical Physiology, 5th ed. Philadelphia, W. B. Saunders Company, 1976, pp. 1000–1002; 1019–1035; 1036–1068.

Hager, D. C., and Hollingsworth, D. B.: Fluid and electrolyte imbalances. In Jones, D. A., Dunbar, C. F., and Jirovec, M. M.: Medical-Surgical Nursing, A Conceptual Approach. New York, McGraw-Hill Book Company, 1978, p. 445.

Hamilton, H. (ed.): Monitoring Fluids and Electrolytes Precisely. Nursing 79 Books. Horsham, Pa., Intermed Communications, Inc., 1978.

Jirovec, M. M., and Nolan, J. W.: The concepts of fluid and electrolyte dynamics. *In* Jones, D. A., Dunbar, C. F., and Jirovec, M. M.: Medical-Surgical Nursing, A Conceptual Approach. New York, McGraw-Hill Book Company, 1978, p. 423.

Kee, J.: Fluids and Electrolytes With Clinical Applications: A Programmed Approach, 2nd ed. New York, John Wiley & Sons, Inc., 1978.

Leaf, A.: Posterior pituitary. *In* Beeson, P. B., McDermott, W., and Wyngaarden, J. B. (eds.): Cecil Textbook of Medicine, 15th ed. Philadelphia, W. B. Saunders Company, 1979, p. 2109.

Liddle, G. W.: Adrenal cortex. *In* Beeson, P. B., McDermott, W., and Wyngaarden, J. B. (eds.): Cecil Textbook of Medicine, 15th ed. Philadelphia, W. B. Saunders Company, 1979, p. 2144.

Luckmann, J., and Sorensen, K. C.: Medical-Surgical Nursing, A Psychophysiologic Approach, 2nd ed. Philadelphia, W. B. Saunders Company, 1980, pp. 171–227.

Metheny, N. M., and Snively, W. D.: Nurses' Handbook of Fluid Balance, 3rd ed. Philadelphia, J. B. Lippincott Company, 1979.

Pflanzer, R. G., and Tanner, G. A.: Acid-base regulation. *In* Selkurt, E. E. (ed.): Basic Physiology for the Health Sciences. Boston, Little, Brown & Company, 1975, p. 519.

Reed, G. M., and Sheppard, V. F.: Regulation of Fluid and Electrolyte Balance: A Programmed Instruction in Clinical Physiology, 2nd ed. Philadelphia, W. B. Saunders Company, 1977.

Schwartz, W. B.: Disorders of fluid, electrolyte, and acid-base balance. *In* Beeson, P. B., McDermott, W., and Wyngaarden, J. B. (eds.): Cecil Textbook of Medicine, 15th ed. Philadelphia, W. B. Saunders Company, 1979, p. 1950.

Selkurt, E. E.: Body water and electrolyte composition and their regulation. *In* Selkurt, E. E. (ed.): Basic Physiology for the Health Sciences. Boston, Little, Brown & Company, 1975, p. 487.

Soltis, B.: Fluid and electrolyte imbalance. *In* Phipps, W. J., Long, B. C., and Woods, N. F.

(eds.): Medical-Surgical Nursing, Concepts and Clinical Practice. St. Louis, The C. V. Mosby Company, 1979, p. 299.

Stroot, V. R., Lee, C. A., and Schaper, C. A.: Fluids and Electrolytes: A Practical Approach, 2nd ed. Philadelphia, F. A. Davis Company, 1977.

Weldy, N. J.: Body Fluids and Electrolytes, A Programmed Presentation, 3rd ed. St. Louis, The C. V. Mosby Company, 1980.

Articles

Bay, W. H., and Ferris, T. F.: Hypernatremia and hyponatremia: Disorders of tonicity. Geriatrics, *31*:53, 1976.

Bransome, E. D., Jr.: Polyuria and water intoxication: Disorders of antidiuretic hormone. Consultant, *18*:29, 1977.

Del Bueno, G. J.: Electrolyte imbalance: How to recognize and respond to it. Part 1. RN, *38*:52, 1975.

Gill, J. R.: Edema. Annu. Rev. Med., *21*:273, 1970.

Keyes, J.: Basic mechanisms in acid-base homeostasis. Heart Lung, *5*:239, 1976.

Keyes, J.: Blood gas analysis and the assessment of acid-base status. Heart Lung, *5*:247, 1976.

Khokhar, N.: Inappropriate secretion of antidiuretic hormone. Postgrad. Med., *62*:73, 1977.

Lancour, J.: ADH and aldosterone: How to recognize their effects. Nursing 78, *8*:36, 1978.

Lee, C. A., Stroot, V. R., and Schaper, C. A.: What to do when acid-base problems hang in the balance. Nursing 75, *5*:32, 1975.

Manzi, C. C.: Edema: How to tell if it's a danger signal. Nursing 77, *7*:66, 1977.

Nugent, C. A.: Answers to questions on the differential diagnosis of hypercalcemia. Hosp. Med., *14*:106, 1978.

Oakes, A., and Morrow, H.: Understanding blood gases. Nursing 73, *3*:15, 1973.

Randall, H. T.: Fluid, electrolyte, and acid-base balance. Surg. Clin. North Am., *56*:1019, 1976.

Reed, G. M.: Confused about potassium? Here's a clear and concise guide. Nursing 74, *4*:20, 1974.

Sharer, J. E.: Reviewing acid-base balance. Am. J. Nurs., *75*:980, 1975.

Sieger, P.: The physiologic approach to acid-base balance. Med. Clin. North Am., *57*:863, 1973.

Tripp, A.: Hyper- and hypocalcemia. Am. J. Nurs., *76*:1142, 1976.

Index

Page numbers in *italics* indicate an illustration, and page numbers followed by (t) indicate a table.